Molecular Mechanisms in the Nervous System

Molecular Mechanisms in the Nervous System

Editor: Jenna Stephenson

AMERICAN
MEDICAL PUBLISHERS
www.americanmedicalpublishers.com

AMERICAN
MEDICAL PUBLISHERS
www.americanmedicalpublishers.com

Cataloging-in-Publication Data

Molecular mechanisms in the nervous system / edited by Jenna Stephenson.
p. cm.
Includes bibliographical references and index.
ISBN 979-8-88740-278-9
1. Molecular neurobiology. 2. Molecular biology. 3. Neurobiology. 4. Nervous system--Diseases--Molecular aspects.
5. Neurology. I. Stephenson, Jenna.
QP356.2 .M65 2023
591.188--dc23

American Medical Publishers,
41 Flatbush Avenue,
1st Floor, New York,
NY 11217, USA

ISBN 979-8-88740-278-9 (Hardback)

Contents

Preface

Every book is initially just a concept; it takes months of research and hard work to give it the final shape in which the readers receive it. In its early stages, this book also went through rigorous reviewing. The notable contributions made by experts from across the globe were first molded into patterned chapters and then arranged in a sensibly sequential manner to bring out the best results.

The nervous system consists of all of the nerve cells in the human body. It is responsible for signal transmission between the brain and other organs of the body. It receives information from the senses, interprets it and sets off reactions, such as muscle contraction or feeling pain. The peripheral nervous system (PNS) and the central nervous system (CNS) are the two major components of the nervous system. The CNS is made up of the spinal cord and the brain, while PNS is primarily made up of nerves which are bundles of axons or fibers that link the CNS to every other organ and tissue in the body. The nervous system also comprises glia, which are non-neuron cells and perform significant functions to make the nervous system function properly. This book outlines the molecular mechanisms in the nervous system in detail. Its extensive content provides the readers with a thorough understanding of the subject.

It has been my immense pleasure to be a part of this project and to contribute my years of learning in such a meaningful form. I would like to take this opportunity to thank all the people who have been associated with the completion of this book at any step.

Editor

1

Hox gene regulation in the central nervous system of *Drosophila*

Maheshwar Gummalla*[1,2†], *Sandrine Galetti*[1], *Robert K. Maeda*[1]* and *François Karch*[1]

[1] Department of Genetics and Evolution, University of Geneva, Geneva, Switzerland
[2] Institute of Biochemistry, University of Medicine – University of Göttingen, Göttingen, Germany

Correspondence:
Robert K. Maeda and François Karch, Department of Genetics and Evolution, University of Geneva, 30 quai Ernest Ansermet, 1211 Geneva 4, Switzerland
e-mail: robert.maeda@unige.ch; francois.karch@unige.ch

†Present address:
Maheshwar Gummalla, Institute of Biochemistry, University of Medicine – University of Göttingen, Göttingen, Germany

Hox genes specify the structures that form along the anteroposterior (AP) axis of bilateria. Within the genome, they often form clusters where, remarkably enough, their position within the clusters reflects the relative positions of the structures they specify along the AP axis. This correspondence between genomic organization and gene expression pattern has been conserved through evolution and provides a unique opportunity to study how chromosomal context affects gene regulation. In *Drosophila,* a general rule, often called "posterior dominance," states that Hox genes specifying more posterior structures repress the expression of more anterior Hox genes. This rule explains the apparent spatial complementarity of Hox gene expression patterns in *Drosophila*. Here we review a noticeable exception to this rule where the more-posteriorly expressed *Abd-B* Hox gene fails to repress the more-anterior *abd-A* gene in cells of the central nervous system (CNS). While *Abd-B* is required to repress ectopic expression of *abd-A* in the posterior epidermis, *abd-A* repression in the posterior CNS is accomplished by a different mechanism that involves a large 92 kb long non-coding RNA (lncRNA) encoded by the intergenic region separating *abd-A* and *Abd-B* (the iab8ncRNA). Dissection of this lncRNA revealed that *abd-A* is repressed by the lncRNA using two redundant mechanisms. The first mechanism is mediated by a microRNA (mir-iab-8) encoded by intronic sequence within the large *iab8*-ncRNA. Meanwhile, the second mechanism seems to involve transcriptional interference by the long iab-8 ncRNA on the *abd-A* promoter. Recent work demonstrating CNS-specific regulation of genes by ncRNAs in *Drosophila,* seem to highlight a potential role for the *iab-8*-ncRNA in the evolution of the *Drosophila* Hox complexes.

Keywords: Hox genes, *abd-A*, ncRNA, miRNA, bithorax-complex

Hox CLUSTERS

Hox genes specify the structures that form along the anteroposterior (AP) axis of bilateria. They are strikingly conserved between invertebrates and vertebrates. This conservation extends past the gene sequences and into their relative positioning along the chromosome, as Hox genes are generally found in clusters (or complexes) in which the individual Hox genes are aligned along the chromosome in the same order as the structures they specify along the AP axis (McGinnis and Krumlauf, 1992). While this correspondence between genomic organization and body axis is suggestive of a fundamental mechanism of activation that has been conserved through evolution, thus far, no common overlying principle can completely explain the evolutionary conservation of the collinear alignment of the genes. In fact, clustering does not seem to be absolutely necessary for proper Hox gene regulation in *Drosophila,* the place where Hox genes were first discovered. Indeed, the Hox gene cluster in fruit flies has been split at different location during the evolution of the *Drosophila* lineage (Lewis et al., 2003; Negre et al., 2003; Negre and Ruiz, 2007). In *D. melanogaster*, the Hox genes have been split into two clusters separated between the *Antennapedia* (*Antp*) and *Ultrabithorax* (*Ubx*) Hox genes (forming the *Antp* complex, and the bithorax complex, BX-C). Meanwhile, in *Drosophila virilis*, the complex is split between the *Ubx* and *abd-A* genes (Von Allmen et al., 1996). However, the fact that the *Drosophila* Hox complex has been split does not mean that the remaining collinear arrangement of the *Drosophila* Hox genes plays no role in their regulation. In fact, based on genetic rearrangement experiments, we know that the collinear arrangement of the *Drosophila* Hox genes is important for their proper expression (Maeda and Karch, 2010). Thus, the breaks found in the *Drosophila* Hox complexes may be exceptional cases of rearrangements that bypassed deleterious effects.

Based on our current understanding of Hox gene regulation in vertebrates and invertebrates, it now seems likely that at least some of the reason for preserving collinearity diverged during the evolutionary history of the two lineages. In mammals, collinearity seems to be preserved primarily due to the sharing of distal enhancer elements. Within the mouse Hoxd cluster, for example, it has been shown that Hox gene expression is controlled by shared remote enhancers located, 5′ and 3′ to the Hox complex. This sharing of enhancers presumably provides evolutionary pressure to keep the Hox genes clustered. Furthermore, it seems that distance from these enhancers controls the timing and ultimate location of Hox gene expression, providing pressure to preserve collinearity. However, this is not the case in invertebrates. In *Drosophila*, Hox gene expression is controlled by gene-specific enhancers located within the complex itself. It is perhaps for this reason that invertebrate Hox complexes are generally larger than their vertebrate counterparts and why the *Drosophila* Hox complex could be split in two.

Work on non-coding RNAs (ncRNAs) has provided an additional aspect regarding the conservation of the Hox gene clusters. Two microRNA genes (miRNA) have been found at similar positions within the Hox clusters of vertebrates and arthropods (Lagos-Quintana et al., 2003). The conserved miR-10 miRNA lies between the *Drosophila* Hox genes *Deformed* and *Sex-comb-reduced*. These fly Hox genes correspond to mammalian orthologs *Hox4* and *Hox5*, respectively. Remarkably, the vertebrate miR-10b miRNA can be found between the *Hox4* and *Hox5* paralogs in the *HoxB* complex. A second miRNA gene in vertebrates (miR-196) is located between the *Hox9* and *Hox10* paralogs in the *HoxA* complex. These genes correspond to the fly genes *abd-A* and *Abd*-B. As in the case of miR10, a miRNA gene is found at a similar location in arthropods, though the primary sequence of the miRNA genes differ between the two lineages. In *Drosophila*, this miRNA gene is transcribed on both strands, giving rise to *miR-iab-4* on one strand, and *miR-iab-8* on the other strand. The *miR-iab-8* template is embedded in a very large transcription unit of >92 kb (the iab-8ncRNA). Recent work from our lab on the *iab-8*-ncRNA has led to a number of interesting results, and provide additional reasons for the preservation of Hox clustering.

THE BITHORAX COMPLEX

Hox genes were discovered through mutations that affect the identities of the segments that form along the AP axis of the fly. Many of these mutations were identified within the posterior Hox complex of the fly, called the BX-C (Lewis, 1978 for review, see Maeda and Karch, 2006). The BX-C encodes three Hox genes, *Ubx*, *abd-A*, and *Abd-B* (**Figure 1**), which are responsible for the identities of parasegments 8 to 13. These parasegments form the posterior thorax and all the abdominal segments of the fly (posterior T2, T3 and all eight abdominal segments A1–A8)[1]. Before the molecular genetic era, classical genetic analysis revealed

[1]An explanation of some *Drosophila* nomenclature. The segmental boundaries visible in the adult fly do not correspond to the reiterated units that form during the early stages of embryogenesis. In embryogenesis, the embryos is subdivided into units that are slightly shifted relative to the adult segments. These units are called parasegments, with one parasegement being composed of cells giving rise to the posterior part of one adult segment and the anterior part of the next segments (Martinez-Arias and Lawrence, 1985). For example, parasegment 5 (PS5) is makes up of the posterior part of the second thoracic segment (T2) and the anterior part of the third thoracic segment (T3). It is for this reason that we will generally refer to embryonic patterns in parasegmental nomenclature and adult patterns in segmental

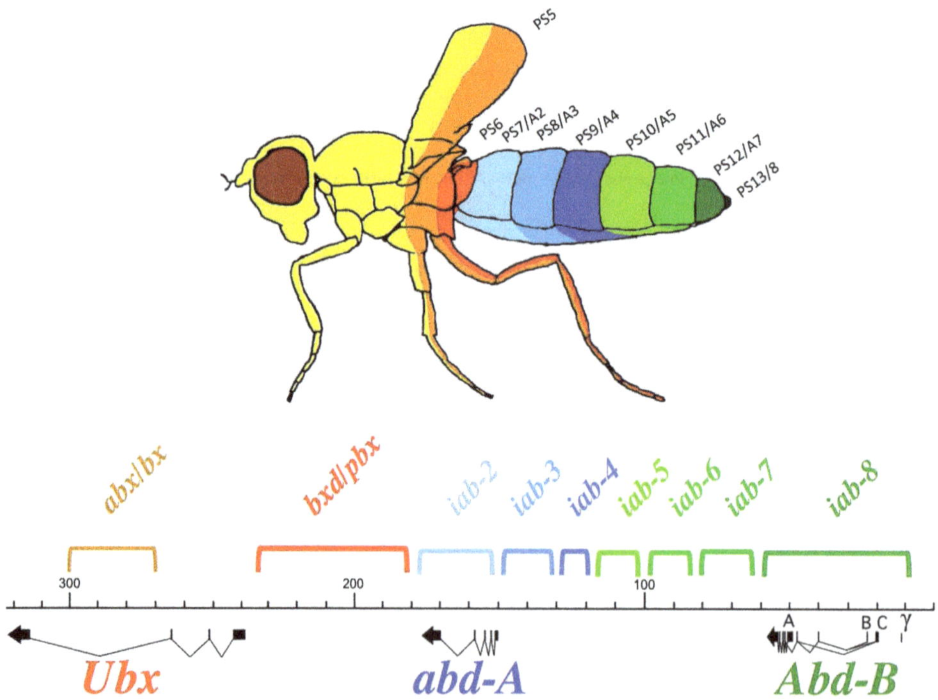

FIGURE 1 | Synopsis of the BX-C. The genomic region of the BX-C is marked off in kilobases according to the numbering of (Martin et al., 1995). The three transcription units *Ubx*, *abd-A*, and *Abd-B* with their exons marked as thick lines and the arrows showing the transcription polarity are drawn below the DNA map. The horizontal and colored brackets above the DNA line indicate the extends of the segment-specific *cis*-regulatory regions with the following color code. Orange and red (*abx/bx* and *bxd/pb*) regulate expression of *Ubx* in PS5/T3 and PS6/A1, respectively. The blue *iab-2*, *iab-3*, and *iab-4* regions regulate *abd-A* expression in PS7/A2, PS8/A3, and PS9/A4. Finally, the green *iab-5*, *iab-6*, *iab-7*, and *iab-8* regulate *Abd-B* expression in PS10/A5, PS11/A6, PS12/A7, and PS13/A8, respectively. These segmental boundaries are depicted with the same colors on the fly above the BX-C map. Note that the parasegmental boundaries are visible in the thoracic segments where PS5 corresponds to the posterior part of T2 and the anterior part of T3. PS6 corresponds to posterior T3 and anterior A1.

the existence of mutations that affect the identities of each of the segments under the control of the BX-C. These mutations defined nine segment-specific functions. By genetic mapping, Ed Lewis discovered that these nine segments-specific functions are aligned along the chromosome in the same order as the segments they specify along the AP axis. This was the first identification of colinearity. Molecular analysis later revealed that the BX-C encoded only three, homeotic genes and that the genetically identified segment-specific functions were probably regulatory in nature. This was confirmed by antibody staining in mutant embryos. Antibody staining showed that *Ubx*, *abd-A*, and *Abd-B* are expressed in overlapping domains in the posterior half of the embryo (see also below). These expression patterns are intricate and finely tuned from one parasegment to the next (see for example **Figure 2**). By staining various mutant embryos it was shown that the segment-specific functions correspond to *cis*-regulatory regions that regulate the expression of *Ubx*. *abd-A*, or *Abd-B* in a parasegment-specific fashion. Thus the *abx/bx* and *bxd/pbx cis*-regulatory regions direct *Ubx* expression in PS5 and PS6, respectively. Similarly the *iab-2* through *iab-4 cis*-regulatory regions direct the parasegment-specific expression patterns of *abd-A* in PS7, PS8, and PS9 (**Figures 1** and **2**; for review, see Maeda and Karch, 2006). And finally, the *iab-5* trough *iab-8 cis*-regulatory regions regulate *Abd-B* in PS10 to PS13, respectively. Thus, the collinearity that exists in flies extends beyond the genes themselves to the *cis*-regulatory elements that drive the Hox gene expression.

nomenclature. For the abdominal segments however, as their posterior compartment is not visible in adult fly (being folded under the anterior half) there is a fairly direct correlation between parasegmental and visible segmental borders. Thus, for the sake of simplicity, we will often simply refer both parasegments and segments simultaneously (i.e., the second abdominal segment will be referred to (A2/PS7).

Antp Ubx, abd-A, AND *Abd-B* Hox GENES ARE EXPRESSED IN BROAD DOMAINS

Like in vertebrates, most *Drosophila* Hox genes are expressed in broad domains along the AP axis. This is the case for the *Antp* gene that specifies the identity of PS4. While its segmental specification role is restricted to this single parasegments, *Antp* remains expressed in all the more posterior parasegments, until PS12 (Hafen et al., 1984) Similarly, the *Ubx* gene that specifies PS5 and PS6 identities remains expressed up to PS12 (White and Wilcox, 1984; Akam and Martinez-Arias, 1985; Beachy et al., 1985). Finally, *abd-A* that specifies PS7 to PS9 remains expressed up to PS12 (Karch et al., 1990; Macias et al., 1990; see **Figure 2B**). Thus these three Hox genes remain expressed posterior to the parasegments

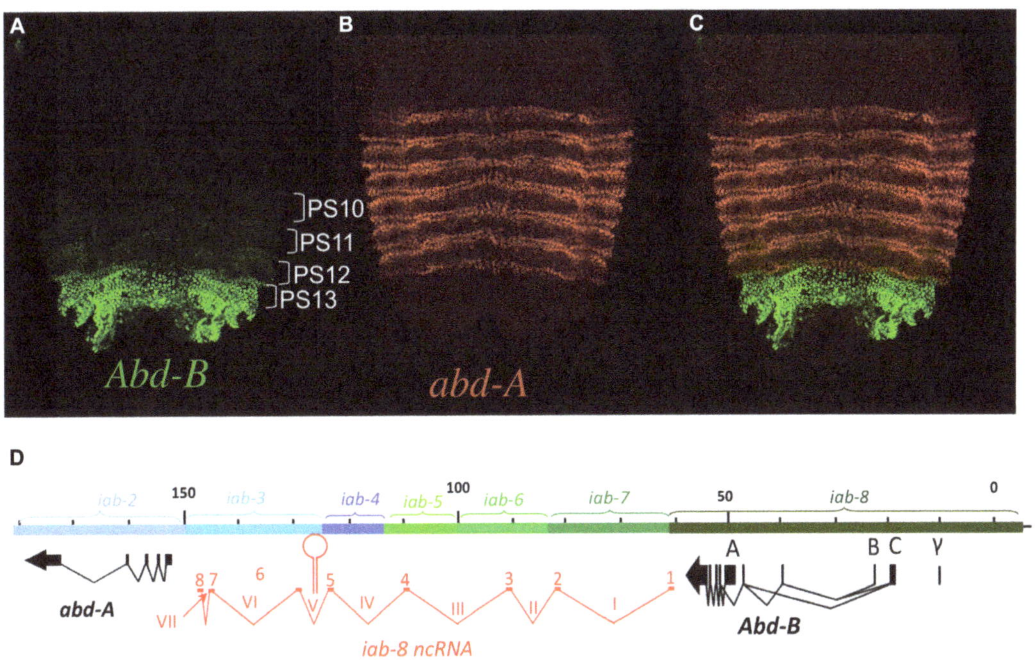

FIGURE 2 | *abd-A* and *Abd-B* are expressed in broad domains. Panels **A**, **B**, and **C** show pelts of stage 13 embryos. In these preparations, embryos were cut along the dorsal midline and flattened on a slide. Anterior is at the top. In stage 13 embryos, Hox gene expression is mostly visible in the epidermis with *abd-A* displayed in red and *Abd-B* in green. In panel **A**, *Abd-B* appears in a graded fashion from PS10 to PS13 (parasegments are marked by brackets). In these parasegments, *Abd-B* is produced from promoter A under the regulation of, respectively the *iab-5, iab-6, iab-7,* and *iab-8* regulatory regions (see also text). In PS14 an alternative form of *Abd-B* is produced from promoters B, C, and γ. The *abd-A* expression pattern in PS7 to PS12 is shown in panel **B**. Both *abd-A* and *Abd-B* are displayed in panel **C**. Note that their overall expression domains appear complementary to each other. Original observations published in (Celniker et al., 1990; Karch et al., 1990; Gummalla et al., 2012) The abdominal part of the BX-C is shown in panel **D** with the same map coordinates as in **Figure 1** (Martin et al., 1995) and with the same color code for the *abd-A*, *Abd-B* genes and their respective regulatory domains. The structure of the *iab-8 ncRNA* is shown in red under te DNA map. Introns are numbered with latin numbers and exons with regular numbering. Note that the polarity of transcription is the same as that for *abd-A* and *Abd-B*. Note also the presence of one exon for each of the *iab cis*-regulatory regions to the exception of 2 exons in *iab-3*. The location of miRiab-4/iab-8 in intron V is shown.

they specify respectively (though, in each parasegment, expression is limited to a subset of cells, see below).

Abd-B organization is a bit more complex than its counterparts of the BX-C, *Ubx*, and *abd*-A. While *Abd-B* is also expressed in a broad domain (**Figure 2A**), it is expressed as a parasegmental step-wise gradient and plays a visible specification role in all the parasegments where it is expressed (from PS10/A5 to PS13/A8; Kuziora and McGinnis, 1988; Celniker et al., 1990; Delorenzi and Bienz, 1990). Also, there is an alternatively spliced, truncated form of *Abd-B* originating from upstream promoters (B, C, and γ). This alternatively spliced isoform produces a truncated protein called *Abd-B*^{r}, which is expressed in PS14 (see **Figures 2D, 4E, 5B, 6A, 8A or 9A**) and where it plays a role in specifying PS14 identity (see below for more details).

TRANSCRIPTIONAL POSTERIOR DOMINANCE OF Hox GENES

Looking at the overall parasegment-specific expression pattern of *Ubx* and *abd-A*, or that of *abd-A* and *Abd-B* (**Figure 2**), their respective expression domains appear complementary to each other. These complementary appearances result from a general rule referred as to as "posterior dominance" in which a posterior Hox gene represses the expression of the immediately adjacent anterior Hox gene. For instances, *abd-A* represses *Ubx* in PS7 to PS12 (Struhl and White, 1985), and *Abd-B* represses *abd-A* in PS10 to PS13 (Karch et al., 1990). It should be noted that *abd-A* repression is not easily visible in PS10, PS11, and PS12, as *Abd-B* is expressed in only a few cells in these parasegments. A similar negative, *trans*-regulatory interaction exists between *Ubx* and *Antp*, the Hox gene responsible for PS4 specification. In this case, *Ubx* is known to repress *Antp* (Hafen et al., 1984; Carroll et al., 1986).

As a result of these negative cross-regulatory interactions, each parasegement is a mosaic of cells expressing different combinations of Hox genes. In Peifer et al. (1987) proposed that parasegmental identity was the readout of the unique mosaicism in each parasegments. This model predicts that each cell within a parasegment expresses a single Hox gene. In order to test his hypothesis, we carefully reexamined Hox gene expression in the *Drosophila* embryo using confocal microscopy analysis with antibodies directed against *Ubx*, *abd-A*, and *Abd-B*. The general rule that a given Hox gene represses expression of the immediately anterior expressed Hox gene appears mostly true. However, there is a notable exception with *abd-A* and *Abd-B* in the central nervous system (CNS), where both proteins are found co-expressed in many cells (**Figure 3**). Interestingly, we often found that cells with the highest levels of Abd-A protein also express high levels of Abd-B protein (**Figure 3**).

Abd-B DOES NOT REPRESS *abd-A* IN THE EMBRYONIC CENTRAL NERVOUS SYSTEM

The finding of cells expressing both *abd-A* and *Abd-B* contradicted the posterior transcriptional dominance rule of Hox genes as established by previous experiments. This prompted us to reexamine some of these experiments in more detail. Previously, it was shown that in the absence of *Abd-B* protein, *abd-A* protein becomes ectopically expressed in more posterior parasegments (Karch et al., 1990). This finding supported the idea that *Abd-B* and the posterior dominance rule restricted *abd-A* to more anterior abdominal parasegments. When we examined *Abd-B* null mutants in detail, we found that while we do indeed observe an extension of *abd-A* expression in PS13 in the epidermis, expression in the CNS remains unaffected (**Figure 4B**). This can, perhaps, be more easily seen in *Abd-B*^{D14} mutants (*Abd-B*^{D14}; **Figure 5**). As mentioned above, the *Abd-B* transcription unit displays some complexity, harboring multiple promoters (marked A, B, C, and γ; **Figures 1–8**; Zavortink and Sakonju, 1989; Boulet et al., 1991). Transcription initiating from the A promoter encodes the long isoform of the *Abd-B* protein referred as to the "m" isoform (for morphogenetic function; Casanova et al., 1986). The ABD-B m isoform is expressed from PS10/A5 to PS13/A8, thereby assigning identities to these parasegments/segments. Promoters B, C, and γ are only active in PS14. Splicing of these transcripts lead to the generation of a shorter isoform of *Abd-B* lacking the N terminal sequences of the m isoform. This shorter isoform is referred as to the "r" isoform (for regulatory function; Casanova et al., 1986; Kuziora and McGinnis, 1988; Boulet et al., 1991). In *Abd-B*^{D14}, a deletion removes the "A" promoter along with the N-terminal coding sequences of the ABD-B m isoform (Karch et al., 1985; Zavortink and Sakonju, 1989). As a consequence, there is no detectable expression of *Abd-B* in PS10 through PS13 (**Figure 5**). In agreement with this observation, the few emerging escaper flies have their fifth through eighth abdominal segments transformed into the fourth abdominal segment (Karch et al., 1985). In PS14, however, note the presence of the truncated "r" ABD-B isoform that is encoded by transcripts initiating from the B, C, and γ promoters. While *Abd-B* is absent in PS10-13, there is no extension of *abd-A* expression in the CNS into PS13 in the context of the *Abd-B*^{D14} mutant background (as illustrated by the gap between the red and green staining in **Figure 4**). This indicates that *Abd-B* is probably not responsible (or at least, not exclusively responsible) for *abd-A* repression in PS13.

We further confirmed this finding by asking if ectopic *Abd-B* could repress *abd-A* in the CNS. If PS13 like levels of *Abd-B* could repress *abd-A*, then ectopically activating *Abd-B* to PS13

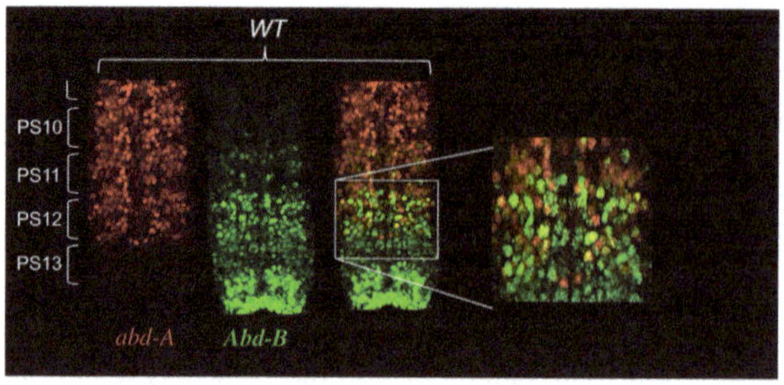

FIGURE 3 | *abd-A* and *Abd-B* are both co-expressed in some cells of the central nervous system. CNS of stage 15 embryos stained for *abd-A* (red) and *Abd-B* (green) were dissected and mounted on a slide with anterior on top. Parasegments boundaries are shown. Note the presence of neurons in PS10 to PS12 expressing both proteins as seen by the yellow color. Often the neurons expressing high level of *abd-A* also express *Abd-B*. (original observation published in Gummalla et al., 2012).

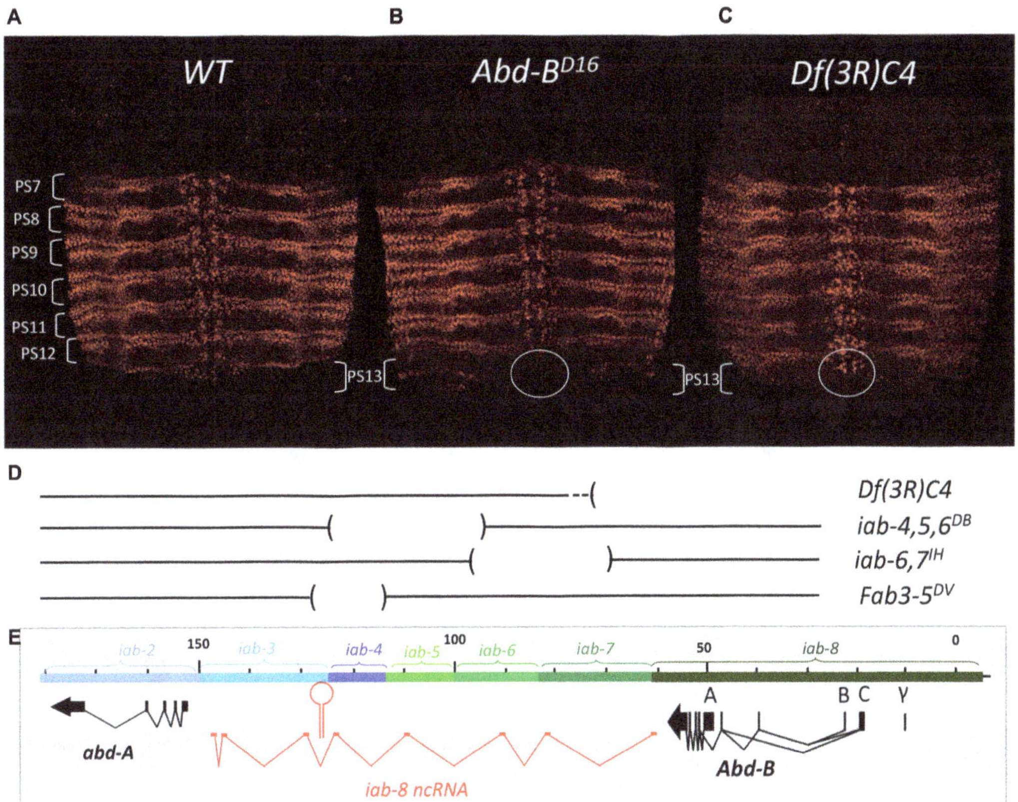

FIGURE 4 | *abd-A* expansion in PS13 in *Abd-B* mutant context is restricted to the epidermis. Pelts of stage 15 embryos stained for *abd-A* were prepared as in **Figure 1**. The WT expression pattern from PS7 to PS12 is shown in panel **A**. Panel **B** shows the pattern of *abd-A* expression in a homozygous *Abd-B*^{D16} mutant embryo. Note the expansion of *abd-A* expression in PS13 in the epidermis. In the CNS, however, (circled) there is no expansion. Panel **C** shows a homozygous *Df(3R)C4* mutant embryo in which *abd-A* expansion in PS13 occurs in both epidermis and CNS (circled; original observation published in Gummalla et al., 2012). Panel **D** depicts the extend of the various deficiencies we used in our unsuccessful attempts to locate a second discrete repressive mechanism (see page 13). Panel **E**, same as panel **D** in **Figure 2**.

levels in another PS, should repress *abd-A* expression. To do this, we used the *Fab-8*^{205} mutation (Barges et al., 2000). *Fab-8*^{205} is a mutation that removes a *cis*-regulatory domain boundary between *iab-7* and *iab-8*. Through a mechanism that is too complex to explain here, this deletion results in *iab-8*, normally driving PS13 levels of *Abd-B* expression, being activated in PS12. As expected of such a mutation, *Fab-8*^{205} results in a homeotic transformation of PS12/A7 into PS13/A8. Staining of *Fab-8*^{205} for *abd-A* showed normal levels of *abd-A* protein in PS12, indicating that PS13 levels of Abd-B cannot repress *abd-A* in the CNS(data not shown).

abd-A DEREPRESSION IN MUTATIONS EFFECTING A LONG-NON-CODING RNA

Based on these results, two possibilities can be imagined to account for the lack of *abd-A* expression in PS13 of the CNS. The simplest possibility is that *abd-A* may not be expressed in PS13 simply because it is never turned on. This would imply that the *iab cis*-regulatory domains act differently on *abd-A* in the epidermis versus the CNS. Alternatively, the lack of *abd-A* in PS13 of the CNS could results from a different, not-yet-identified repressive mechanism.

Mutation analysis points to the latter hypothesis as being correct. *Df(3R)C4* is a large deficiency that removes the entire *Abd-B* transcription unit as well as *iab-8* and about half of the of *iab-7* (**Figure 4D**). Staining for *abd-A* protein in *Df(3R)C4* embryos demonstrates that *abd-A* can be expressed in the CNS of PS13 (**Figure 4C**), suggesting that a repressive mechanism is involved in limiting *abd-A* expression. As we know *Abd-B* is not involved in this repression, we must assume that *Df(3R)C4* must delete additional sequences essential for the this second repressive mechanism. Previously, a large, 92 kb ncRNA spanning the intergenic region between *abd-A* and *Abd-B* was discovered emanating from a region in *iab-8* near the *Fab-8* boundary (see below and **Figures 2D, 4E, 5B, 6A, 8A,** and **9A**). We wondered if this long non-coding RNA (lncRNA), called the *iab-8*-ncRNA, could be involved in *abd-A* repression. As the promoter for the *iab-8*-ncRNA mapped to a region in *iab-8* just next to the *Fab-8* boundary, we examined *abd-A* expression in a larger *Fab-8* deletion (*Fab-8*^{64}) that also removes the ncRNA promoter. Interestingly, we found that in *Fab-8*^{64} mutants, we could see ectopic *abd-A* in PS13 even though *Abd-B* was expressed in both PS12 and PS13 at PS13 levels (**Figure 8C**). In fact, the levels of *abd-A* protein in PS13 resembled the levels of expression

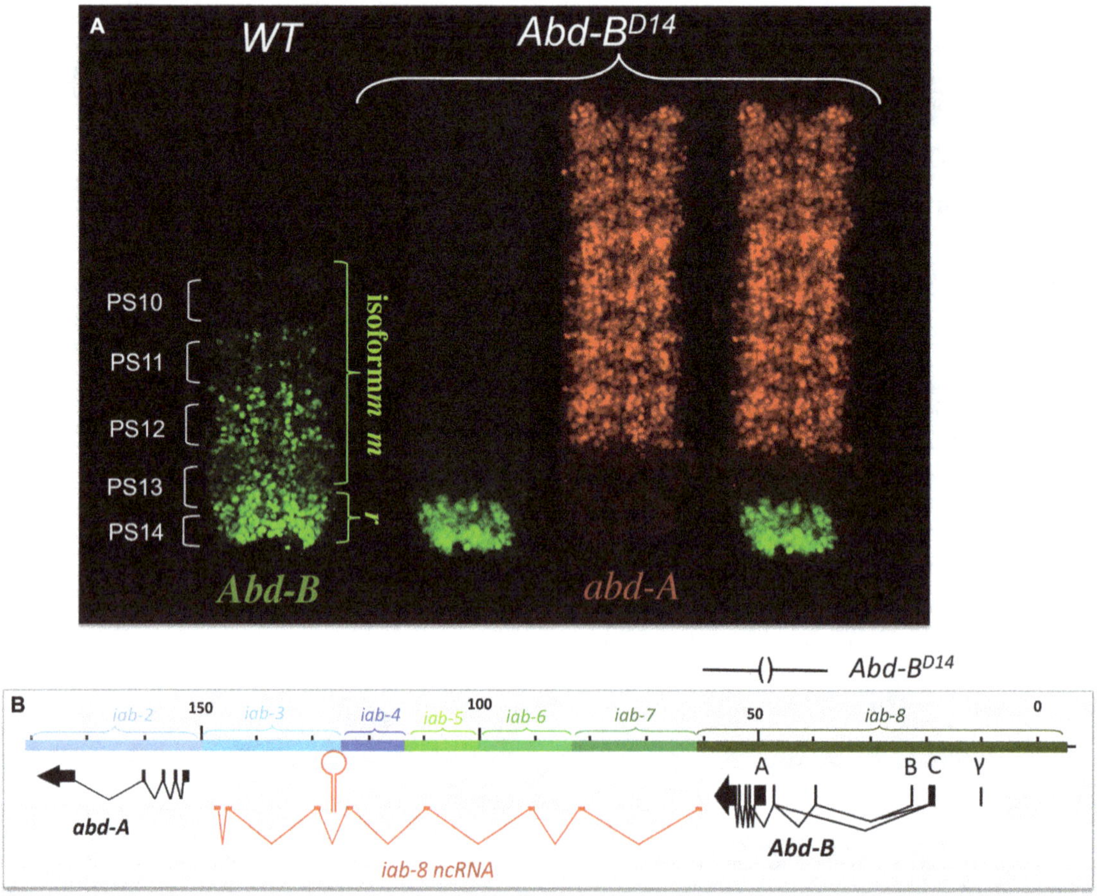

FIGURE 5 | *abd-A* is still repressed in the CNS of *Abd-B*^{D14} mutant embryo. *Abd-B*^{D14} removes the promoter A of the *Abd-B* transcription unit (indicated above panel **B**). As the A promoter is regulated by the *iab-5*, *iab-6*, *iab-7*, and *iab-8* regulatory domains, there is no *Abd-B* expression in PS10 to PS13 (see panel **A**). In PS14, however, a truncated version of *Abd-B* (cross-reacting with the antibody) is expressed in PS14 from the B, C, and γ promoters (panel **A**). This result indicates the existence of alternate mechanism(s) (than *Abd-B* repression) to keep *abd-A* off in PS13 (original observation published in Gummalla et al., 2012).

normally seen in PS12. Thus, these results pointed to the long *iab-8* ncRNA as the probable source of *abd-A* repression in PS13 of the CNS.

THE iab-8 ncRNA TRANSCRIPTION UNIT AND THE miR-iab-8 GENE

The first evidence for the existence of a large transcription unit spanning the *abd-A/Abd-B* intergenic region arose with the emergence of *in situ* hybridization techniques. Already, Sanchez-Herrero and Akam (1989) noticed the presence of a signal at the posterior end of the embryos detected with many large genomic probes. Then, several studies reported similar embryonic expression patterns in the CNS and epidermis in PS13 and 14 with strand-specific probes detecting transcripts oriented from *Abd-B* toward *abd-A* (Bae et al., 2002; Drewell et al., 2002; Hogga and Karch, 2002; Rank et al., 2002; Schmitt et al., 2005). The similarity between the expression patterns reported in these various studies was evident, but it was only in 2008 that it became clear that they reflected the existence of a very large transcription unit active in PS13 and PS14 (Bender, 2008). In Bender (2008) used gene conversion to generate a surgical deletion of a miRNA located between *abd-A* and *Abd-B*. At the time, it was known that the miRNA was expressed from both DNA strands and were called miR iab3-4 and miR iab 4-3 respectively, based on the orientation of the transcription unit producing the miRNA. The deletion created was only 45 nucleotides long (henceforth called Δ*miRNA*) to remove only the sequence encoding the two miRNAs. Although both miRNAs were predicted to target the *Ubx* and *abd-A* Hox genes, flies homozygous for the deletion did not harbor any segmental abnormalities, indicating that both miRNAs probably do not have a strict "homeotic function." While the body structure and anatomy of these flies appeared completely normal, both females and males deleted for these miRNAs are sterile. However, this sterility does not seem to stem from a physical problem with their reproductive organs (gonads and/or the genitalia). Instead, the sterility phenotype present in Δ*miRNA* flies seems to stem from a neuronal defect that makes them either unable to copulate (males) or unable to deposit eggs (females).

In as much as the miRNA gene is transcribed on both strands, Bender (2008) used a classical complementation test to determine

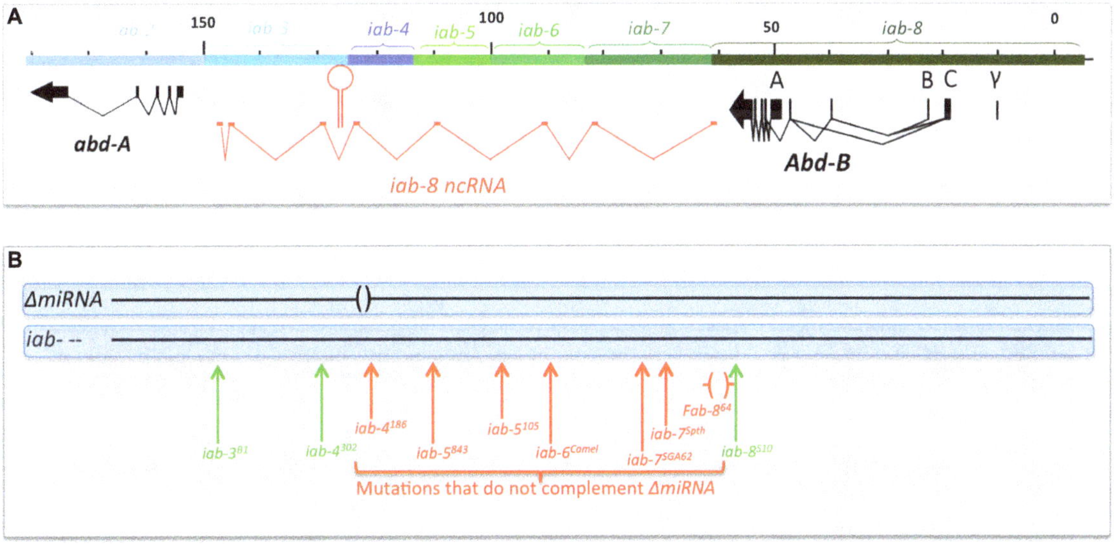

FIGURE 6 | Chromosomal breaks to the right of the miR-iab-8 fail to complement Δ*miRNA*. Panel **A** shows the genomic map of the abdominal region of the BX-C as described in **Figure 2**. Panel **B** symbolizes the two homologs chromosomes of heterozygotes between Δ*miRNA* and various rearrangement breakpoints that disrupt the abdominal region of the BX-C. Breaks in red fail to complement the sterility phenotype of ΔmiRNA, while break in green are fully fertile over ΔmiRNA. The *Fab-8*^{64} deletion removing the promoter of the iab-8 ncRNA is indicated by red brackets.

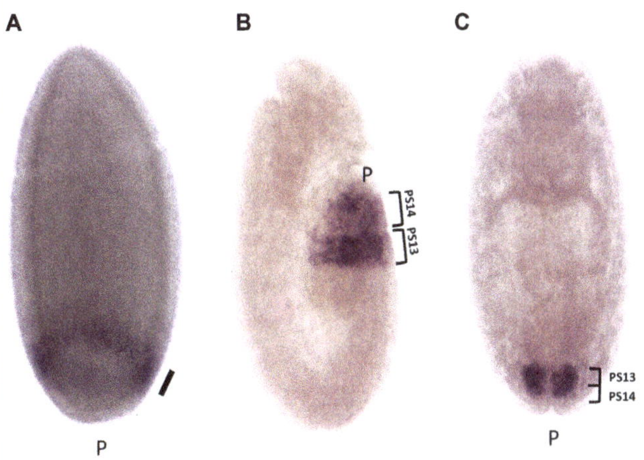

FIGURE 7 | Expression pattern of the *iab-8 ncRNA*. Embryos were hybridized with a strand-specific probe derived from the *iab-6* region, to detect transcription in the same polarity than *abd-A* and *Abd-B*. Panel **A** shows an embryo 3 h after fertilization at the cellular blastoderm stage. **A** uniform band is visible at the posterior end of the embryo (shown by the thick oblique bar). At this stage, transient transcription from the *iab-6* regulatory regions is detectable in PS11 (oblique arrow). At the elongated germ band stage **(B)**, transcription is visible in the epidermis in PS13 and PS14. Panel **C** show a stage 15 embryo, after germ band contraction. Transcription is restricted to the CNS in PS13 and PS14 (original observation published in Bender, 2008).

if the sterility resulted from failure in the production of one or the other (or both) miRNA. Drawing from the vast collections of bithorax alleles that interrupt the chromosomal continuity of the abdominal region of the BX-C, he determined that a 65 kb-long region between the miRNAs and *Abd-B* was required for the production of the miRNA (**Figure 6B**), as any chromosomal break within this region (the red vertical arrows in **Figure 6B**) failed to complement Δ*miRNA*. Breaks further to the left of the site of the miRNAs (**Figure 6B**) or to the right of *Fab-8*^{64} (green vertical arrows) are fertile when in *trans* to Δ*miRNA*. These observations indicate that the sterility phenotype is caused by loss of the miRNA produced from sense stand (relative to *abd-A* and *Abd-B* transcription) and define the region of DNA required for the production of this template RNA that spans from the region just downstream of the *Abd-B* transcription unit and extending to, at least, the site of the miRNA. As the position of the promoter lies within the *iab-8* regulatory domain, the transcript was named the *iab-8*-ncRNA and the miRNA was renamed miR-*iab-8* (Bender, 2008). RACE and RNAseq data later led to the precise definition of the *iab-8*-ncRNA as a 92 kb-long transcription unit spanning the entire *abd-A-Abd-B* intergenic region (Enderle et al., 2011; Graveley et al., 2011; Gummalla et al., 2012). Remarkably, the pri-miRNA transcript is spiced, with an exon derived from each of the *iab cis*-regulatory domains. A comparison with the genomic sequence data from 13 *Drosophila* species revealed that the transcript is conserved. Intriguingly, it is not the exonic sequences that are the most conserved, but the intron/exon junctions, as if it was the act of spicing that matters for the function of the *iab-8*-ncRNA. At present, there is no hint at the function of the spliced product or at the role of spicing in the function of the *iab-8*-ncRNA and/or miR-*iab-8*.

The expression pattern of the *iab-8*-ncRNA (and thus miR-*iab-8*) is consistent with the location of the promoter in *iab-8*, which controls the expression of *Abd-B* in PS13. The *iab-8*-ncRNA transcripts first appear at the posterior end of the embryo 3 h after fertilization, at the cellular blastoderm stage (**Figure 7A**). When

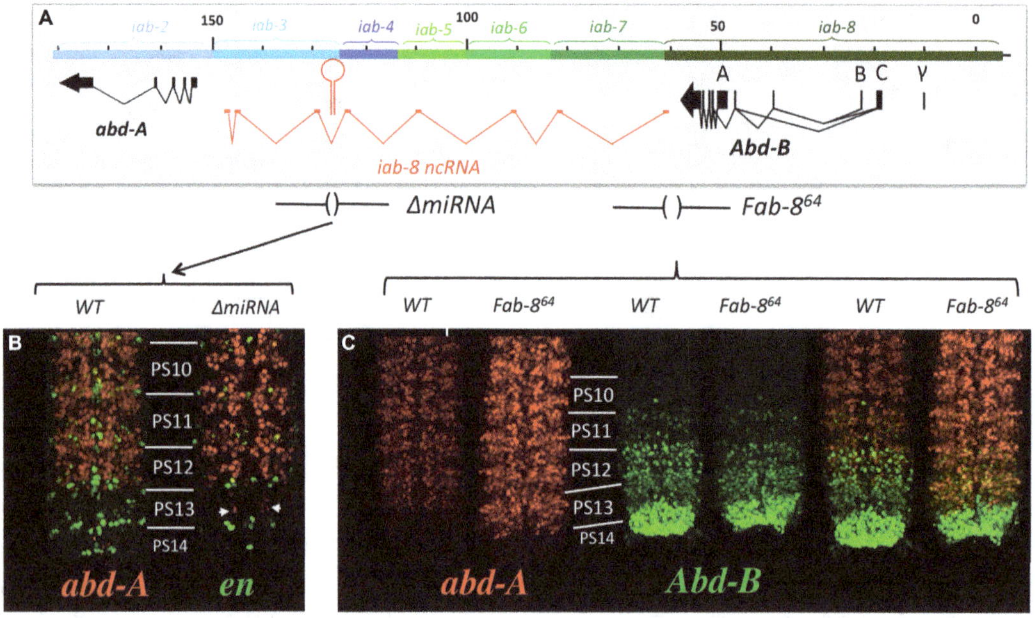

FIGURE 8 | *abd-A* is only de-repressed in a few cells in PS13 in Δ*miRNA*. Panel **A** shows the genomic map of the abdominal region of the BX-C as described in **Figure 2** with the ΔmiRNA deletion drawn above. CNSs were dissected out from stage 15 embryos Note in panel **B** that *abd-A* is de-repressed in only few neurons in PS13. Panel **C** show the *abd-A*(red) and *Abd-B* (green) expression patterns in WT and *Fab-8*^{64} homozygotes. Note the complete de-repression of *abd-A* in PS13 (original observation published in Gummalla et al., 2012).

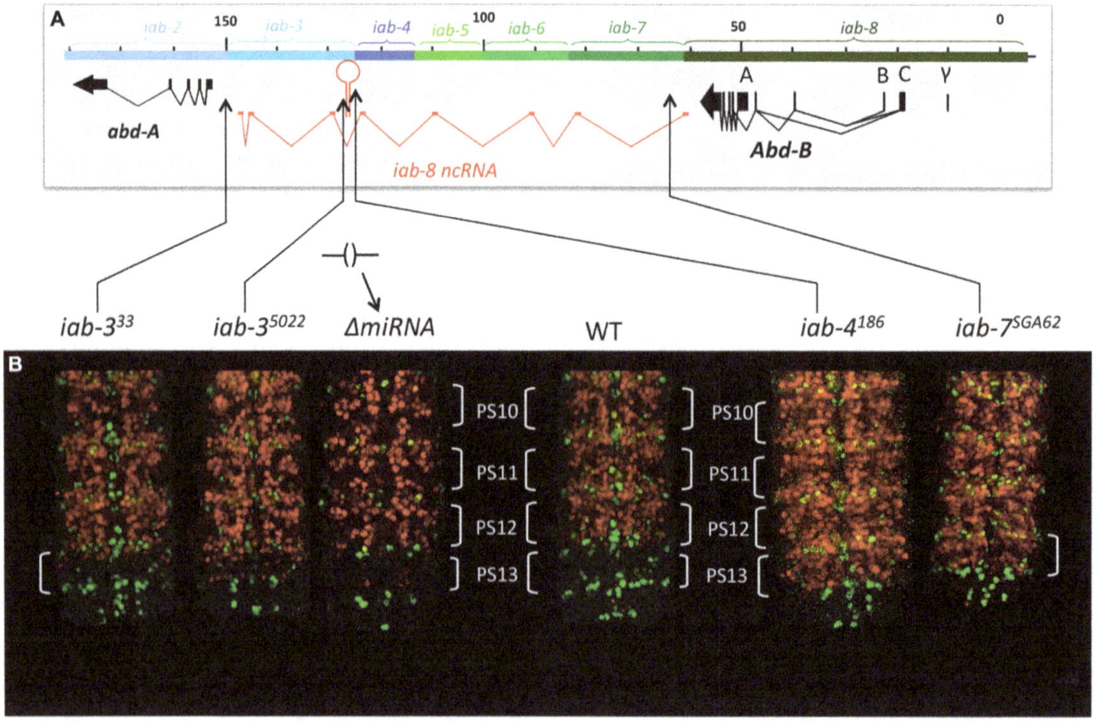

FIGURE 9 | *abd-A* expression in the CNS in mutant that truncate the iab-8 ncRNA. Panel **A**, show the molecular map of the abdominal region of the BX-C as in the figure above. The various rearrangement breaks truncating the iab-8ncRNA are shown below the map, along with the ΔmiRNA. Panel **B** show the posterior CNS of embryos that were stained for *abd-A* (red) and *engrailed* (*en*, green). The *engrailed* stripes mark each of the parasegments. Note that rearrangements disrupting the iab-8ncRNA upstream from miR-iab-8 lead to a complete de-repression of *abd-A* in the CNS in PS13 (*iab-6*^{186}, *iab-7*^{SGA62}). Rearrangements breaks disrupting the iab-8-ncRNA downstream from the site of miR-iab-8 result in only a partial de-repression of *abd-A* in PS13. A ΔmiRNA CNS is also shown for comparisons (original observation published in Gummalla et al., 2012).

the first signs of segmentation are visible (during germband elongation, **Figure 7B**), expression is restricted to PS13 and PS14 and mostly visible in the epidermis. After germband retraction, at the developmental stage where the nerve chord become visible, expression decays rapidly in the epidermis and become predominantly expressed in the CNS in PS13 and PS14, where it remains until for some time (**Figure 7C**). In fact, PS13/14 expression can even be seen in the CNS of third instar larvae (unpublished).

miR-iab-8 REPRESSES *abd-A* IN THE CNS IN PS13, BUT THIS IS NOT THE WHOLE STORY

Several features of miR-*iab-8* made it the prime candidate to be the repressor of *abd-A* expression in PS13 of the CNS. First, bioinformatics analysis predicted *abd-A* as a probable target of miR-*iab-8*. Second, it was strongly expressed in the cells where *abd-A* is repressed (PS13 of the CNS). Third, deletion of its promoter leads to a strong derepression of abd-A. And finally, reporter and ectopic expression studies showed that the *abd-A* 3′ UTR could in fact be targeted by the miRNA for translational repression (Stark et al., 2008; Tyler et al., 2008). Based on these findings, it seemed obvious that deletion of the miRNA would lead to *abd-A* derepression.

Examining *abd-A* expression in the CNS of Δ*miRNA* mutant embryos showed that there is indeed a misexpression of *abd-A* in animals lacking miR-*iab8*. Surprisingly, however, this misexpression is limited to only a few neurons (**Figure 8B**). Furthermore, the misexpression appears stochastic as the pattern of derepression varies between different nerve chords. This observation was unexpected as the deletion of the promoter caused much more drastic derepression (**Figure 8C**). Based on this result, we hypothesized the existence of a second, partially redundant mechanism involving the *iab-8*-ncRNA to keep *abd-A* repressed.

SEARCHING FOR A SECOND REPRESSION MECHANISM

As mentioned earlier, deletion of the *iab-8*-ncRNA promoter resulted in a complete derepression of *abd-A* in PS13. We used this phenotype to map additional elements in the *iab-8-ncRNA* that were important for *abd-A* repression. To do this, we first stained embryos, homozygous for various internal deficiencies in the *iab-8*-ncRNA sequence, thinking that if something like a second miRNA existed in the transcript, we might be able to identify it in this manner (Mihaly et al., 2006). Unfortunately, all deficiencies tested, with the exception of *Fab-3-5^{DV}*, which removes the iab-8-miRNA, show no phenotype in this assay (see **Figure 4D** for the extend of the deficiencies). It must be noted, however, that while most of the ncRNA sequence has been tested by deletion analysis, we have no deficiencies spanning the 3′ end of the RNA (a region of about 15 kb) that do not also remove the *abd-A* promoter.

Therefore, to continue this analysis, we next decided to stain embryos from flies homozygous for chromosomal rearrangements that break the continuity of the *iab-8*-ncRNA. Using these lines, we found that all breaks lying in between the miRNA and its promoter showed complete derepression of *abd-A* in PS13 of the CNS (**Figure 9**). For example, break *iab-4^{186}*, which breaks just upstream if the miRNA, shows a complete derepression of *abd-A* in PS13 of the CNS, much like an *iab-8*-ncRNA promoter deletion. Meanwhile, breaks lying between the miRNA and its 3′ end, which presumably still make the miRNA, showed a much milder, but visible derepression of *abd-A* in PS13 (**Figure 9**). This phenotype was reminiscent of Δ*miRNA* embryos (see, for example *iab-3^{5022}* in **Figure 9**). Based on the 3′-most rearrangement that causes a derepression of abd-A, we can limit the area where this second element must lie to a sequence of, at most, 5 kb (due to the resolution of the mutation mapping). This area contains two exons of the lncRNA and lies just 5′ to the *abd-A* transcriptional start site.

As stated above, we have no deficiencies covering most of this area that do not also remove the *abd-A* promoter. Therefore, we have had difficulty identifying the exact mechanism of this repression. However, a number of observations make us believe that the second mechanism does not involve a diffusible molecule, but simply depends on the transcription of the region around the *abd-A* promoter. First, no miRNAs have been predicted bioinformatically, or found from any miRNA screens, derived from the area in question. Second, although the transcript is spliced and polyadenylated, no known polypeptides are encoded by this transcript. Here, it must be noted that our colleague, Bender (2008) has studied the resulting cDNA from the spliced *iab-8*-ncRNA transcript in the fly. While he has found a conserved sequence in the eighth exon that could encode a micropeptide (Gummalla et al., 2012), overexpression of the *iab-8* cDNA has no affect on *abd-A* expression.

Based on our mapping experiments, we know that the second repressive function must be located in the last ~5 kb of the *iab-8*-ncRNA. Much of this sequence makes up the final two exons of the *iab-8*-ncRNA, whose spliced product seems to play no role in *abd-A* regulation. As this region also includes the upstream promoter area of *abd-A*, we wondered if the act of transcribing this area could provide the repressive function. This was a difficult thing to test because of the lack of genetic tools in the area. Still, we thought about what such a mechanism would imply. We reasoned that diffusible molecules should work both in *cis* and in *trans*, meaning that if one copy of the element is mutated, the product of the other copy of the element should be able to compensate for its loss, since it is a diffusible molecule. Indeed, loss of one copy of the *iab-8*-miRNA shows no effect on *abd-A* expression (it is recessive). However, if the mechanism was transcription across the *abd-A* promoter, then this mode of repression should only worked in *cis*, as the wild-type copy of the element on one chromosome should not be able to compensate for its loss on the other. We tested this by staining heterozygous rearrangement break mutants whose breaks were downstream of the miRNA. In all of the lines previously shown to derepress *abd-A* as homozygotes, we observed weaker but still noticeable derepression of *abd-A* as heterozygotes (**Figure 10**). The fact that a deficiency that removes the entire BX-C (including the *abd-A* and the *iab-8*-ncRNA) does not show a similar phenotype (Gummalla et al., 2012) means that this derepression is not due to simple haploinsufficiency for this second element and points to a *cis*-dominant effect, consistent with our model that transcription across the *abd-A* promoter causes *abd-A* repression.

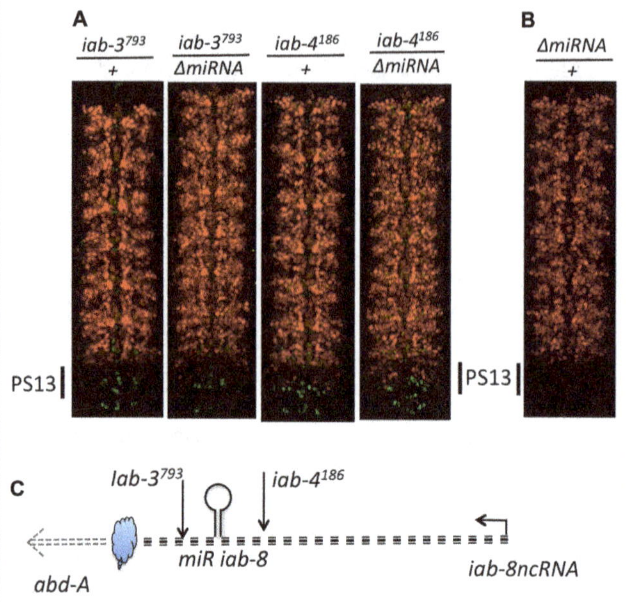

FIGURE 10 | Haplo-insufficiency of breaks disrupting the iab-8 ncRNA. Panel **A** show CNSs stained for *abd-A* (red) and *engrailed* (green) from embryos heterozygous for mutations disrupting the iab-8ncRNA. Panel **B** dispalys a CNS from a heterozygous ΔmiRNA/+ embryo. Note that while one dose of miR-iab-8 is sufficient to keep *abd-A* repressed in PS13 **(B)**, de-repression of *abd-A* in PS13 is observed in each of the four genotypes displayed in panel **A**. Panel **C** summarizes the relative positions of the *trans*-acting repression mechanism (miRiab-8) and *cis*-acting repression mechanism symbolized as a cloud. The level of de-repressions depends on the position of the disrupting break (upstream or downstream of miRiab-8). De-repression increases when the disrupting break is over ΔmiRNA. In *iab-4*^{186}/Δ*miRNA* PS13 *abd-A* expression reaches a level as if only one of the two homologs produces *abd-A*.

This type of repressive mechanism is generally called transcriptional interference. Although some instances of this phenomenon have been reported in metazoans, it has mostly been observed in yeast where one gene is inhibited by the transcription of its promoter region by a polymerase transcribing from an upstream gene (Greger and Proudfoot, 1998; Martens et al., 2005; Kim et al., 2012). This is very similar to the situation we observe at the *abd-A* locus, where the *iab-8*-ncRNA, though its promoter lies 93 kb away, is transcribed across the intervening sequence until within about 1 kb of the *abd-A* transcriptional start site. Though we have not proved this, we imagine that this transcription would then prevent promoter proximal enhancer elements from initiating transcription at the *abd-A* promoter.

A RETURN TO POSTERIOR DOMINANCE AND EVOLUTIONARY CONSIDERATIONS

We started this review by explaining how *abd-A* regulation in the CNS seems to break the posterior dominance rule of the *Drosophila* Hox genes. Now, with this new data, we realize that this may not be the case. The transcriptional control of *abd-A* by the *iab-8*-ncRNA can simply be viewed as a modified example of posterior dominance. In this case, the repression occurs not through a transcription factor, but through two, completely different mechanisms: a miRNA-based repression mechanism and what is most likely a transcriptional interference-based repression mechanism. If we think of the *iab-8*-ncRNA as a Hox complex "gene," then a more-posterior "gene" is still inhibiting a more anterior Hox gene, which fits with the posterior dominance rule.

The transcriptional interference model also provides another reason to explain the clustering of Hox genes in the fly. Transcriptional interference relies on having two genes in close proximity, so that the transcription of one interferes with the promoter of the other. Here, this seems to have been accomplished by the transcription of a lncRNA interfering with the promoter of the *abd-A* gene. The fact that loss of the ncRNA causes sterility and that it is initiated from a promoter in the *iab-8 cis*-regulatory domain (which controls *Abd-B* expression) means that there will be selective pressure to keep the *abd-A* and *Abd-B* genes clustered.

But why create such a complex mechanism to control *abd-A* expression in PS13 and 14 of the CNS? Although we cannot truly answer this question, we can provide some thoughts on the issue. First, we must assume that, in the CNS, there is a reason to eliminate the standard cross-regulatory interactions between *Abd-B* and *abd*-A to allow co-expression of the two Hox genes in the same cell. While fate mapping work has been extensively done in the CNS, we have not identified all of the neurons that express *abd-A*, or *Abd-B* or both, to know if the combinatorial expression of Hox genes leads to modification of cell fate. However, having said that, we do have some indication that co-expressing at least some Hox genes might affect cell viability. Work from the lab of Alex Gould showed that expression of *abd-A* in larval abdominal neuroblasts was required for the cessation cell division and eventual apoptosis of these cells (Bello et al., 2003). This work stemmed from the idea that there must be something to control neuroblast division in the brain, and from the initial observation that the there were ~10× fewer neuroblasts in the abdominal segments than in the thoracic segments. Based on the abdominal localization of this phenomenon, Bello et al. (2003) asked if *abd-A* could mediate this loss of neuroblasts. Their experiments showed both that the loss of *abd-A* in abdominal neuroblast led to an increase in the pool of neuroblasts and that the ectopic expression of *abd-A* in thoracic neuroblasts led to a decrease in the pool of neuroblasts. These phenotypes eventually could all be attributed to a pulse of *abd-A* expression during the third instar stage that caused the neuroblasts to undergo apoptosis. As the loss of neuroblasts affects A1–A7, it seems likely that *abd-A* and *Abd-B* might have to be expressed in the same cell to have this phenomenon occur in A5–A7.

Next, we must ask why this new type of regulation happens in the CNS. As it turns out, regulation by miRNAs may be a common feature for neuronal genes in *Drosophila*. Work by the Levine lab has shown that the function of the common pan-neuronal gene ELAV is to bind to the 3′ UTR sequences of certain transcripts and to prevent normal polyadenylation. The result of this activity is the extension of 3′ UTR sequences for many neuronal genes (Hilgers et al., 2011, 2012). In agreement with this finding it has been long known that many Hox genes with extended 3′ UTR (*Antp, Ubx, abd-A*, and *Abd-B*) are specifically expressed in the nervous system (Garber et al., 1983; Scott et al., 1983; Akam and Martinez-Arias, 1985; Kuziora and McGinnis, 1988; O'Connor et al., 1988). Supporting this work, the lab of Claudio Alonso has recently shown that many Hox genes, including *abd-A*, possess CNS-specific 3′ UTR extensions. The result of these extensions is often an increase in the number of miRNA target sites. In the case of *abd-A*, the extension adds two additional targets for the *iab-8*-miRNA. Alonso and colleagues propose that these 3′ extensions could indicate a need to lose miRNA regulation in the epidermis or a need to augment miRNA regulation in the CNS (Thomsen et al., 2010). The fact that the *iab-8*-ncRNA is expressed primarily in the CNS would definitely support the latter hypothesis with regards to *abd-A* regulation.

Lastly, we must discuss why such a long transcript has been conserved to perform these functions when a much smaller transcript might be able to do the same. Indeed a transcript starting just upstream of the miRNA could, if expressed in the right place, perform the same function. We know, for example, that artificially starting a transcript downstream of the actual *iab-8*-ncRNA promoter can inhibit *abd-A* expression in anterior segments (Gummalla, 2011). However, if the *iab-8*-ncRNA is required only in the posterior parasegments, then how could such a smaller RNA be expressed only in PS13 and 14 within the context of a more-anterior *cis*-regulatory domain. Although gene regulation in the BX-C is a little too complex to explain in this review, we can say that, in general, promoters located in a specific *cis*-regulatory domain, gain regulation by that *cis*-regulatory domain. Thus, a promoter located in *iab-4* would probably be expressed in a pattern driven by the *iab-4 cis*-regulatory domain (meaning that expression would start in PS9/A4) and would be expressed too anterior to be viable. Of course, one could simply imagine the cells of the CNS making a specific transcription factor or miRNA from another locus to inhibit *abd-A* expression in certain places, but then the issue becomes a matter of cost from where the system originated. Given that the fly has a system to elongate neuronal transcripts to provide more miRNA targets, and has a perfect place to obtain PS13 and 14 expression, we imagine that it was simpler to evolve the current ncRNA system than a secondary repressor. Given the large amount of ncRNAs currently being found in the cells of most organisms, it now seems clear that the energetic cost of transcription is probably not prohibitively high.

But this all assumes that transcriptional interference was added after the other mechanisms of Hox gene repression. This is still far from clear. It is possible that the first Hox genes were regulated by transcriptional interference. This is not an absurd notion to entertain. We know that the Hox genes were probably derived from tandem duplication events. Based on the similarity in construction of different *cis*-regulatory domains it seems likely that they too were made by duplication events happening later in evolution of an ancestral *cis*-regulatory region. Thus, the ancestral Hox complex contained just two very similar Hox genes, each probably controlled by small *cis*-regulatory domains. Each gene would probably express in a very similar pattern, having been duplicated from the same gene. Assuming a perfect duplication event, then the only differing feature with regards to these genes would be a slight difference in location on the chromosome and their neighboring genes. One can therefore imagine that if the 5′ gene could interfere with the transcription of its downstream brother, then this could have been one of the first events differentiating the two genes and allowing divergent functions to evolve.

ACKNOWLEDGMENTS

We thank Eva Favre Benjamin Barendun and Jorge Faustino for excellent technical assistance. This work was supported by the State of Geneva, the Swiss National Fund for Research and the Fonds Claraz.

REFERENCES

Akam, M. E., and Martinez-Arias, A. (1985). The distribution of *Ultrabithorax* transcripts in *Drosophila* embryos. *EMBO J.* 4, 1689–1700.

Bae, E., Calhoun, V. C., Levine, M., Lewis, E. B., and Drewell, R. A. (2002). Characterization of the intergenic RNA profile at abdominal-A and abdominal-B in the *Drosophila* bithorax complex. *Proc. Natl. Acad. Sci. U.S.A.* 99, 16847–16852. doi: 10.1073/pnas.222671299

Barges, S., Mihaly, J., Galloni, M., Hagstrom, K., Müller, M., Shanower, G., et al. (2000). The Fab-8 boundary defines the distal limit of the bithorax complex iab-7 domain and insulates iab-7 from initiation elements and a PRE in the adjacent iab-8 domain. *Development* 127, 779–790.

Beachy, P. A., Helfand, S. L., and Hogness, D. S. (1985). Segmental distribution of bithorax complex proteins during *Drosophila* development. *Nature* 313, 545–551. doi: 10.1038/313545a0

Bello, B. C., Hirth, F., and Gould, A. P. (2003). A pulse of the *Drosophila* Hox protein abdominal-A schedules the end of neural proliferation via neuroblast apoptosis. *Neuron* 37, 209–219. doi: 10.1016/S0896-6273(02)01181-9

Bender, W. (2008). MicroRNAs in the *Drosophila* bithorax complex. *Genes Dev.* 22, 14–19. doi: 10.1101/gad.1614208

Boulet, A., Lloyd, A., and Sakonju, S. (1991). Molecular definition of the morphogenetic and regulatory functions and the *cis*-regulatory elements of the *Drosophila* Abd-B homeotic gene. *Development* 111, 393–405.

Carroll, S. B., Laymon, R. A., McCutcheon, M. A., Riley, P. D., and Scott, M. P. (1986). The localization and regulation of Antennapedia protein expression in *Drosophila* embryos. *Cell* 47, 113–122. doi: 10.1016/0092-8674(86)90372-7

Casanova, J., Sanchez-Herrero, E., and Morata, G. (1986). Identification and characterization of a parasegment specific regulatory element of the abdominal-B gene of *Drosophila. Cell* 47, 627–636. doi: 10.1016/0092-8674(86)90627-6

Celniker, S. E., Sharma, S., Keelan, D. J., and Lewis, E. B. (1990). The molecular genetics of the bithorax complex of *Drosophila: cis-* regulation in the abdominal-B domain. *EMBO J.* 9, 4277–4286.

Delorenzi, M., and Bienz, M. (1990). Expression of abdominal-B homeoproteins in *Drosophila* embryos. *Development* 108, 323–329.

Drewell, R. A., Bae, E., Burr, J., and Lewis, E. B. (2002). Transcription defines the embryonic domains of *cis*-regulatory activity at the *Drosophila* bithorax complex. *Proc. Natl. Acad. Sci. U.S.A.* 99, 16853–16858. doi: 10.1073/pnas.222671199

Enderle, D., Beisel, C., Stadler, M. B., Gerstung, M., Athri, P., and Paro, R. (2011). Polycomb preferentially targets stalled promoters of coding and noncoding transcripts. *Genome Res.* 21, 216–226. doi: 10.1101/gr.114348.110

Garber, R. L., Kuroiwa, A., and Gehring, W. J. (1983). Genomic and cDNA clones of the homeotic locus *Antennapedia* in *Drosophila. EMBO J.* 2, 2027–2036.

Graveley, B. R., Brooks, A. N., Carlson, J. W., Duff, M. O., Landolin, J. M., Yang, L., et al. (2011). The developmental transcriptome of *Drosophila melanogaster. Nature* 471, 473–479. doi: 10.1038/nature09715

Greger, I. H., and Proudfoot, N. J. (1998). Poly(A) signals control both transcriptional termination and initiation between the tandem GAL10 and GAL7 genes of *Saccharomyces cerevisiae. EMBO J.* 17, 4771–4779. doi: 10.1093/emboj/17.16.4771

Gummalla, M. (2011). *abd-A regulation by the iab-8 noncoding RNA.* Ph.D. thesis, Thesis no. 4379, Faculty of Science, University of Geneva, Geneva.

Gummalla, M., Maeda, R. K., Castro Alvarez, J. J., Gyurkovics, H., Singari, S., Edwards, K. A., et al. (2012). abd-A regulation by the iab-8 noncoding RNA. *PLoS Genet.* 8:e1002720. doi: 10.1371/journal.pgen.1002720

Hafen, E., Levine, M., and Gehring, W. J. (1984). Regulation of *Antennapedia* transcript distribution by the bithorax complex in *Drosophila. Nature* 307, 287–289. doi: 10.1038/307287a0

Hilgers, V., Lemke, S. B., and Levine, M. (2012). ELAV mediates 3' UTR extension in the *Drosophila* nervous system. *Genes Dev.* 26, 2259–2264. doi: 10.1101/gad.199653.112

Hilgers, V., Perry, M. W., Hendrix, D., Stark, A., Levine, M., and Haley, B. (2011). Neural-specific elongation of 3' UTRs during *Drosophila* development. *Proc. Natl. Acad. Sci. U.S.A.* 108, 15864–15869. doi: 10.1073/pnas.1112672108

Hogga, I., and Karch, F. (2002). Transcription through the iab-7 *cis*-regulatory domain of the bithorax complex interferes with maintenance of Polycomb-mediated silencing. *Development* 129, 4915–4922.

Karch, F., Bender, W., and Weiffenbach, B. (1990). abdA expression in *Drosophila* embryos. *Genes Dev.* 4, 1573–1587. doi: 10.1101/gad.4.9.1573

Karch, F., Weiffenbach, B., Peifer, M., Bender, W., Duncan, I., Celniker, S., et al. (1985). The abdominal region of the bithorax complex. *Cell* 43, 81–96. doi: 10.1016/0092-8674(85)90014-5

Kim, T., Xu, Z., Clauder-Munster, S., Steinmetz, L. M., and Buratowski, S. (2012). Set3 HDAC mediates effects of overlapping noncoding transcription on gene induction kinetics. *Cell* 150, 1158–1169. doi: 10.1016/j.cell.2012.08.016

Kuziora, M. A., and McGinnis, W. (1988). Different transcripts of the *Drosophila* Abd-B gene correlate with distinct genetic sub-functions. *EMBO J.* 7, 3233–3244.

Lagos-Quintana, M., Rauhut, R., Meyer, J., Borkhardt, A., and Tuschl, T. (2003). New microRNAs from mouse and human. *RNA* 9, 175–179. doi: 10.1261/rna.2146903

Lewis, E. B. (1978). A gene complex controlling segmentation in *Drosophila. Nature* 276, 565–570. doi: 10.1038/276565a0

Lewis, E. B., Pfeiffer, B. D., Mathog, D. R., and Celniker, S. E. (2003). Evolution of the homeobox complex in the Diptera. *Curr. Biol.* 13, R587–R588. doi: 10.1016/S0960-9822(03)00520-7

Macias, A., Casanova, J., and Morata, G. (1990). Expression and regulation of the abd-A gene of *Drosophila. Development* 110, 1197–1207.

Maeda, R. K., and Karch, F. (2006). The ABC of the BX-C: the bithorax complex explained. *Development* 133, 1413–1422. doi: 10.1242/dev.02323

Maeda, R. K., and Karch, F. (2010). *Cis*-regulation in the *Drosophila* bithorax complex. *Adv. Exp. Med. Biol.* 689, 17–40. doi: 10.1007/978-1-4419-6673-5_2

Martens, J. A., Wu, P. Y., and Winston, F. (2005). Regulation of an intergenic transcript controls adjacent gene transcription in *Saccharomyces cerevisiae. Genes Dev.* 19, 2695–2704. doi: 10.1101/gad.1367605

Martin, C. H., Mayeda, C. A., Davis, C. A., Ericsson, C. L., Knafels, J. D., Mathog, D. R., et al. (1995). Complete sequence of the bithorax complex of *Drosophila. Proc. Natl. Acad. Sci. U.S.A.* 92, 8398–8402. doi: 10.1073/pnas.92.18.8398

Martinez-Arias, A., and Lawrence, P. (1985). Parasegments and compartments in the *Drosophila* embryo. *Nature* 313, 639–642. doi: 10.1038/313639a0

McGinnis, W., and Krumlauf, R. (1992). Homeobox genes and axial patterning. *Cell* 68, 283–302. doi: 10.1016/0092-8674(92)90471-N

Mihaly, J., Barges, S., Sipos, L., Maeda, R., Cleard, F., Hogga, I., et al. (2006). Dissecting the regulatory landscape of the Abd-B gene of the bithorax complex. *Development* 133, 2983–2993. doi: 10.1242/dev.02451

Negre, B., Ranz, J. M., Casals, F., Caceres, M., and Ruiz, A. (2003). A new split of the Hox gene complex in *Drosophila*: relocation and evolution of the gene labial. *Mol. Biol. Evol.* 20, 2042–2054. doi: 10.1093/molbev/msg238

Negre, B., and Ruiz, A. (2007). HOM-C evolution in *Drosophila*: is there a need for Hox gene clustering? *Trends Genet.* 23, 55–59. doi: 10.1016/j.tig.2006.12.001

O'Connor, M. B., Binari, R., Perkins, L. A., and Bender, W. (1988). Alternative RNA products from the *Ultrabithorax* domain of the bithorax complex. *EMBO J.* 7, 435–445.

Peifer, M., Karch, F., and Bender, W. (1987). The bithorax complex: control of segmental identity. *Genes Dev.* 1, 891–898. doi: 10.1101/gad.1.9.891

Rank, G., Prestel, M., and Paro, R. (2002). Transcription through intergenic chromosomal memory elements of the *Drosophila* bithorax complex correlates with an epigenetic switch. *Mol. Cell. Biol.* 22, 8026–8034. doi: 10.1128/MCB.22.22.8026-8034.2002

Sanchez-Herrero, E., and Akam, M. (1989). Spatially ordered transcription of regulatory DNA in the bithorax complex of *Drosophila. Development* 107, 321–329.

Schmitt, S., Prestel, M., and Paro, R. (2005). Intergenic transcription through a polycomb group response element counteracts silencing. *Genes Dev.* 19, 697–708. doi: 10.1101/gad.326205

Scott, M. P., Weiner, A. J., Hazelrigg, T. I., Polisky, B. A., Pirrotta, V., Scalenghe, F., et al. (1983). The molecular organization of the *Antennapedia* locus of *Drosophila. Cell* 35, 763–776. doi: 10.1016/0092-8674(83)90109-5

Stark, A., Bushati, N., Jan, C. H., Kheradpour, P., Hodges, E., Brennecke, J., et al. (2008). A single Hox locus in *Drosophila* produces functional microRNAs from opposite DNA strands. *Genes Dev.* 22, 8–13. doi: 10.1101/gad.1613108

Struhl, G., and White, R. A. (1985). Regulation of the *Ultrabithorax* gene of *Drosophila* by other bithorax complex genes. *Cell* 43, 507–519. doi: 10.1016/0092-8674(85)90180-1

Thomsen, S., Azzam, G., Kaschula, R., Williams, L. S., and Alonso, C. R. (2010). Developmental RNA processing of 3'UTRs in Hox mRNAs as a context-dependent mechanism modulating visibility to microRNAs. *Development* 137, 2951–2960. doi: 10.1242/dev.047324

Tyler, D. M., Okamura, K., Chung, W. J., Hagen, J. W., Berezikov, E., Hannon, G. J., et al. (2008). Functionally distinct regulatory RNAs generated by bidirectional transcription and processing of microRNA loci. *Genes Dev.* 22, 26–36. doi: 10.1101/gad.1615208

Von Allmen, G., Hogga, I., Spierer, A., Karch, F., Bender, W., Gyurkovics, H., et al. (1996). Splits in fruitfly Hox gene complexes. *Nature* 380, 116. doi: 10.1038/380116a0

White, R. A., and Wilcox, M. (1984). Protein products of the bithorax complex in *Drosophila. Cell* 39, 163–171. doi: 10.1016/0092-8674(84)90202-2

Zavortink, M., and Sakonju, S. (1989). The morphogenetic and regulatory functions of the *Drosophila* abdominal- B gene are encoded in overlapping RNAs transcribed from separate promoters. *Genes Dev.* 3, 1969–1981. doi: 10.1101/gad.3.12a.1969

2

microRNAs in axon guidance

Archana N. Iyer*[1]*, Anaïs Bellon*[2] *and Marie-Laure Baudet*[1]**

[1] *Center for Integrative Biology, University of Trento, Trento, Italy*
[2] *Department of Physiology, Development and Neuroscience, University of Cambridge, Cambridge, UK*

Brain wiring is a highly intricate process in which trillions of neuronal connections are established. Its initial phase is particularly crucial in establishing the general framework of neuronal circuits. During this early step, differentiating neurons extend axons, which reach their target by navigating through a complex environment with extreme precision. Research in the past 20 years has unraveled a vast and complex array of chemotropic cues that guide the leading tip of axons, the growth cone, throughout its journey. Tight regulation of these cues, and of their receptors and signaling pathways, is necessary for the high degree of accuracy required during circuit formation. However, little is known about the nature of regulatory molecules or mechanisms fine-tuning axonal cue response. Here we review recent, and somewhat fragmented, research on the possibility that microRNAs (miRNAs) could be key fine-tuning regulatory molecules in axon guidance. miRNAs appear to shape long-range axon guidance, fasciculation and targeting. We also present several lines of evidence suggesting that miRNAs could have a compartmentalized and differential action at the cell soma, and within axons and growth cones.

****Correspondence:***
Marie-Laure Baudet, Center for Integrative Biology, University of Trento, Via delle Regole, 101, Trento 38123, Italy
e-mail: marielaure.baudet@unitn.it

Keywords: miRNAs, axon guidance, axon, growth cone, neuron, development

INTRODUCTION

Brain wiring occurs during the development of the nervous system and ensures the formation of a highly complex network of inter-communicating neurons. For these circuits to be established, neurons form remarkably accurate connections with their target cells. Initially, neurons send out cell protrusions called axons, which navigate a complex environment to reach their exact targets: a process known as axon guidance (or "pathfinding"). How do axons know where to go? Specific molecules present along the pathway act as signposts to guide axons to their final destination by either repelling or attracting the leading tip of the axon—the growth cone. These guidance cues are also capable of promoting axon fasciculation, i.e., the bundling of axons together, and interactions between axons and their substrate (Tessier-Lavigne and Goodman, 1996). Over the past two decades, genetic, biochemical and cell culture analysis have unraveled four major families of guidance molecules, which can be classified into four families: Ephrins, Semaphorins, Slits, and Netrins (Dickson, 2002). More recent works demonstrated that some morphogens, growth factors, and cell-adhesion molecules also have guidance function (Kolodkin and Tessier-Lavigne, 2011). Cue-mediated signaling leads to complex remodeling of the cytoskeleton in growth cones, which in turn regulates its directional steering and interactions with other axons, cells, and the environment (Dent et al., 2011).

The nervous system contains up to a few billions of neurons depending on the species, and each neuron is at the core of a highly complex connectome, which can receive and project to up to hundreds of thousands of synaptic partners. The startling complexity of this system has long confronted neuroscientists with the incongruity of the seemingly inadequate size of the genome of roughly 20,000 defined genes. Alternative splicing is thought to partly account for such complexity, since it can generate hundreds of isoforms from a single coding gene (Schmucker et al., 2000; Li et al., 2007). In addition to this, the non-coding regulatory regions of the transcriptome, or "dark matter" (Johnson et al., 2005), is increasingly thought to account for the complexity of the neuronal connectome at the molecular level. This includes a growing number of families of small RNAs, primarily the microRNAs (miRNAs).

miRNAs are a class of small ~22 nt non-coding RNAs that have emerged, in recent years, as key post-transcriptional regulators in most eukaryotic cells. They do so by specifically binding to mRNA through partial complementarity, thereby inhibiting transcript translation, and/or stability (Bartel, 2009). Since the discovery of the first miRNA, *lin*-4, more than 20 years ago in *C. elegans* (Lee et al., 1993; Wightman et al., 1993), hundreds of new miRNAs have been identified (Griffiths-Jones, 2004; Griffiths-Jones et al., 2008; Kozomara and Griffiths-Jones, 2011, 2013) (www.miRbase.org). Importantly, the nervous system is the site of an intricate "miRNnome," as numerous miRNAs are enriched or specifically expressed there in time and place (Johnston and Hobert, 2003; Krichevsky et al., 2003; Chang et al., 2004b; Hsieh, 2012; Zou et al., 2013). Recent large-scale studies have further revealed that individual miRNAs fine-tune the expression of hundreds of transcripts (Baek et al., 2008; Selbach et al., 2008; Guo et al., 2010). The regulatory potential of miRNAs in developing organisms, and particularly in the nervous system, thus appears infinite. The roles of miRNAs in promoting the complexity and accuracy required for circuit formation, and axon guidance in particular, has however just started to emerge.

Here, we review a small, but compelling body of research suggesting that miRNAs are important players in axon guidance. We first examine the roles of miRNAs in key steps of axon pathfinding, namely long-range guidance, fasciculation, and targeting. We then expose some evidence which points toward the possibility that miRNAs might have a compartmentalized action in projecting neurons, in the soma, axon, or growth cone.

ROLES OF miRNAs IN AXON GUIDANCE

LONG-RANGE GUIDANCE

In the initial phase of axon navigation, axons must first polarize, and subsequently navigate through a complex cellular terrain containing guidance cue-expressing "guidepost" cells. Neuronal or glial cells can take on the role of guidepost cells and act as substrates or intermediary targets for the growing axon. This enables axons to extend in a directed manner rather than by passive adhesion in a step-wise manner, using mechanisms that are highly conserved in both vertebrates and invertebrates (Raper and Mason, 2010). miRNAs could impact the transcriptome of projection neurons, regulating the expression of molecules that transduce cue signaling. Alternatively, they could affect guidepost cells to regulate directly or indirectly cue expression. In this section, we review a few recent findings on different model systems suggesting multiple roles and sites for miRNA action, which regulates both the navigating neuron and its environment.

Pinter and Hindges (2010) were the first to report that miRNAs, as a class of molecules, are important for long-range axon navigation using mice retinal ganglion cells (RGCs) as a model. RGCs are the only projection neurons of the retina and convey visual information to higher brain centers. In wild type monocular species, almost all RGC axons decussate at the optic chiasm, a midline structure. Whereas in binocular species, such as mice, some axons do not cross at the chiasm, but remain ipsilateral. The midline is thus an important choice point. The authors observed that, in absence of most miRNAs, many contralateral-projecting RGC axons failed to cross at the chiasm, and instead, aberrantly navigated ipsilaterally or overshot the midline. The molecular mechanisms leading to this phenotype is unknown to date. To abolish miRNAs function, Pinter and Hindges used mutants mice where Dicer, a key enzyme responsible for the maturation of most miRNAs (Bernstein et al., 2001; Grishok et al., 2001; Ketting et al., 2001; Knight and Bass, 2001), was conditionally ablated in Rx-expressing cells including RGCs and cells forming the optic chiasm. Depletion of miRNAs in these mutants could, therefore, either lead to impaired cue expression by guidepost cells at the midline, or to altered sensitivity of RGC growth cones to midline cues following misexpression of their cognate receptors or associated signaling molecules. Several ligand-receptor pairs are known to mediate midline crossing in mice: ephrin-B2/EphB1 (Nakagawa et al., 2000; Williams et al., 2003) Slit 1/2/Robo 1/2 (Plump et al., 2002; Plachez et al., 2008) VEGF164/Neuropilin-1 (Erskine et al., 2011), Sema 6D/Nr-CAM, and Plexin A1 (Kuwajima et al., 2012). Their direct or indirect regulation by miRNAs is however unknown to date except for Neuropilin-1 (Baudet et al., 2012; Cui et al., 2012; Zhang et al., 2012) and Robo 1 and 2 (Alajez et al., 2011; Fish et al., 2011; Yang et al., 2012). Of interest, miR-218 was documented to target Slit receptors Robo 1 and 2 in non-neural cells such as cancer cells (Alajez et al., 2011; Fish et al., 2011; Yang et al., 2012) suggesting it might also play a role in neurons including axons where it is also expressed (Sasaki et al., 2013). Overall, this study is the first *in vivo* evidence to show that miRNAs may impact projecting neurons, guidepost cells, or both.

miR-9 was also recently documented to regulate the long-range guidance of thalamocortical (TCAs) and corticofugal axons (CFAs) tracts (Shibata et al., 2011). Both tracts cross the telencephalon and navigate through the internal capsule, a telencephalic structure, before reaching their final destination (Molnár et al., 2012). Migration of guidepost cells called "corridor cells" to the internal capsule is a crucial event in TCA and CFA pathfinding. These cells create a permissive corridor within the medial ganglionic eminence (MGE), a telencephalic region, normally non-permissive to the growth of TCAs, and thus enable these axons to cross the telencephalon prior to reaching their final destination (López-Bendito et al., 2006). To address the roles of miR-9 specifically in telencephalic development, Shibata, and colleagues generated miR-9-2/3 double mutant mice lacking two of the three miR-9 pre-cursors, namely miR-9-2, and miR-9-3 (Shibata et al., 2011). In miR-9-2/3 double mutants, CFAs and TCAs were severely misrouted. CFAs poorly innervated the internal capsule. Similarly, TCAs failed to reach this region, and instead aberrantly projected into the hypothalamus, an area that they normally avoid. The deregulated molecular mechanisms leading to this phenotype are unclear, and likely to be complex. Evidence suggests that the TCA and CFA aberrant projections might be attributed to impaired patterning of corridor cells, although the possibility that miR-9 acts cell-autonomously in these projecting tracts cannot be excluded. Indeed, the topographical distribution of corridor cells within the telencephalon was affected; corridor neurons were expanded or dispersed in mutant animals. In addition, corridor cell markers islet-1 and Meis2 (predicted targets of miR-9) expression appeared to be qualitatively up-regulated in miR-9-2/3 double mutant mice. The mechanistic implication of this dysregulation on the pathfinding defects observed is, however, unclear. Thus, these data suggest that miR-9 may ensure the proper development of corridor cells and in turn the accurate projection of TCA and CFA to this intermediate target. Together, this study points to the interesting possibility that long-range axon guidance defects might indirectly rise from miRNA-induced impaired patterning of guidepost cells.

Finally, *lin*-4 was recently reported to also regulate long-range guidance of the axonal projection of anterior ventral microtubule (AVM) neurons in *C. elegans* larvae (Zou et al., 2012). In wild type animals, AVM axons project to the nerve ring, a neuropil considered as the *C. elegans*' brain. Before projecting anteriorly toward their target, AVM neurons are guided by two chemotropic cues that, together, orient the axons ventrally toward the midline. SLT-1 (Slit) repels AVM axons, preventing them from projecting dorsally, and UNC-6 (Netrin) attracts AVM axons ventrally (Chang et al., 2004a). The authors examined whether *lin*-4, a miRNA expressed in AVM during axon pathfinding, is important for UNC-6-mediated axon guidance. *lin*-4 was found to inhibit UNC-6 signaling during AVM axon guidance (Zou et al., 2012). Importantly, *lin*-4 acted cell-autonomously, at least in part, and specifically in post-migrating neurons. LIN-14, a transcription factor and well-described target of *lin*-4, is also expressed in AVM neurons. LIN-14 was found to mediate *lin*-4 action on AVM guidance and to potentiate UNC-6 mediated attraction of AVM axons by acting on UNC-40 (DCC) receptors. Surprisingly, *lin-14* did not alter *unc-40* promoter activity. Instead, it enhanced UNC-40 protein expression via an unknown mechanism, shifting its distribution from the confined perinuclear region to the whole cell. Intriguingly, *lin-4* and *lin-14* are broadly expressed in *C. elegans*, and both are found in several UNC-40 guided neurons. This suggests that a *lin-4/lin-14* based conserved regulatory pathway might modulate UNC-6-mediated axon attraction of other tracts. In addition, miR-125, a *lin-4* ortholog, is also present in neurons of vertebrates (Sempere et al., 2004; Smirnova et al., 2005), indicating that this ancient microRNA may have conserved its guidance function. Overall, this study revealed that *lin-4* regulates cue-mediated attraction by modulating the signaling pathway of a receptor to guidance cue. Importantly, it also provided evidence that miRNAs can act cell-autonomously to modulate axon guidance to the midline. In summary, a few studies have revealed that miRNAs regulate long-range axon navigation, acting cell autonomously on projecting neurons, and possibly on guidepost cells.

FASCICULATION

Pioneers axons begin their pathfinding journey in an environment devoid of axons and are the first to establish connection with the target. Follower axons arise at a later time point in development and can progress along the pathway through axon-axon contact, thereby using topographical information provided by pioneers (Pittman et al., 2008). The process by which those co-extending axons form tight bundles is called fasciculation and is thought to be mediated by various classes of molecules including neural cell adhesion molecules (NCAM) but also guidance cues (Huber et al., 2005; Luxey et al., 2013). As reviewed below, some evidence suggests that miRNAs could play a role in the formation of these fasciculated bundles.

Giraldez et al. (2005) reported that Maternal Zygotic (MZ) Dicer zebrafish mutants, devoid of maternal and embryonic sources of Dicer, exhibit several defasciculated axon tracts. Specifically, fasciculation of the post-optic commissure and hindbrain axonal scaffold, formed by longitudinal and commissural tracts, were severely disrupted in the absence of most miRNAs. Although defasciculation can lead to aberrant axonal trajectory (Huber et al., 2005), projections were correctly established at least for longitudinal hindbrain axons. In addition, early patterning and fate specification was preserved in these animals. This suggests that these defects may be linked to altered molecular programs specifically in these projecting neurons, although impaired cue expression within the axonal environment cannot be formally ruled-out. Interestingly, exogenous miR-430 family members partly rescued this phenotype. This suggests that members of this family, or other uncharacterized miRNAs, may alter the expression or signaling of molecules mediating bundling of these tracts. Such molecules may include Sema3D and its cognate receptor Neuropilin-1A, which is known to promote fasciculation of hindbrain longitudinal axons in zebrafish (Wolman et al., 2004; Kwok et al., 2012). A defasciculation phenotype of RGC axons was also observed in Rx-conditional Dicer knockout mice (Pinter and Hindges, 2010). In these animals, RGC axons failed to form a tight bundle within the retina. In addition at the midline, axons that aberrantly projected ipsilaterally were defasciculated, while axons overshooting the chiasm formed a secondary defasciculated tract. Interestingly, Sema 3D, Plexin A-1, Nr-CAM, Slit1, and 2 are implicated in the fasciculation of RGC axons (Ringstedt et al., 2000; Plump et al., 2002; Kuwajima et al., 2012) suggesting that their signaling might be derailed in Dicer mutants. Overall, miRNAs appear to regulate fasciculation, although the molecular mechanisms and the nature of the miRNAs involved are still largely elusive.

AXON TARGETING

After their long journey, axons reach their final destinations. Targeting of axons to their exact partner is absolutely essential, as it ensures proper circuit formation. This process is highly complex and requires several classes of molecules that promote defasciculation and specific entry within the target region, restricts any further elongation but also prevent axons from exiting the target-area. Cue-mediated restriction of the target-area is a highly regulated process in which miRNAs have been recently shown to play a role (Baudet et al., 2012).

Using *Xenopus laevis*, Baudet et al. (2012) uncovered a miRNA based signaling pathway that regulates axon targeting of RGCs to the optic tectum. Knockdown of miR-124 neither altered the birth of RGCs nor the general progression of their differentiation. However, it appeared to affect post-mitotic RGCs axon projection. While long-range guidance was unaffected, a subset of axons failed to appropriately stall within the optic tectum. Instead, they invaded Sema3A expressing territories in the ventral border, normally repellent to these axons at this stage. The effect of miR-124 is likely to be cell-autonomous, as straying axons were observed both when miR-124 was knocked down in cells of the central nervous system (which include RGCs and tectal cells), and also when knocked down at a later developmental stage in retinal cells. In addition, growth cone responsiveness to Sema3A was impaired in miR-124 morphants. The authors also elucidated the molecular pathway mediating miR-124-regulated Sema3A repulsion. miR-124 indirectly promoted the expression of Neuropilin-1, a Sema3A receptor, at the growth cone, since its depletion decreased Neuropilin-1 levels within growth cones *in vitro* and axons *in vivo*. miR124 regulated Neuropilin-1 via the silencing of its conserved target coREST, a cofactor of the global neuronal repressor REST (RE1-silencing transcription factor). Indeed, knockdown of coREST rescued Neuropilin-1 levels at the growth cone, and also growth cone responsiveness to Sema3A, in miR-124 morphants *in vitro*. Overall, this study uncovered a complex mechanism whereby miR-124 ensures RGC axonal response to Sema3A, at the right time and place, by dynamically inhibiting coREST repression of Neuropilin-1 within maturing RGCs. It also revealed for the first time that a miRNA regulates axon guidance (targeting) *in vivo*.

CONCLUSION

In summary, several studies have together revealed the function of miRNAs in axonal navigation to their final destinations using central nervous system projections as model (**Table 1**, **Figure 1**) (Giraldez et al., 2005; Pinter and Hindges, 2010; Shibata et al.,

Table 1 | List miRNAs and their target involved in guidance.

miRNA	mRNA	Age	Species	Neuron type	Phenotype*	References
lin-4	LIN-14	L1 and L2 stage	*C. elegans*	AVM	Impaired long-range guidance	Zou et al., 2012
miR-124	CoREST	St 24,32,40	*X. laevis*	RGC	Impaired targeting	Baudet et al., 2012
miR-134	Xlimk1	St 22	*X. laevis*	Spinal	Loss of BDNF-induced growth cone turning	Han et al., 2011

**upon loss of function.*
Abbreviations: AVM, Anterior Ventral Microtubule; RGC, Retinal Ganglion Cells; st, stage; X, Xenopus.

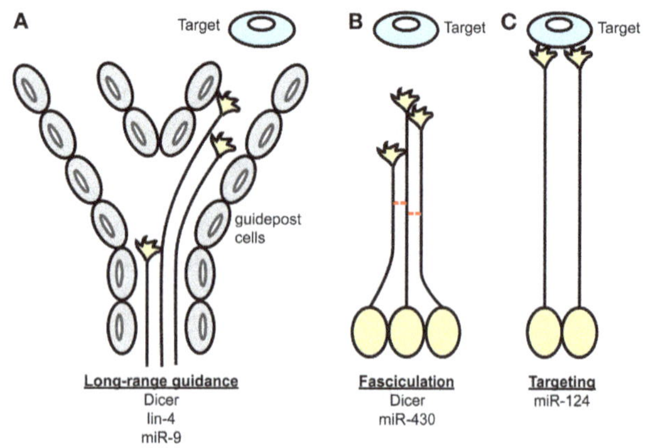

FIGURE 1 | Key processes of axon guidance regulated by miRNAs. During axon pathfinding toward a target, miRNAs regulate **(A)** the long-range guidance of axons by acting within projection neurons and/or guidepost cells located along permissive corridors or at the midline, **(B)** the fasciculation of axons in a given tract, and **(C)** the restriction of the axonal targeting area. The components of the miRNA pathway involved in each process are specified under each scheme.

2011; Baudet et al., 2012; Zhang et al., 2013; Chiu et al., 2014). Earlier work took a broad approach, and knocked down the entire pool of miRNAs using a Dicer loss-of-function strategy (Giraldez et al., 2005; Pinter and Hindges, 2010). This was particularly important at that time to determine whether miRNAs, as a class of molecules, are involved in axon guidance. Although striking phenotypes were observed suggesting the importance of miRNAs in this process, the full extent of miRNAs' implication in guidance maybe somewhat underestimated for several reasons. miRNA turn-over varies, and some can be particularly stable for a long time following ablation of Dicer (Schaefer et al., 2007). In addition, recent studies have shown that miRNAs can be synthesized via a Dicer-independent mechanism (Cheloufi et al., 2010; Cifuentes et al., 2010; Yang et al., 2010)—although, only one miRNA, miR-451, is documented to employ this non-canonical pathway (Yang et al., 2010). Of interest, Dicer is also involved in small interfering (si) RNA processing from various sources such as small nuclear (sn) RNA and viral double stranded (ds) RNA (Bernstein et al., 2001; Grishok et al., 2001; Ketting et al., 2001; Knight and Bass, 2001; Li et al., 2002). Dicer loss-of-function in these initial analyses (Giraldez et al., 2005; Pinter and Hindges, 2010) could thus impair this processing also. The importance of these additional roles has yet to be demonstrated in neurons however. Later studies went on to unravel the roles of individual miRNAs in axon guidance. New insight has come from those that have explored the cell-autonomous roles of miRNAs *in vivo*; for instance directly in projecting neurons (Baudet et al., 2012; Zou et al., 2012). Future research *in vivo* should however reveal additional functions of miRNAs, and their associated mechanisms of action. In particular, it is unknown whether miRNAs modulate cue expression in the pathway, either by acting directly on post-transcriptional regulation of transcripts expressed in guidepost cells, or on their patterning. However, gaining future insight will be complicated by the fact that this field has several pitfalls. High level of redundancy of miRNA function exists, especially for those miRNAs derived from the same family (Choi et al., 2008) or the same polycistron (Ventura et al., 2008) making the identification of individual guidance miRNAs particularly difficult. Deciphering the molecular mechanisms at play represents also a hurdle, since miRNAs are often part of complex molecular networks. Overcoming these challenges will thus be crucial in the future elucidation of miRNA function in guidance.

COMPARTMENTALIZED ACTION OF miRNAs

Numerous miRNAs appear to be differentially distributed within organisms, tissues, and cells. This is particularly true for the nervous system where miRNAs are enriched and specifically located in different regions and cell types (Krichevsky et al., 2003; Landgraf et al., 2007; Pichardo-Casas et al., 2012). Intriguingly, differential distribution is also observed at the subcellular level. Specific miRNAs are found to be enriched at synapses and dendrites compared to the cell soma (Siegel et al., 2009). This is perhaps not surprising considering that neurons are highly polarized cells with compartmentalized mRNA repertoires (Taylor et al., 2009; Zivraj et al., 2010; Gumy et al., 2011; Kaplan et al., 2013) implying that different compartments may have different regulatory requirements. Recent data have emerged suggesting that miRNAs are localized and might function within different subcellular location of projection neurons. For instance, some miRNAs may act within soma, affecting targets that have a global range of action; whilst others may have a more restricted, compartmentalized action within axons, and possibly, restricted to growth cones. The following section presents data summarizing these two possibilities.

SOMATIC ROLES OF miRNAs

Aforementioned studies have provided evidence that at least two specific miRNAs are likely to act primarily within the neuronal cell body during axon guidance. miR-124 in *Xenopus* (Baudet et al., 2012) and *lin*-4 in *C.elegans* (Zou et al., 2013) have somatic distribution within RGCs and AVM, respectively. *lin*-4 ortholog miR-125b is enriched in axons of the superior cervical ganglion (SCG) in mice (Natera-Naranjo et al., 2010) however, suggesting that the subcellular distribution might be cell or species specific. In contrast, miR-124 is enriched in the perinuclear cell soma of various neurons, compared to axons, synapses, or dendrites (Kye et al., 2007; Siegel et al., 2009; Natera-Naranjo et al., 2010), suggesting that this miRNA might have a conserved site of action. In addition, the molecular nature of the miR-124 and *lin*-4 targets strongly suggest restricted action within cell bodies, as both targets are transcription factors: coREST (Baudet et al., 2012) and *lin*-14 (Zou et al., 2012). Taken together, this suggests that miR-124 and *lin*-4 acts within neuronal cell soma of projecting neurons to regulate axonal pathfinding.

miRNAs were first described as heterochronic genes regulating the developmental timing of many *C.elegans* cell lineages (Lee et al., 1993; Wightman et al., 1993; Reinhart et al., 2000). Their roles as timers also occur in vertebrates including in neuronal lineages (Decembrini et al., 2009; Cremisi, 2013; La Torre et al., 2013). Intriguingly, miRNAs might also function as timers in in post-mitotic neurons during later developmental events (Olsson-Carter and Slack, 2010; Baudet et al., 2012; Zou et al., 2012) but also following terminal differentiation (Chiu and Chang, 2013; Zou et al., 2013). In particular, *lin*-4 and miR-124 were reported to affect the developmental aging of post-mitotic differentiating neurons during the period of axon elongation and guidance. As mentioned above, miR-124 regulates Sema3A-mediated RGC axon targeting within the tectum through transcriptional de-repression of Neuropilin-1 by coREST silencing (Baudet et al., 2012). Importantly, RGC axons gain responsiveness to Sema3A over time, as they navigate along the pathway, and this onset of responsiveness is due to the increase in Neuropilin-1 expression at the growth cone (Campbell et al., 2001). Remarkably, miR-124 may act as a timer, regulating the timetable of neuropilin-1 expression. Indeed, Baudet et al. (2012) showed series of evidence suggesting that a temporal increase of miR-124 in differentiating RGCs, during the period of guidance, accelerates the clearance of coREST transcripts, which progressively releases the transcriptional repression on Neuropilin-1. In turn, Neuropilin-1 protein levels increase at the growth cone over time. All-in-all, miR-124 indirectly determines the time at which Neuropilin-1 is expressed above a level that is necessary for growth cones to gain sensitivity to Sema3A. This mechanism enables growth cones to respond appropriately to this repellent at the right time and place.

Similarly to RGC growth cones, AVM axons progressively switch and lose responsiveness to UNC-6 toward the end of the axon guidance period (Zou et al., 2013). This loss-of-sensitivity is thought to enable axons to subsequently proceed with synaptogenesis (Zou et al., 2013). *C. elegans lin*-4 is a well acknowledged regulator of developmental timing, affecting numerous cell types (Chalfie et al., 1981; Lee et al., 1993; Wightman et al., 1993). In AVM neurons, *lin*-4, like miR-124, displays a clear dynamic temporal regulation suggesting it might also regulate developmental timing in these cells. Importantly, it starts being expressed in AVM neurons only after cell fate determination and cell migration has occurred. Moreover, the 3'UTR activity of its target, *lin*-14, is also down-regulated overtime in these cells (Zou et al., 2013). This indicates that it could act as a timer to promote neuronal differentiation and axon guidance.

Two different molecular pathways have thus been uncovered, where miRNAs appear to endorse a timer function by regulating a switch in growth cone responsiveness over time. The regulatory mechanisms leading to the dynamic expression of these two miRNAs is however unknown. It would be interesting to investigate whether a master clock, regulating this common timetable of growth cone sensitivity, exists upstream that regulate the temporal expression of these miRNAs.

LOCAL ROLES OF miRNAs AT THE GROWTH CONE

The growth cone is a subcellular compartment that can function with a great deal of independence from the cell body, since severed growth cones can navigate on their own along the pathway for a few hours (Harris et al., 1987) and possess all the machinery necessary to respond to cues (Vitriol and Zheng, 2012). Remarkably, growth cones and axons are packed with complex and dynamically changing mRNA repertoires (Taylor et al., 2009; Zivraj et al., 2010). mRNA translation is also shown to mediate growth cone turning in response to several cues (Jung and Holt, 2011). Interestingly, mRNA regulation has emerged as an important mechanism to promote crisp growth cone steering (Jung et al., 2011). However, the identity of key molecular players, their modes of action, and the mechanisms employed by extracellular signals to modulate mRNA translation, are largely unknown. miRNAs may thus be important post-transcriptional regulators for growth cone behavior (Jung et al., 2011), since they ensure that proteins are expressed at precise levels, at the right time and place (Bartel, 2009; Ebert and Sharp, 2012). Although this has yet to be demonstrated, a few lines of evidence support this possibility.

miRNA profiling within axons

Recent studies have profiled miRNAs directly within developing distal axons (also comprising growth cones) using different technical approaches and biological systems (Natera-Naranjo et al., 2010; Sasaki et al., 2013; Hancock et al., 2014). These have revealed that a complex miRNome exists in distal axons and that several miRNAs are enriched (or depleted) in this compartment (**Table 2**). As suggested (Hancock et al., 2014), this would be consistent with the differential expression of axonal mRNA repertoires at different developmental stages or in different species (Zivraj et al., 2010; Gumy et al., 2011). High throughput profiling of miRNAs have yet to be documented. However, in these studies, several miRNAs were also detected in growth cones by fluorescent *in situ* hybridization: miR-16 and miR-221 in SCG neurons (Natera-Naranjo et al., 2010), miR-532 and miR-181a-1* in E16 cortical neurons and in dissociated hippocampal neurons (Sasaki et al., 2013) and miR-132 in E13.5 DRG explants culture (Hancock et al., 2014). Importantly the list and number of enriched axonal miRNAs, in all three studies, is strikingly different. Several reasons might explain these results. First, miRNAs might be differentially distributed in axons depending on the species (rat vs. mouse), cell type (SCG, cortical, and DRG neurons) and developmental stage (P3, E16, E13.5). Second, these differences may be due to different axonal culture (compartmentalized chamber vs. neuronal ball) and profiling methodologies

Table 2 | List of miRNAs enriched or depleted in axons, or present in growth cones during axon development.

miRNAs	Age	Species	Neuron type	Enriched/Depleted in axons[a]	Method used	References
let-7c	P3[c]	Rat	SCG	Enriched	Microarray and qRT-PCR	Natera-Naranjo et al., 2010
let-7-e	E13.5[d]	Mouse	DRG	Enriched	qRT-PCR	Hancock et al., 2014
let-7-i	E13.5[d]	Mouse	DRG	Depleted	qRT-PCR	Hancock et al., 2014
miR-9	E16[d]	Mouse	Cortical	Depleted	Multiplex qRT-PCR	Sasaki et al., 2013
miR-9[a]	E17[d]	Mouse	Cortical	Present	qRT-PCR	Dajas-Bailador et al., 2012
miR-15b	P3[c]	Rat	SCG	Enriched	Microarray and qRT-PCR	Natera-Naranjo et al., 2010
miR-16[b]	P3[c]	Rat	SCG	Enriched	Microarray and qRT-PCR	Natera-Naranjo et al., 2010
miR-16	E13.5[d]	Mouse	DRG	Depleted	qRT-PCR	Hancock et al., 2014
miR-17	E13.5[d]	Mouse	DRG	Enriched	qRT-PCR	Hancock et al., 2014
miR-18a	E18	Rat	Cortical	Enriched	RT-PCR	Zhang et al., 2013
miR-19a	E18	Rat	Cortical	Enriched	RT-PCR	Zhang et al., 2013
miR-19b	E13.5[d]	Mouse	DRG	Enriched	qRT-PCR	Hancock et al., 2014
miR-23a	P3[c]	Rat	SCG	Enriched	Microarray and qRT-PCR	Natera-Naranjo et al., 2010
miR-23b	P3[c]	Rat	SCG	Enriched	Microarray and qRT-PCR	Natera-Naranjo et al., 2010
miR-24	P3[c]	Rat	SCG	Enriched	Microarray and qRT-PCR	Natera-Naranjo et al., 2010
miR-24	E13.5[d]	Mouse	DRG	Enriched	qRT-PCR	Hancock et al., 2014
miR-26a	P3[c]	Rat	SCG	Enriched	Microarray and qRT-PCR	Natera-Naranjo et al., 2010
miR-29a	E13.5[d]	Mouse	DRG	Enriched	qRT-PCR	Hancock et al., 2014
miR-30b	E13.5[d]	Mouse	DRG	Enriched	qRT-PCR	Hancock et al., 2014
miR-30c	E13.5[d]	Mouse	DRG	Enriched	qRT-PCR	Hancock et al., 2014
miR-34b-3p	E13.5[d]	Mouse	DRG	Depleted	qRT-PCR	Hancock et al., 2014
miR-92	E18	Rat	Cortical	Enriched	RT-PCR	Zhang et al., 2013
miR-103	P3[c]	Rat	SCG	Enriched	Microarray and qRT-PCR	Natera-Naranjo et al., 2010
miR-106a	E13.5[d]	Mouse	DRG	Enriched	qRT-PCR	Hancock et al., 2014
miR-124	P3[c]	Rat	SCG	Depleted	Microarray and qRT-PCR	Natera-Naranjo et al., 2010
miR-125a-5p	E13.5[d]	Mouse	DRG	Enriched	qRT-PCR	Hancock et al., 2014
miR- 125b	P3[c]	Rat	SCG	Enriched	Microarray and qRT-PCR	Natera-Naranjo et al., 2010
miR-127	P3[c]	Rat	SCG	Enriched	Microarray and qRT-PCR	Natera-Naranjo et al., 2010
miR-132[b]	E13.5[d]	Mouse	DRG	Enriched	qRT-PCR	Hancock et al., 2014
miR-134[a]	St22	*Xen.*	Spinal	Present	qRT-PCR, FISH	Han et al., 2011
miR-135a	E16[d]	Mouse	Cortical	Depleted	Multiplex qRT-PCR	Sasaki et al., 2013
miR-137	E16[d]	Mouse	Cortical	Depleted	Multiplex qRT-PCR	Sasaki et al., 2013
miR-138	E13.5[d]	Mouse	DRG	Enriched	qRT-PCR	Hancock et al., 2014
miR-181a-1[b]	E16[d]	Mouse	Cortical	Enriched	Multiplex qRT-PCR	Sasaki et al., 2013
miR-182	E13.5[d]	Mouse	DRG	Enriched	qRT-PCR	Hancock et al., 2014
miR-185	P3[c]	Rat	SCG	Enriched	Microarray and qRT-PCR	Natera-Naranjo et al., 2010
miR-191	E13.5[d]	Mouse	DRG	Enriched	qRT-PCR	Hancock et al., 2014
miR-195	E16[d]	Mouse	Cortical	Depleted	Multiplex qRT-PCR	Sasaki et al., 2013
miR-196c	E13.5[d]	Mouse	DRG	Depleted	qRT-PCR	Hancock et al., 2014
miR-204	P3[c]	Rat	SCG	Enriched	Microarray and qRT-PCR	Natera-Naranjo et al., 2010
miR-206	P3[c]	Rat	SCG	Depleted	Microarray and qRT-PCR	Natera-Naranjo et al., 2010
miR-218	E16[d]	Mouse	Cortical	Depleted	Multiplex qRT-PCR	Sasaki et al., 2013
miR-221[b]	P3[c]	Rat	SCG	Enriched	Microarray and qRT-PCR	Natera-Naranjo et al., 2010
miR-296	E16[d]	Mouse	Cortical	Depleted	Multiplex qRT-PCR	Sasaki et al., 2013
miR-297	P3[c]	Rat	SCG	Depleted	Microarray and qRT-PCR	Natera-Naranjo et al., 2010
miR-320	P3[c]	Rat	SCG	Enriched	Microarray and qRT-PCR	Natera-Naranjo et al., 2010
miR-328	E16[d]	Mouse	Cortical	Depleted	Multiplex qRT-PCR	Sasaki et al., 2013
miR-328	E13.5[d]	Mouse	DRG	Enriched	qRT-PCR	Hancock et al., 2014
miR-329	P3[c]	Rat	SCG	Enriched	Microarray and qRT-PCR	Natera-Naranjo et al., 2010
miR-342-3p	E13.5[d]	Mouse	DRG	Enriched	qRT-PCR	Hancock et al., 2014
miR-361	E16[d]	Mouse	Cortical	Enriched	Multiplex qRT-PCR	Sasaki et al., 2013

(Continued)

Table 2 | Continued

miRNAs	Age	Species	Neuron type	Enriched/Depleted in axons[a]	Method used	References
miR-379	E16[d]	Mouse	Cortical	Depleted	Multiplex qRT-PCR	Sasaki et al., 2013
miR-382	P3[c]	Rat	SCG	Enriched	Microarray and qRT-PCR	Natera-Naranjo et al., 2010
miR-384-5p	E13.5[d]	Mouse	DRG	Enriched	qRT-PCR	Hancock et al., 2014
miR-423	E16[d]	Mouse	Cortical	Depleted	Multiplex qRT-PCR	Sasaki et al., 2013
miR-434-3p	E16[d]	Mouse	Cortical	Depleted	Multiplex qRT-PCR	Sasaki et al., 2013
miR-434-3p	E13.5[d]	Mouse	DRG	Enriched	qRT-PCR	Hancock et al., 2014
miR-484	E13.5[d]	Mouse	DRG	Enriched	qRT-PCR	Hancock et al., 2014
miR-495	E13.5[d]	Mouse	DRG	Enriched	qRT-PCR	Hancock et al., 2014
miR-532[b]	E16[d]	Mouse	Cortical	Enriched	Multiplex qRT-PCR	Sasaki et al., 2013
miR-541	P3[c]	Rat	SCG	Enriched	Microarray and qRT-PCR	Natera-Naranjo et al., 2010
miR-680	E13.5[d]	Mouse	DRG	Enriched	qRT-PCR	Hancock et al., 2014
miR-685	E16[d]	Mouse	Cortical	Enriched	Multiplex qRT-PCR	Sasaki et al., 2013
miR-709	E16[d]	Mouse	Cortical	Enriched	Multiplex qRT-PCR	Sasaki et al., 2013
miR-720	E16[d]	Mouse	Cortical	Enriched	Multiplex qRT-PCR	Sasaki et al., 2013

[a]miRNA detected ("present") in axons and growth cones.
[b]miRNAs enriched in axons and detected in growth cones by fluorescent in situ hybridization.
[c]neuron cultured for 3–10 days in vitro.
[d]neurons cultured for 4 days in vitro.
Abbreviations: E, embryonic day; DRG, Dorsal Root Ganglion; SCG, Superior Cervical Ganglion; st, stage; P, postnatal day; Xen., Xenopus.

(microarray/qRT-PCR vs. multiplex qRT-PCR). Third, they may be due to limited coverage of the known mature miRNAs to date (miRbase release 19), and the different cut-off values used for analyses. In addition in the first two studies, the majority of miRNAs appear to be distributed in both cell body and axonal compartments, suggesting that most miRNAs might not have a preferred site of action (Natera-Naranjo et al., 2010; Sasaki et al., 2013). Intriguingly, the presence of miRNAs in axons and growth cones, and to some extent differentially expressed miRNAs derived from the same polycistron (Natera-Naranjo et al., 2010; Kaplan et al., 2013; Zhang et al., 2013), suggest that a mechanism of transport similar to that speculated for dendrites exists (Kosik, 2006). Mature miRNAs could thus be translocated along axons to growth cones either as individual molecules, as precursors, or within ribonucleoparticle bound to their targets and components of the silencing machinery. For instance, pre-miR-134 was recently documented to localize to dendrites through DEAH-box helicase DHX36-mediated transport (Bicker et al., 2013). Overall, these findings point to the possibility that miRNAs might be transported to and function within growth cones to modulate steering.

Table 3 | Reports of miRNA processing machinery in neurons.

RISC component	Species	Neuron type	Age	References
Dicer	Rat	DRG	E15[a]	Hengst et al., 2006
	Rat	Cortical	E18	Zhang et al., 2013
	Rat	SCG	P3[b]	Aschrafi et al., 2008
	Mouse	DRG	E13.5[b]	Hancock et al., 2014
ago2	Rat	Cortical	E18	Zhang et al., 2013
	Mouse	DRG	E13.5[b]	Hancock et al., 2014
ago3	Rat	DRG	E15[b]	Hengst et al., 2006
ago4	Rat	DRG	E15[b]	Hengst et al., 2006
GW-182	Mouse	Cortical	E17[b]	Dajas-Bailador et al., 2012

[a]neurons cultured for 3–7 days in vitro; [b]neurons cutlured for 3 days in vitro.
Abbreviations: DIV, Days in vitro; DRG, Dorsal Root Ganglion; SCG, Superior Cervical Ganglion.

miRNA RISC machinery is present in growth cones

Several studies have demonstrated the silencing machinery RISC (RNA-induced silencing complex) is present and functional in growth cone, further supporting a potential role of miRNA in growth cones. Argonautes (ago) are the catalytic components of RISC. Four Ago proteins are reported in vertebrates (mammals), each binding a similar repertoire of miRNA and mRNA targets (Meister, 2013). While ago 2 was reported to induce mRNA target cleavage with perfect complementarity with a given miRNA, the roles of ago1, 3, and 4 are still elusive. Another RISC component, GW182 protein family (TNRC6 in mammals), coordinates all downstream steps in gene silencing (Pfaff et al., 2013). Key molecules for small RNA-mediated silencing such as ago2 (Zhang et al., 2013; Hancock et al., 2014), ago 3 and 4 (Hengst et al., 2006), eIF2c (Eukaryotic Initiation Factor 2C) (Aschrafi et al., 2008) and GW182 (Dajas-Bailador et al., 2012) were detected in the embryonic and perinatal distal axons, and/or growth cones of various cell types (**Table 3**). In addition, one study also revealed that RISC is functional in distal axons (Hengst et al., 2006). Exogenous siRNA directed against RhoA, a small GTPase protein led to the decrease in RhoA transcript and RhoA immunoreactivity in distal axons. Importantly, FITC-labeled siRNA was not detected in proximal axons, and no RhoA mRNA knockdown was detected in the somatodendritic compartment. Taken together, these data revealed that exogenous siRNA-induced silencing exists in distal axons (Hengst et al., 2006). It would be interesting to explore whether RISC can also mediate endogenous miRNA action in this compartment, and most specifically in growth cones. Intriguingly, the RISC component Dicer is also detected in distal axons, including growth cones (Hengst et al., 2006; Zhang et al., 2013; Hancock et al., 2014). This suggests that, as in dendrites (Bicker et al., 2013), pre-miRNAs could be transported and processed into mature miRNAs, in this compartment. Axonal transfection of pre-miR-338 and pre-miR-16 indeed result in a substantial increase in their concomitant mature form in axons, suggesting that miRNA processing does occur in distal axons (Aschrafi et al., 2008; Kar et al., 2013). Several key components are thus present in growth cones and/or distal axons, and RNA interference occurs in this compartment, suggesting that miRNAs are likely to be functional there. The documented presence of RISC components Armitage, MOV10 and Dicer (Lugli et al., 2005; Ashraf et al., 2006; Banerjee et al., 2009) in pre- and post-synaptic compartments underscore that miRNAs may have broader subcellular sites of action in polarized cells like neurons.

Do miRNAs play a local role in growth cone turning?

The presence of RISC within growth cones suggests that miRNAs could act locally within this compartment and shape the local transcriptome during axon guidance. In particular, miRNAs could regulate local translation, known to play a role in growth cone steering in response to some cues (Jung et al., 2011). Although this has yet to be clearly demonstrated, recent studies suggest that it might be the case.

miRNAs are known to regulate outgrowth in development and following injury (Wu and Murashov, 2013; Chiu et al., 2014). miRNA-mediated silencing of mRNA was recently reported to occur locally within axons to modulate outgrowth. Axonal miRNAs were initially documented to inhibit the translation of cytoskeletal regulatory molecules locally (Dajas-Bailador et al., 2012; Hancock et al., 2014). Using mice cortical neurons, Dajas-Bailador et al. (2012) first revealed that a miRNA, miR-9, modulates the translational repression of exogenous Map1b (microtubule-associated protein 1b) 3′UTR, which has a key role in the regulation of dynamic microtubules. Short BDNF stimulation modulated miR-9 expression, while inhibition of miR-9 affected axonal growth only when applied locally in axons, suggesting that BDNF affects this developmental process via local, miRNA-mediated translational control of a cytoskeletal regulator. Further support for such local mechanisms came in a recent study from Flanagan's group (Hancock et al., 2014). Hancock and colleagues reported that axon-enriched miR-132 promotes embryonic DRG axon outgrowth by targeting endogenous p120RasGAP (Rasa1), a protein involved in cytoskeletal regulation (Hancock et al., 2014). Interestingly, miR-132-induced increase in axonal Rasa1 protein level was dependent on local protein synthesis, as it was abolished in the presence of translation inhibitor applied to severed axons (Hancock et al., 2014). This demonstrated that miR-132 acts indeed within this cell compartment to regulate target translation, removing the possibility of cross-talk with the cell body. Of note, Rasa 1 was previously reported to mediate responsiveness to chemotropic cues but here, miR-132 activity did not change upon stimulation by a few guidance molecules suggesting that these findings may not be strictly transposed to the guidance field (Hancock et al., 2014). In addition, axonal miRNAs were also recently documented to promote outgrowth by silencing axonal transcripts other than cytoskeletal regulators. Using 3d rat SCG neurons, Kar and colleagues reported that axon abundant miR-16 reduces the levels of the eukaryotic translation initiation factors eIF2B2 and eIF4G2 mRNAs, specifically within axons without affecting the levels of these transcripts in the soma (Kar et al., 2013). Interestingly, axonal miR-16 reduced outgrowth, and siRNA-mediated decrease in eIF2B2 and eIF4G2 levels in axons lead to inhibition of local protein synthesis and reduced axon extension. Together, this suggests that miR-16 might regulate elongation by modulating the axonal protein synthetic system. Finally using rat E18 cortical neurons, Zhang et al. (2013) documented that axonal miR-19a, a member of the miR-17-92 cluster, regulates axon outgrowth via PTEN (phosphatase and tensin homolog), a negative regulator of the PI3K/mTOR signaling pathway. Importantly, axonal miR-19a regulates PTEN protein levels specifically within axons and not at the cell soma suggesting compartmentalized action for this miRNA. Local regulation of mRNA by miRNA has thus been reported in axons in a biological context of elongation.

The possibility that miRNA-mediated regulation of growth cone turning via local regulation of mRNA is further supported by a recent study. Several years ago, miR-134 was shown to locally modulate the size of dendritic spines of rat hippocampal cells (Schratt et al., 2006). This miRNA keeps Limk1, a kinase regulating actin polymerization, in a dormant untranslated state, and releases its repression in response to extracellular BDNF stimulation. Limk1 is thus translated, resulting in spine size increase (Schratt et al., 2006). Zheng's group recently investigated whether this mechanism is conserved in growth cones of *X. laevis* spinal neurons, where they detected this miRNA (Han et al., 2011). Similar to dendritic spines, miR-134 was found to be important for BDNF-induced growth cone attraction. In addition, miR-134 appeared to regulate protein synthesis in response to this cue, as loss- and gain-of-function of miR-134 in the whole embryo blocked protein synthesis dependent turning response of growth cones. The effect of this miRNAs on spinal neuron cell bodies cannot be formally excluded, since miR-134 was knocked down or overexpressed in whole embryos, and not exclusively in axons. Limk1, also detected in spinal growth cones, was confirmed as a *bona fide* target of miR-134 in *Xenopus* by *in vivo* luciferase assay. This suggests that Limk1 may mediate miR-134 regulation of BDNF-induced growth cone attraction. All-in-all, this study provided the first evidence, that growth cone turning can be modulated by miRNAs. It also indicated that conserved miRNA-based local control may exist in neuronal compartments, enabling the acute regulation of cytoskeletal dynamics in response to external stimuli.

Based on these recent findings, one could speculate that several possible mechanisms of mRNA regulation in growth cones exist during steering. On the one hand miRNAs could silence translation, keeping the transcript dormant until a cue is encountered, and a newly synthesized protein is asymmetrically required.

Similar mechanisms of action are also reported in dendrites (Schratt et al., 2006; Siegel et al., 2009) suggesting they could be conserved across neuronal compartments. On the other end, cue-induced activation of miRNAs could lead to the inhibition of transcript translation and/or stability, when newly synthesized protein(s) are no longer required for guidance. In particular, such silencing could arrest cue-induced translation of mRNA, thereby terminating growth cone response to a given chemotropic cue. Furthermore, an asymmetric rise in local mRNA translation of a cytoskeletal protein was reported to occur at the growth cone on the side of cue exposure (Leung et al., 2006). From this, one could finally conceive that miRNAs may have an asymmetric function in this compartment, allowing silencing to occur on one side of the growth cone, and translation on the other. This putative mechanism might be unique to growth cones, as opposed to dendrites or synapses, to support directional steering.

CONCLUSIVE REMARKS AND PERSPECTIVES

In conclusion, recent studies have uncovered that miRNAs are hitherto unsuspected, important regulatory molecules in axon guidance (**Figure 1**) (Giraldez et al., 2005; Pinter and Hindges, 2010; Han et al., 2011; Shibata et al., 2011; Baudet et al., 2012; Zou et al., 2012). These have revealed that miRNAs are likely to have widespread and important roles, affecting different species and several projections, and when knocked out, result in varying degrees of severity in guidance errors. The studies have also shown that miRNAs are likely to regulate both guidance response to cues or cue expression. In particular, miRNAs can specifically modulate growth cone steering (Han et al., 2011; Baudet et al., 2012). To do so, they can act cell-autonomously to fine-tune the molecular make-up of projection neurons, thereby affecting their responsiveness to cues. This regulation may take place at the soma, via transcription factor regulation, which in turn, modulates expression levels of receptors to cues (Baudet et al., 2012; Zou et al., 2012). miRNAs are also suspected to act locally, and affect downstream signaling molecules of various nature including axon cytoskeleton (Han et al., 2011; Dajas-Bailador et al., 2012; Kar et al., 2013; Hancock et al., 2014). Although the evidence is more elusive, miRNAs could also modulate brain patterning, and thereby control either the presence of guidepost cells or the expression of guidance cues at key topographical locations (Pinter and Hindges, 2010; Shibata et al., 2011) (**Figures 1, 2**).

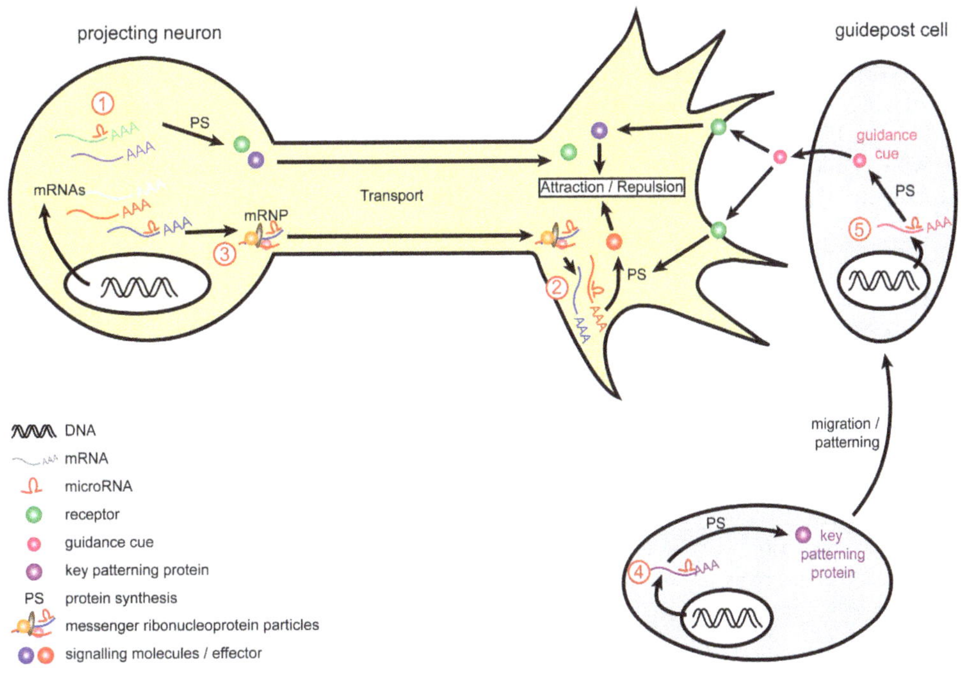

FIGURE 2 | Model of miRNA-mediated regulation of axon guidance. During pathfinding, tight regulation of mRNAs occurs to ensure protein expression of guidance molecules at the right time and place, and enable accurate growth cone steering. Within projection neurons, transcripts are translated into the cell body and are subsequently transported within the axon to the growth cone to mediate guidance cue-induced signaling. Alternatively, mRNAs associate into messenger ribonucleoprotein particles (mRNPs) to be transported to the growth cone, where they can be locally translated. Retrograde transport of transcripts from growth cones to cell soma also exists (not represented here). miRNAs are speculated to act at multiple level. They may regulate transcripts translation and stability (1) within the cell body as suggested for miR-124 and lin-4 (Baudet et al., 2012; Zhang et al., 2013) or (2) directly within growth cones as suggested for miR-134 (Han et al., 2011) and by the presence of RISC within this compartment (**Table 3**). (3) As speculated (Kosik, 2006), miRNAs may translocate along the axons alone or within mRNPs (shown here) and/or be transported as pre-miRNAs and locally produced within growth cones. Guidepost cells are important partners for projection neurons, as they provide them with positional information through the expression of guidance cues. The regulation of guidepost cell transcriptome is thus of crucial importance to ensure the correct patterning of these cells and also the delivery of the right guidance cue at the right place. miRNAs could act by directly regulating the expression of guidance cues within guidepost cells (4) or by indirectly regulating molecules involved in the patterning of these cells (5), as suggested for miR-9 (Shibata et al., 2011).

Guidance molecules appear to have pleiotropic roles and as such, are involved in several processes outside of the nervous system development. In particular, they are now acknowledged regulators of the immune and cardiovascular systems, including of vascular development, and angiogenesis (Adams and Eichmann, 2010; Kumanogoh and Kikutani, 2013). Guidances cues are also involved in pathological processes such as cancer and tumor progression (Chédotal, 2007; Mehlen et al., 2011). miRNAs, as key post-transcriptional regulator in most eukaryotic cells, are also implicated in these physiological and pathophysiological processes (Croce, 2009; Xiao and Rajewsky, 2009; Small and Olson, 2011) suggesting a possible mechanistic link between the two class of molecules outside of the nervous system. Importantly, several miRNAs modulate guidance cues and their receptors in cells other than neurons, including cancer cell lines but also in endothelial cells (**Table 4**) (Baudet et al., 2013). This raises the intriguing possibility that a given miRNA may regulate the same guidance molecules in different cellular contexts.

miRNAs may have conserved important developmental roles, including axon guidance, throughout evolution. Indeed, miRNAs appear to regulate pathfinding in several species, ranging from *Drosophila* and *C. elegans* to mice and guidance miRNAs affect the same pathway in different species (e.g., the visual pathway of lower vertebrate Baudet et al., 2012 vs. higher vertebrates Pinter and Hindges, 2010). Moreover, a specific miRNA, miR-9, regulates guidance of different tracts (Shibata et al., 2011). Interestingly, two of the four miRNAs involved in guidance, miR-124, lin-4/miR-125, are highly conserved, and considered as ancient miRNAs with neural-like function (Christodoulou et al., 2010).Unsurprisingly, these miRNAs appear to have multifactorial neural action, and besides regulating guidance, also modulate earlier developmental events such as neurogenesis, cell fate determination, lineage progression, and later events such as synaptogenesis (Gao, 2010).

Table 4 | List of miRNAs regulating guidance molecules in non-neuronal cells.

miRNA	Target	Cell type	References
miR-9	Neuropilin-1	Endothelial cells	Cui et al., 2012
miR 27a/b	Sema 6a	Endothelial cells	Urbich et al., 2012
miR-34	Sema 4b	Cardiomyoblast H9c2 cells	Bernardo et al., 2012
miR-181b	Neuropilin-1	Endothelial cells	Cui et al., 2012
miR-210	EphrinA3	U2OS ostesarcoma cell line	Fasanaro et al., 2008
miR-210	EphrinA3	293T cells	Pulkkinen et al., 2008
miR-214	Plexin -B1	HeLa cells	Qiang et al., 2011
miR-218	Robo1	Human breast cancer cells	Yang et al., 2012
miR-218	Robo1	Nasopharyngeal carcinoma	Alajez et al., 2011
miR-218	Robo1 and 2	HeLa cells	Fish et al., 2011
miR-218	Robo1 and 2	COS cells	Small et al., 2010
miR-218	Robo1	Human gastric cell lines	Tie et al., 2010
miR-320	Neuropilin-1	Colorectal cancer cells	Zhang et al., 2012
miR-331-3p	Neuropilin-2	Glioblastoma multiforme	Epis et al., 2009

Guidance miRNAs appear to have a delicate regulatory action on guidance signaling pathways. The three miRNAs, for which signaling mechanisms have been uncovered, fine-tune the levels of their endogenous (Baudet et al., 2012; Zou et al., 2012) or exogenous targets (Han et al., 2011). This is very much in agreement with recent evidence that miRNAs do not act as off-switches, as originally thought from earlier studies in *C. elegans*, but rather as a rheostat, which fine-tunes protein output to functional levels (Baek et al., 2008; Selbach et al., 2008; Bartel, 2009; Guo et al., 2010). It is thus particularly interesting that mRNAs translated in the growth cone give rise to only small increases in protein levels (Jung et al., 2011), consistent with the hypothesis that miRNAs might be responsible for this. miRNAs may thus provide an additional layer of gene regulation in projection neurons, to ensure that guidance molecules are expressed at the right time and place, supporting the high level of precision critical for axon guidance.

Navigating growth cones are exposed to a myriad of cues along their pathway, and it appears that cross-talk exists between these cues and miRNAs. miRNAs can intrinsically alter the way growth cones respond to a cue, modulating the levels of their cognate receptor (Baudet et al., 2012; Zou et al., 2012). Conversely, cues also modulate miRNA's silencing potential at the growth cone. For instance, they are suspected to repress miRNA-mediated silencing, leading to local protein translation and growth cone steering (Han et al., 2011). Cues can induce a rise in miRNA levels in axons, which in turn leads to increased post-transcriptional gene silencing (Dajas-Bailador et al., 2012). The exact signaling mechanisms mediating cue-regulated miRNA action are unknown. One possibility, as has been previously shown in dendrites (Schratt et al., 2006), includes phosphorylation and activation of mTOR pathway, which is a suspected global regulator of translational activity in growth cones (Jung et al., 2012). Furthermore, cues or any external stimulus affecting the neuronal projection could also shape the miRNA repertoire of the whole neuron or specifically that of the growth cone. External stimuli were reported to either activate Dicer (Lugli et al., 2005) or degrade the RISC component (MOV10) (Banerjee et al., 2009) at the synapse- another neuronal compartment. In addition, neuronal activity was also shown to regulate miRNA turnover rate, by modulating their transcription or promoting their decay (Krol et al., 2010a), which in turn can affect dendritic remodeling (Fiore et al., 2009). A similar cue-mediated regulation of miRNA levels is conceivable in axons of projecting neurons.

Recent evidence has revealed that miRNA function could be modulated by different means. For instance, RNA-binding proteins (RNA-BP) were shown to either act in concert with miRNAs to promote silencing or, on the contrary, to compete for binding sites (Krol et al., 2010b). For instance miR-125a and Fragile X mental retardation protein (FMRP) were revealed to act cooperatively at the 3′UTR of PSD-95 mRNA to inhibit translation of this transcript within synapses (Muddashetty et al., 2011). miRNAs can also actively regulate RNA-BP in neurons (Fiore et al.,

2009). RNA-BPs play important roles in developing projection neurons, ensuring mRNA transport and translational repression (Hörnberg and Holt, 2013). It is therefore conceivable that these two classes of molecules act in a coordinated manner to modulate transcript levels during axon guidance. In addition, other classes of non-coding RNAs, such as endogenous circular miRNA (Hansen et al., 2013; Memczak et al., 2013) and long-non-coding RNAs, have emerged as important regulators of miRNA action, acting as decoy or sponges that sequester, and thus buffer miRNAs in the cell (Salmena et al., 2011). Such endogenous competing RNAs (ceRNAs) might also include transcripts of protein-coding genes, whose miRNA-mediated silencing does not affect their function (Seitz, 2009; Salmena et al., 2011). In projection neurons, these ceRNAs could modulate miRNA access to their target transcript, providing an additional layer of regulation, and enabling fine-tuning of their translation. However, their existence and function in cells during axon guidance is yet to be demonstrated.

In conclusion, while the body of work reviewed here has just started to reveal the role of miRNAs in axon guidance, future research promises to unravel how these key regulatory molecules are embedded in the molecular network that enables axons to navigate to their targets with extreme precision.

ACKNOWLEDGMENTS

The authors thank Giovanni Stefani (University of Trento, Italy), Hosung Jung (Yonsei University College of Medicine, Korea) and ASK Scientific (askscientific.com) for their valuable comments on the manuscript. Archana N. Iyer is a recipient of a University of Trento PhD studentship, Anaïs Bellon of EMBO and Human Frontier Fellowships. Marie-Laure Baudet of a G. Armenise-Harvard Foundation Career Development grant, and of a University of Trento start-up grant.

REFERENCES

Adams, R. H., and Eichmann, A. (2010). Axon guidance molecules in vascular patterning. *Cold Spring Harb. Perspect. Biol.* 2:a001875. doi: 10.1101/cshperspect.a001875

Alajez, N. M., Lenarduzzi, M., Ito, E., Hui, A. B., Shi, W., Bruce, J., et al. (2011). MiR-218 suppresses nasopharyngeal cancer progression through downregulation of survivin and the SLIT2-ROBO1 pathway. *Cancer Res.* 71, 2381–2391. doi: 10.1158/0008-5472.CAN-10-2754

Aschrafi, A., Schwechter, A. D., Mameza, M. G., Natera-Naranjo, O., Gioio, A. E., and Kaplan, B. B. (2008). MicroRNA-338 regulates local cytochrome c oxidase IV mRNA levels and oxidative phosphorylation in the axons of sympathetic neurons. *J. Neurosci.* 28, 12581–12590. doi: 10.1523/JNEUROSCI.3338-08.2008

Ashraf, S. I., McLoon, A. L., Sclarsic, S. M., and Kunes, S. (2006). Synaptic protein synthesis associated with memory is regulated by the RISC pathway in Drosophila. *Cell* 124, 191–205. doi: 10.1016/j.cell.2005.12.017

Baek, D., Villén, J., Shin, C., Camargo, F. D., Gygi, S. P., and Bartel, D. P. (2008). The impact of microRNAs on protein output. *Nature* 455, 64–71. doi: 10.1038/nature07242

Banerjee, S., Neveu, P., and Kosik, K. S. (2009). A coordinated local translational control point at the synapse involving relief from silencing and MOV10 degradation. *Neuron* 64, 871–884. doi: 10.1016/j.neuron.2009.11.023

Bartel, D. P. (2009). MicroRNAs: target recognition and regulatory functions. *Cell* 136, 215–233. doi: 10.1016/j.cell.2009.01.002

Baudet, M.-L., Bellon, A., and Holt, C. E. (2013). Role of microRNAs in Semaphorin function and neural circuit formation. *Semin. Cell Dev. Biol.* 24, 146–155. doi: 10.1016/j.semcdb.2012.11.004

Baudet, M.-L., Zivraj, K. H., Abreu-Goodger, C., Muldal, A., Armisen, J., Blenkiron, C., et al. (2012). miR-124 acts through CoREST to control onset of Sema3A sensitivity in navigating retinal growth cones. *Nat. Neurosci.* 15, 29–38. doi: 10.1038/nn.2979

Bernardo, B. C., Gao, X.-M., Winbanks, C. E., Boey, E. J. H., Tham, Y. K., Kiriazis, H., et al. (2012). Therapeutic inhibition of the miR-34 family attenuates pathological cardiac remodeling and improves heart function. *Proc. Natl. Acad. Sci.* 109, 17615–17620. doi: 10.1073/pnas.1206432109

Bernstein, E., Caudy, A. A., Hammond, S. M., and Hannon, G. J. (2001). Role for a bidentate ribonuclease in the initiation step of RNA interference. *Nature* 409, 363–366. doi: 10.1038/35053110

Bicker, S., Khudayberdiev, S., Weiß, K., Zocher, K., Baumeister, S., and Schratt, G. (2013). The DEAH-box helicase DHX36 mediates dendritic localization of the neuronal precursor-microRNA-134. *Genes Dev.* 27, 991–996. doi: 10.1101/gad.211243.112

Campbell, D. S., Regan, A. G., Lopez, J. S., Tannahill, D., Harris, W. A., and Holt, C. E. (2001). Semaphorin 3A elicits stage-dependent collapse, turning, and branching in Xenopus retinal growth cones. *J. Neurosci.* 21, 8538–8547.

Chalfie, M., Horvitz, H. R., and Sulston, J. E. (1981). Mutations that lead to reiterations in the cell lineages of C. *elegans*. *Cell* 24, 59–69. doi: 10.1016/0092-8674(81)90501-8

Chang, C., Yu, T. W., Bargmann, C. I., and Tessier-Lavigne, M. (2004a). Inhibition of netrin-mediated axon attraction by a receptor protein tyrosine phosphatase. *Science* 305, 103–106. doi: 10.1126/science.1096983

Chang, S., Johnston, R. J., Frøkjaer-Jensen, C., Lockery, S., and Hobert, O. (2004b). MicroRNAs act sequentially and asymmetrically to control chemosensory laterality in the nematode. *Nature* 430, 785–789. doi: 10.1038/nature02752

Chédotal, A. (2007). Chemotropic axon guidance molecules in tumorigenesis. *Prog. Exp. Tumor Res.* 39, 78–90. doi: 10.1159/000100048

Cheloufi, S., Dos Santos, C. O., Chong, M. M. W., and Hannon, G. J. (2010). A dicer-independent miRNA biogenesis pathway that requires Ago catalysis. *Nature* 465, 584–589. doi: 10.1038/nature09092

Chiu, H., Alqadah, A., and Chang, C. (2014). The role of microRNAs in regulating neuronal connectivity. *Front. Cell. Neurosci.* 7:283. doi: 10.3389/fncel.2013.00283

Chiu, H., and Chang, C. (2013). Rejuvenating nerve cells in adults. *Aging (Albany, NY)* 5, 485–486.

Choi, P. S., Zakhary, L., Choi, W.-Y., Caron, S., Alvarez-Saavedra, E., Miska, E. A., et al. (2008). Members of the miRNA-200 family regulate olfactory neurogenesis. *Neuron* 57, 41–55. doi: 10.1016/j.neuron.2007.11.018

Christodoulou, F., Raible, F., Tomer, R., Simakov, O., Trachana, K., Klaus, S., et al. (2010). Ancient animal microRNAs and the evolution of tissue identity. *Nature* 463, 1084–1088. doi: 10.1038/nature08744

Cifuentes, D., Xue, H., Taylor, D. W., Patnode, H., Mishima, Y., Cheloufi, S., et al. (2010). A novel miRNA processing pathway independent of Dicer requires Argonaute2 catalytic activity. *Science* 328, 1694–1698. doi: 10.1126/science.1190809

Cremisi, F. (2013). MicroRNAs and cell fate in cortical and retinal development. *Front. Cell. Neurosci.* 7:141. doi: 10.3389/fncel.2013.00141

Croce, C. M. (2009). Causes and consequences of microRNA dysregulation in cancer. *Nat. Rev. Genet.* 10, 704–714. doi: 10.1038/nrg2634

Cui, Y., Han, Z., Hu, Y., Song, G., Hao, C., Xia, H., et al. (2012). MicroRNA-181b and microRNA-9 mediate arsenic-induced angiogenesis via NRP1. *J. Cell. Physiol.* 227, 772–783. doi: 10.1002/jcp.22789

Dajas-Bailador, F., Bonev, B., Garcez, P., Stanley, P., Guillemot, F., and Papalopulu, N. (2012). microRNA-9 regulates axon extension and branching by targeting Map1b in mouse cortical neurons. *Nat. Neurosci.* 15, 697–699. doi: 10.1038/nn.3082

Decembrini, S., Bressan, D., Vignali, R., Pitto, L., Mariotti, S., Rainaldi, G., et al. (2009). MicroRNAs couple cell fate and developmental timing in retina. *Proc. Natl. Acad. Sci. U.S.A.* 106, 21179–2184. doi: 10.1073/pnas.0909167106

Dent, E. W., Gupton, S. L., and Gertler, F. B. (2011). The growth cone cytoskeleton in axon outgrowth and guidance. *Cold Spring Harb. Perspect. Biol.* 3:a001800. doi: 10.1101/cshperspect.a001800

Dickson, B. J. (2002). Molecular mechanisms of axon guidance. *Science* 298, 1959–1964. doi: 10.1126/science.1072165

Ebert, M. S., and Sharp, P. A. (2012). Roles for MicroRNAs in conferring robustness to biological processes. *Cell* 149, 515–524. doi: 10.1016/j.cell.2012.04.005

Epis, M. R., Giles, K. M., Barker, A., Kendrick, T. S., and Leedman, P. J. (2009). miR-331-3p regulates ERBB-2 expression and androgen receptor signaling in prostate cancer. *J. Biol. Chem.* 284, 24696–24704. doi: 10.1074/jbc.M109.030098

Erskine, L., Reijntjes, S., Pratt, T., Denti, L., Schwarz, Q., Vieira, J. M., et al. (2011). VEGF signaling through neuropilin 1 guides commissural axon crossing at the optic chiasm. *Neuron* 70, 951–965. doi: 10.1016/j.neuron.2011.02.052

Fasanaro, P., D'Alessandra, Y., Di Stefano, V., Melchionna, R., Romani, S., Pompilio, G., et al. (2008). MicroRNA-210 modulates endothelial cell response to hypoxia and inhibits the receptor tyrosine kinase ligand Ephrin-A3. *J. Biol. Chem.* 283, 15878–15883. doi: 10.1074/jbc.M800731200

Fiore, R., Khudayberdiev, S., Christensen, M., Siegel, G., Flavell, S. W., Kim, T.-K., et al. (2009). Mef2-mediated transcription of the miR379-410 cluster regulates activity-dependent dendritogenesis by fine-tuning Pumilio2 protein levels. *EMBO J.* 28, 697–710. doi: 10.1038/emboj.2009.10

Fish, J. E., Wythe, J. D., Xiao, T., Bruneau, B. G., Stainier, D. Y. R., Srivastava, D., et al. (2011). A Slit/miR-218/Robo regulatory loop is required during heart tube formation in zebrafish. *Development* 138, 1409–1419. doi: 10.1242/dev.060046

Gao, F.-B. (2010). Context-dependent functions of specific microRNAs in neuronal development. *Neural Dev.* 5, 25. doi: 10.1186/1749-8104-5-25

Giraldez, A. J., Cinalli, R. M., Glasner, M. E., Enright, A. J., Thomson, J. M., Baskerville, S., et al. (2005). MicroRNAs regulate brain morphogenesis in zebrafish. *Science* 308, 833–838. doi: 10.1126/science.1109020

Griffiths-Jones, S. (2004). The microRNA Registry. *Nucleic Acids Res.* 32, D109–D111. doi: 10.1093/nar/gkh023

Griffiths-Jones, S., Saini, H. K., van Dongen, S., and Enright, A. J. (2008). miRBase: tools for microRNA genomics. *Nucleic Acids Res.* 36, D154–D158. doi: 10.1093/nar/gkm952

Grishok, A., Pasquinelli, A. E., Conte, D., Li, N., Parrish, S., Ha, I., et al. (2001). Genes and mechanisms related to RNA interference regulate expression of the small temporal RNAs that control C. *elegans developmental timing. Cell* 106, 23–34. doi: 10.1016/S0092-8674(01)00431-7

Gumy, L. F., Yeo, G. S. H., Tung, Y.-C. L., Zivraj, K. H., Willis, D., Coppola, G., et al. (2011). Transcriptome analysis of embryonic and adult sensory axons reveals changes in mRNA repertoire localization. *RNA* 17, 85–98. doi: 10.1261/rna.2386111

Guo, H., Ingolia, N. T., Weissman, J. S., and Bartel, D. P. (2010). Mammalian microRNAs predominantly act to decrease target mRNA levels. *Nature* 466, 835–840. doi: 10.1038/nature09267

Han, L., Wen, Z., Lynn, R. C., Baudet, M.-L., Holt, C. E., Sasaki, Y., et al. (2011). Regulation of chemotropic guidance of nerve growth cones by microRNA. *Mol. Brain* 4, 40. doi: 10.1186/1756-6606-4-40

Hancock, M. L., Preitner, N., Quan, J., and Flanagan, J. G. (2014). MicroRNA-132 Is Enriched in Developing Axons, Locally Regulates Rasa1 mRNA, and Promotes Axon Extension. *J. Neurosci.* 34, 66–78. doi: 10.1523/JNEUROSCI.3371-13.2014

Hansen, T. B., Jensen, T. I., Clausen, B. H., Bramsen, J. B., Finsen, B., Damgaard, C. K., et al. (2013). Natural RNA circles function as efficient microRNA sponges. *Nature* 495, 384–388. doi: 10.1038/nature11993

Harris, W. A., Holt, C. E., and Bonhoeffer, F. (1987). Retinal axons with and without their somata, growing to and arborizing in the tectum of Xenopus embryos: a time-lapse video study of single fibres *in vivo*. *Development* 101, 123–133.

Hengst, U., Cox, L. J., Macosko, E. Z., and Jaffrey, S. R. (2006). Functional and selective RNA interference in developing axons and growth cones. *J. Neurosci.* 26, 5727–5732. doi: 10.1523/JNEUROSCI.5229-05.2006

Hörnberg, H., and Holt, C. (2013). RNA-binding proteins and translational regulation in axons and growth cones. *Front. Neurosci.* 7:81. doi: 10.3389/fnins.2013.00081

Hsieh, J. (2012). Orchestrating transcriptional control of adult neurogenesis. *Genes Dev.* 26, 1010–1021. doi: 10.1101/gad.187336.112

Huber, A. B., Kania, A., Tran, T. S., Gu, C., De Marco Garcia, N., Lieberam, I., et al. (2005). Distinct roles for secreted semaphorin signaling in spinal motor axon guidance. *Neuron* 48, 949–964. doi: 10.1016/j.neuron.2005.12.003

Johnson, J. M., Edwards, S., Shoemaker, D., and Schadt, E. E. (2005). Dark matter in the genome: evidence of widespread transcription detected by microarray tiling experiments. *Trends Genet.* 21, 93–102. doi: 10.1016/j.tig.2004.12.009

Johnston, R. J., and Hobert, O. (2003). A microRNA controlling left/right neuronal asymmetry in Caenorhabditis elegans. *Nature* 426, 845–849. doi: 10.1038/nature02255

Jung, H., and Holt, C. E. (2011). Local translation of mRNAs in neural development. *Wiley Interdiscip. Rev. RNA* 2, 153–165. doi: 10.1002/wrna.53

Jung, H., O'Hare, C. M., and Holt, C. E. (2011). Translational regulation in growth cones. *Curr. Opin. Genet. Dev.* 21, 458–464. doi: 10.1016/j.gde.2011.04.004

Jung, H., Yoon, B. C., and Holt, C. E. (2012). Axonal mRNA localization and local protein synthesis in nervous system assembly, maintenance and repair. *Nat. Rev. Neurosci.* 13, 308–324. doi: 10.1038/nrn3274

Kaplan, B. B., Kar, A. N., Gioio, A. E., and Aschrafi, A. (2013). MicroRNAs in the axon and presynaptic nerve terminal. *Front. Cell. Neurosci.* 7:126. doi: 10.3389/fncel.2013.00126

Kar, A. N., MacGibeny, M. A., Gervasi, N. M., Gioio, A. E., and Kaplan, B. B. (2013). Intra-axonal synthesis of eukaryotic translation initiation factors regulates local protein synthesis and axon growth in rat sympathetic neurons. *J. Neurosci.* 33, 7165–7174. doi: 10.1523/JNEUROSCI.2040-12.2013

Ketting, R. F., Fischer, S. E., Bernstein, E., Sijen, T., Hannon, G. J., and Plasterk, R. H. (2001). Dicer functions in RNA interference and in synthesis of small RNA involved in developmental timing in C. *elegans. Genes Dev.* 15, 2654–2659. doi: 10.1101/gad.927801

Knight, S. W., and Bass, B. L. (2001). A role for the RNase III enzyme DCR-1 in RNA interference and germ line development in Caenorhabditis elegans. *Science* 293, 2269–2271. doi: 10.1126/science.1062039

Kolodkin, A. L., and Tessier-Lavigne, M. (2011). Mechanisms and molecules of neuronal wiring: a primer. *Cold Spring Harb. Perspect. Biol.* 3:a001727. doi: 10.1101/cshperspect.a001727

Kosik, K. S. (2006). The neuronal microRNA system. *Nat. Rev. Neurosci.* 7, 911–920. doi: 10.1038/nrn2037

Kozomara, A., and Griffiths-Jones, S. (2011). miRBase: integrating microRNA annotation and deep-sequencing data. *Nucleic Acids Res.* 39, D152–D157. doi: 10.1093/nar/gkq1027

Kozomara, A., and Griffiths-Jones, S. (2013). miRBase: annotating high confidence microRNAs using deep sequencing data. *Nucleic Acids Res.* 42, D68–D73. doi: 10.1093/nar/gkt1181

Krichevsky, A. M., King, K. S., Donahue, C. P., Khrapko, K., and Kosik, K. S. (2003). A microRNA array reveals extensive regulation of microRNAs during brain development. *RNA* 9, 1274–1281. doi: 10.1261/rna.5980303

Krol, J., Busskamp, V., Markiewicz, I., Stadler, M. B., Ribi, S., Richter, J., et al. (2010a). Characterizing light-regulated retinal microRNAs reveals rapid turnover as a common property of neuronal microRNAs. *Cell* 141, 618–631. doi: 10.1016/j.cell.2010.03.039

Krol, J., Loedige, I., and Filipowicz, W. (2010b). The widespread regulation of microRNA biogenesis, function and decay. *Nat. Rev. Genet.* 11, 597–610. doi: 10.1038/nrg2843

Kumanogoh, A., and Kikutani, H. (2013). Immunological functions of the neuropilins and plexins as receptors for semaphorins. *Nat. Rev. Immunol.* 13, 802–814. doi: 10.1038/nri3545

Kuwajima, T., Yoshida, Y., Takegahara, N., Petros, T. J., Kumanogoh, A., Jessell, T. M., et al. (2012). Optic chiasm presentation of Semaphorin6D in the context of Plexin-A1 and Nr-CAM promotes retinal axon midline crossing. *Neuron* 74, 676–690. doi: 10.1016/j.neuron.2012.03.025

Kwok, J. C. F., Yuen, Y.-L., Lau, W.-K., Zhang, F.-X., Fawcett, J. W., Chan, Y.-S., et al. (2012). Chondroitin sulfates in the developing rat hindbrain confine commissural projections of vestibular nuclear neurons. *Neural Dev.* 7, 6. doi: 10.1186/1749-8104-7-6

Kye, M.-J., Liu, T., Levy, S. F., Xu, N. L., Groves, B. B., Bonneau, R., et al. (2007). Somatodendritic microRNAs identified by laser capture and multiplex RT-PCR. *RNA* 13, 1224–1234. doi: 10.1261/rna.480407

Landgraf, P., Rusu, M., Sheridan, R., Sewer, A., Iovino, N., Aravin, A., et al. (2007). A mammalian microRNA expression atlas based on small RNA library sequencing. *Cell* 129, 1401–1414. doi: 10.1016/j.cell.2007.04.040

La Torre, A., Georgi, S., and Reh, T. A. (2013). Conserved microRNA pathway regulates developmental timing of retinal neurogenesis. *Proc. Natl. Acad. Sci. U.S.A.* 110, E2362–E2370. doi: 10.1073/pnas.1301837110

Lee, R. C., Feinbaum, R. L., and Ambros, V. (1993). The *C. elegans* heterochronic gene lin-4 encodes small RNAs with antisense complementarity to lin-14. *Cell* 75, 843–854. doi: 10.1016/0092-8674(93)90529-Y

Leung, K.-M., van Horck, F. P. G., Lin, A. C., Allison, R., Standart, N., and Holt, C. E. (2006). Asymmetrical beta-actin mRNA translation in growth cones mediates attractive turning to netrin-1. *Nat. Neurosci.* 9, 1247–1256. doi: 10.1038/nn1775

Li, H., Li, W. X., and Ding, S. W. (2002). Induction and suppression of RNA silencing by an animal virus. *Science* 296, 1319–1321. doi: 10.1126/science.1070948

Li, Q., Lee, J.-A., and Black, D. L. (2007). Neuronal regulation of alternative premRNA splicing. *Nat. Rev. Neurosci.* 8, 819–831. doi: 10.1038/nrn2237

López-Bendito, G., Cautinat, A., Sánchez, J. A., Bielle, F., Flames, N., Garratt, A. N., et al. (2006). Tangential neuronal migration controls axon guidance: a role for neuregulin-1 in thalamocortical axon navigation. *Cell* 125, 127–142. doi: 10.1016/j.cell.2006.01.042

Lugli, G., Larson, J., Martone, M. E., Jones, Y., and Smalheiser, N. R. (2005). Dicer and eIF2c are enriched at post-synaptic densities in adult mouse brain and are modified by neuronal activity in a calpain-dependent manner. *J. Neurochem.* 94, 896–905. doi: 10.1111/j.1471-4159.2005.03224.x

Luxey, M., Jungas, T., Laussu, J., Audouard, C., Garces, A., and Davy, A. (2013). Eph:ephrin-B1 forward signaling controls fasciculation of sensory and motor axons. *Dev. Biol.* 383, 264–274. doi: 10.1016/j.ydbio.2013.09.010

Mehlen, P., Delloye-Bourgeois, C., and Chédotal, A. (2011). Novel roles for Slits and netrins: axon guidance cues as anticancer targets? *Nat. Rev. Cancer* 11, 188–197. doi: 10.1038/nrc3005

Meister, G. (2013). Argonaute proteins: functional insights and emerging roles. *Nat. Rev. Genet.* 14, 447–459. doi: 10.1038/nrg3462

Memczak, S., Jens, M., Elefsinioti, A., Torti, F., Krueger, J., Rybak, A., et al. (2013). Circular RNAs are a large class of animal RNAs with regulatory potency. *Nature* 495, 333–338. doi: 10.1038/nature11928

Molnár, Z., Garel, S., López-Bendito, G., Maness, P., and Price, D. J. (2012). Mechanisms controlling the guidance of thalamocortical axons through the embryonic forebrain. *Eur. J. Neurosci.* 35, 1573–1585. doi: 10.1111/j.1460-9568.2012.08119.x

Muddashetty, R. S., Nalavadi, V. C., Gross, C., Yao, X., Xing, L., Laur, O., et al. (2011). Reversible inhibition of PSD-95 mRNA translation by miR-125a, FMRP phosphorylation, and mGluR signaling. *Mol. Cell* 42, 673–688. doi: 10.1016/j.molcel.2011.05.006

Nakagawa, S., Brennan, C., Johnson, K. G., Shewan, D., Harris, W. A., and Holt, C. E. (2000). Ephrin-B regulates the Ipsilateral routing of retinal axons at the optic chiasm. *Neuron* 25, 599–610. doi: 10.1016/S0896-6273(00)81063-6

Natera-Naranjo, O., Aschrafi, A., Gioio, A. E., and Kaplan, B. B. (2010). Identification and quantitative analyses of microRNAs located in the distal axons of sympathetic neurons. *RNA* 16, 1516–1529. doi: 10.1261/rna.1833310

Olsson-Carter, K., and Slack, F. J. (2010). A developmental timing switch promotes axon outgrowth independent of known guidance receptors. *PLoS Genet.* 6: e1001054. doi: 10.1371/journal.pgen.1001054

Pfaff, J., Hennig, J., Herzog, F., Aebersold, R., Sattler, M., Niessing, D., et al. (2013). Structural features of Argonaute-GW182 protein interactions. *Proc. Natl. Acad. Sci. U.S.A.* 110, E3770–E3779. doi: 10.1073/pnas.1308510110

Pichardo-Casas, I., Goff, L. A., Swerdel, M. R., Athie, A., Davila, J., Ramos-Brossier, M., et al. (2012). Expression profiling of synaptic microRNAs from the adult rat brain identifies regional differences and seizure-induced dynamic modulation. *Brain Res.* 1436, 20–33. doi: 10.1016/j.brainres.2011.12.001

Pinter, R., and Hindges, R. (2010). Perturbations of microRNA function in mouse dicer mutants produce retinal defects and lead to aberrant axon pathfinding at the optic chiasm. *PLoS ONE* 5:e10021. doi: 10.1371/journal.pone.0010021

Pittman, A. J., Law, M.-Y., and Chien, C.-B. (2008). Pathfinding in a large vertebrate axon tract: isotypic interactions guide retinotectal axons at multiple choice points. *Development* 135, 2865–2871. doi: 10.1242/dev.025049

Plachez, C., Andrews, W., Liapi, A., Knoell, B., Drescher, U., Mankoo, B., et al. (2008). Robos are required for the correct targeting of retinal ganglion cell axons in the visual pathway of the brain. *Mol. Cell. Neurosci.* 37, 719–730. doi: 10.1016/j.mcn.2007.12.017

Plump, A. S., Erskine, L., Sabatier, C., Brose, K., Epstein, C. J., Goodman, C. S., et al. (2002). Slit1 and Slit2 cooperate to prevent premature midline crossing of retinal axons in the mouse visual system. *Neuron* 33, 219–232. doi: 10.1016/S0896-6273(01)00586-4

Pulkkinen, K., Malm, T., Turunen, M., Koistinaho, J., and Ylä-Herttuala, S. (2008). Hypoxia induces microRNA miR-210 *in vitro* and *in vivo* ephrin-A3 and neuronal pentraxin 1 are potentially regulated by miR-210. *FEBS Lett.* 582, 2397–2401. doi: 10.1016/j.febslet.2008.05.048

Qiang, R., Wang, F., Shi, L.-Y., Liu, M., Chen, S., Wan, H.-Y., et al. (2011). Plexin-B1 is a target of miR-214 in cervical cancer and promotes the growth and invasion of HeLa cells. *Int. J. Biochem. Cell Biol.* 43, 632–641. doi: 10.1016/j.biocel.2011.01.002

Raper, J., and Mason, C. (2010). Cellular strategies of axonal pathfinding. *Cold Spring Harb. Perspect. Biol.* 2:a001933. doi: 10.1101/cshperspect.a001933

Reinhart, B. J., Slack, F. J., Basson, M., Pasquinelli, A. E., Bettinger, J. C., Rougvie, A. E., et al. (2000). The 21-nucleotide let-7 RNA regulates developmental timing in Caenorhabditis elegans. *Nature* 403, 901–906. doi: 10.1038/35002607

Ringstedt, T., Braisted, J. E., Brose, K., Kidd, T., Goodman, C., Tessier-Lavigne, M., et al. (2000). Slit inhibition of retinal axon growth and its role in retinal axon pathfinding and innervation patterns in the diencephalon. *J. Neurosci.* 20, 4983–4991.

Salmena, L., Poliseno, L., Tay, Y., Kats, L., and Pandolfi, P. P. (2011). A ceRNA hypothesis: the Rosetta Stone of a hidden RNA language? *Cell* 146, 353–358. doi: 10.1016/j.cell.2011.07.014

Sasaki, Y., Gross, C., Xing, L., Goshima, Y., and Bassell, G. J. (2013). Identification of axon-enriched MicroRNAs localized to growth cones of cortical neurons. *Dev. Neurobiol.* 74, 397–406. doi: 10.1002/dneu.22113

Schaefer, A., O'Carroll, D., Tan, C. L., Hillman, D., Sugimori, M., Llinas, R., et al. (2007). Cerebellar neurodegeneration in the absence of microRNAs. *J. Exp. Med.* 204, 1553–1558. doi: 10.1084/jem.20070823

Schmucker, D., Clemens, J. C., Shu, H., Worby, C. A., Xiao, J., Muda, M., et al. (2000). Drosophila Dscam is an axon guidance receptor exhibiting extraordinary molecular diversity. *Cell* 101, 671–684. doi: 10.1016/S0092-8674(00)80878-8

Schratt, G. M., Tuebing, F., Nigh, E. A., Kane, C. G., Sabatini, M. E., Kiebler, M., et al. (2006). A brain-specific microRNA regulates dendritic spine development. *Nature* 439, 283–289. doi: 10.1038/nature04367

Seitz, H. (2009). Redefining microRNA targets. *Curr. Biol.* 19, 870–873. doi: 10.1016/j.cub.2009.03.059

Selbach, M., Schwanhäusser, B., Thierfelder, N., Fang, Z., Khanin, R., and Rajewsky, N. (2008). Widespread changes in protein synthesis induced by microRNAs. *Nature* 455, 58–63. doi: 10.1038/nature07228

Sempere, L. F., Freemantle, S., Pitha-Rowe, I., Moss, E., Dmitrovsky, E., and Ambros, V. (2004). Expression profiling of mammalian microRNAs uncovers a subset of brain-expressed microRNAs with possible roles in murine and human neuronal differentiation. *Genome Biol.* 5:R13. doi: 10.1186/gb-2004-5-3-r13

Shibata, M., Nakao, H., Kiyonari, H., Abe, T., and Aizawa, S. (2011). MicroRNA-9 regulates neurogenesis in mouse telencephalon by targeting multiple transcription factors. *J. Neurosci.* 31, 3407–3422. doi: 10.1523/JNEUROSCI.5085-10.2011

Siegel, G., Obernosterer, G., Fiore, R., Oehmen, M., Bicker, S., Christensen, M., et al. (2009). A functional screen implicates microRNA-138-dependent regulation of the depalmitoylation enzyme APT1 in dendritic spine morphogenesis. *Nat. Cell Biol.* 11, 705–716. doi: 10.1038/ncb1876

Small, E. M., and Olson, E. N. (2011). Pervasive roles of microRNAs in cardiovascular biology. *Nature* 469, 336–342. doi: 10.1038/nature09783

Small, E. M., Sutherland, L. B., Rajagopalan, K. N., Wang, S., and Olson, E. N. (2010). MicroRNA-218 regulates vascular patterning by modulation of Slit-Robo signaling. *Circ. Res.* 107, 1336–1344. doi: 10.1161/CIRCRESAHA.110.227926

Smirnova, L., Gräfe, A., Seiler, A., Schumacher, S., Nitsch, R., and Wulczyn, F. G. (2005). Regulation of miRNA expression during neural cell specification. *Eur. J. Neurosci.* 21, 1469–1477. doi: 10.1111/j.1460-9568.2005.03978.x

Taylor, A. M., Berchtold, N. C., Perreau, V. M., Tu, C. H., Li Jeon, N., and Cotman, C. W. (2009). Axonal mRNA in uninjured and regenerating cortical mammalian axons. *J. Neurosci.* 29, 4697–4707. doi: 10.1523/JNEUROSCI.6130-08.2009

Tessier-Lavigne, M., and Goodman, C. S. (1996). The molecular biology of Axon guidance. *Science* 274, 1123–1133. doi: 10.1126/science.274.5290.1123

Tie, J., Pan, Y., Zhao, L., Wu, K., Liu, J., Sun, S., et al. (2010). MiR-218 inhibits invasion and metastasis of gastric cancer by targeting the Robo1 receptor. *PLoS Genet.* 6:e1000879. doi: 10.1371/journal.pgen.1000879

Urbich, C., Kaluza, D., Frömel, T., Knau, A., Bennewitz, K., Boon, R. A., et al. (2012). MicroRNA-27a/b controls endothelial cell repulsion and angiogenesis by targeting semaphorin 6A. *Blood* 119, 1607–1616. doi: 10.1182/blood-2011-08-373886

Ventura, A., Young, A. G., Winslow, M. M., Lintault, L., Meissner, A., Erkeland, S. J., et al. (2008). Targeted deletion reveals essential and overlapping functions of the miR-17 through 92 family of miRNA clusters. *Cell* 132, 875–886. doi: 10.1016/j.cell.2008.02.019

Vitriol, E. A., and Zheng, J. Q. (2012). Growth cone travel in space and time: the cellular ensemble of cytoskeleton, adhesion, and membrane. *Neuron* 73, 1068–1081. doi: 10.1016/j.neuron.2012.03.005

Wightman, B., Ha, I., and Ruvkun, G. (1993). Posttranscriptional regulation of the heterochronic gene lin-14 by lin-4 mediates temporal pattern formation in C. *elegans. Cell* 75, 855–862. doi: 10.1016/0092-8674(93)90530-4

Williams, S. E., Mann, F., Erskine, L., Sakurai, T., Wei, S., Rossi, D. J., et al. (2003). Ephrin-B2 and EphB1 mediate retinal axon divergence at the optic chiasm. *Neuron* 39, 919–935. doi: 10.1016/j.neuron.2003.08.017

Wolman, M. A., Liu, Y., Tawarayama, H., Shoji, W., and Halloran, M. C. (2004). Repulsion and attraction of axons by semaphorin3D are mediated by different neuropilins *in vivo*. *J. Neurosci.* 24, 8428–8435. doi: 10.1523/JNEUROSCI.2349-04.2004

Wu, D., and Murashov, A. K. (2013). MicroRNA-431 regulates axon regeneration in mature sensory neurons by targeting the Wnt antagonist Kremen1. *Front. Mol. Neurosci.* 6:35. doi: 10.3389/fnmol.2013.00035

Xiao, C., and Rajewsky, K. (2009). MicroRNA control in the immune system: basic principles. *Cell* 136, 26–36. doi: 10.1016/j.cell.2008.12.027

Yang, J.-S., Maurin, T., Robine, N., Rasmussen, K. D., Jeffrey, K. L., Chandwani, R., et al. (2010). Conserved vertebrate mir-451 provides a platform for Dicer-independent, Ago2-mediated microRNA biogenesis. *Proc. Natl. Acad. Sci. U.S.A.* 107, 15163–15168. doi: 10.1073/pnas.1006432107

Yang, L., Li, Q., Wang, Q., Jiang, Z., and Zhang, L. (2012). Silencing of miRNA-218 promotes migration and invasion of breast cancer via Slit2-Robo1 pathway. *Biomed. Pharmacother.* 66, 535–540. doi: 10.1016/j.biopha.2012.04.006

Zhang, Y., He, X., Liu, Y., Ye, Y., Zhang, H., He, P., et al. (2012). microRNA-320a inhibits tumor invasion by targeting neuropilin 1 and is associated with liver metastasis in colorectal cancer. *Oncol. Rep.* 27, 685–694. doi: 10.3892/or.2011.1561

Zhang, Y., Ueno, Y., Liu, X. S., Buller, B., Wang, X., Chopp, M., et al. (2013). The MicroRNA-17-92 cluster enhances axonal outgrowth in embryonic cortical neurons. *J. Neurosci.* 33, 6885–6894. doi: 10.1523/JNEUROSCI.5180-12.2013

Zivraj, K. H., Tung, Y. C. L., Piper, M., Gumy, L., Fawcett, J. W., Yeo, G. S. H., et al. (2010). Subcellular profiling reveals distinct and developmentally regulated repertoire of growth cone mRNAs. *J. Neurosci.* 30, 15464–15478. doi: 10.1523/JNEUROSCI.1800-10.2010

Zou, Y., Chiu, H., Domenger, D., Chuang, C.-F., and Chang, C. (2012). The lin-4 microRNA targets the LIN-14 transcription factor to inhibit netrin-mediated axon attraction. *Sci. Signal.* 5, ra43. doi: 10.1126/scisignal.2002437

Zou, Y., Chiu, H., Zinovyeva, A., Ambros, V., Chuang, C.-F., and Chang, C. (2013). Developmental decline in neuronal regeneration by the progressive change of two intrinsic timers. *Science* 340, 372–376. doi: 10.1126/science.1231321

3

Novel ncRNAs transcribed by Pol III and elucidation of their functional relevance by biophysical approaches

Paola Gavazzo[1]*, Massimo Vassalli[1], Delfina Costa[2] and Aldo Pagano[2,3]

[1] Institute of Biophysics, National Research Council (CNR), Genoa, Italy
[2] Department of Experimental Medicine, University of Genoa, Genoa, Italy
[3] IRCCS Azienda Ospedaliera Universitaria San Martino-IST, Genoa, Italy

In the last decade the role of non coding (nc) RNAs in neurogenesis and in the onset of neurological diseases has been assessed by a multitude of studies. In this scenario, approximately 30 small RNA polymerase (pol) III–dependent ncRNAs were recently identified by computational tools and proposed as regulatory elements. The function of several of these transcripts was elucidated *in vitro* and *in vivo* confirming their involvement in cancer and in metabolic and neurodegenerative disorders. Emerging biophysical technologies together with the introduction of a physical perspective have been advantageous in regulatory RNA investigation providing original results on: (a) the differentiation of neuroblastoma (NB) cells towards a neuron-like phenotype triggered by Neuroblastoma Differentiation Marker 29 (NDM29) ncRNA; (b) the modulation of A-type K^+ current in neurons induced by the small ncRNA 38A and (c) the synthesis driven by 17A ncRNA of a GABAB2 receptor isoform unable to trigger intracellular signaling. Moreover, the application of Single Cell Force Spectroscopy (SCFS) to these studies suggests a correlation between the malignancy stage of NB and the micro-adhesive properties of the cells, allowing to investigate the molecular basis of such a correlation.

***Correspondence:**
Paola Gavazzo, Institute of Biophysics, National Research Council (CNR), Via De Marini 6, 16149 Genoa, Italy
e-mail: gavazzo@ge.ibf.cnr.it

Keywords: RNA polymerase III, non-coding RNA, neuroblastoma, single cell force spectroscopy (SCFS), patch clamp

REGULATORY RNAs TRANSCRIBED BY POL III

In the last few years polymerase (pol) III stepped in the limelight as a complex machinery that synthesizes a bulk of transcripts much higher than expected. Indeed, since 2007, a very active synthesis of non coding RNAs (ncRNAs) with regulatory features has been demonstrated (Pagano et al., 2007) and subsequently strengthened by further studies (Barski et al., 2010; Moqtaderi et al., 2010; Oler et al., 2010). These studies showed that pol III machinery is not to be considered as almost exclusively engaged in the synthesis of tRNAs and 5S ribosomal RNA, as this protein complex may transcribe in a cell type-/cell stage-specific manner a significant amount of small RNAs with regulatory features (Bruzzone et al., 2012; Garritano et al., 2012). Since pol III machinery does not bind elongation factors, the length of these RNAs ranges from 70 to 350 nucleotides. Coherently with heterogeneity in length, a lack of shared secondary structures indicates that a peculiar molecular organization is not the common hallmark of this set of noncoding molecules (Pagano et al., 2007). Since many of these transcripts map in introns of protein-coding genes in antisense configuration, it is possible to hypothesize that their function in cis may be devoted to the regulation of mRNA maturation and splicing. However, a correlation between genomic localization and alternative splicing sites has not been documented yet and the molecular details of the mechanism of splicing control are still elusive.

In the recent past, the functional analysis of a panel of these RNAs disclosed their crucial roles in several physiopathological processes where they impact strongly on the determination of a cell fate. Interestingly, a significant fraction of the newly identified molecules plays a role in the nervous system and/or in the determination of a neuron-like phenotype (Castelnuovo et al., 2010; Massone et al., 2011a, 2012; Ciarlo et al., 2013; Penna et al., 2013). To this aim, a wide panel of molecular markers are often used to characterize the phenotype of the cell and to determine the functional role of the over-/down-regulation of a ncRNA of interest. However, the profile obtained solely by the analysis of biomolecular markers is often over-esteemed, as the expression of a limited set of genes characteristic of a differentiation stage does not ensure the concomitant achievement of a corresponding functional phenotype. In this scenario, the analysis of functional parameters (such as biophysical determinations of specific conductances in the study of the phenotype of neural-like cells) is auspicable in order to better characterize the differentiation stage.

CELL DIFFERENTIATION AND MALIGNANCY REGRESSION TRIGGERED BY 29A (NDM29) OVEREXPRESSION IN NEUROBLASTOMA: ANALYSIS OF MEMBRANE CONDUCTANCES

In a recent study a ncRNA the overexpression of which leads to the differentiation of strongly malignant neuroblastoma (NB) cells was identified (Castelnuovo et al., 2010). This series of experiments disclosed the key role played by a pol III-transcribed ncRNA (Neuroblastoma Differentiation Marker 29, NDM29) in differentiation and malignancy and suggested a novel way to control cell differentiation. Indeed, NDM29 ncRNA exhibits a tight control of NB cell differentiation leading, ultimately, to the restriction of the malignant potential. Engineered SKNBE2 cell clones harboring extra copies of the NDM29 units have been generated and the most active in overexpressing NDM29 ncRNA (S1 clone) has been selected for detailed experiments. A panel of experiments *in vitro*, further strengthened by evidences obtained *in vivo*, demonstrated that a series of parameters that characterize the differentiation stages were directly influenced by the level of expression of NDM29 RNA. S1 cell model exhibits a scarcely malignant phenotype confirmed by modifications in cell morphology, elongation of cell cycle, increase of cell adhesiveness, decrease of tumorigenic potential *in vivo*. Since the differentiation of NB cells is characterized by the acquisition of a neuron-like phenotype, the analysis of possible membrane conductance modifications related to NDM29-triggered S1 differentiation has been performed (Gavazzo et al., 2011). To this aim it was decided to apply electrophysiology, the most reliable and sensitive approach to get straightforward information about the electrical activity of cells. Interestingly, whole–cell patch-clamp recordings assessed that stable overexpression of NDM29 in S1 cells actively promotes the acquisition of electrophysiological features typical of neuronal cells, such as a sizeable increase of inward Tetrodotoxin-sensitive voltage-activated Na^+ current (**Figure 1A**) and the capability to generate overshooting active action potentials (**Figure 1B**), a typical hallmark of neurons which makes them excitable. S1 firing events in particular show amplitude and duration typical of mature neurons (average amplitude 49.14 ± 5.33 mV, duration at half amplitude 6.38 ± 0.66 ms). However, such events are never spontaneous nor multiple. All these changes are correlated with the hyperpolarization of resting potential, that shifts from −35 mV in Mock to −43 mV in S1, a discrepancy commonly observed between a cancerous and highly proliferating cell and its differentiated counterpart (Gavazzo et al., 2011).

As a consequence of overexpressing NDM29, S1 cells synthesize and assemble functional $GABA_A$ ionotropic receptors, the most important inhibitory neurotrasmitter receptors in central nervous systems (CNS) of humans (**Figures 1C, D**). $GABA_A$ receptors are heteropentamers assembled from the combination of 16 different subunits (α 1–6, β 1–3, γ 1–3, δ, ϵ, π, ρ) with a minimal requirement for 2α, 2β and 1γ or δ subunit to be functional. A combination of Real Time Reverse Transcription-Polymerase Chain Reaction (RT-PCR) experiments, electrophysiological recordings and pharmacological analysis have assessed that S1-SKNBE2 cells are likely to express a major amount of α1 subunit, together with β1 and β3 and γ1 and 2, giving rise to receptors mainly composed by $\alpha_1\beta_n\gamma_n$, which is known to be the most abundant and widespread combination in the CNS (Laurie et al., 1992). $GABA_A$ receptors in fact accomplish their function in the brain, where they are involved in higher CNS functions and implicated in a variety of neurological disorders such as epilepsy, anxiety, Huntington disease, schizophrenia (D'Hulst et al., 2009). The availability of a cell clone stably expressing $GABA_A$ receptors of known composition acquires a valuable relevance, since these proteins are the target of important drugs such as benzodiazepines, barbiturates, neuroactive steroids and convulsivants, the effects of which are selectively modulated by specific subtypes of receptors. Hence S1 cells are an attractive tool in pharmacological research focused to the identification of new drug molecules for therapeutic purposes.

In conclusion, a sustained expression of NDM29 ncRNA supports a well-coordinated differentiation process of NB cells toward a neuron-like phenotype, togheter with a reduction of malignancy. A direct relationship seems to link the level of NDM29 and phenotype modifications, as also suggested from results obtained with the S2-SKNBE2 engineered clone, expressing NDM29 at intermediate level with respect to S1 and Mock and showing an intermediate phenotype as well (Castelnuovo et al., 2010).

ALTERATION OF NEURONAL ACTIVITY INDUCED BY THE SMALL NON CODING MOLECULES 38A/B AND 17A: A POSSIBLE CONNECTION WITH NEURODEGENERATION

Neuron excitability is mediated by the combination of voltage- and neurotrasmitter—gated ion channels, whose simultaneous activity shapes the variety of electrical behaviors observed in neural cells. A-type K^+current (I_A) is mainly mediated by the Kv4 subfamily of voltage-gated K^+ channels and has been shown to take part in the control of slow repetitive firing as well as in contributing to integrate hippocampal electrical signal to associative events such as long term potentiation (LTP) and depression (LTD; Holmqvist et al., 2002). I_A current is generally characterized by a fast inactivation that can be modulated by the presence of the K^+-channel interacting protein 4 (KCNIP4), expressed in different splicing isoforms, with the canonical splice variant I detectable in all the brain compartments, whereas the variant IV is only localized in globus pallidus and basal forebrain neurons (Trimmer and Rhodes, 2004). The combination of Kv4 α subunits with KCNIP4 variant IV is associated with a remarkable slowing down of the I_A—inactivation and with a reduction of membrane expression of Kv4 channels as well (Baranauskas, 2004). Notably, one of the human RNA regulatory transcripts driven by pol III, 38A RNA, maps an intron of KCNIP4 gene and its expression drives the synthesis of the alternative variant IV. This was verified in the NDM29 overexpressing SKNBE2 clone S1 previously described. The cells, due to their neural phenotype, are usually endowed with at least a component of I_A current, that is suppressed after cells are transiently transfected with 38A (Massone et al., 2011a).

I_A K^+ current behavior was assessed in mouse neurons. The bioinformatic search for pol III-driven regulatory RNAs in the mouse genome provided a set of transcriptional units, which are considered putative functional homologs of their human counterparts. 38B RNA (the murine counterpart of 38A) was selected and I_A current recorded from hippocampal neurons transfected with a plasmid overexpressing 38B RNA. The results showed a strong reduction of the fast component of the current, with the constant of inactivation at +50 mV shifting to 250 ms from the 55 ms of the native neurons (Bruzzone et al., 2012). Again, the overexpression of 38B leads to the impairment of the balance between different KCNIP4 splice variants.

The alteration of excitatory properties of neurons has often been correlated with neurological disorders and in this framework

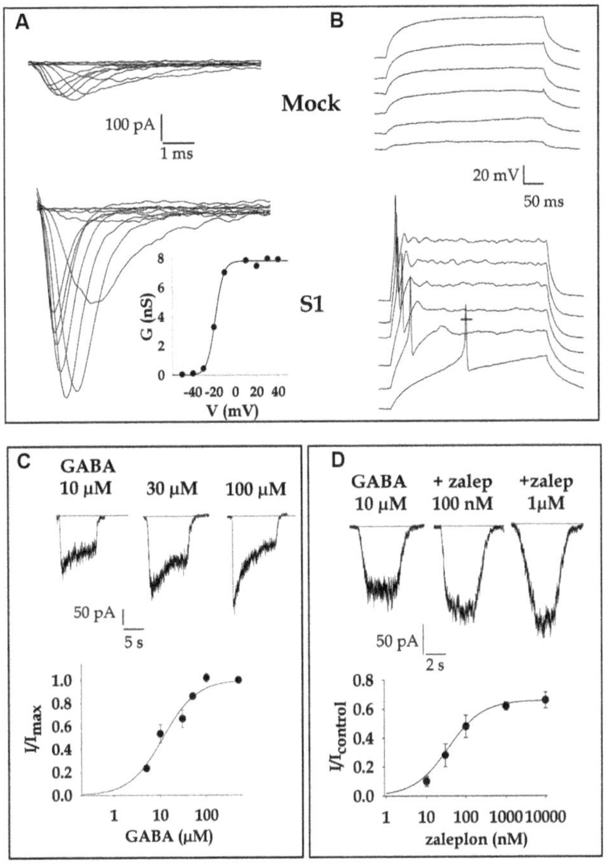

FIGURE 1 | Electrophysiological profile of NB SKNBE2 cells is modified from NDM29 overexpression. (A) Fast inward voltage-gated Na^+ current is drastically enhanced in cells stably overexpressing NDM29 (S1 clone, average value of current density at −10 mV = 43 ± 7 pA/pF) respect to untransfected cells (Mock clone, average value = 7.7 ± 1.7 pA/pF). Current were elicited by step depolarization from −50 mV to +40 mV in 10 mV increments from a holding potential (V_h) = −90 mV. Bath solution contained (mM): 140 NaCl, 5.4 KCl, 2 $CaCl_2$, 1 $MgCl_2$ 10 Hepes (4-(2-hydroxyethyl)-1-piperazineethanesulfonic acid), 10 Glucose, pH 7.3 adjusted with NaOH. The intracellular pipette solution contained (mM): 50 CsCl, 80 CsF, 11 ethylene glycol tetraacetic acid (EGTA), 1 $CaCl_2$, 1 $MgCl_2$, 10 Hepes, pH 7.3 adjusted with Trizma Base. In the inset the activation curve calculated from the above S1 cell traces is shown. Reversal potential of Na^+ was set to +90 mV and experimental points were fitted with a Boltzman equation (see Gavazzo et al., 2011). The potential value at which the conductance is half of the maximum value ($V_{1/2}$) was estimated −19 mV for this representative cell. **(B)** Current clamp recordings, obtained passing depolarizing current in 10 pA steps, showed overshooting action potentials in S1 cell, but only a passive response in Mock. **(C)** GABA-gated currents in S1 cell were activated clamping the cell at a potential of −60 mV and applying for a short time (2 s) increasing concentrations of the neurotransmitter every 40 s. The normalized dose-response curve of GABA-activated current is shown below. Fitting the experimental points, the concentration of GABA eliciting half maximal current amplitude (EC50) was estimated = 11.4 μM. **(D)** Pharmacological analysis of S1 current allowed to identify the subunit composition of the functional $GABA_A$ receptors. Cell were challenged with GABA alone or in the presence of several drugs (Gavazzo et al., 2011). Among all zaleplon, a compound that binds the benzodiazepine site of the α1 subunit containing receptors, potentiated the current with a EC50 = 25 nM. (Adapted from Gavazzo et al., 2011 with permission).

the effect of 38A RNA on the nervous system is also detrimental for several reasons. First of all, the suppression of the fast component of the K^+ current alters the I_A activity, which plays an essential role for neuron firing and stabilization of higher functions associated to brain plasticity and memory, such as LTP. Secondly, biochemical evidence suggests that KCNIP4 unusual variant IV loses the ability to interact with Presenilin 2, affecting its role in the gamma secretase complex and possibly favoring the secretion of the neurotoxic insoluble form of beta amiloid peptide x-42 (Massone et al., 2011a).

The investigation of the molecular mechanisms adopted by ncRNAs to accomplish their regulatory function provides at least another example of alternative protein synthesis dependent on the activity of a pol III-transcribed RNA which, ultimately, leads to the impairment of GABA B2 metabotropic receptor signaling. 17A ncRNA maps in intron 3 of G-protein-coupled receptor 51 (GPR51) gene that undergoes extensive alternative splicing giving rise to several isoforms of GABA B2 receptor endowed with different biological activities. Only the canonical splice variant A is able to form heterodimers with the GABA B1 subunit and, through a second messenger system, to regulate the intracellular 3′-5′- cyclic adenosine monophosphate (cAMP) accumulation and the activation of specific K^+ channels. It has been recently shown (Massone et al., 2011b) that the overexpression of 17A RNA in human neuroblastoma cell line-differentiated (SH-SY5Y) NB cells drives to the production of the GABA B2 receptor variant B which suppresses intracellular signaling. This was demonstrated recording the inward rectifying K^+ current in SH-SY5Y cells untransfected or after transfection with a plasmid harboring extra 17A transcriptional units. Challenging cells with baclofen, a selective GABA B agonist, and with the antagonist [(2S)-3-[[(1S)-1-(3,4-Dichlorophenyl)ethyl]amino]-2-hydroxypropyl](phenylmethyl)phosphinic acid hydrochloride (CGP55845), it was possible to assess that functionally active receptors are expressed in control cells, while this functionality is suppressed by 17A RNA overexpression.

Presynaptic GABAB receptors have been shown to inhibit high-voltage activated Ca^{2+} channels in the brain, causing a reduction of neurotransmitter release in the synaptic cleft; moreover they are responsible of the slow inhibitory post-synaptic current (IPSC) mediated by the activation of inwardly rectifying K^+ channels (Kir3) with the consequent hyperpolarization of the postsynaptic membrane. In this scenario, it is reasonable to speculate that the impairment of their activity might correlate with neural disorders. Indeed, 17A RNA, usually expressed in human brain, is upregulated in cerebral tissue derived from Alzheimer's patients suggesting its possible direct or indirect involvement in the etiology of the disease or in a pathway acting concomitantly (Massone et al., 2011b).

SINGLE CELL FORCE SPECTROSCOPY: A POTENTIAL TOOL FOR CANCER STADIATION

It is common knowledge that substantial variations of cell adhesion properties go along the process of tumorigenesis and often discriminate among different cellular components of tumor nodules (Okegawa et al., 2004). In this context several assays aimed at quantitatively evaluating the cell adhesion properties are suitable for the analysis of tumor cells and are usually accompanied by the analysis of colony growth efficiency in semisolid media in order to assess the tumorigenic potential of cancer cells. Although this approach offers the appropriate way to quantitatively determine cell malignancy, it does not provide any information about the class of molecules that drive this phenotype and might provide a prognostic tool.

Recently, a novel spectroscopic approach based on the application of an Atomic Force Microscope (AFM) was addressed, in order to extract high sensitivity mechanical information from single cells. An AFM is a device in which a micrometer-sized cantilever, with a sharp tip on top, is brought into contact with a sample that is moved under the tip. While scanning the sample, the cantilever deflects following the profile, thus giving information on the three dimensional morphology of the sample with a resolution limited by the tip radius that can be cast as low as 1–2 nm. Nevertheless, before being a microscope, the AFM touches the sample, thus experiencing and measuring the interaction force with high sensitivity. In the last decade this aspect of the instrument was largely stressed and many relevant results were obtained on single molecule biomechanics (Kellermayer and Grama, 2002; Sbrana et al., 2011) and their interaction (Weisel et al., 2003), but also on larger systems, such as bacteria or unicellular organisms (Pletikapic et al., 2012).

In particular, the force spectroscopy feature of the AFM was exploited to measure the mechanical properties of single cells (Papi et al., 2013), mainly by using non sharp tips (to avoid huge pressures, potentially damaging living cells), gluing a micrometer-sized sphere on top of the cantilever or even attaching the cell itself, to directly probe the interaction with the substrate (Canale et al., 2013). In a standard AFM-based single cell force spectroscopy (SCFS) experiment, the cantilever is approached to the cell with a constant speed while measuring the interaction force (**Figure 2A**, region 1) that increases upon contact with the cell membrane. The shape of the indentation curve (**Figure 2A**, region 2) carries information about the mechanical properties of the cell, mainly the elasticity, in terms of Young's modulus (Loparic et al., 2010). After a short delay (typically 1–5 s), the cantilever is thus moved away and a characteristic pattern is recorded (**Figure 2A**, region 3) from which several adhesion-related quantitative parameters can be extracted (see notes in **Figure 2A**).

As suggested, the detailed analysis of the force versus displacement pattern obtained from SCFS measurements can lead to the determination of single-cell mechanical parameters that can be measured over a population, obtaining a relevant distribution to be compared among samples in different biological stages. This approach proved helpful in characterizing the biomechanical properties of single cancer cells (Suresh, 2007), but it can also be extended, from a biophysical point of view, to address the comprehension of the underlying molecular mechanisms. As an example, SCFS has been recently applied to the characterization of the SKNBE2 NB cells described above (Mescola et al., 2012). Noteworthy, it was possible to show a statistically relevant difference in several parameters including, for instance, the DW value between cells expressing lower (Mock) or higher levels of NDM29 (S1 clone), as shown in **Figure 2B**, red bars. The novelty of the measurements performed with SCFS is that they provide a quantitative information of the adhesiveness of the probed cells that directly reflects their microscale molecular properties. To assess this interpretation, a comparison was carried out with Human Embryonic Kidney (HEK) cells before and after the treatment with cytoskeleton-affecting drugs. In fact, cytoskeleton is known to be strongly modified by the onset of a cancerous stage (Yamaguchi and Condeelis, 2007) and, specifically for NB, the microtubule network was identified as a major target. By treating HEK cells with colchicine (affecting microtubule polimerization) or cytochalasin D (damaging the microfilament network) it is possible to observe the effect of a change in a selected molecular component that reflects on the whole DW of the cell (**Figure 2B**, yellow bars). Interestingly, the value of DW showed to decrease, with respect to control, when cells were treated against microtubules, while it increased after treatment against microfilaments. Interestingly, Mock cells, which adopt a cancerous phenotype associated with a loss in microtubules stability (Van de Water and Olmstebd, 1980), showed a lower DW with respect to S1 cells. This result, as a reference example, highlights the ability of SCFS measurements to infer about the molecular origin of the observed physiological state.

SUMMARY AND PERSPECTIVES

The regulatory effects of ncRNAs often impact on relevant biological aspects of the cell such as stemness, differentiation and

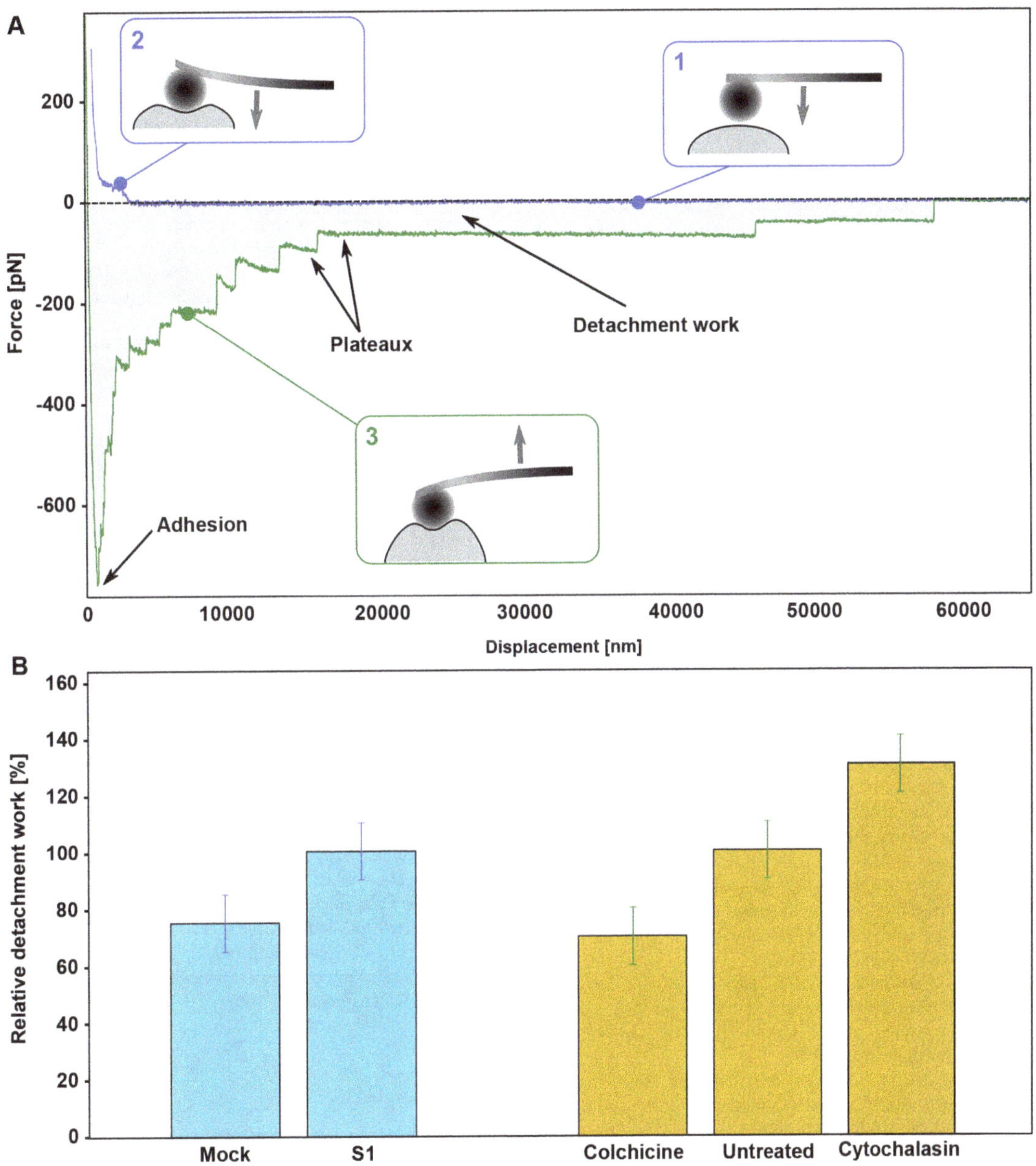

FIGURE 2 | (A) Typical SCFS experiment output showing approach (blue) and retract (green) curves on a Human Embryonic Kidney (HEK) cell. The main features of the curve contributing to the definition of mechanical parameters are highlighted. Among all, of particular interest are the adhesion (force value of the maximal adhesion force) and the detachment work (DW) (the gray area between the approach and retract curve). **(B)** Histogram of the relative DW on a statistical set of cells, both from SKNBE2 (blu bars) and HEK (yellow bars) cells (Adapted from Mescola et al., 2012 with permission).

tumorigenic potential. Therefore, the availability of techniques that can correlate the identification of novel genetic transcriptional units with specific phenotypic treats is of crucial importance. A general advancement of the use of biomolecular markers at both RNA and protein levels has been developed with the final aim to precisely trace the phenotypic hallmarks of specific cell and/or differentiation stages; however, in our view, this biochemical approach is not sufficient and a misinterpretation of biological data is often possible. In this context the association of functional tests that unequivocally draw the capacity of the cell to exert the biological activities peculiar of a specific stage is always enlightening. Since the vast majority of pol III transcripts here described exert crucial roles in "neuro-specific" pathways, the biophysical approach with electrophysiology traditionally represents the golden method for its unique ability to directly monitor the activity of the cell. On the other side the application of SCFS in cellular biology is only at its beginning but many results indicate that it is a promising technique to bridge the gap between physiological state and molecular determinants starting from a new perspective, based on the mechanical fingerprint of individual cells.

ACKNOWLEDGMENTS

The authors are grateful to Dr. Francesca Spanò for proofreading.

REFERENCES

Baranauskas, G. (2004). Cell-type-specific splicing of KChIP4 mRNA correlates with slower kinetics of A-type current. *Eur. J. Neurosci.* 20, 385–391. doi: 10.1111/j.1460-9568.2004.03494.x

Barski, A., Cheopelev, I., Liko, D., Cuddapah, S., Fleming, A. B., Birch, J., et al. (2010). Pol II and its associated epigenetic marks are present at Pol III-transcribed noncoding RNA genes. *Nat. Struct. Mol. Biol.* 17, 629–634. doi: 10.1030/nsmb.1806

Bruzzone, M. J., Gavazzo, P., Massone, S., Balbi, C., Villa, F., Conti, A., et al. (2012). The Murine PSE/TATA-dependent transcriptome: evidence of functional homologies with its human counterpart. *Int. J. Mol. Sci.* 13, 14813–14827. doi: 10.3390/ijms131114813

Canale, C., Petrelli, A., Salerno, M., Diaspro, A., and Dante, S. (2013). A new quantitative experimental approach to investigate single cell adhesion on multi-functional substrates. *Biosens. Bioelectron.* 48, 172–179. doi: 10.1016/j.bios.2013.04.015

Castelnuovo, M., Massone, S., Tasso, R., Fiorino, G., Gatti, M., Robello, M., et al. (2010). An Alu-like RNA promotes cell differentiation and reduces malignancy of human neuroblastoma cells. *FASEB J.* 24, 4033–4046. doi: 10.1096/fj.10-157032

Ciarlo, E., Massone, S., Penna, I., Nizzari, M., Gigoni, A., Dieci, G., et al. (2013). An intronic ncRNA-dependent regulation of SORL1 expression affecting Aβ formation is upregulated in post-mortem Alzheimer's disease brain samples. *Dis. Model. Mech.* 6, 424–433. doi: 10.1242/dmm.009761

D'Hulst, C., Atack, J., and Kooy, F. R. (2009). The complexity of the $GABA_A$ receptor shapes unique pharmacological profiles. *Drug Discov. Today* 14, 866–874. doi: 10.1016/j.drudis.2009.06.009

Garritano, S., Gigoni, A., Costa, D., Malatesta, P., Florio, T., Cancedda, R., et al. (2012). A novel collection of snRNA-like promoters with tissue-specific transcription properties. *Int. J. Mol. Sci.* 13, 11323–11332. doi: 10.3390/ijms130911323

Gavazzo, P., Vella, S., Marchetti, C., Nizzari, M., Cancedda, R., and Pagano, A. (2011). Acquisition of neuron-like electrophysiological properties in neuroblastoma cells by controlled expression of NDM29 ncRNA. *J. Neurochem.* 119, 989–1001. doi: 10.1111/j.1471-4159.2011.07492.x

Holmqvist, M. H., Cao, J., Hernandez-Pineda, R., Jacobson, M. D., Carroll, K. I., Sung, M. A., et al. (2002). Elimination of fast inactivation in Kv4 A-type potassium channels by an auxiliary subunit domain. *Proc. Natl. Acad. Sci. U S A* 99, 1035–1040. doi: 10.1073/pnas.022509299

Kellermayer, M. S. Z., and Grama, L. (2002). Stretching and visualizing titin molecules: combining structure, dynamics and mechanics. *J. Muscle Res. Cell Motil.* 23, 499–511. doi: 10.1023/A:1023414624092

Laurie, D. J., Seeburg, P. H., and Wisden, W. (1992). The distribution of thirteen GABA-A receptor subunit mRNAs in the rat brain. III. Embryonic and postnatal development. *J. Neurosci.* 12, 4151–4172.

Loparic, M., Wirz, D., Daniels, A. U., Raiteri, R., Vanlandingham, M. R., Guex, G., et al. (2010). Micro- and nanomechanical analysis of articular cartilage by indentation-type atomic force microscopy: validation with a gel-microfiber composite. *Biophys. J.* 98, 2731–2740. doi: 10.1016/j.bpj.2010.02.013

Massone, S., Ciarlo, E., Vella, S., Nizzari, M., Florio, T., Russo, C., et al. (2012). NDM29, a RNA polymerase III-dependent non coding RNA, promotes amyloidogenic processing of APP and amyloid β secretion. *Biochim. Biophys. Acta* 1823, 1170–1177. doi: 10.1016/j.bbamcr.2012.05.001

Massone, S., Vassallo, I., Castelnuovo, M., Fiorino, G., Gatta, E., Robello, M., et al. (2011a). RNA polymerase III drives alternative splicing of the potassium channel-interacting protein contributing to brain complexity and neurodegeneration. *J. Cell Biol.* 193, 851–866. doi: 10.1083/jcb.201011053

Massone, S., Vassallo, I., Fiorino, G., Castelnuovo, M., Barbieri, F., Borghi, R., et al. (2011b). 17A, a novel non-coding RNA, regulates GABA B alternative splicing and signaling in response to inflammatory stimuli and in Alzheimer disease. *Neurobiol. Dis.* 41, 308–317. doi: 10.1016/j.nbd.2010.09.019

Mescola, A., Vella, S., Scotto, M., Gavazzo, P., Canale, C., Diaspro, A., et al. (2012). Probing cytoskeleton organisation of neuroblastoma cells with single-cell force spectroscopy. *J. Mol. Recognit.* 25, 270–277. doi: 10.1002/jmr.2173

Moqtaderi, Z., Wang, J., Raha, D., White, R. J., Snyder, M., Weng, Z., et al. (2010). Genomic binding profiles of functionally distinct RNA polimerase III transcription complexes in human cells. *Nat. Struct. Mol. Biol.* 17, 635–640. doi: 10.1038/nsmb.1794

Okegawa, T., Pong, R. C., Li, Y., and Hsieh, J. T. (2004). The role of cell adhesion molecules in cancer progression and its application in cancer therapy. *Acta Biochim. Pol.* 51, 445–457.

Oler, A. J., Alla, R. K., Robetrs, D. N., Hollenhorst, P. C., Chandler, K. J., Cassiday, P. A., et al. (2010). Human RNA polimerase III transcriptomes and relationships to Pol II promoter chromatin and enhancer-binding factors. *Nat. Struct. Mol. Biol.* 17, 620–628. doi: 10.1038/nsmb.1801

Pagano, A., Castelnuovo, M., Tortelli, F., Ferrari, R., Dieci, G., and Cancedda, R. (2007). New small nuclear RNA gene-like transcriptional units as sources of regulatory transcripts. *PLoS Genet.* 3:e1. doi: 10.1371/journal.pgen.0030001

Papi, M., Maiorana, A., Douet, C., Maulucci, G., Parasassi, T., Brunelli, R., et al. (2013). Viscous forces are predominant in the zona pellucida mechanical resistance. *Appl. Phys. Lett.* 102, 43703–43704. doi: 10.1063/1.4789503

Penna, I., Vassallo, I., Nizzari, M., Russo, D., Costa, D., Menichini, P., et al. (2013). A novel snRNA-like transcript affects amyloidogenesis and cell cycle progression through perturbation of Fe65L1 (APBB2) alternative splicing. *Biochim. Biophys. Acta* 1833, 1511–1526. doi: 10.1016/j.bbamcr.2013.02.020

Pletikapic, G., Berquand, A., Mišic, R. T., and Svetlicic, V. (2012). Quantitative nanomechanical mapping of marine diatom in seawater using peak force tapping atomic force microscopy. *J. Phycol.* 48, 174–185. doi: 10.1111/j.1529-8817.2011.01093.x

Sbrana, F., Lorusso, M., Canale, C., Bochicchio, B., and Vassalli, M. (2011). Effect of chemical cross-linking on the mechanical properties of elastomeric peptides studied by single molecule force spectroscopy. *J. Biomech.* 44, 2118–2122. doi: 10.1016/j.jbiomech.2011.05.028

Suresh, S. (2007). Biomechanics and biophysics of cancer cells. *Acta Mater.* 55, 3989–4014. doi: 10.1016/j.actamat.2007.04.022

Trimmer, J. S., and Rhodes, K. J. (2004). Localization of voltage-gated ion channels in mammalian brain. *Ann. Rev. Physiol.* 66, 477–519. doi: 10.1146/annurev.physiol.66.032102.113328

Van de Water, L., and Olmstebd, J. B. (1980). The quantitation of tubulin in neuroblastoma cells by radioimmunoassay. *J. Biol. Chem.* 255, 10744–10751.

Weisel, J. W., Shuman, H., and Litvinov, R. I. (2003). Protein–protein unbinding induced by force: single-molecule studies. *Curr. Opin. Struct. Biol.* 13, 227–235. doi: 10.1016/S0959-440X(03)00039-3

Yamaguchi, H., and Condeelis, J. (2007). Regulation of the actin cytoskeleton in cancer cell migration and invasion. *Biochim. Biophys. Acta* 1773, 642–652. doi: 10.1016/j.bbamcr.2006.07.001

4

Micro spies from the brain to the periphery: new clues from studies on microRNAs in neuropsychiatric disorders

Elisabetta Maffioletti*[1,2], *Daniela Tardito*[3], *Massimo Gennarelli*[1,2] and *Luisella Bocchio-Chiavetto*[4]

[1] Genetic Unit, IRCCS Centro S. Giovanni di Dio Fatebenefratelli, Brescia, Italy
[2] Department of Molecular and Translational Medicine, University of Brescia, Brescia, Italy
[3] Dipartimento di Scienze Farmacologiche e Biomolecolari, Università degli Studi di Milano, Milano, Italy
[4] Neuropsychopharmacology Unit, IRCCS Centro S. Giovanni di Dio Fatebenefratelli, Brescia, Italy

Correspondence:
Luisella Bocchio-Chiavetto, Neuropsychopharmacology Unit, IRCCS Centro S. Giovanni di Dio Fatebenefratelli, Via Pilastroni 4, 25125 Brescia, Italy
e-mail: lbocchio@fatebenefratelli.it

microRNAs (miRNAs) are small non-coding RNAs (20–22 nucleotides) playing a major role in post-transcriptional regulation of gene expression. miRNAs are predicted to regulate more than 50% of all the protein-coding genes. Increasing evidence indicates that they may play key roles in the biological pathways that regulate neurogenesis and synaptic plasticity, as well as in neurotransmitter homeostasis in the adult brain. In this article we review recent studies suggesting that miRNAs may be involved in the pathophysiology of neuropsychiatric disorders and in the action of psychotropic drugs, in particular by analyzing the contribution of genomic studies in patients' peripheral tissues. Alterations in miRNA expression have been observed in schizophrenia, bipolar disorder, major depression, Parkinson's disease, Alzheimer's disease and other neuropsychiatric conditions. In particular, intriguing findings concern the identification of disease-associated miRNA signatures in peripheral tissues, or modifications in miRNA profiles induced by drug treatments. Furthermore, genetic variations in miRNA sequences and miRNA-related genes have been described in neuropsychiatric diseases. Overall, though still at a preliminary stage, several lines of evidence indicate an involvement of miRNAs in both the pathophysiology and pharmacotherapy of neuropsychiatric disorders. In this regard, the data obtained in peripheral tissues may provide further insights into the etiopathogenesis of several brain diseases and contribute to identify new biomarkers for diagnostic assessment improvement and treatment personalization.

Keywords: microRNA, schizophrenia, major depression, bipolar disorder, Alzheimer disease, Parkinson disease, genetic variation, SNP

INTRODUCTION

microRNAs (miRNAs) are a large family of conserved small (20–22 nucleotides) non-coding RNAs, with a key role in the post-transcriptional regulation of gene expression. In mammals, miRNAs are predicted to control the activity of ~50% of all the protein-coding genes. Their discovery dates back to 1993 with the identification of lin-4, a small ribonucleotide molecule involved in the regulation of "larva to adult switch" in *C. elegans* (Lee et al., 1993). miRBase, the primary online repository for all miRNA sequences, continuously upgrades the data on newly identified miRNAs and nowadays, at its 20th release (June 2013), it annotates 2578 human mature miRNAs and 1872 precursors (Kozomara and Griffiths-Jones, 2014; http://www.mirbase.org) (**Figure 1**).

miRNAs are transcribed in the nucleus by RNA polymerase II to primary miRNA (pri-miRNA) transcripts, double-stranded stem loop structures of 100–1000 nucleotides in length, then processed to >60–70 nucleotide precursors (pre-miRNAs), by a complex containing the RNAse-III type endonuclease Drosha and its cofactor DGCR8, as well as other cofactors. Pre-miRNAs are then exported in the cytoplasm by exportin-5 and cleaved in a ~20 bp miRNA/miRNA* duplex by the RNase-III type enzyme Dicer and its cofactor TRBP. In mammals, Dicer is supported by Argonaute 2 (Ago2), a RNaseH-like endonuclease that cleaves the 3′ arms of pre-miRNAs, thus generating mature miRNAs. The "right" strand of the miRNA duplex is then loaded into the RNA-induced silencing complex (RISC), whereas the other strand (miRNA*) is released and degraded, although in some cases both strands can associate with RISC to target distinct sets of mRNAs (Schwarz et al., 2003; Davis and Hata, 2009; Breving and Esquela-Kerscher, 2010; Krol et al., 2010; O'Carroll and Schaefer, 2012) (**Figure 2**).

miRNAs regulate protein synthesis post-transcriptionally by base-pairing to target mRNAs. Generally, miRNAs inhibit protein synthesis either by repressing translation or by inducing deadenylation and degradation of target mRNAs, but were also reported to activate translation (Chekulaeva and Filipowicz, 2009; Huntzinger and Izaurralde, 2011). Individual miRNAs have the potential to target hundreds of different mRNAs, and a single mRNA can be modulated by several different miRNAs, thus implying a coordinate and fine-tuned regulation of protein expression in a cell and even in particular cell compartments (Krol et al., 2010; O'Carroll and Schaefer, 2012).

Many miRNAs are expressed in a tissue-specific or developmental stage-specific manner, thereby contributing to cell type-specific profiles of protein expression. Functional studies indicate

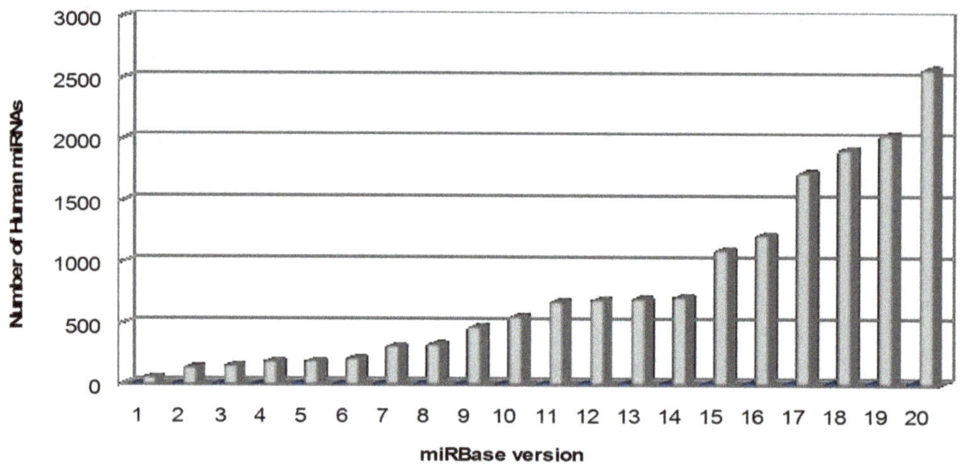

FIGURE 1 | Overtime trend in the number of human microRNAs annotated in miRBase. The number of mature human microRNAs annotated in miRBase database (Kozomara and Griffiths-Jones, 2014; http://www.mirbase.org) is continuously growing, starting from few dozens in the first release (2002) to more than 2500 in the last release (version 20, June 2013).

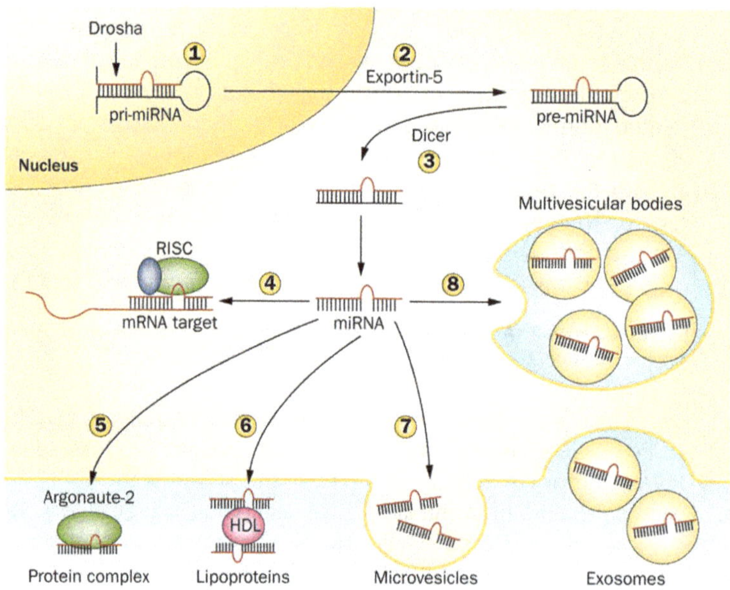

FIGURE 2 | Mechanisms regulating microRNA processing and release. Pri-miRNAs are cleaved in the nucleus by Drosha (1) to generate pre-miRNAs, then exported in the cytoplasm by Exportin-5 (2) and further cleaved by Dicer to produce 21–23 nucleotide duplexes (3). One strand of the miRNA duplex can either associate to the RISC complex and guide translational repression of target mRNAs (4) or be released by the cells. In the latter case, the mature miRNA binds to RNA-binding proteins, such as Argonaute-2 (5) or to lipoproteins (6). Alternatively, miRNAs can be loaded in microvesicles formed by plasma membrane blebbing (7) or in exosomes that are released in the extracellular space upon exocytic fusion of multivesicular bodies with the plasma membrane (8). Abbreviations: miRNA, microRNA; pre-miRNA, miRNA precursor; pri-miRNA, primary miRNA transcript; RISC, RNA-induced silencing complex. Figure reprinted by permission from Macmillan Publishers Ltd: Nature Reviews Endocrinology, Guay C. and Regazzi R. Circulating microRNAs as novel biomarkers for diabetes mellitus. 9, 513–521 (September 2013).

that miRNAs participate in the regulation of almost every cellular process and therefore it is not surprising that changes in their expression or function are associated with many human pathologies (Sayed and Abdellatif, 2011; Chan and Kocerha, 2012; Pasquinelli, 2012), as cancer (Farazi et al., 2013; Profumo and Gandellini, 2013) and cardiovascular diseases (Madrigal-Matute et al., 2013; Papoutsidakis et al., 2013).

In the past few years growing evidence has supported a key role for miRNAs in central nervous system (CNS) development and homeostasis. It has been reported that almost 50% of all the identified miRNAs are expressed in the human brain, with putative target genes regulating synaptogenesis and other basic neuronal processes (Ziats and Rennert, 2013). A role for miRNAs in neurogenesis, neuronal differentiation and survival, as well as in neuroplasticity, is now well established, although further work is needed to better clarify these aspects (Smalheiser and Lugli, 2009; Siegel et al., 2011; Olde Loohuis et al., 2012).

The unique mode of functioning of miRNAs, that is, the ability of a single miRNA to target several different mRNAs often belonging to specific functional networks, has prompted research toward the study of the potential involvement of miRNAs in the pathogenesis and pharmacotherapy of neurologic and psychiatric disorders (Kolshus et al., 2013; Tardito et al., 2013).

First evidence in post-mortem brain studies showed an overall decrease of miRNA expression in the prefrontal cortex (PFC) of schizophrenic (SCZ) subjects (Perkins et al., 2005, 2007; Miller et al., 2012). Other authors described an increase in miRNA expression in temporal regions of SCZ patients, associated to a dysregulation of the biogenesis cofactor DGCR8, *inter alia* mapped in the 22q11 Di George syndrome critical region, one of the candidate susceptibility loci for SCZ (Beveridge et al., 2008, 2010). Elevated miRNA expression and DICER1 mRNA increase were observed also by Santarelli et al. (2011) in dorsolateral PFC of SCZ post-mortem brains. Furthermore, alterations in miRNA levels were evidenced in post-mortem PFC from bipolar patients (BD) (Kim et al., 2010; Moreau et al., 2011). Notably, most of the differentially expressed miRNAs were downregulated in both the SCZ and BD groups relative to controls, in line with previous results (Perkins et al., 2007), but only a few of them were in common among the various studies. More recently, Banigan et al. (2013) reported an increase in exosomal miRNA content in SCZ post-mortem brains. Finally, an overall decrease in miRNA expression was observed in PFC of depressed suicide committers, with significant modifications of 21 miRNAs (Smalheiser et al., 2012).

Regarding a possible involvement of miRNAs in the action of psychotropic drugs, Zhou et al. (2009) showed that chronic treatment with mood stabilizers induced significant modifications of miRNA expression in the rat hippocampus. The effects of lithium on miRNA expression were confirmed also by a study in lymphoblastoid cell lines (LCLs) from BD patients (Chen et al., 2009). First preclinical studies on antidepressant drug effects suggested a role for miR-16 in the mechanism of action of fluoxetine; specifically, miR-16 appeared to create new serotonin sources in the brain through the switch of noradrenergic neurons toward a serotonergic phenotype (Baudry et al., 2010). Treatments with fluoxetine and desipramine, two antidepressants with a different primary mechanism of action, were reported to induce early and time-associated miRNA modulation in rat hippocampus (Pelizzari et al., 2012). Acute treatment with ketamine (an NMDA receptor antagonist shown to induce a rapid and sustained antidepressant effect), electroconvulsive shock therapy and chronic fluoxetine treatment were described to reverse the changes in rat hippocampal miRNA expression induced by early life stress (O'Connor et al., 2013). In a genome-wide miRNA investigation conducted on LCLs screened for growth inhibition by paroxetine, Oved et al. (2012) observed a differential expression of 6 miRNAs in paroxetine-sensitive cells, suggesting that these miRNAs could represent tentative SSRI response biomarkers. Finally, a modulation of small subsets of miRNAs regulating metabolic pathways was also reported after treatment with different antipsychotics, supporting possible associations with drug side effects (Santarelli et al., 2013).

Accumulating evidence indicates also in Alzheimer's disease (AD) brains a dysregulation of specific miRNAs, several of which potentially involved in the regulation of key disease genes (see for review: Junn and Mouradian, 2012; Tan et al., 2013). Among them, particularly interesting is the miR-29 cluster, which was significantly downregulated in AD patients in whom BACE-1 (β-amyloid cleavage enzyme 1) protein was aberrantly increased (Hébert et al., 2008; Nunez-Iglesias et al., 2010). Moreover, a decrease of miR-107 in AD brains was reported, paralleled by an increase of BACE-1 mRNA levels (Wang et al., 2008a, 2011; Nelson and Wang, 2010). Another dysregulated miRNA in AD brains is miR-132, which was described to be differentially expressed also in frontotemporal lobar degeneration (FTLD), together with 2 other miRNAs belonging to the same cluster (miR-132* and miR-212) (Chen-Plotkin et al., 2012; Hébert et al., 2013). Among the top target mRNAs of both miR-132 and miR-212 there is TMEM106B, a gene linked to FTLD by a genome-wide association study (GWAS) (Van Deerlin et al., 2010). Concerning Parkinson's disease (PD), decreased brain expression levels of miR-34b and miR-34c were observed (Miñones-Moyano et al., 2011), potentially affecting key pathways in PD pathogenesis, such as mitochondrial dysfunction, and reducing DJ1 and Parkin levels. Moreover, miR-133 was identified as deficient in PD midbrain tissue showing neuronal loss (Kim et al., 2007). Also *in vitro* studies supported the involvement of miRNAs in PD; as an example, miR-7 and miR-153 were shown to downregulate the expression of α-synuclein, one of the key genes implicated in PD etiopathogenesis (Junn et al., 2009; Doxakis, 2010).

MicroRNAs AS BIOMARKERS IN PERIPHERAL TISSUES

Besides their presence in cells, miRNAs were also observed in a highly stable, cell-free form (Cortez et al., 2011). Indeed, a number of studies have detected miRNAs in several peripheral biological matrices, including whole blood, plasma, serum, cerebrospinal fluid (CSF), saliva, and others (Cogswell et al., 2008; Mitchell et al., 2008; Park et al., 2009; Hanke et al., 2010; Zubakov et al., 2010).

Although it is clear that miRNAs function as a mechanism for post-transcriptional regulation, it has not been conclusively proven whether their presence in body fluids is simply a by-product of cell degradation or whether are they actively secreted into the body fluids to mediate intercellular gene regulation. A body of evidence supports the hypothesis that miRNAs can be actively and selectively secreted; for example, miR-1246 and miR-451 were found to be released by the breast cancer cell line MCF-7, but not by the non-malignant mammary epithelial breast cell line (Pigati et al., 2010). Also in support of active secretion is the appropriate packaging of miRNAs to facilitate circulation and to protect them from degradation in body fluids. miRNAs in serum are resistant to circulating ribonucleases and severe physicochemical conditions, such as extended storage, freeze-thawing and extreme pH (Chen et al., 2008; Mitchell et al., 2008). As described in **Figure 2**, there are three known ways by which miRNAs are packaged: in lipid microvesicles, such as exosomes and apoptotic bodies; bound by RNA-binding proteins, such as nucleophosmin 1 and Argonaute 2; and associated with high-density lipoproteins (Wang et al., 2010a; Arroyo et al., 2011). Similarly to hormones and cytokines, secreted miRNAs might serve as signaling molecules of cell-to-cell communication (Valadi et al., 2007), and their packaging also facilitates their transfer between individuals, as exemplified by the case of immune-related miRNAs in breast milk in the first 6 months of lactation, showing that packaged miRNAs could be absorbed orally and not digested (Iguchi et al., 2010).

Recently, studies suggested that miRNAs in plasma and serum might derive from circulating blood cells under healthy conditions, but could be released from pathological tissues during an illness (Chen et al., 2008; Fichtlscherer et al., 2010). The correlation between circulating miRNAs and tissue miRNAs suggests that miRNAs in human fluids might serve as biomarkers for various diseases (Skog et al., 2008; Laterza et al., 2009; Zeng et al., 2011). Some of the innate properties of miRNAs make them highly attractive as potential biomarkers: miRNAs can be readily detected in small volume samples using specific and sensitive quantitative real-time PCR (qRT-PCR), and their levels in plasma and serum are stable. Moreover, blood collection is a common and easy clinical procedure, and different individuals within the same species display similar levels of circulating miRNAs. However, a prerequisite to use circulating miRNAs as diagnostic and prognostic biomarkers is the ability to quantify them in different matrices (plasma, serum, CSF, whole blood) with an adequate sensitivity and precision. The quality of miRNA measurements with different techniques might be associated to many variables, including those related to preanalytic variants, such as specimen collection, RNA extraction efficiency and technical issues related to data analysis and normalization (Kroh et al., 2010). For example, there is a risk of cellular contamination during CSF collection with lumbar puncture and plasma and serum preparation; moreover, the anticoagulant used might influence the results of the analyses, since heparin impedes a qRT-PCR step (Boeckel et al., 2013). Furthermore, there may be an individual variability in both the protein and lipid content in serum and plasma specimens that could affect the efficiency of RNA extraction. Finally, there is no consensus on suitable small RNA reference genes that could be used as internal controls for normalization in different biological fluids (Mitchell et al., 2008; Kroh et al., 2010).

GENETIC VARIANTS IN microRNA-RELATED GENES

Two major classes of genetic variants in miRNA-related genes have been documented: single nucleotide polymorphisms (SNPs) and copy number variations (CNVs). SNPs are small genetic variations in chromosomal DNA sequences in which a single nucleotide is substituted by one of the other three nucleotides. SNPs are the most common form of variation present in the human genome (~10–30 million SNPs with a frequency >1% in the human population, occurring on average every 100–300 bases). The availability of high-throughput technologies investigating the genome led to the demonstration that a large number of genomic sequences, many of which encompass entire genes, vary in copy number among individuals. These deletions and duplications, referred to as CNVs, are more common in the general population than ever imagined before. Beside population-specific, common CNVs, there are rare, disease-causing CNVs, which constitute an important class of genetic variability in mendelian and multifactorial disorders. Both SNPs and CNVs in miRNA-related genes are underrepresented compared with the reference human genome, suggesting possible negative selection (Duan et al., 2009; Felekkis et al., 2011; Marcinkowska et al., 2011). In contrast, the number of miRNA target genes in polymorphic CNVs is higher than in non-CNV regions, suggesting that genes integral to polymorphic CNVs are more likely to be regulated by miRNAs, in order to counteract their expression changes due to copy number variability of the region in which they reside (Felekkis et al., 2011). Multiple cancer studies show that miRNAs integral to CNVs demonstrate gain or loss at the genomic level, and are associated with expression changes for ~10–20% of miRNAs (Schiffman et al., 2011; Shim et al., 2012).

Genetic variants in miRNA-related genes include variations in miRNA/pri-/pre-miRNA sequences, in miRNA biogenesis and machinery genes, as well as in the 3′-UTR of target genes, where mature miRNAs are bound. Therefore, these variants can affect the transcription of pri-miRNAs, the processing and maturation of pre-miRNAs and miRNA-mRNA interaction.

The initial demonstration that miRNA-related genetic variants can affect disease phenotype was given by Abelson et al. (2005), who found that a mutation in miR-189 binding site of SLITRK1 gene was associated with Tourette's syndrome. Since then, several studies have identified associations between polymorphisms, mainly SNPs, influencing miRNA function and different human disorders, going from PD to multiple forms of cancer (Sethupathy and Collins, 2008).

The identification of miRNA SNPs has greatly improved in the last few years. The first efforts aimed at the selection of these variants were conducted by Muiños-Gimeno et al. (2010) and by Duan et al. (2009), who respectively identified 24 and 187 SNPs in miRNA/pre-miRNA sequences, employing the by now old miRBase versions 7.1 and 13.0. More recently, thanks to the 1000 genomes project (http://www.1000genomes.org), many other variants have been identified; so far, more than 1000 miRNA SNP have been annotated (Han and Zheng, 2013). Many online databases collecting miRNA SNPs, more or less up-to-date, are available; some of them also offer information about the association with various diseases [see for example MicroSNiPer (http://epicenter.ie-freiburg.mpg.de/services/microsniper/), Patrocles (http://www.patrocles.org/), Polymirts (http://compbio.uthsc.edu/miRSNP/) and mirSNP (http://202.38.126.151/hmdd/mirsnp/search/)].

In this narrative review we present a wide overview of recent studies analyzing both disease alterations in miRNA expression levels in patients' peripheral matrices and associations with miRNA-related genetic variants.

EXPRESSION STUDIES IN HUMAN PERIPHERAL TISSUES

EXPRESSION STUDIES IN PSYCHIATRIC DISORDERS

Schizophrenia

Gardiner et al. (2012) analyzed the global miRNA expression in peripheral blood mononuclear cells (PBMCs) from SCZ patients compared to healthy controls and identified an expression profile significantly associated with SCZ; many of the differentially-expressed miRNAs were found to be part of a large cluster on the imprinted DLK1-DIO3 region on chromosome 14q, suggesting a possible significant underlying genetic or epigenetic alteration associated with this disease. To gain an appreciation of the biological implications of the disease-associated changes, the authors also examined predicted miRNA targets, identifying many pathways related to neural functions, such as axon guidance, regulation of the actin cytoskeleton, long-term potentiation, long-term depression, neuroactive ligand–receptor interaction, focal adhesion and neurotrophins. A similar study was conducted by Lai et al. (2011) by evaluating miRNA expression profiles in white blood cells (WBCs) from SCZ subjects. A 7-miRNA signature was significantly associated with SCZ diagnosis and its clinical characteristics, such as symptoms, neurocognitive performances and neurophysiological functions, showing a high discriminating accuracy. The predicted target genes for the identified miRNAs were shown to pertain to pathways involved in nervous system development and function, such as cyclin-dependent kinase 5 (Cdk5), Notch and dopamine receptor signaling. A candidate miRNA approach was instead employed by Shi et al. (2012), who measured in SCZ patients' serum the levels of 9 miRNAs, selected on the basis of previously published studies, since they had been shown to be implicated in SCZ or predicted to target SCZ-related genes. Among them, 5 were shown to be differentially expressed. Changes in miRNA expression were also observed to be induced by and/or implicated in effective antipsychotic treatment: 2 miRNAs were downregulated after a 1-year treatment with risperidone in plasma from first-episode SCZ patients, all of which had achieved remission (Liu et al., 2013).

Bipolar disorder

Only one expression study was conducted on BD for one candidate miRNA (Rong et al., 2011). In plasma from drug-free manic patients, miR-134 was shown to be downregulated compared to controls; consistently, its level increased after a 4-weeks treatment with different combinations of antypsychotics and/or mood stabilizers. Both in drug-free and in medicated patients (2 and 4 weeks), miR-134 levels were negatively correlated with manic symptoms, assessed through BRMS scores.

Major depression and anxiety

The first study on peripheral miRNA expression in drug-free patients suffering from MD was conducted by Bocchio-Chiavetto et al. (2013), by evaluating the changes in global miRNA levels in whole blood after a 12-weeks effective treatment with the antidepressant drug escitalopram (a SSRI). A modulation was observed for 30 miRNAs; interestingly, target gene prediction and pathways analysis showed that these miRNAs might be implicated in several pathways associated with brain functions, such as neuroactive ligand–receptor interaction, axon guidance, long-term potentiation and depression, supporting the hypothesis of their involvement in the antidepressant mechanism. Belzeaux et al. (2012), by means of a global analysis, reported a differential expression of 14 miRNAs in PBMCs from non drug-free MD patients compared to controls. Putative interactions between the dysregulation in miRNAs and in mRNAs, identified through a parallel expression analysis, have been subsequently recognized. Moreover, after an effective 8-weeks treatment with different classes of antidepressant drugs, in mono- or polytherapy, a modulation was observed for 8 miRNAs. Finally, Li et al. (2013) reported in the serum of MD patients an upregulation of 2 miRNAs which had been previously described to decrease *in vitro* protein levels of brain-derived neurotrophic factor (BDNF), a neurotrophin widely implicated in MD.

Although no expression study on anxiety-related disorder in human peripheral tissues is available, it was reported that stressful conditions due to academic examination induce an enhancement in blood levels of specific miRNAs, in particular miR-16, miR-144/144* and miR-26b (Katsuura et al., 2012; Honda et al., 2013).

Table 1 summarizes the above-reported expression studies in psychiatric disorders, with indication of samples, methodologies, and main results.

EXPRESSION STUDIES IN NEUROLOGIC DISORDERS

Alzheimer's disease and other dementias

Because of its proximity to the brain parenchyma and the free exchange with the brain extracellular space, the biochemical composition of CSF provides information of the brain chemistry; this has determined the introduction of CSF biomarker analysis into routine clinical practice for AD (Blennow and Zetterberg, 2013). A first study conducted in CSF from AD patients identified 60 miRNAs as differentially expressed compared to healthy individuals, both upregulated and downregulated (Cogswell et al., 2008). Interestingly, these AD-specific miRNAs are linked to immunity-related pathways, in particular innate immunity and T cell activation and differentiation, which have been widely described to be altered in AD (Boutajangout and Wisniewski, 2013; Monsonego et al., 2013). In 2012, other CSF-derived miRNAs were described as differentially expressed in AD (Alexandrov et al., 2012), but contrasting results were reported by a recent study that showed an opposite alteration of some of the same miRNAs (Kiko et al., 2013). An interesting finding concerns the role played by let-7b, which was found to be increased in AD subjects. The intrathecal injection of let-7b into the CSF of mice resulted in neurodegeneration, an effect thought to be due to the activation of toll-like receptor (TLR) 7, since knock-out mice lacking TLR7 were resistant to neurodegeneration (Lehmann et al., 2012). Finally, a downregulation of miR-146 was detected in CSF from AD patients (Müller et al., 2014).

However, CSF is a not a readily accessible tissue and this may restrict the study sample sizes; to overcome these limitations, a number of researches was grounded on the analysis of peripheral blood and its derived products, which can be more easily obtained and potentially enable researchers to achieve larger samples. A first global investigation conducted on PBMCs led to the identification of 4 miRNAs upregulated in AD patients (Schipper et al., 2007). Still in PBMCs, a downregulation of miR-590-3p was described. Intriguingly, this miRNA is strongly predicted to target the heterogeneous nuclear ribonucleoprotein (hnRNP) A1, which is involved in the maturation of amyloid precursor protein (APP). The mRNA levels of hnRNPA1 were observed to be negatively correlated with miR-590-3p levels, supporting the hypothesis that

Table 1 | microRNA expression studies in psychiatric disorders.

Disease	Sample	Tissue	Method	Main finding	Reference
Schizophrenia	112 SCZ vs. 76 CTRL	PBMCs	miRNA array Illumina (miRBase v. 9.1), qRT-PCR	↓ miR-31, miR-99b, miR-107, miR-134, miR-431, miR-433, miR-487b	Gardiner et al., 2012
	90 SCZ vs. 60 CTRL	WBCs	TaqMan Low Density Array v. 1.0	↑ miR-34a, miR-449a, miR-548d, miR-564, miR-572 and miR-652 ↓ miR-432	Lai et al., 2011
	115 SCZ vs. 40 CTRL	Serum	qRT-PCR	↑ let-7g, miR-181b, miR-219-2-3p, miR-1308 ↓ miR-195	Shi et al., 2012
	40 first-episode SCZ	Plasma	qRT-PCR	↓ miR-365 and miR-520c-3p after a 1-year treatment with risperidone	Liu et al., 2013
Bipolar disorder	21 BD vs. 21 CTRL	Plasma	qRT-PCR	In BD vs. ctrl: ↓ miR-134 ↑ miR-134 after a 4-weeks treatment (different combinations of antypsychotics and/or mood stabilizers)	Rong et al., 2011
Major depression	10 MD	Peripheral blood	TaqMan Array Human MicroRNA A+B Cards Set v. 3.0	30 miRNAs differentially expressed after a 12-weeks treatment with escitalopram: ↑ let-7d, let-7e, let-7f, let-7g, miR-22*, miR-26a, miR-26b, miR-29b-2*, miR-30d, miR-103, miR-106b*, miR-128, miR-130b*, miR-132, miR-140-3p, miR-183, miR-191, miR-335, miR-361-5p, miR-374b, miR-494, miR-500, miR-502-3p, miR-505*, miR-574-3p, miR-589, miR-629, miR-664 ↓ miR-770-5p, miR-34c-5p	Bocchio-Chiavetto et al., 2013
	9 MD vs. 9 CTRL	PBMCs	TaqMan Array Human MicroRNA A+B Cards Set v. 3.0	In MD vs. ctrl: ↑ miR-107, miR-133a, miR-148a, miR-425-3p, miR-494, miR-579, miR-589, miR-652, miR-941 ↓ miR-200c, miR-381, miR-517b, miR-636, miR-1243 After an 8-weeks treatment (different classes of antidepressant drugs): ↑ miR-20b-3p, miR-133a, miR-145, miR-409-3p, miR-410, miR-433, miR-485-3p ↓ miR-331-5p	Belzeaux et al., 2012
	40 MD vs. 40 CTRL	Serum	qRT-PCR	↑ miR-132 and miR-182	Li et al., 2013

BD, bipolar disorder patients; CTRL, healthy controls; MD, major depression patients; PBMCs, peripheral blood mononuclear cells; SCZ, schizophrenia patients; WBCs, white blood cells.

this miRNA acts as a regulator of hnRNPA1, therefore influencing APP production (Villa et al., 2011). Another study on candidate miRNAs, previously found to be reduced in post-mortem brain cortices of AD patients (Geekiyanage and Chan, 2011), described a downregulation of 4 of these (among them, miR 29a/b) in the serum of individuals suffering from mild cognitive impairment (MCI) or AD (Geekiyanage et al., 2012). This consistency of results indicates that peripheral blood and its derivatives represent valid tissues to study miRNAs in CNS diseases, as they could reflect brain alterations. Interestingly, miR-29a/b had been previously shown to target BACE1/beta-secretase, which mediates the cleavage of APP producing β-amyloid peptide (Hébert et al., 2008). A serum alteration of 3 miRNAs was reported by an independent study on a wide sample of AD patients and controls (105 vs. 150 subjects) (Tan et al., 2014). Sheinerman et al. (2012) identified in plasma two sets of miRNA pairs differentiating early AD and MCI patients from healthy controls with good sensitivity and specificity. Finally, a very recent study employed a next-generation sequencing (NGS) technique to screen the entire miRNome in whole peripheral blood from AD patients (Leidinger et al., 2013).

Through this comprehensive approach, 140 miRNAs were identified as differentially expressed in AD patients vs. control subjects. Moreover, a panel of 12 miRNAs (see **Table 2**) allowed to distinguish with high diagnostic accuracy (sensitivity and specificity >92%) between AD patients and healthy controls, and also between AD patients and patients affected by other neuropsychiatric disorders, including MCI, PD, as well as SCZ, MD, and BD.

Parkinson's disease

A first study conducted on peripheral blood from PD patients revealed a decrease in the expression levels of 3 miRNAs; moreover, subjects treated with levodopa/carbidopa vs. untreated showed higher levels of other 2 miRNAs (Margis et al., 2011). A subsequent study analyzing miRNA expression profiles in PBMCs identified 4 differentially-expressed miRNAs. Interestingly, many of the predicted target genes revealed an overepresentation in pathways previously linked to PD, as well as in novel pathways (Martins et al., 2011). Finally, through RNA-seq other miRNAs were discovered to be differentially expressed in leukocytes from PD patients and, consistently, after deep brain stimulation (DBS) some of them were modulated in the opposite direction (Soreq et al., 2013).

Table 2 summarizes the above-reported expression studies in neurological disorders, with indication of samples, methodologies, and main results.

CLUES FROM EXPRESSION STUDIES: CONVERGING RESULTS AND METHODOLOGICAL ISSUES

On the basis of the above-reported results on patients' peripheral matrices, a differential expression of a set of miRNAs emerges, supporting a role for miRNAs as key common players for different psychiatric and neurologic diseases. Moreover, many of these observations converge with results obtained in cerebral tissues from both humans and preclinical models.

miR-134 was reported to be decreased in PBMCs and plasma respectively of SCZ and BD patients (Rong et al., 2011; Gardiner et al., 2012); its alteration, although with an opposite direction, was observed also in SCZ post-mortem brains (Santarelli et al., 2011), supporting a role of this miRNA in the illness pathogenesis. Moreover, miR-134 was increased within a set of miRNA associated to AD and MCI diagnosis in comparison to control subjects (Sheinerman et al., 2012). miR-134 is a brain actively regulated miRNA mainly localized in dendritic spines, with a major role in the regulation of synaptic proteins and neuronal plasticity, in terms of memory and cognitive functions, through a CREB-BDNF mediated mechanism (Gao et al., 2010a; Jimenez-Mateos et al., 2012; Bicker et al., 2013). Moreover, miR-134 is a fine-tuning regulator of embryonic neurodevelopment and neuronal differentiation both *in vitro* and *in vivo* (Gaughwin et al., 2011).

miR-26a and **miR-26b** were found altered in peripheral blood of MD patients during antidepressant treatment (Bocchio-Chiavetto et al., 2013), in AD patients (Leidinger et al., 2013) and PD patients (Margis et al., 2011), as well as in students experiencing pre-examination stress (Honda et al., 2013). Both miRNAs can regulate the expression of the neurotrophin BDNF, a main player of adult brain neurogenesis and synaptic plasticity maintenance (Caputo et al., 2011). A dysregulation of miR-26b was observed also in SCZ and AD post-mortem brains (Perkins et al., 2007; Absalon et al., 2013).

An increase in **miR-34a** peripheral blood cell content was observed in SCZ (Lai et al., 2011) and AD patients (Schipper et al., 2007), while antidepressant treatments were able to decrease **miR-34c**-5p in the blood of MD patients (Bocchio-Chiavetto et al., 2013). miR-34c levels were elevated in the hippocampus of AD patients and corresponding mouse models, suggesting that this miRNA could be a marker for the onset of cognitive disturbances (Zovoilis et al., 2011). In contrast, a downregulation of miR-34 was reported in CSF and plasma from AD patients (Kiko et al., 2013). Moreover, an alteration of miR-34a was evidenced also in the PFC of SCZ post-mortem brains (Kim et al., 2010). Basic studies indicated that Drosophila miR-34 has a role in age-associated events, aging, and neurodegeneration (Liu et al., 2012a). Experiments with antagomiRs revealed that targeting miR-34a might increase neuronal survival and reduce death and apoptosis in a rat model of temporal lobe epilepsy (Hu et al., 2012). Moreover, *in vitro* experiments showed that ectopic expression of miR-34a downregulates the endogenous activity-regulated, cytoskeleton-associated protein Arc, a crucial factor for experience-dependent synaptic plasticity and long-term memory in mammals (Wibrand et al., 2012). Finally, studies in mice models indicated a role for miR-34a in the central stress response and suggested this miRNA as a potential target for the treatment of stress-related disorders (Haramati et al., 2011).

miR-107 was found increased in PBMCs from MD subjects (Belzeaux et al., 2012), but decreased in PBMCs of SCZ (Gardiner et al., 2012) and in blood of AD patients (Leidinger et al., 2013). Reduced levels of miR-107 were found also in AD post-mortem brains (Nelson and Wang, 2010) and a recent study in SCZ post-mortem brains correlated the expression levels of miR-107 with a loss in the expression of cortical muscarinic receptors (CHRM1), observed in the 25% of patient tissues (Scarr et al., 2013). Moreover, altered miR-107 were associated with cytoskeletal pathology in a transgenic mouse model of AD and with granulin/progranulin expression regulation *in vivo* and *in vitro*, with implications for brain disorders (Wang et al., 2008a, 2010b).

miRNAs of the let-7 family (**let-7b**, **let-7d-3p**, **let-7f**, **let-7g**) were found dysregulated in different peripheral tissues of SCZ patients (Shi et al., 2012), AD patients (Schipper et al., 2007; Cogswell et al., 2008; Lehmann et al., 2012; Leidinger et al., 2013) and modulated by antidepressant treatment (Bocchio-Chiavetto et al., 2013), supporting their involvement in mental disorder etiology and treatment. In this regard, studies in animal models indicated a neurodegenerative effect of let-7b (Lehmann et al., 2012) and a negative regulation of the cortical muscarinic acetylcholine receptor levels (M1) (Creson et al., 2011).

Other studies indicated an increase of **miR-181b** in serum of SCZ patients (Shi et al., 2012) and in PBMCs of AD patients (Schipper et al., 2007). In parallel, an upregulated expression of this miRNA was reported in the temporal cortex of SCZ post-mortem brains, with a concomitant downregulation of its main neural target genes, the calcium sensor gene visinin-like 1 (VSNL1) and the ionotropic AMPA glutamate receptor subunit (GRIA2), suggesting possible effects on gene expression in

Table 2 | microRNA expression studies in neurologic disorders.

Disease	Sample	Tissue	Method	Main finding	Reference
Alzheimer's disease	10 AD vs. 10 CTRL	CSF	qRT-PCR	60 miRNAs differentially expressed; in the first positions: ↑ let-7f, miR-105, miR-125a, miR-135a, miR-138 ↓ miR-10a, miR-10b, miR-126, miR-126*, miR-127	Cogswell et al., 2008
	6 AD vs. 6 CTRL	CSF	Fluorescent miRNA array, LED-Northern dot blot	↑ miR-9, miR-125b, miR-146a, miR-155	Alexandrov et al., 2012
	13 AD vs. 11 CTRL	CSF	qRT-PCR	↑ let-7b	Lehmann et al., 2012
	20 AD vs. 22 CTRL	CSF	qRT-PCR	↓ miR-146	Müller et al., 2014
	10 AD vs. 10 CTRL	CSF, plasma	qRT-PCR	In CSF: ↓ miR-34a, miR-125b, miR-146a ↑ miR-29a, miR-29b In plasma: ↓ miR-34a, miR-146a	Kiko et al., 2013
	16 AD vs. 16 CTRL	PBMCs	MMChip, qRT-PCR	↑ miR-34a, miR-181b, miR-200a, let-7f	Schipper et al., 2007
	287 AD vs. 344 CTRL	PBMCs	qRT-PCR	↓ miR-590-3p	Villa et al., 2011
	7 AD, 7 MCI vs. 7 CTRL	Serum	qRT-PCR	↓ miR-137, miR-181c, miR-9, miR-29a/b	Geekiyanage et al., 2012
	105 AD vs. 150 CTRL	Serum	qRT-PCR	↓ miR-125b, miR-181c ↑ miR-9	Tan et al., 2014
	20 early AD, 20 MCI vs. 20 CTRL	Plasma	qRT-PCR	Two sets of miRNA pairs differentiating early AD and MCI from controls: 1) miR-128/miR-491-5p, miR-132/miR-491-5p and mir-874/miR-491-5p 2) miR-134/miR-370, miR-323-3p/miR-370 and miR-382/miR-370	Sheinerman et al., 2012
	106 AD vs. 22 CTRL	Peripheral blood	NGS (with Illumina HiSeq 2000), qRT-PCR	↑ brain-miR-112, brain-miR-161, let-7d-3p, miR-5010-3p, miR-26a-5p, miR-1285-5p, miR-151a-3p ↓ miR-103a-3p. miR-107, miR-532-5p, miR-26b-5p, let-7f-5p	Leidinger et al., 2013
Parkinson's disease	15 PD vs. 8 CTRL	Peripheral blood	qRT-PCR	In PD vs. ctrl: ↓ miR-1, miR-22*, miR-29 In treated with levodopa/carbidopa vs. untreated PD: ↑ miR-16-2*, miR-26a-2*	Margis et al., 2011
	19 PD vs. 13 CTRL	PBMCs	miRCURY LNA microRNA Array v. 10.0, qRT-PCR	↓ miR-116*, miR-32, miR-101 ↑ miR-15	Martins et al., 2011
	7 PD vs. 6 CTRL	WBCs	RNA-seq (with Applied Biosystems SOLiD sequencer)	In PD vs. ctrl: ↓ miR-320a/b/c, miR-769, miR-92b, miR-16 ↑ miR-199b, miR-1274b, miR-21, miR-150, miR-671, miR-1249, miR-20a, miR-18b*, miR-378c, miR-4293 In PD after DBS: ↓ miR-4293, miR-378c, miR-18b*, miR-20a, miR-1249, miR-424*, miR-210, miR-93 ↑ miR-4317, miR-143, miR-424	Soreq et al., 2013

AD, Alzheimer's disease patients; CSF, cerebrospinal fluid; CTRL, healthy controls; MCI, mild cognitive impairment patients; PBMCs, peripheral blood mononuclear cells; PD, Parkinson's disease patients; WBCs, white blood cells.

patients (Beveridge et al., 2008). A role of miR-181b in mental pathologies could be also linked to its involvement in neuroprotection (Peng et al., 2013) and in NMDA receptor-dependent plasticity response in mature neurons (van Spronsen et al., 2013).

Elevated levels of **miR-9** were reported in the CSF of AD patients (Alexandrov et al., 2012), whereas lower levels were observed in serum of patients with the same pathology (Geekiyanage et al., 2012). miR-9 is widely expressed in the mammalian brain and can play a role in different neuronal functions, ranging from early neurogenesis and differentiation to dendritic morphogenesis and synaptic plasticity in the adult brain (Gao, 2010b), as well as in neurotoxic mechanisms, since the expression of miR-9 is downregulated by β-amyloid in hippocampal cell cultures (Schonrock et al., 2010).

Finally, alterations in peripheral levels of **miR-132** were recently associated to MD and AD/MCI diagnosis (Sheinerman et al., 2012; Li et al., 2013), as well as to the effects of antidepressant therapy (Bocchio-Chiavetto et al., 2013). These data are consistent with the observations obtained in AD and FTLD post-mortem brains (Hébert et al., 2013; Lau et al., 2013), confirming in patients' tissues the substantial role played by miR-132 in basic mechanisms of synaptic plasticity. In particular, miR-132 is one of the main mediators of the beneficial effects of the neurotrophin BDNF on CNS neurons (Numakawa et al., 2011) and it is implicated in brain response to stress stimuli (Shaltiel et al., 2013), as well as in the regulation of cognitive function as learning and memory formation (Hansen et al., 2013).

Generally speaking, miRNAs in body fluids were measured both as single candidates using qRT-PCR methods and by the employment of "whole-genome" approaches, through different miRNA profiling techniques. In the reviewed studies, the most used technologies were microarrays for the simultaneous analysis of, at most, about 900 miRNAs (Schipper et al., 2007; Alexandrov et al., 2012; Gardiner et al., 2012) and qRT-PCR arrays which can detect about 750 miRNAs (Belzeaux et al., 2012; Bocchio-Chiavetto et al., 2013). Microarray technologies permit a lower cost miRNA profiling, compared to qRT-PCR arrays, but they require the subsequent validation of the most significant results through qRT-PCR; this can be money- and time-consuming, particularly in large study samples. Two studies (Leidinger et al., 2013; Soreq et al., 2013) analyzed miRNA profiles with small RNA NGS, which virtually allows the detection of all the miRNAs and other small RNAs expressed in a given sample. NGS techniques were employed also in basic examinations to characterize miRNA whole expression in different biofluids, highlighting the presence of more than 500 and 400 miRNAs, respectively in serum and CSF of healthy subjects (Burgos et al., 2013).

It is still an open question whether and how miRNA levels in the periphery (such as in CSF, serum, plasma, blood, lymphoblasts etc.) may reflect brain modifications, and this issue generally concerns all the potential peripheral biomarkers in psychiatric and neurologic disorders. A first evidence has suggested a possible correlation between central and peripheral levels, since miRNAs could pass through biological membranes in free-form or into microvesicles. In this regard, tumor-specific microvesicles containing miRNAs at altered levels were detected in the serum of patients affected by glioblastomas (Skog et al., 2008) and brain-specific miRNAs quantified in plasma were proposed as biomarkers for brain injury in animal models (Laterza et al., 2009). Finally the levels of miR-210, described as significantly decreased in the blood of stroke patients, showed a correlation between brain and blood in ischemic mice (Zeng et al., 2011).

A major reason for the lack of conclusive data might be attributed to the low number of studies which have explored brain-periphery correlation, also due to the difficulties in getting concomitant brain and peripheral samples of the same human subjects. This problem could be overcome by the employment of animal models; however, these studies are limited, since the number of annotated miRNAs is widely different between species (miRBase 20th release, June 2013: 2578 mature miRNAs in humans, 728 in rats and 1908 in mice).

GENETIC VARIANTS IN microRNA-RELATED GENES IN PSYCHIATRIC AND NEUROLOGIC DISORDERS

SINGLE NUCLEOTIDE POLYMORPHISMS IN microRNA MATURE SEQUENCES OR PRECURSORS

The most considerable findings about an involvement of SNPs located in miRNA mature sequences or precursors in neuropsychiatric disorders come from studies on SCZ. Hansen et al. (2007) identified an association between a SNP located in the brain-expressed mir-206 (rs17578796) and the disease. Few years later, an analysis of SNPs in miRNAs mapping on the X chromosome, conducted on male SCZ subjects, led to the identification of 8 ultra-rare variants in 8 distinct miRNA genes (3 precursor and 5 mature miRNA sequences) in 4% of the analyzed patients (Feng et al., 2009). In a Chinese population, a SNP located in pre-mir-30e (ss178077483) was later detected to be associated to SCZ (Xu et al., 2010a), and the same research group described an association of this variant also with MD (Xu et al., 2010b). In a GWAS of substantial size on SCZ, the strongest finding was with rs1625579, a SNP located within an intron of the non-protein coding gene AK094607, which contains the primary transcript for miR-137, a known regulator of neuronal development (Ripke et al., 2011). However, the polymorphism resides more than 8 kilobases away from the pri-miR-137. In subsequent studies the same variant was associated with specific SCZ/psychosis endophenotypes, characterized by severe cognitive deficits and negative symptoms, rather then with the disease itself (Cummings et al., 2013; Green et al., 2013). Another recent study suggested a possible functional explanation for this SNP, showing an association between the risk genotype and reduced expression levels of miR-137 in the dorsolateral PFC of healthy subjects; interestingly, this corresponded to increased levels of the miR-137 target gene TCF4, a SCZ candidate gene (Guella et al., 2013).

Small evidence is available for MD; in addition to the above-mentioned study on pre-mir-30e (ss178077483) (Xu et al., 2010b), so far only another investigation has been conducted, revealing an association between a SNP in pre-mir-182 and late insomnia in MD patients, thus suggesting that this variant could be involved in the alteration of circadian rhythms described in depressed patients (Saus et al., 2010).

Finally, two SNPs, respectively located in mir-22 (rs6502892) and mir-339 (rs11763020), were associated to panic disorder. Interestingly, functional studies showed that mir-22 is a regulator of candidate genes for panic disorder (BDNF, HTR2C, MAOA and RGS2), suggesting a possible contribution of its genetic variants in the development of this disease (Muiños-Gimeno et al., 2011).

SINGLE NUCLEOTIDE POLYMORPHISMS IN microRNA TARGET GENES

Genetic variants in miRNA target genes, in particular in their 3′-UTR, are equally important as SNPs in miRNA mature sequences or precursors, since they can alter the complementarity between mRNA and miRNA, therefore influencing their binding.

Concerning psychiatric diseases, a SNP (rs3822674) in the complexin 2 gene (CPLX2), associated with altered cognition in SCZ subjects, was described to affect miR-498 binding and gene expression (Begemann et al., 2010). Interestingly, an allelic variant of rs11122396 in the 3′-UTR of disrupted-in-schizophrenia-1 (DISC-1) gene, which had been associated to schizophrenia through a rare haplotype (Hennah et al., 2003), has recently been brought to the forefront thanks to a functional study showing that this variant disrupts miR-135b-5p binding, leading to elevated DISC-1 levels (Rossi et al., 2013). Finally, 3 other SNPs (rs17110432, rs11178988 and rs11178989) in the 3′-UTR of TBC1D15 gene were reported as associated to SCZ and predicted to affect miRNA binding (Liu et al., 2012b).

Another significant association was detected between allelic variants of rs1653625 in the purinergic receptor P2X gene (P2RX7) and MD; this SNP resides in a putative miRNA target site (Rahman et al., 2010). In patients affected by obsessive-compulsive disorder (OCD), a SNP (rs28521337) located in a functional target site for miR-485-3p, in the truncated isoform of neurotrophin-3 receptor gene (NTRK3), was associated with hoarding, a particular endophenotype of the disease (Muiños-Gimeno et al., 2009).

Evidence in this field is available also for neurodegenerative diseases: a study conducted on FTLD with TDP-43 inclusions (FTLD-TDP) by Rademakers et al. (2008) unveiled a functional effect for the high-risk allele of rs5848 in progranulin gene (GRN), which promotes a more efficient binding of miR-659, resulting in augmented translational inhibition of GRN. Similarly, rs1050283 in the oxidized LDL receptor 1 gene (OLR1), which acts as a risk factor for sporadic AD, was hypothesized to influence miR369-3p binding (Serpente et al., 2011). Moreover, other previously known AD-associated genetic variants in the 3′-UTR of APP were empirically shown to influence miRNA binding, both by inhibiting (T117C, effect on miR-147) or increasing it (A454G, effect on miR-20a), and therefore inversely affecting APP levels (Delay et al., 2011).

An association was also detected between PD and rs12720208 in the 3′-UTR of fibroblast growth factor 20 (FGF20) gene. The risk allele was described to disrupt a binding site for miR-433, increasing FGF20 levels *in vitro* and *in vivo*, and the increase was correlated with α-synuclein overexpression, which had previously been implicated in PD pathophysiology (Wang et al., 2008b), though a later study failed to confirm the association of this SNP with PD (de Mena et al., 2010).

SINGLE NUCLEOTIDE POLYMORPHISMS IN microRNA PROCESSING GENES

Genetic variants affecting genes implicated in miRNA biogenesis and processing are extremely relevant, since they can exert pleiotropic effects on a multitude of miRNAs.

So far, only two studies have inquired into this important topic; the first one investigated the possible association between MD and 3 SNPs located in 3 miRNA processing genes (DGCR8, DICER, and GEMIN4). Variants of rs3757 in DGCR8 and rs636832 in AGO1 were associated with an increased risk for this disease (He et al., 2012). The second study evaluated 6 SNPs in 5 miRNA processing genes (DGCR8, DICER, GEMIN4, DROSHA, and AGO1) in SCZ subjects. The same above-mentioned variant in DGCR8 was found to be associated also with SCZ, together with rs3742330 in DICER (Zhou et al., 2013). Interestingly, an elevated expression of DGCR8 was observed in PFC of SCZ patients (Santarelli et al., 2011); rs3757 is located in the 3′-UTR of this gene, possibly affecting the regulation of its expression by miRNAs and resulting in an overall increase in miRNA production.

Table 3 summarizes all the above-reported genetic studies in psychiatric and neurologic disorders, with indication of samples and main results.

CONCLUSIONS

The research on miRNA involvement in psychiatric and neurologic disorders has grown up in the last years, supporting a role of miRNAs in several neuropsychiatric conditions and suggesting a possible usefulness of these small non-coding RNAs as disease-related biomarkers.

However, the continuously growing number of annotated miRNAs, as described in **Figure 1**, implies a major complexity in the global interpretation of the current available results, since many newly discovered miRNAs have not been sufficiently studied yet. New investigations will be welcome to clarify the role played by the already known miRNAs and to identify new critical ones. Moreover, some technical issues have to be resolved. A reliable and reproducible quantification of miRNAs is essential to compare results arising from different studies and, given that many experimental variables can affect miRNA measurement, all the related technical procedures should be carefully optimized and standardized. Till then, the transferability of these studies to the clinical practice will be inevitably limited. Finally, there is still a lack of data about the origin of miRNAs in blood and also whether they accurately reflect miRNA activity in the brain; further studies to elucidate these aspects are needed (Kolshus et al., 2013).

Concerning genetic studies on miRNA-related genes, we are still in an embryonic stage, but the recent annotation of new miRNA SNPs paves the way to a growing research in this field. The study of miRNA CNVs is an even more unexplored area; new investigations on these topics are strongly advisable to widen the knowledge on the genetic bases of psychiatric and neurologic diseases. Great help for these investigations is likely to come from the new NGS technologies, allowing a faster and cheaper scan of the whole genome than ever before.

Table 3 | Genetic studies on microRNA-related genes in psychiatric and neurologic disorders.

	Sample	Main finding	Reference
SNPs in miRNAs	840 SCZ vs. 1476 CTRL (Scandinavian)	rs17578796 (in mir-206) associated with SCZ	Hansen et al., 2007
	193 SCZ vs. 191 CTRL (Caucasian, all males)	Eight ultra-rare variants on X chromosome identified in 4% of SCZ patients: 32 A>G in pre-mir-18b, 8 C>T in pre-mir-505, 13 C>G in pre-mir-502, 11 G>A in let-7f-2, 7 C>T in mir-188-3p, 8 G>A in mir-325-3p, 15 C>T in mir-660, 13 C>T in mir-509-3p	Feng et al., 2009
	456 SCZ vs. 453 CTRL (Chinese)	ss178077483 (in pre-mir-30e) associated with SCZ	Xu et al., 2010a
	Discovery stage: 9394 SCZ vs. 12462 CTRL; replication stage: 8442 SCZ vs. 21397 CTRL (European-ancestry)	rs1625579 (in a putative primary transcript for mir-137) associated with SCZ	Ripke et al., 2011
	617 SCZ vs. 764 CTRL (Australian)	rs1625579 (in a putative primary transcript for mir-137) associated with a specific SCZ phenotype	Green et al., 2013
	821 SCZ/BD/SCHIZOAFFECTIVE vs. 171 CTRL (Irish)	rs1625579 (in a putative primary transcript for mir-137) associated with a specific psychosis phenotype	Cummings et al., 2013
	1088 MD vs. 1102 CTRL (Chinese)	ss178077483 (in pre-mir-30e) associated with MD	Xu et al., 2010b
	359 MD vs. 341 CTRL (Spanish)	rs76481776 (in pre-mir-182) associated with late insomnia MD	Saus et al., 2010
	200 panic disorder vs. 340 CTRL (Spanish)	rs6502892 (in mir-22) and rs11763020 (in mir-339) associated with panic disorder	Muiños-Gimeno et al., 2011
SNPs in miRNA target genes	1071 SCZ (Caucasian)	rs3822674 (in CPLX2 gene) associated with altered cognition in SCZ subjects, affecting miR-498 binding and gene expression	Begemann et al., 2010
	607 SCZ vs. 1128 CTRL (Finnish)	rs11122396 in DISC-1 gene associated to SCZ through a rare haplotype	Hennah et al., 2003
	746 SCZ vs. 1599 CTRL (Chinese)	rs17110432, rs11178988 and rs11178989) in TBC1D15 gene associated to SCZ, possibly affecting miRNA binding	Liu et al., 2012b
	171 MD+BD vs. 178 CTRL (Hungarian)	rs1653625 (in a putative miRNA-target site in P2RX7 gene) associated with MD	Rahman et al., 2010
	153 OCD (Spanish)	rs28521337 (in a target site for miR-485-3p in the truncated isoform of NTRK3 gene) associated with hoarding phenotype of OCD	Muiños-Gimeno et al., 2009
	59 FTLD vs. 433 CTRL (ethnicity not specified)	rs5848 (in GRN gene) associated with FTLD, enhancing miR-659 binding and translational inhibition of GRN	Rademakers et al., 2008
	453 AD vs. 393 CTRL (Italian)	rs1050283 (in OLR1 gene) associated with AD, possibly influencing miR-369-3p binding	Serpente et al., 2011
	1089 PD vs. 1165 CTRL (ethnicity not specified)	rs12720208 (in FGF20 gene) associated with PD, disrupting miR-433 binding and increasing FGF20 levels	Wang et al., 2008b
SNPs in miRNA processing genes	252 SCZ vs. 256 CTRL (Chinese)	rs3757 (in DGCR8 gene) and rs3742330 (in DICER gene) associated with SCZ	Zhou et al., 2013
	314 MD vs. 252 CTRL (Chinese)	rs3757 (in DGCR8 gene) and rs636832 (in AGO1 gene) associated with MD	He et al., 2012

BD, bipolar disorder patients; CTRL, healthy controls; FTLD, frontotemporal lobar degeneration; MD, major depression patients; OCD, obsessive-compulsive disorder patients; SCZ, schizophrenia patients.

In general, the scientific community has great expectations for the use of miRNA measures and genetic data as non-invasive biomarkers for the diagnosis, prognosis, and therapeutic appraisal of many illnesses. The fact that differential expression levels of peripheral miRNAs have been associated with several disease processes and to similar modifications in brain tissues suggests the potential for using them as a new generation of biomarkers in neuropsychiatric conditions and opens new avenues for the treatment of these disorders.

ACKNOWLEDGMENTS

This work was supported by grants from the Cariplo Foundation (MICROMOOD Project 2009-2701) and from the Italian Ministry of Health (Ricerca Corrente). We want to thank Dr. Carlo Maj for his help.

REFERENCES

Abelson, J. F., Kwan, K. Y., O'Roak, B. J., Baek, D. Y., Stillman, A. A., Morgan, T. M., et al. (2005). Sequence variants in SLITRK1 are associated with Tourette's syndrome. *Science* 310, 317–320. doi: 10.1126/science.1116502

Absalon, S., Kochanek, D. M., Raghavan, V., and Krichevsky, A. M. (2013). MiR-26b, upregulated in Alzheimer's disease, activates cell cycle entry, tau-phosphorylation, and apoptosis in postmitotic neurons. *J. Neurosci.* 33, 14645–14659. doi: 10.1523/JNEUROSCI.1327-13.2013

Alexandrov, P. N., Dua, P., Hill, J. M., Bhattacharjee, S., Zhao, Y., and Lukiw, W. J. (2012). microRNA (miRNA) speciation in Alzheimer's disease (AD) cerebrospinal fluid (CSF) and extracellular fluid (ECF). *Int. J. Biochem. Mol. Biol.* 3, 365–373.

Arroyo, J. D., Chevillet, J. R., Kroh, E. M., Ruf, I. K., Pritchard, C. C., Gibson, D. F., et al. (2011). Argonaute2 complexes carry a population of circulating microRNAs independent of vesicles in human plasma. *Proc. Natl. Acad. Sci. U.S.A.* 108, 5003–5008. doi: 10.1073/pnas.1019055108

Banigan, M. G., Kao, P. F., Kozubek, J. A., Winslow, A. R., Medina, J., Costa, J., et al. (2013). Differential expression of exosomal microRNAs in prefrontal cortices of schizophrenia and bipolar disorder patients. *PLoS ONE* 8:e48814. doi: 10.1371/journal.pone.0048814

Baudry, A., Mouillet-Richard, S., Schneider, B., Launay, J. M., and Kellermann, O. (2010). miR-16 targets the serotonin transporter: a new facet for adaptive responses to antidepressants. *Science* 329, 1537–1541. doi: 10.1126/science.1193692

Begemann, M., Grube, S., Papiol, S., Malzahn, D., Krampe, H., Ribbe, K., et al. (2010). Modification of cognitive performance in schizophrenia by complexin 2 gene polymorphisms. *Arch. Gen. Psychiatry* 67, 879–888. doi: 10.1001/archgenpsychiatry.2010.107

Belzeaux, R., Bergon, A., Jeanjean, V., Loriod, B., Formisano-Tréziny, C., Verrier, L., et al. (2012). Responder and nonresponder patients exhibit different peripheral transcriptional signatures during major depressive episode. *Transl. Psychiatry* 2, e185. doi: 10.1038/tp.2012.112

Beveridge, N. J., Gardiner, E., Carroll, A. P., Tooney, P. A., and Cairns, M. J. (2010). Schizophrenia is associated with an increase in cortical microRNA biogenesis. *Mol. Psychiatry* 15, 1176–1189. doi: 10.1038/mp.2009.84

Beveridge, N. J., Tooney, P. A., Carroll, A. P., Gardiner, E., Bowden, N., Scott, R. J., et al. (2008). Dysregulation of miRNA 181b in the temporal cortex in schizophrenia. *Hum. Mol. Genet.* 17, 1156–1168. doi: 10.1093/hmg/ddn005

Bicker, S., Khudayberdiev, S., WeißK., Zocher, K., Baumeister, S., and Schratt, G. (2013). The DEAH box helicase DHX36 mediates dendritic localization of the neuronal precursor-microRNA-134. *Genes Dev.* 27, 991–996. doi: 10.1101/gad.211243.112

Blennow, K., and Zetterberg, H. (2013). The application of cerebrospinal fluid biomarkers in early diagnosis of Alzheimer disease. *Med. Clin. North Am.* 97, 369–376. doi: 10.1016/j.mcna.2012.12.012

Bocchio-Chiavetto, L., Maffioletti, E., Bettinsoli, P., Giovannini, C., Bignotti, S., Tardito, D., et al. (2013). Blood microRNA changes in depressed patients during antidepressant treatment. *Eur. Neuropsychopharmacol.* 23, 602–611. doi: 10.1016/j.euroneuro.2012.06.013

Boeckel, J. N., Thomé C. E., Leistner, D., Zeiher, A. M., Fichtlscherer, S., and Dimmeler, S. (2013). Heparin selectively affects the quantification of microRNAs in human blood samples. *Clin. Chem.* 59, 1125–1127. doi: 10.1373/clinchem.2012.199505

Boutajangout, A., and Wisniewski, T. (2013). The innate immune system in Alzheimer's disease. *Int. J. Cell Biol.* 2013, 576383. doi: 10.1155/2013/576383

Breving, K., and Esquela-Kerscher, A. (2010). The complexities of microRNA regulation: mirandering around the rules. *Int. J. Biochem. Cell Biol.* 42, 1316–1329. doi: 10.1016/j.biocel.2009.09.016

Burgos, K. L., Javaherian, A., Bomprezzi, R., Ghaffari, L., Rhodes, S., Courtright, A., et al. (2013). Identification of extracellular miRNA in human cerebrospinal fluid by next-generation sequencing. *RNA* 19, 712–722. doi: 10.1261/rna.036863.112

Caputo, V., Sinibaldi, L., Fiorentino, A., Parisi, C., Catalanotto, C., Pasini, A., et al. (2011). Brain derived neurotrophic factor (BDNF) expression is regulated by microRNAs miR 26a and miR-26b allele-specific binding. *PLoS ONE* 6:e28656. doi: 10.1371/journal.pone.0028656

Chan, A. W., and Kocerha, J. (2012). The path to microRNA therapeutics in psychiatric and neurodegenerative disorders. *Front. Genet.* 3:82. doi: 10.3389/fgene.2012.00082

Chekulaeva, M., and Filipowicz, W. (2009). Mechanisms of miRNA-mediated post-transcriptional regulation in animal cells. *Curr. Opin. Cell Biol.* 21, 452–460. doi: 10.1016/j.ceb.2009.04.009

Chen, H., Wang, N., Burmeister, M., and McInnis, M. G. (2009). MicroRNA expression changes in lymphoblastoid cell lines in response to lithium treatment. *Int. J. Neuropsychopharmacol.* 12, 975–981. doi: 10.1017/S1461145709000029

Chen, X., Ba, Y., Ma, L., Cai, X., Yin, Y., Wang, K., et al. (2008). Characterization of microRNAs in serum: a novel class of biomarkers for diagnosis of cancer and other diseases. *Cell Res.* 18, 997–1006. doi: 10.1038/cr.2008.282

Chen-Plotkin, A. S., Unger, T. L., Gallagher, M. D., Bill, E., Kwong, L. K., Volpicelli-Daley, L., et al. (2012). TMEM106B, the risk gene for frontotemporal dementia, is regulated by the microRNA-132/212 cluster and affects progranulin pathways. *J. Neurosci.* 32, 11213–11227. doi: 10.1523/JNEUROSCI.0521-12.2012

Cogswell, J. P., Ward, J., Taylor, I. A., Waters, M., Shi, Y., Cannon, B., et al. (2008). Identification of miRNA changes in Alzheimer's disease brain and CSF yields putative biomarkers and insights into disease pathways. *J. Alzheimers Dis.* 14, 27–41.

Cortez, M. A., Bueso-Ramos, C., Ferdin, J., Lopez-Berestein, G., Sood, A. K., and Calin, G. A. (2011). MicroRNAs in body fluids–the mix of hormones and biomarkers. *Nat. Rev. Clin. Oncol.* 8, 467–477. doi: 10.1038/nrclinonc.2011.76

Creson, T. K., Austin, D. R., Shaltiel, G., McCammon, J., Wess, J., Manji, H. K., et al. (2011). Lithium treatment attenuates muscarinic M(1) receptor dysfunction. *Bipolar Disord.* 13, 238–249. doi: 10.1111/j.1399-5618.2011.00915.x

Cummings, E., Donohoe, G., Hargreaves, A., Moore, S., Fahey, C., Dinan, T. G., et al. (2013). Mood congruent psychotic symptoms and specific cognitive deficits in carriers of the novel schizophrenia risk variant at MIR-137. *Neurosci. Lett.* 532, 33–38. doi: 10.1016/j.neulet.2012.08.065

Davis, B. N., and Hata, A. (2009). Regulation of microRNA biogenesis: a miRiad of mechanisms. *Cell Commun. Signal.* 7, 18. doi: 10.1186/1478-811X-7-18

Delay, C., Calon, F., Mathews, P., and Hébert, S. S. (2011). Alzheimer-specific variants in the 3′UTR of Amyloid precursor protein affect microRNA function. *Mol. Neurodegener.* 6, 70. doi: 10.1186/1750-1326-6-70

de Mena, L., Cardo, L. F., Coto, E., Miar, A., Díaz, M., Corao, A. I., et al. (2010). FGF20 rs12720208 SNP and microRNA-433 variation: no association with Parkinson's disease in Spanish patients. *Neurosci. Lett.* 479, 22–25. doi: 10.1016/j.neulet.2010.05.019

Doxakis, E. (2010). Post-transcriptional regulation of alpha-synuclein expression by mir-7 and mir-153. *J. Biol. Chem.* 285, 12726–12734. doi: 10.1074/jbc.M109.086827

Duan, S., Mi, S., Zhang, W., and Dolan, M. E. (2009). Comprehensive analysis of the impact of SNPs and CNVs on human microRNAs and their regulatory genes. *RNA Biol.* 6, 412–425. doi: 10.4161/rna.6.4.8830

Farazi, T. A., Hoell, J. I., Morozov, P., and Tuschl, T. (2013). MicroRNAs in human cancer. *Adv. Exp. Med. Biol.* 774, 1–20. doi: 10.1007/978-94-007-5590-1_1

Felekkis, K., Voskarides, K., Dweep, H., Sticht, C., Gretz, N., and Deltas, C. (2011). Increased number of microRNA target sites in genes encoded in CNV regions. Evidence for an evolutionary genomic interaction. *Mol. Biol. Evol.* 14, 2421–2424. doi: 10.1093/molbev/msr078

Feng, J., Sun, G., Yan, J., Noltner, K., Li, W., Buzin, C. H., et al. (2009). Evidence for X-chromosomal schizophrenia associated with microRNA alterations. *PLoS ONE* 4:e6121. doi: 10.1371/journal.pone.0006121

Fichtlscherer, S., De Rosa, S., Fox, H., Schwietz, T., Fischer, A., Liebetrau, C., et al. (2010). Circulating microRNAs in patients with coronary artery disease. *Circ. Res.* 107, 677–684. doi: 10.1161/CIRCRESAHA.109.215566

Gao, F. B. (2010b). Context-dependent functions of specific microRNAs in neuronal development. *Neural Dev.* 5, 25. doi: 10.1186/1749-8104-5-25

Gao, J., Wang, W. Y., Mao, Y. W., Gräff, J., Guan, J. S., Pan, L., et al. (2010a). A novel pathway regulates memory and plasticity via SIRT1 and miR-134. *Nature.* 466, 1105–1109. doi: 10.1038/nature09271

Gardiner, E., Beveridge, N. J., Wu, J. Q., Carr, V., Scott, R. J., Tooney, P. A., et al. (2012). Imprinted DLK1-DIO3 region of 14q32 defines a schizophrenia-associated miRNA signature in peripheral blood mononuclear cells. *Mol. Psychiatry* 17, 827–840. doi: 10.1038/mp.2011.78

Gaughwin, P., Ciesla, M., Yang, H., Lim, B., and Brundin, P. (2011). Stage-specific modulation of cortical neuronal development by Mmu-miR-134. *Cereb. Cortex* 21, 1857–1869. doi: 10.1093/cercor/bhq262

Geekiyanage, H., and Chan, C. (2011). MicroRNA-137/181c regulates serine palmitoyltransferase and in turn amyloid β, novel targets in sporadic Alzheimer's disease. *J. Neurosci.* 31, 14820–14830. doi: 10.1523/JNEUROSCI.3883-11.2011

Geekiyanage, H., Jicha, G. A., Nelson, P. T., and Chan, C. (2012). Blood serum miRNA: non-invasive biomarkers for Alzheimer's disease. *Exp. Neurol.* 235, 491–496. doi: 10.1016/j.expneurol.2011.11.026

Green, M. J., Cairns, M. J., Wu, J., Dragovic, M., Jablensky, A., Tooney, P. A., et al. (2013). Genome-wide supported variant MIR137 and severe negative symptoms predict membership of an impaired cognitive subtype of schizophrenia. *Mol. Psychiatry.* 18, 774–780. doi: 10.1038/mp.2012.84

Guay, C., and Regazzi, R. (2013). Circulating microRNAs as novel biomarkers for diabetes mellitus. *Nat. Rev. Endocrinol.* 9, 513–521. doi:10.1038/nrendo.2013.86

Guella, I., Sequeira, A., Rollins, B., Morgan, L., Torri, F., van Erp, T. G., et al. (2013). Analysis of miR-137 expression and rs1625579 in dorsolateral prefrontal cortex. *J. Psychiatr. Res.* 47, 1215–1221. doi: 10.1016/j.jpsychires.2013.05.021

Han, M., and Zheng, Y. (2013). Comprehensive analysis of single nucleotide polymorphisms in human microRNAs. *PLoS ONE* 8:e78028. doi: 10.1371/journal.pone.0078028

Hanke, M., Hoefig, K., Merz, H., Feller, A. C., Kausch, I., Jocham, D., et al. (2010). A robust methodology to study urine microRNA as tumor marker: microRNA-126 and microRNA 182 are related to urinary bladder cancer. *Urol. Oncol.* 28, 655–661. doi: 10.1016/j.urolonc.2009.01.027

Hansen, K. F., Karelina, K., Sakamoto, K., Wayman, G. A., Impey, S., and Obrietan, K. (2013). miRNA-132: a dynamic regulator of cognitive capacity. *Brain Struct. Funct.* 218, 817–831. doi: 10.1007/s00429-012-0431-4

Hansen, T., Olsen, L., Lindow, M., Jakobsen, K. D., Ullum, H., Jonsson, E., et al. (2007). Brain expressed microRNAs implicated in schizophrenia etiology. *PLoS ONE* 2:e873. doi: 10.1371/journal.pone.0000873

Haramati, S., Navon, I., Issler, O., Ezra-Nevo, G., Gil, S., Zwang, R., et al. (2011). MicroRNA as repressors of stress-induced anxiety: the case of amygdalar miR-34. *J. Neurosci.* 31, 14191–14203. doi: 10.1523/JNEUROSCI.1673-11.2011

Hébert, S. S., Horré, K., Nicolaï, L., Papadopoulou, A. S., Mandemakers, W., Silahtaroglu, A. N., et al. (2008). Loss of microRNA cluster miR-29a/b-1 in sporadic Alzheimer's disease correlates with increased BACE1/beta-secretase expression. *Proc. Natl. Acad. Sci. U.S.A.* 105, 6415–6420. doi: 10.1073/pnas.0710263105

Hébert, S. S., Wang, W. X., Zhu, Q., and Nelson, P. T. (2013). A study of small RNAs from cerebral neocortex of pathology-verified Alzheimer's disease, dementia with lewy bodies, hippocampal sclerosis, frontotemporal lobar dementia, and non demented human controls. *J. Alzheimers. Dis.* 35, 335–348. doi: 10.3233/JAD-122350

He, Y., Zhou, Y., Xi, Q., Cui, H., Luo, T., Song, H., et al. (2012). Genetic variations in microRNA processing genes are associated with susceptibility in depression. *DNA Cell Biol.* 31, 1499–1506. doi: 10.1089/dna.2012.1660

Hennah, W., Varilo, T., Kestilä, M., Paunio, T., Arajärvi, R., Haukka, J., et al. (2003). Haplotype transmission analysis provides evidence of association for DISC1 to schizophrenia and suggests sex-dependent effects. *Hum. Mol. Genet.* 12, 3151–3159. doi: 10.1093/hmg/ddg341

Honda, M., Kuwano, Y., Katsuura-Kamano, S., Kamezaki, Y., Fujita, K., Akaike, Y., et al. (2013). Chronic academic stress increases a group of microRNAs in peripheral blood. *PLoS ONE* 8:e75960. doi: 10.1371/journal.pone.0075960

Hu, K., Xie, Y. Y., Zhang, C., Ouyang, D. S., Long, H. Y., Sun, D. N., et al. (2012). MicroRNA expression profile of the hippocampus in a rat model of temporal lobe epilepsy and miR-34a-targeted neuroprotection against hippocampal neurone cell apoptosis post-status epilepticus. *BMC Neurosci.* 13:115. doi: 10.1186/1471-2202-13-115

Huntzinger, E., and Izaurralde, E. (2011). Gene silencing by microRNAs: contributions of translational repression and mRNA decay. *Nat. Rev. Genet.* 12, 99–110. doi: 10.1038/nrg2936

Iguchi, H., Kosaka, N., and Ochiya, T. (2010). Secretory microRNAs as a versatile communication tool. *Commun. Integr. Biol.* 3, 478–481. doi: 10.4161/cib.3.5.12693

Jimenez-Mateos, E. M., Engel, T., Merino-Serrais, P., McKiernan, R. C., Tanaka, K., Mouri, G., et al. (2012). Silencing microRNA-134 produces neuroprotective and prolonged seizure-suppressive effects. *Nat. Med.* 18, 1087–1094. doi: 10.1038/nm.2834

Junn, E., Lee, K. W., Jeong, B. S., Chan, T. W., Im, J. Y., and Mouradian, M. M. (2009). Repression of alpha-synuclein expression and toxicity by microRNA-7. *Proc. Natl. Acad. Sci. U.S.A.* 106, 13052–13057. doi: 10.1073/pnas.0906277106

Junn, E., and Mouradian, M. M. (2012). MicroRNAs in neurodegenerative diseases and their therapeutic potential. *Pharmacol. Ther.* 133, 142–150. doi: 10.1016/j.pharmthera.2011.10.002

Katsuura, S., Kuwano, Y., Yamagishi, N., Kurokawa, K., Kajita, K., Akaike, Y., et al. (2012). MicroRNAs miR-144/144* and miR-16 in peripheral blood are potential biomarkers for naturalistic stress in healthy Japanese medical students. *Neurosci. Lett.* 516, 79–84. doi: 10.1016/j.neulet.2012.03.062

Kiko, T., Nakagawa, K., Tsuduki, T., Furukawa, K., Arai, H., and Miyazawa, T. (2013). MicroRNAs in plasma and cerebrospinal fluid as potential markers for Alzheimer's disease. *J. Alzheimers Dis.* 39, 253–259. doi: 10.3233/JAD-130932

Kim, A. H., Reimers, M., Maher, B., Williamson, V., McMichael, O., McClay, J. L., et al. (2010). MicroRNA expression profiling in the prefrontal cortex of individuals affected with schizophrenia and bipolar disorders. *Schizophr. Res.* 124, 183–191. doi: 10.1016/j.schres.2010.07.002

Kim, J., Inoue, K., Ishii, J., Vanti, W. B., Voronov, S. V., Murchison, E., et al. (2007). MicroRNA feedback circuit in midbrain dopamine neurons. *Science* 317, 1220–1224. doi: 10.1126/science.1140481

Kolshus, E., Dalton, V. S., Ryan, K. M., and McLoughlin, D. M. (2013). When less is more - microRNAs and psychiatric disorders. *Acta Psychiatr. Scand.* doi: 10.1111/acps.12191. [Epub ahead of print].

Kozomara, A., and Griffiths-Jones, S. (2014). miRBase: annotating high confidence microRNAs using deep sequencing data. *Nucleic Acids Res.* 42, D68–D73. doi: 10.1093/nar/gkt1181

Kroh, E. M., Parkin, R. K., Mitchell, P. S., and Tewari, M. (2010). Analysis of circulating microRNA biomarkers in plasma and serum using quantitative reverse transcription-PCR (qRT-PCR). *Methods* 50, 298–301. doi: 10.1016/j.ymeth.2010.01.032

Krol, J., Loedige, I., and Filipowicz, W. (2010). The widespread regulation of microRNA biogenesis, function and decay. *Nat. Rev. Genet.* 11, 597–610. doi: 10.1038/nrg2843

Lai, C. Y., Yu, S. L., Hsieh, M. H., Chen, C. H., Chen, H. Y., Wen, C. C., et al. (2011). MicroRNA expression aberration as potential peripheral blood biomarkers for schizophrenia. *PLoS ONE* 6:e21635. doi: 10.1371/journal.pone.0021635

Laterza, O. F., Lim, L., Garrett-Engele, P. W., Vlasakova, K., Muniappa, N., Tanaka, W. K., et al. (2009). Plasma MicroRNAs as sensitive and specific biomarkers of tissue injury. *Clin. Chem.* 55, 1977–1983. doi:10.1373/clinchem.2009.131797

Lau, P., Bossers, K., Janky, R., Salta, E., Frigerio, C. S., Barbash, S., et al. (2013). Alteration of the microRNA network during the progression of Alzheimer's disease. *EMBO Mol. Med.* 5, 1613–1634. doi: 10.1002/emmm.201201974

Lee, R. C., Feinbaum, R. L., and Ambros, V. (1993). The, C. elegans heterochronic gene lin-4 encodes small RNAs with antisense complementarity to lin-14. *Cell* 75, 843-854. doi:10.1016/0092-8674(93)90529-Y

Lehmann, S. M., Krüger, C., Park, B., Derkow, K., Rosenberger, K., Baumgart, J., et al. (2012). An unconventional role for miRNA: let-7 activates Toll-like receptor 7 and causes neurodegeneration. *Nat. Neurosci.* 15, 827–835. doi: 10.1038/nn.3113

Leidinger, P., Backes, C., Deutscher, S., Schmitt, K., Mueller, S. C., Frese, K., et al. (2013). A blood based 12-miRNA signature of Alzheimer disease patients. *Genome Biol.* 14, R78. doi: 10.1186/gb-2013-14-7-r78

Li, Y. J., Xu, M., Gao, Z. H., Wang, Y. Q., Yue, Z., Zhang, Y. X., et al. (2013). Alterations of serum levels of BDNF-related miRNAs in patients with depression. *PLoS ONE* 8:e63648. doi: 10.1371/journal.pone.0063648

Liu, C., Zhang, F., Li, T., Lu, M., Wang, L., Yue, W., et al. (2012b). MirSNP, a database of polymorphisms altering miRNA target sites, identifies miRNA-related SNPs in GWAS SNPs and eQTLs. *BMC Genomics* 13:661. doi: 10.1186/1471-2164-13-661

Liu, N., Landreh, M., Cao, K., Abe, M., Hendriks, G. J., Kennerdell, J. R., et al. (2012a). The microRNA miR-34 modulates ageing and neurodegeneration in Drosophila. *Nature* 482, 519–523. doi: 10.1038/nature10810

Liu, S., Yuan, Y. B., Guan, L. L., Wei, H., Cheng, Z., Han, X., et al. (2013). MiRNA-365 and miRNA-520c-3p respond to risperidone treatment in first-episode schizophrenia after a 1 year remission. *Chin. Med. J. (Engl.).* 126, 2676–2680.

Madrigal-Matute, J., Rotllan, N., Aranda, J. F., and Fernández-Hernando, C. (2013). MicroRNAs and atherosclerosis. *Curr. Atheroscler. Rep.* 15, 322. doi: 10.1007/s11883-013-0322-z

Marcinkowska, M., Szymanski, M., Krzyzosiak, W. J., and Kozlowski, P. (2011). Copy number variation of microRNA genes in the human genome. *BMC Genomics* 14:183. doi: 10.1186/1471-2164-12-183

Margis, R., Margis, R., and Rieder, C. R. (2011). Identification of blood microRNAs associated to Parkinsonis disease. *J. Biotechnol.* 152, 96–101. doi: 10.1016/j.jbiotec.2011.01.023

Martins, M., Rosa, A., Guedes, L. C., Fonseca, B. V., Gotovac, K., Violante, S., et al. (2011). Convergence of miRNA expression profiling, α-synuclein interacton and GWAS in Parkinson's disease. *PLoS ONE* 6:e25443. doi: 10.1371/journal.pone.0025443

Miller, B. H., Zeier, Z., Xi, L., Lanz, T. A., Deng, S., Strathmann, J., et al. (2012). MicroRNA-132 dysregulation in schizophrenia has implications for both neurodevelopment and adult brain function. *Proc. Natl. Acad. Sci. U.S.A.* 109, 3125–3130. doi: 10.1073/pnas.1113793109

Miñones-Moyano, E., Porta, S., Escaramís, G., Rabionet, R., Iraola, S., Kagerbauer, B., et al. (2011). MicroRNA profiling of Parkinson's disease brains identifies early downregulation of miR-34b/c which modulate mitochondrial function. *Hum. Mol. Genet.* 20, 3067–3078. doi: 10.1093/hmg/ddr210

Mitchell, P. S., Parkin, R. K., Kroh, E. M., Fritz, B. R., Wyman, S. K., Pogosova-Agadjanyan, E. L., et al. (2008). Circulating microRNAs as stable blood-based markers for cancer detection. *Proc. Natl. Acad. Sci. U.S.A.* 105, 10513–10518. doi: 10.1073/pnas.0804549105

Monsonego, A., Nemirovsky, A., and Harpaz, I. (2013). CD4 T cells in immunity and immunotherapy of Alzheimer's disease. *Immunology* 139, 438–446. doi: 10.1111/imm.12103

Moreau, M. P., Bruse, S. E., David-Rus, R., Buyske, S., and Brzustowicz, L. M. (2011). Altered microRNA expression profiles in postmortem brain samples from individuals with schizophrenia and bipolar disorder. *Biol. Psychiatry* 69, 188–193. doi: 10.1016/j.biopsych.2010.09.039

Muiños-Gimeno, M., Espinosa-Parrilla, Y., Guidi, M., Kagerbauer, B., Sipilä, T., Maron, E., et al. (2011). Human microRNAs miR-22, miR-138-2, miR-148a, and miR-488 are associated with panic disorder and regulate several anxiety candidate genes and related pathways. *Biol. Psychiatry* 69, 526–533. doi: 10.1016/j.biopsych.2010.10.010

Muiños-Gimeno, M., Guidi, M., Kagerbauer, B., Martín-Santos, R., Navinés, R., Alonso, P., et al. (2009). Allele variants in functional MicroRNA target sites of the neurotrophin-3 receptor gene (NTRK3) as susceptibility factors for anxiety disorders. *Hum. Mutat.* 30, 1062–1071. doi: 10.1002/humu.21005

Muiños-Gimeno, M., Montfort, M., Bayés, M., Estivill, X., and Espinosa-Parrilla, Y. (2010). Design and evaluation of a panel of single-nucleotide polymorphisms in microRNA genomic regions for association studies in human disease. *Eur. J. Hum. Genet.* 18, 218–226. doi: 10.1038/ejhg.2009.165

Müller, M., Kuiperij, H. B., Claassen, J. A., Küsters, B., and Verbeek, M. M. (2014). MicroRNAs in Alzheimer's disease: differential expression in hippocampus and cell-free cerebrospinal fluid. *Neurobiol. Aging* 35, 152–158. doi: 10.1016/j.neurobiolaging.2013.07.005

Nelson, P. T., and Wang, W. X. (2010). MiR-107 is reduced in Alzheimer's disease brain neocortex: validation study. *J. Alzheimers Dis.* 21, 75–79. doi: 10.3233/JAD-2010-091603

Numakawa, T., Richards, M., Adachi, N., Kishi, S., Kunugi, H., and Hashido, K. (2011). MicroRNA function and neurotrophin BDNF. *Neurochem. Int.* 59, 551–558. doi: 10.1016/j.neuint.2011.06.009

Nunez-Iglesias, J., Liu, C. C., Morgan, T. E., Finch, C. E., and Zhou, X. J. (2010). Joint genome-wide profiling of miRNA and mRNA expression in Alzheimer's disease cortex reveals altered miRNA regulation. *PLoS ONE* 5:e8898. doi: 10.1371/journal.pone.0008898

O'Carroll, D., and Schaefer, A. (2012). General principals of miRNA biogenesis and regulation in the brain. *Neuropsychopharmacology* 38, 39–54. doi: 10.1038/npp.2012.87

O'Connor, R. M., Grenham, S., Dinan, T. G., and Cryan, J. F. (2013). microRNAs as novel antidepressant targets: converging effects of ketamine and electroconvulsive shock therapy in the rat hippocampus. *Int. J. Neuropsychopharmacol.* 16, 1885–1892. doi: 10.1017/S1461145713000448

Olde Loohuis, N. F., Kos, A., Martens, G. J., Van Bokhoven, H., Nadif Kasri, N., and Aschrafi, A. (2012). MicroRNA networks direct neuronal development and plasticity. *Cell. Mol. Life Sci.* 69, 89–102. doi: 10.1007/s00018-011-0788-1

Oved, K., Morag, A., Pasmanik-Chor, M., Oron-Karni, V., Shomron, N., Rehavi, M., et al. (2012). Genome-wide miRNA expression profiling of human lymphoblastoid cell lines identifies tentative SSRI antidepressant response biomarkers. *Pharmacogenomics* 13, 1129–1139. doi: 10.2217/pgs.12.93

Papoutsidakis, N., Deftereos, S., Kaoukis, A., Bouras, G., Giannopoulos, G., Theodorakis, A., et al. (2013). MicroRNAs and the heart: small things do matter. *Curr. Top. Med. Chem.* 13, 216–230. doi: 10.2174/1568026611313020009

Park, N. J., Zhou, H., Elashoff, D., Henson, B. S., Kastratovic, D. A., Abemayor, E., et al. (2009). Salivary microRNA: discovery, characterization, and clinical utility for oral cancer detection. *Clin. Cancer Res.* 15, 5473–5477. doi: 10.1158/1078-0432.CCR-09-0736

Pasquinelli, A. E. (2012). MicroRNAs and their targets: recognition, regulation and an emerging reciprocal relationship. *Nat. Rev. Genet.* 13, 271–282. doi: 10.1038/nrg3162

Pelizzari, M., Tardito, D., Mallei, A., Corna, S., Treccani, G., Bocchio-Chiavetto, L., et al. (2012). Analysis of miRNome expression profiles in hippocampus of rats treated with antidepressants. *Eur. Neuropsychopharmacol.* 22, S101–S102. doi: 10.1016/S0924-977X(12)70108-6

Peng, Z., Li, J., Li, Y., Yang, X., Feng, S., Han, S., et al. (2013). Downregulation of miR-181b in mouse brain following ischemic stroke induces neuroprotection against ischemic injury through targeting heat shock protein A5 and ubiquitin carboxyl-terminal hydrolase isozyme L1. *J. Neurosci. Res.* 91, 1349–1362. doi: 10.1002/jnr.23255

Perkins, D. O., Jeffries, C. D., Jarskog, L. F., Thomson, J. M., Woods, K., Newman, M. A., et al. (2007). microRNA expression in the prefrontal cortex of individuals with schizophrenia and schizoaffective disorder. *Genome Biol.* 8, R27. doi: 10.1186/gb-2007-8-2-r27

Perkins, D. O., Jeffries, C., and Sullivan, P. (2005). Expanding the 'central dogma': the regulatory role of nonprotein coding genes and implications for the genetic liability to schizophrenia. *Mol. Psychiatry* 10, 69–78. doi: 10.1038/sj.mp.4001577

Pigati, L., Yaddanapudi, S. C., Iyengar, R., Kim, D. J., Hearn, S. A., Danforth, D., et al. (2010). Selective release of microRNA species from normal and malignant mammary epithelial cells. *PLoS ONE* 5:e13515. doi: 10.1371/journal.pone.0013515

Profumo, V., and Gandellini, P. (2013). MicroRNAs: cobblestones on the road to cancer metastasis. *Crit. Rev. Oncog.* 18, 341–355. doi: 10.1615/CritRevOncog.2013007182

Rademakers, R., Eriksen, J. L., Baker, M., Robinson, T., Ahmed, Z., Lincoln, S. J., et al. (2008). Common variation in the miR-659 binding-site of GRN is a major risk factor for TDP43-positive frontotemporal dementia. *Hum. Mol. Genet.* 17, 3631–3642. doi: 10.1093/hmg/ddn257

Rahman, O. A., Sasvari-Szekely, M., Szekely, A., Faludi, G., Guttman, A., and Nemoda, Z. (2010). Analysis of a polymorphic microRNA target site in the purinergic receptor P2RX7 gene. *Electrophoresis* 31, 1790–1795. doi: 10.1002/elps.200900664

Ripke, S., Sanders, A. R., Kendler, K. S., Levinson, D. F., Sklar, P., Holmans, P. A., et al. (2011). Genome-wide association study identifies five new schizophrenia loci. *Nat. Genet.* 43, 969–976. doi: 10.1038/ng.940

Rong, H., Liu, T. B., Yang, K. J., Yang, H. C., Wu, D. H., Liao, C. P., et al. (2011). MicroRNA-134 plasma levels before and after treatment for bipolar mania. *J. Psychiatr. Res.* 45, 92–95. doi: 10.1016/j.jpsychires.2010.04.028

Rossi, M., Kilpinen, H., Muona, M., Surakka, I., Ingle, C., Lahtinen, J., et al. (2013). Allele-specific regulation of DISC1 expression by miR-135b-5p. *Eur. J. Hum. Genet.* doi: 10.1038/ejhg.2013.246. [Epub ahead of print].

Santarelli, D. M., Beveridge, N. J., Tooney, P. A., and Cairns, M. J. (2011). Upregulation of dicer and microRNA expression in the dorsolateral prefrontal cortex Brodmann area 46 in schizophrenia. *Biol. Psychiatry* 69, 180–187. doi: 10.1016/j.biopsych.2010.09.030

Santarelli, D. M., Liu, B., Duncan, C. E., Beveridge, N. J., Tooney, P. A., Schofield, P. R., et al. (2013). Gene-microRNA interactions associated with antipsychotic mechanisms and the metabolic side effects of olanzapine. *Psychopharmacology* 227, 67–78. doi: 10.1007/s00213-012-2939-y

Saus, E., Soria, V., Escaramís, G., Vivarelli, F., Crespo, J. M., Kagerbauer, B., et al. (2010). Genetic variants and abnormal processing of pre-miR-182, a circadian clock modulator, in major depression patients with late insomnia. *Hum. Mol. Genet.* 19, 4017–4025. doi: 10.1093/hmg/ddq316

Sayed, D., and Abdellatif, M. (2011). MicroRNAs in development and disease. *Physiol. Rev.* 91, 827–887. doi: 10.1152/physrev.00006.2010

Scarr, E., Craig, J. M., Cairns, M. J., Seo, M. S., Galati, J. C., Beveridge, N. J., et al. (2013). Decreased cortical muscarinic M1 receptors in schizophrenia are associated with changes in gene promoter methylation, mRNA and gene targeting microRNA. *Transl. Psychiatry* 3, e230. doi: 10.1038/tp.2013.3

Schiffman, J. D., Lorimer, P. D., Rodic, V., Jahromi, M. S., Downie, J. M., Bayerl, M. G., et al. (2011). Genome wide copy number analysis of paediatric Burkitt lymphoma using formalin-fixed tissues reveals a subset with gain of chromosome 13q and corresponding miRNA over expression. *Br. J. Haematol.* 14, 477–486. doi: 10.1111/j.1365-2141.2011.08883.x

Schipper, H. M., Maes, O. C., Chertkow, H. M., and Wang, E. (2007). MicroRNA expression in Alzheimer blood mononuclear cells. *Gene Regul. Syst. Bio.* 1, 263–274.

Schonrock, N., Ke, Y. D., Humphreys, D., Staufenbiel, M., Ittner, L. M., Preiss, T., et al. (2010). Neuronal microRNA deregulation in response to Alzheimer's disease amyloid-beta. *PLoS ONE* 5:e11070. doi: 10.1371/journal.pone.0011070

Schwarz, D. S., Hutvágner, G., Du, T., Xu, Z., Aronin, N., and Zamore, P. D. (2003). Asymmetry in the assembly of the RNAi enzyme complex. *Cell* 115, 199–208. doi: 10.1016/S0092-8674(03)00759-1

Serpente, M., Fenoglio, C., Villa, C., Cortini, F., Cantoni, C., Ridolfi, E., et al. (2011). Role of OLR1 and its regulating hsa-miR369-3p in Alzheimer's disease: genetics and expression analysis. *J. Alzheimers Dis.* 26, 787–793. doi: 10.3233/JAD-2011-110074

Sethupathy, P., and Collins, F. S. (2008). MicroRNA target site polymorphisms and human disease. *Trends Genet.* 24, 489–497. doi: 10.1016/j.tig.2008.07.004

Shaltiel, G., Hanan, M., Wolf, Y., Barbash, S., Kovalev, E., Shoham, S., et al. (2013). Hippocampal microRNA-132 mediates stress-inducible cognitive deficits through its acetylcholinesterase target. *Brain Struct. Funct.* 218, 59–72. doi: 10.1007/s00429-011-0376-z

Sheinerman, K. S., Tsivinsky, V. G., Crawford, F., Mullan, M. J., Abdullah, L., and Umansky, S. R. (2012). Plasma microRNA biomarkers for detection of mild cognitive impairment. *Aging (Albany NY).* 4, 590–605.

Shi, W., Du, J., Qi, Y., Liang, G., Wang, T., Li, S., et al. (2012). Aberrant expression of serum miRNAs in schizophrenia. *J. Psychiatr. Res.* 46, 198–204. doi: 10.1016/j.jpsychires.2011.09.010

Shim, S. M., Nam, H. Y., Lee, J. E., Kim, J. W., Han, B. G., and Jeon, J. P. (2012). MicroRNAs in human lymphoblastoid cell lines. *Crit. Rev. Eukaryot. Gene. Expr.* 14, 189–196. doi: 10.1615/CritRevEukarGeneExpr.v22.i3.20

Siegel, G., Saba, R., and Schratt, G. (2011). microRNAs in neurons: manifold regulatory roles at the synapse. *Curr. Opin. Genet. Dev.* 21, 491–497. doi: 10.1016/j.gde.2011.04.008

Skog, J., Würdinger, T., van Rijn, S., Meijer, D. H., Gainche, L., Sena-Esteves, M., et al. (2008). Glioblastoma microvesicles transport RNA and proteins that promote tumour growth and provi.de diagnostic biomarkers. *Nat. Cell Biol.* 10, 1470–1476. doi: 10.1038/ncb1800

Smalheiser, N. R., and Lugli, G. (2009). microRNA regulation of synaptic plasticity. *Neuromolecular Med.* 11, 133–140. doi: 10.1007/s12017-009-8065-2

Smalheiser, N. R., Lugli, G., Rizavi, H. S., Torvik, V. I., Turecki, G., and Dwivedi, Y. (2012). MicroRNA expression is down-regulated and reorganized in prefrontal cortex of depressed suicide subjects. *PLoS ONE* 7:e33201. doi: 10.1371/journal.pone.0033201

Soreq, L., Salomonis, N., Bronstein, M., Greenberg, D. S., Israel, Z., Bergman, H., et al. (2013). Small RNA sequencing-microarray analyses in Parkinson leukocytes reveal deep brain stimulation induced splicing changes that classify brain region transcriptomes. *Front. Mol. Neurosci.* 6:10. doi: 10.3389/fnmol.2013.00010

Tan, L., Yu, J. T., Hu, N., and Tan, L. (2013). Non-coding RNAs in Alzheimer's disease. *Mol. Neurobiol.* 47, 382–393. doi: 10.1007/s12035-012-8359-5

Tan, L., Yu, J. T., Liu, Q. Y., Tan, M. S., Zhang, W., Hu, N., et al. (2014). Circulating miR-125b as a biomarker of Alzheimer's disease. *J. Neurol. Sci.* 336, 52–56. doi: 10.1016/j.jns.2013.10.002

Tardito, D., Mallei, A., and Popoli, M. (2013). Lost in translation. New unexplored avenues for neuropsychopharmacology: epigenetics and microRNAs. *Expert Opin. Investig. Drugs* 22, 217–233. doi: 10.1517/13543784.2013.749237

Valadi, H., Ekström, K., Bossios, A., Sjöstrand, M., Lee, J. J., and Lötvall, J. O. (2007). Exosome mediated transfer of mRNAs and microRNAs is a novel mechanism of genetic exchange between cells. *Nat. Cell Biol.* 9, 654–659. doi: 10.1038/ncb1596

Van Deerlin, V. M., Sleiman, P. M., Martinez-Lage, M., Chen-Plotkin, A., Wang, L. S., Graff-Radford, N. R., et al. (2010). Common variants at 7p21 are associated with frontotemporal lobar degeneration with TDP-43 inclusions. *Nat. Genet.* 42, 234–239. doi: 10.1038/ng.536

van Spronsen, M., van Battum, E. Y., Kuijpers, M., Vangoor, V. R., Rietman, M. L., Pothof, J., et al. (2013). Developmental and activity-dependent miRNA expression profiling in primary hippocampal neuron cultures. *PLoS ONE* 8:e74907. doi: 10.1371/journal.pone.0074907

Villa, C., Fenoglio, C., De Riz, M., Clerici, F., Marcone, A., Benussi, L., et al. (2011). Role of hnRNP-A1 and miR-590-3p in neuronal death: genetics and expression analysis in patients with Alzheimer disease and frontotemporal lobar degeneration. *Rejuvenation Res.* 14, 275–281. doi: 10.1089/rej.2010.1123

Wang, G., van der Walt, J. M., Mayhew, G., Li, Y. J., Züchner, S., Scott, W. K., et al. (2008b). Variation in the miRNA-433 binding site of FGF20 confers risk for Parkinson disease by overexpression of alpha-synuclein. *Am. J. Hum. Genet.* 82, 283–289. doi: 10.1016/j.ajhg.2007.09.021

Wang, K., Zhang, S., Weber, J., Baxter, D., and Galas, D. J. (2010a). Export of microRNAs and microRNA-protective protein by mammalian cells. *Nucleic Acids Res.* 38, 7248–7259. doi: 10.1093/nar/gkq601

Wang, W. X., Huang, Q., Hu, Y., Stromberg, A. J., and Nelson, P. T. (2011). Patterns of microRNA expression in normal and early Alzheimer's disease human temporal cortex: white matter versus gray matter. *Acta Neuropathol.* 121, 193–205. doi: 10.1007/s00401-010-0756-0

Wang, W. X., Rajeev, B. W., Stromberg, A. J., Ren, N., Tang, G., Huang, Q., et al. (2008a). The expression of microRNA miR-107 decreases early in Alzheimer's disease and may accelerate disease progression through regulation of beta-site amyloid precursor protein-cleaving enzyme 1. *J. Neurosci.* 28, 1213–1223. doi: 10.1523/JNEUROSCI.5065-07.2008

Wang, W. X., Wilfred, B. R., Madathil, S. K., Tang, G., Hu, Y., Dimayuga, J., et al. (2010b). miR-107 regulates granulin/progranulin with implications for traumatic brain injury and neurodegenerative disease. *Am. J. Pathol.* 177, 334–345. doi: 10.2353/ajpath.2010.091202

Wibrand, K., Pai, B., Siripornmongcolchai, T., Bittins, M., Berentsen, B., Ofte, M. L., et al. (2012). MicroRNA regulation of the synaptic plasticity-related gene Arc. *PLoS ONE* 7:e41688. doi: 10.1371/journal.pone.0041688

Xu, Y., Li, F., Zhang, B., Zhang, K., Zhang, F., Huang, X., et al. (2010a). MicroRNAs and target site screening reveals a pre-microRNA-30e variant associated with schizophrenia. *Schizophr. Res.* 119, 219–227. doi: 10.1016/j.schres.2010.02.1070

Xu, Y., Liu, H., Li, F., Sun, N., Ren, Y., Liu, Z., et al. (2010b). A polymorphism in the microRNA-30e precursor associated with major depressive disorder risk and P300 waveform. *J. Affect. Disord.* 127, 332–336. doi: 10.1016/j.jad.2010.05.019

Zeng, L., Liu, J., Wang, Y., Wang, L., Weng, S., Tang, Y., et al. (2011). MicroRNA-210 as a novel blood biomarker in acute cerebral ischemia. *Front. Biosci. (Elite. Ed.)* 3:330. doi: 10.2741/330

Zhou, R., Yuan, P., Wang, Y., Hunsberger, J. G., Elkahloun, A., Wei, Y., et al. (2009). Evidence for selective microRNAs and their effectors as common long-term targets for the actions of mood stabilizers. *Neuropsychopharmacology* 34, 1395–1405. doi: 10.1038/npp.2008.131

Zhou, Y., Wang, J., Lu, X., Song, X., Ye, Y., Zhou, J., et al. (2013). Evaluation of six SNPs of MicroRNA machinery genes and risk of schizophrenia. *J. Mol. Neurosci.* 49, 594–599. doi: 10.1007/s12031-012-9887-1

Ziats, M. N., and Rennert, O. M. (2013). Identification of differentially expressed microRNAs across the developing human brain. *Mol. Psychiatry.* doi: 10.1038/mp.2013.93. [Epub ahead of print].

5

Emerging bioinformatics approaches for analysis of NGS-derived coding and non-coding RNAs in neurodegenerative diseases

Alessandro Guffanti[1,2]*, Alon Simchovitz[1] and Hermona Soreq[1]*

[1] Laboratory of Molecular Neuroscience, Department of Biological Chemistry, The Edmond and Lily Safra Center of Brain Science, The Hebrew University of Jerusalem, Jerusalem, Israel

[2] Bioinformatics, Genomnia srl, Milano, Italy

***Correspondence:**
Alessandro Guffanti and Hermona Soreq, Laboratory of Molecular Neuroscience, Department of Biological Chemistry, The Edmond and Lily Safra Center of Brain Science, The Hebrew University of Jerusalem, Jerusalem 91904, Israel
e-mail: alessand.guffanti@mail.huji.ac.il; hermona.soreq@mail.huji.ac.il

Neurodegenerative diseases in general and specifically late-onset Alzheimer's disease (LOAD) involve a genetically complex and largely obscure ensemble of causative and risk factors accompanied by complex feedback responses. The advent of "high-throughput" transcriptome investigation technologies such as microarray and deep sequencing is increasingly being combined with sophisticated statistical and bioinformatics analysis methods complemented by knowledge-based approaches such as Bayesian Networks or network and graph analyses. Together, such "integrative" studies are beginning to identify co-regulated gene networks linked with biological pathways and potentially modulating disease predisposition, outcome, and progression. Specifically, bioinformatics analyses of integrated microarray and genotyping data in cases and controls reveal changes in gene expression of both protein-coding and small and long regulatory RNAs; highlight relevant quantitative transcriptional differences between LOAD and non-demented control brains and demonstrate reconfiguration of functionally meaningful molecular interaction structures in LOAD. These may be measured as changes in connectivity in "hub nodes" of relevant gene networks (Zhang et al., 2013). We illustrate here the open analytical questions in the transcriptome investigation of neurodegenerative disease studies, proposing "*ad hoc*" strategies for the evaluation of differential gene expression and hints for a simple analysis of the non-coding RNA (ncRNA) part of such datasets. We then survey the emerging role of long ncRNAs (lncRNAs) in the healthy and diseased brain transcriptome and describe the main current methods for computational modeling of gene networks. We propose accessible modular and pathway-oriented methods and guidelines for bioinformatics investigations of whole transcriptome next generation sequencing datasets. We finally present methods and databases for functional interpretations of lncRNAs and propose a simple heuristic approach to visualize and represent physical and functional interactions of the coding and non-coding components of the transcriptome. Integrating in a functional and integrated vision coding and ncRNA analyses is of utmost importance for current and future analyses of neurodegenerative transcriptomes.

Keywords: neurodegenerative diseases, bioinformatics and computational biology, next-generation sequencing, non-coding RNA, biological networks

INTRODUCTION

Recently emerging bioinformatics analyses of integrated microarray, next generation sequencing (NGS) and genotyping data in brain and peripheral blood cell samples from neurodegenerative disease cases and matched healthy controls consistently reveal changes in gene expression of both protein-coding and small and long regulatory non-coding RNAs (ncRNAs); highlight relevant quantitative transcriptional differences between demented and non-demented control brains and demonstrate reconfiguration of functionally meaningful molecular interaction structures that may be measured as changes of connectivity in "hub nodes" of relevant gene networks (Karni et al., 2009; Zhang et al., 2013). These developments call for constructing complete and coherent tool kits whereby the contributions of these specific groups of transcripts to the initiation and progression of disease will be elucidated.

"Regulatory" ncRNAs predominantly affect the expression and/or functioning of protein-coding genes. NcRNAs show different biogenesis routes and modes of action, and can be broadly classified based on their size. Small RNA species of less than 200 nucleotides include the microRNAs (miRNAs), which have already emerged as important modulators of development, homeostasis and disease by regulating protein levels, mainly at the post-transcriptional stage. Recent evidences suggest that miRNAs may also directly regulate transcription by interaction with the promoter region of divergently transcribed genes (Matsui et al., 2013), suggesting new insights in the complex relationship between small RNAs, longer transcripts and the quantitative ratio between them.

A substantial fraction of longer transcripts (>200 bp) in mammalian genomes do not code for proteins and are usually expressed at a low level. These are classified according to their relative position with respect to the coding gene structure and include long ncRNAs (lncRNAs) and long intergenic ncRNAs (lincRNAs). LncRNAs (also known as processed transcripts) by definition are found within protein-coding genes, overlapping with promoters, exons or introns in either sense or antisense orientations. LincRNAs, on the other hand, are always found in intergenic regions. There is increasing evidence that lncRNAs are involved in brain development and that different lncRNAs are expressed in different neuroanatomic areas, and possibly acting on chromatin; hinting at a regulatory function at the spatio-temporal level of gene expression (Mercer et al., 2008). It is now widely accepted that lncRNAs can have numerous molecular functions, including modulating transcriptional patterns, regulating protein activities, serving structural or organizational roles, altering RNA processing events, and serving as precursors to small RNAs.

The number of lncRNA species increases in genomes of developmentally complex organisms, which highlights the importance of RNA-based levels of control in the evolution of multicellular organisms (Fatica and Bozzoni, 2013). Most common neurodegenerative diseases of the human brain, however, are either not detected in other species, or else they manifest themselves in different ways. Furthermore, a significant fraction of ncRNAs are primate-specific. Taken together, these two pieces of evidence may suggest that the progressive disruption of regulatory lncRNAs plays an important role in neurodegenerative syndromes. However, current systems-level analyses of gene regulatory networks are primarily focused on protein-coding genes, which make up a mere 2% of the human transcriptional output but whose cellular functions are better understood. That highly structured ncRNAs interact with chromatin or provide docking sites for binding proteins or other RNAs suggests that they bridge the gap between protein complexes and sequence information encoded in the genome. This hidden layer of RNA regulatory networks may be central to developmental and homeostatic processes, and its deregulation could be consequently involved in degenerative neurological disorders such as Alzheimer's and Parkinson's disease.

The different and diverse modes of action of regulatory RNAs adds another level of complication, in that such regulation would not necessarily change the observed level of expression of the tested coding transcripts but may block or support their functioning in other upstream or downstream ways. This implies that the customary use of threshold-dependent technologies may miss part of these effects and mask others, and calls for developing threshold-independent analysis modes. Based on all of these considerations, we propose here the concepts and tools for functional investigation of full-transcriptome next-generation sequencing datasets, with focus on both the coding and non-coding ensembles. We examine in a first instance the statistical aspects linked with the evaluation of differential expression in these systems. We then analyze the relevance of ncRNAs in neurodegeneration. We suggest a strategy to implement a network-based integrated exploration of the outcome of differential gene expression analysis. We introduce lncRNAs Finally, we suggest a strategy to integrate and display the coding and ncRNA aspects in a gene network. Such a bioinformatics procedure could be then adapted and applied to original experimental data in late-onset Alzheimer's disease (LOAD) and other neurodegenerative diseases, where complex cell diversities are involved and no drastic transcriptional changes are measured between disease and control as opposed, for instance, to cancer studies.

GUIDELINES FOR TRANSCRIPTOME DIFFERENTIAL EXPRESSION ANALYSIS APPLIED TO NEURODEGENERATIVE DISEASES

Systematic transcriptome study in neurodegenerative diseases such as amyotrophic lateral sclerosis, Parkinson's, and Alzheimer's diseases (AD) has advanced considerably in recent years, alluding to common patterns such as dys-regulation of genes related with neuroinflammation, splicing, intracellular signaling pathways and mitochondrial dysfunctions (Cooper-Knock et al., 2012). In LOAD, the best distinction refers to cognitive deterioration; hence, cognitive stratification of samples may help to identify gradual transcriptome changes along disease progression.

Our laboratory (Barbash and Soreq, 2012) recently proposed a novel strategy to explore brain transcriptome datasets from cognitively stratified patients at different disease stages for unifying the AD molecular patterns involved in disease initiation and progression. Conventional threshold-dependent analysis methods identify transcripts that are drastically modified in AD, ignoring those within-threshold transcripts whose level was only marginally changed. However, if each member of a group of genes relevant to AD etiology is marginally up-regulated, one might expect a relevant pathological state in the observed tissue even in the absence of major gene changes. In this threshold-independent approach, therefore, we compared the distribution of changes in a well-defined gene group with the global distribution of the experiment. This method allows identification of cumulative changes in groups of genes defined by a common parameter: acting in the same pathway, located in the same cellular organelle, and so on. This approach has been applied to the meta analysis of a large number of microarray datasets (Barbash and Soreq, 2012), contributing to the identification of coherent and progressive early onset hippocampal-specific changes in biological processes such as synaptic transmission, protein folding and RNA splicing known to be affected in end stage AD, but for which the dynamics was not yet reported in the literature.

Starting from this background, we reasoned that many relevant gene changes in AD and other neurodegenerative diseases may go unnoticed also in the differential expression analysis of whole transcriptome NGS datasets, which in addition to known exons and transcripts identifies previously unknown regulatory RNAs. There are two main conceptual starting points for the analysis of this kind of data. The older, and widely used, strategy (TopHat/Cufflinks/Cuffdiff) starts from sequence assembly and transcript reconstruction, performs abundance estimation and evaluates differential expression (Trapnell et al., 2010). Cufflinks constructs a parsimonious set of transcripts that "explain" the reads observed in a RNA-seq experiment, doing so by reducing the comparative assembly problem to a mathematical problem (maximum matching in bipartite graphs). It works particularly well with paired reads; and in systems where there is a relevant change in gene expression associated with a relative amount of change in alternative splicing. Nevertheless, apparent changes in neurodegenerative disease transcriptomes may reflect relevant and massive changes in the alternative splicing pattern, while being accompanied by complex modest changes in gene expression (Berson et al., 2012). Therefore, it is doubtful that this algorithm can handle well the kind of analyses that are associated, for instance, with cognitive stratification of LOAD samples.

A second and more recent strategy for the analysis of NGS transcriptome datasets is based on the assumption that the correct distribution for modeling the distribution of reads on the target genome is a binomial negative, and that an "*ad hoc*" normalization method should be employed (Robinson et al., 2010). This method; however does not (yet) provide relevant information on the structural transcript variations, since it is based on read counts associated with each gene, and hence it is insensitive to at least part of the relevant splicing changes associated with the progression of neurodegenerative events. On the other hand, for the same reason, statistical values [false discovery rate (FDR)] will be often reported as non-significant due to the small and widely distributed changes in gene expression that may only be detected by the non-threshold methods. A third analytical strategy consists of using a method very similar to the primary analysis of microarray datasets: perform upper quantile normalization of the values of gene-associated Read Counts per Million (i.e., the read count scaled to 1 million for each sample); evaluate differential expression with an exact *t*-test; and correct multiple testing using the Benjamini–Hochberg approach.

A strategy we propose here for the evaluation of ranked differential gene expression in neurodegenerative diseases, especially in cohorts stratified by cognitive deterioration, is to apply to the same samples two different differential gene expression methods from the three which we have listed above; correlate by sign and compare the Log2 Fold Change values, without in a first instance imposing a statistical threshold or even considering the FDR values; finally, to apply a simple linear model with residual plots to evaluate the statistics and the residuals. Only those genes that show the same sign of variation between two methods, with a Log2FC of at least ± 0.40, should be included in a differentially expressed gene list for the subsequent functional analyses. The statistic (corrected *P*-values) of the method that worked better for the FDR evaluation should confirm the generation of reliable results with this simple strategy. **Figure 1** shows the effect of comparing the same samples (AD vs. non-demented healthy controls) using two different methods: Cufflinks and edgeR vs. Cufflinks and Fisher. The different convergence of methods will produce non-correlated, or correlated, lists of differentially expressed genes with the same sign, when sorted by Fold Change. Examining **Figure 1**, it is readily apparent from the correlation plots and values and from the residuals histogram and normal plot that only analyzing these NGS whole transcriptome datasets with the intersection of edgeR and a method based on upper quantile normalization and Fisher test we will obtain a robust set of differentially expressed genes, upregulated and downregulated. Recent advances in Bayesian methods applied to the analysis of differential expression (Glaus et al., 2012; Bi and Davuluri, 2013) reveal interesting advantages in comparison to the other established methods based on transcript reconstruction or binomial negative read mapping distribution, so they may represent interesting alternatives to the strategy reported here.

Concerning lncRNA transcriptome analyses, important consideration must be given to the choice of reference transcriptome database. A comprehensive specialized lincRNA database has recently become available (Xie et al., 2014; Noncode[1]), and the Ensembl project[2] and related annotation from the BioMart project/Havana group at the Sanger Institute provide effective identification, classification and counting of differentially expressed non-coding transcriptomes associated with Parkinson's disease treatment including an elaborate lincRNA subset (Goedert and Spillantini, 2006). Software capable of local alignments such as the latest version of bowtie2[3] is suggested for ncRNA searches, given the high sequence heterogeneity of these transcripts. Preliminary results of in-house unpublished bioinformatics analyses of whole transcriptomes from early and advanced AD and Control samples identified around 9.900 lncRNA transcripts, of which 600 were differentially expressed in the diseased brains (P value < 0.05 for each comparison). Among these annotated ncRNA transcripts we found antisense RNAs; small nucleolar RNA host genes; transcribed pseudogenes and non-coding transcripts from human leukocyte antigen regions. This example highlights a varied non-canonical transcript panorama, which calls for further functional and integrated transcriptome annotation and functional predictions. Section 5 will introduce some updated approaches to tackle this problem.

THE ROLE OF LONG ncRNAs IN NEURODEGENERATIVE DISEASES

A growing body of evidence links various ncRNAs with neurodegenerative diseases in general and specifically with AD. Both small and long non-coding RNAs are identified as possible suspects in this context by involvement with various neurodegeneration-related processes and proteins; these ncRNAs might be involved both in disease etiology and its progression. Therefore, intensified research of these ncRNAs can assist in both unveiling the mysteries that still remain in the processes underlying various neurodegenerative conditions and in identifying possible candidate target genes for therapeutic interference.

The first example we will describe is that of β-Secretase-1 (BACE1). Cleavage of amyloid precursor protein (APP) to yield the amyloid beta (Aβ) peptide by BACE1 rather than by α-Secretase at a later stage enables the protein's cleavage by γ-Secretase, which causes the formation of characteristic LOAD neuropathology of aggregated amyloid "plaques" (Faghihi et al., 2008). BACE1 mRNA is regulated by both short and lncRNAs. The transcript is subjected to down-regulation by several miRNAs, as well as to up-regulation by the lncRNA BACE1-anti-sense (BACE1-AS;

[1] http://www.noncode.org/

[2] http://www.ensembl.org/info/genome/genebuild/ncrna.html

[3] http://bowtie-bio.sourceforge.net/bowtie2/index.shtml

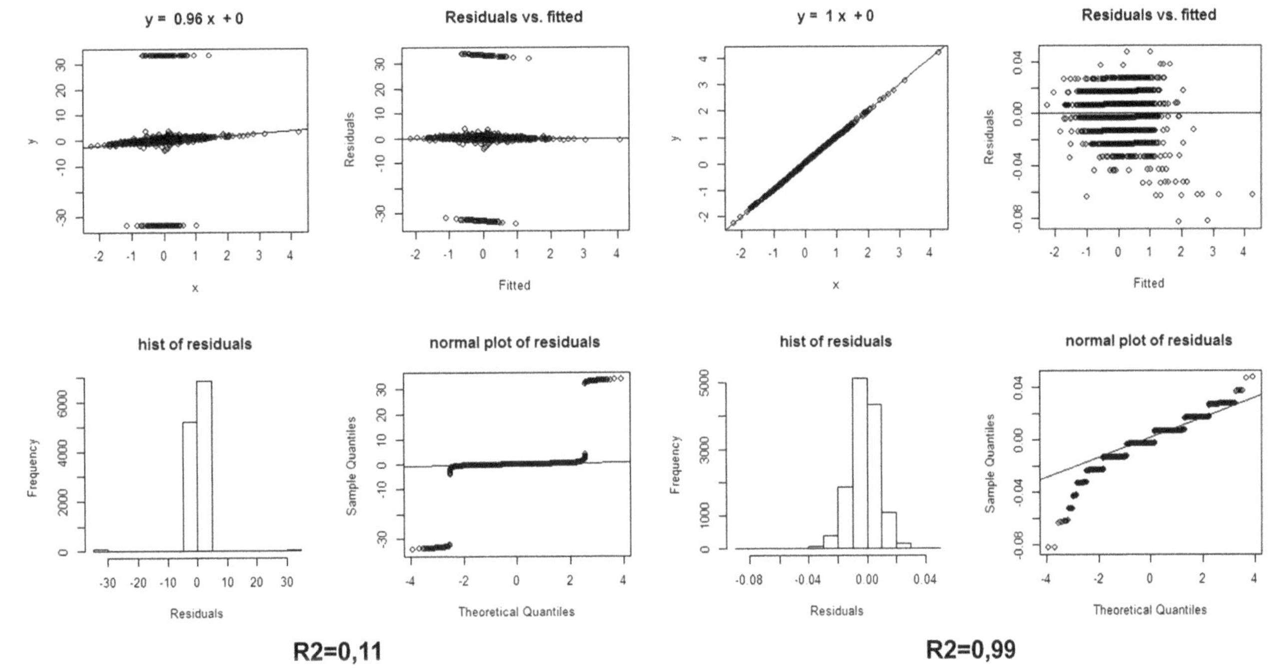

FIGURE 1 | (Left) Statistics on the differential expression results of AD whole transcriptome samples vs. non-demented controls, calculated by edgeR and Cufflink/Cuffdiff, sorted, and compared by Log2 Fold Change only, i.e., without any FDR threshold. (Right) Same statistics on the same samples, using the *Log2 Fold Changes* elaborated with edgeR and the simple Fisher test procedure described in the text. Hist: histogram.

Faghihi et al., 2008). The miRNA mechanism of operation was already described; but BACE1-AS displays a different mechanism of action. Specifically, the non-coding transcript is partially complementary to the coding transcript. The two bind to form a partially double-stranded RNA, increasing BACE1 mRNA stability – and therefore increasing both BACE1 mRNA and protein levels in the cell (Faghihi et al., 2008). Interestingly, both BACE1 and BACE1-AS transcripts are up-regulated in Alzheimer's brains, compared to control brains (Faghihi et al., 2008). Therefore, disruption of the regulatory nature of both short and long transcripts might change BACE1 protein levels, either promoting or interrupting with Aβ aggregates formation and consequently with AD pathology.

Sortilin-related receptor-1 (SORL1) is yet another protein that is connected to AD. This protein's function is still not entirely understood; however, it is believed to be involved in endocytosis, and also in APP recycling. SNPs in this gene have been associated with LOAD, by a possible mechanism of improper recycling of APP that allows the latter's compartmentalization with BACE1, resulting in Aβ formation (Rogaeva et al., 2007). SORL1 was found to be down-regulated in cerebrospinal fluids removed from AD patients (Ma et al., 2009) – However, an ncRNA transcribed in an antisense fashion from intron1 in the SORL1 gene is up-regulated in post-mortem AD brains. This ncRNA, annotated A51, promotes alternative splicing of SORL1, to the formation of a protein with poorer performance in APP localization, elevating Aβ accumulation and aggregation – hence possibly escalating neurodegenerative events and pushing toward the development of AD (Ciarlo et al., 2013).

Another antisense lncRNA which up-regulates protein levels is ubiquitin carboxyl-terminal esterase L1-AS (UCHL1-AS; Carrieri et al., 2012). UCHL1 is a De-Ubiquitinase highly abundant in the brain. A mutation in this gene was identified in a rare form of a familial Parkinson's disease (Leroy et al., 1998), known as PARK5 (Lesage and Brice, 2009). A different mutation was found in a rare progressive neurodegenerative disease (Bilguvar et al., 2013). Both mutations lead to the creation of a loss of function protein (Leroy et al., 1998; Bilguvar et al., 2013), indicating that proper de-ubiquitination and UCHL1 amounts are critical to avoid neurodegenerative deterioration. The UCHL1-AS ncRNA binds in its 5′ Region to the coding transcript's 5′ Region and causes up-regulation of protein levels without affecting mRNA levels (Carrieri et al., 2012). Such change in protein levels might have functional implications, and might have an impact on neurodegenerative pathology without any change in transcript levels.

Another possible aspect of lncRNA involvement in neurodegenerative disease may be in their functioning as competing endogenous RNAs (ceRNA). CeRNAs are transcripts that include miRNA recognition elements (MREs), and are therefore competing with other miRNA targets on miRNA binding, providing a layer of regulation over miRNA function (which is, by itself, regulatory). CeRNAs can be either pseudogenes (Poliseno et al., 2010) or lncRNAs (Cesana et al., 2011). Many lncRNAs with possible MREs have been identified through bioinformatics analyses as being differentially expressed in several neurodegenerative diseases – Huntington's disease (HD), AD and PD (Costa et al., 2012; Soreq et al., 2014). These lncRNAs might each affect multiple miRNAs, and through them many mRNA targets and the expression of many proteins – possibly explaining at least part of the vast transcriptional differences caused by neurodegenerative disease.

A possible emerging therapeutic aspect for ncRNAs can be observed in HD. HD is a severe progressive neurodegenerative disorder, with a known genetic cause – additional CAG nucleotides repeats in the Huntingtin (htt) gene. The disease involves depletion of brain-derived neurotrophic factor (BDNF) in the caudate and putamen nuclei of the striatum, involved in HD pathology (Ferrer et al., 2000). BDNF is weakly transcribed in the striatum, but is rather efficiently transcribed in the cerebral cortex from where it is anterogradely transported to the striatum (Altar et al., 1997). Over-expression of BDNF in the frontal cortex of HD-model mice seems to improve many of the HD symptoms (Gharami et al., 2008). The lncRNA BDNF-AS, also known as BDNF opposing strand (BDNFOS) is an antisense non-coding transcript to BDNF that down-regulates the amount of BDNF (Modarresi et al., 2012). Inhibition of this antisense transcript by small interfering RNA (siRNA) causes up-regulation of BDNF, both *in vitro* (in mouse and human cell lines) and *in vivo* (in mice; Modarresi et al., 2012). Is it possible to use such siRNA to up-regulate BDNF and ameliorate HD symptoms? Time will tell.

GENE NETWORKS AND THEIR APPLICATION IN INTERPRETING WHOLE TRANSCRIPTOME DATASETS: AN APPLICATION TO A NEURODEGENERATION STUDY

The cell is an integrated device made of several thousand types of interacting proteins, each of which is a molecular machine that carries out a specific task with precision. Cells live in a dynamical environment, where different situations require different proteins. For instance, when a cell senses a nutrient, or a risk of damage, it reacts accordingly by synthesizing transport channels or repair proteins. The cell therefore continuously monitors its environment and keeps calculating the amounts at which each type of protein is required. This information-processing function largely determines the rate of production and turnover of each protein, and is primarily carried out by gene networks.

The most familiar gene networks illustrate the dynamics behavior of the cell following exposure to an external signal (input): transcription networks where nodes are genes and edges represent transcriptional regulation of one gene by the protein product of another gene. Other gene networks include signaling pathways; functional interaction (FI) networks and modules; physical interaction networks; biochemical networks and so on. Biologically significant gene networks show a set of features which distinguishes them from random networks: the median number of gene connections must be greater than two; the degree distribution of the gene-to-gene connections must exhibit a tail indicating that many genes are poorly connected while few are highly connected ("gene hubs"); gene-to-gene interconnections must indicate that the network is enriched in "cliques," that is, sets of genes that are all pairwise connected. Such properties of non-random gene-to-gene connections and the structure of these interconnections to form cliques are characteristic of many biological networks (Khanin and Wit, 2006).

Differential equations currently form the most prominent approach for the modeling, analysis and simulation of molecular interaction networks. There is, however, a growing interest in qualitative network analysis approaches, capable of inferring qualitative properties of the system dynamics from the currently available incomplete and non-quantitative data. Non-linear dynamics networks, Boolean networks and graphs are the most popular approaches to qualitative networks, and the last approach is the one mostly used in the applications we present here.

The representation of a gene network (such as a gene regulatory network) as a graph allows the analysis of its structural properties by means of graph-theoretical techniques. The global connectivity properties of the network can, for instance, be described by the average degree and the degree of distribution of the vertices. The degree k of a vertex indicates the number of edges to which it is connected; together with the average k degree and the k degree distribution of the graph, it forms a set of properties that give an indication of the complexity of the graph and allow different types of graphs, and therefore networks, to be distinguished.

A very interesting, comprehensive and recent work compared microarray gene expression datasets between LOAD (376 samples) and control (173 samples) non-demented subjects, using a complex integrated approach (Zhang et al., 2013). Many hundreds of carefully selected brain tissues were profiled both by gene expression analyses using microarrays and by genomic DNA genotype analyses. Gene expression traits showing individual variability in transcript profiles were identified; the correlation (connectivity) strength between differentially expressed genes was calculated, and hierarchical cluster analysis was performed to construct the undirected gene co-expression network. Simultaneously, single nucleotide polymorphisms in brain DNA (eSNPs) were used as causal anchors in the construction of directed relationships among nodes in the network. Comparison of networks in LOAD and non-demented brains was performed to explore any effect on molecular interaction structures associated with the disease. Differentially connected modules in LOAD were investigated for their functional organization, module relevance to clinical outcome, as well as the enrichment of brain eSNPs. Finally, modules were rank-ordered for their strength of the functional enrichment, module correlation to neuropathology, and eSNP enrichment.

While this huge effort could not have detected lncRNAs which may be absent from the employed microarrays, the results highlight interesting functional modules. A module correlated with multiple LOAD clinical covariates was identified as being enriched with immune functions and pathways related to microglia activity. This module includes many classified as members of the complement cascade, such as toll-like receptor signaling, chemokines/cytokines, the Major Histocompatibility Complex, and the Fc-receptor system. This and many other studies on the neuro-inflammation correlates of LOAD supports the notion that targeting genes "located" in the center of the most inter-connected hubs may effectively disrupt disease-related networks for the purpose of therapy.

Another recent computational approach to identify functional network modules possibly implied in AD (Mayburd and Baranova, 2013) starts from gene lists, processed into different tiers of evidence consistently established by enrichment analysis across subsets of the same experiments and across different experiments and platforms. The "Cut-offs" were established through ontological and semantic enrichment, and the resulted shortened gene lists were re-expanded by Ingenuity Pathway Assistant tool[4]. The resulting sub-networks provided the basis for generating mechanistic hypotheses on the AD etiology that were partially validated by literature searches; these were called Compact Disease Model (CDM).

A simple and accessible, yet quite powerful, system for performing functional network analysis starting from gene sets is based on functional protein interaction networks (Wu et al., 2010). The focus here is on biological pathways. Pathway-based hypothesis generation is the basis for several popular data analysis systems, including GOMiner (Zeeberg et al., 2005), Gene Set Enrichment Analysis (Subramanian et al., 2005) and commercial tools such as Ingenuity Systems.

Reactome (Matthews et al., 2009)[5] is an expert-curated, highly reliable knowledgebase of human biological pathways. Pathways in Reactome are described as a series of molecular events that transform one or more input physical entities into one or more output entities in catalyzed or regulated ways by other entities. Entities include small molecules, proteins, complexes, post-translationally modified proteins, and nucleic acid sequences. Each physical entity is assigned a unique accession number and associated with a stable online database. This connects curated data in Reactome with online repositories of genome-scale data such as UniProt and EntrezGenes; ad makes it possible to un-ambiguously associate a position on the genome with a component of the pathway.

In contrast to pathway databases, collections of pairwise relationships among protein and genes offer much higher coverage but can draw in their results a noticeable number of "false" relationships between gene products, since a physical interaction does not obligatorily include a biological relationship. A FI network (Wu et al., 2010) combines curated interactions from Reactome and other pathway databases with un-curated pairwise relationships obtained from physical protein–protein interactions (PPi's) networks in human and model organisms, gene co-expression data, protein domain-domain interactions, protein interactions generated from text mining, and gene ontology (GO) annotations. This approach uses a naive Bayes classifier (NBC) to distinguish high-likelihood FIs from non-functional pairwise relationships as well as outright false positive ones.

Cytoscape (Saito et al., 2012)[6] is an open source software platform for visualizing molecular interaction networks and biological pathways and integrating these networks with annotations, gene expression profiles and other datasets. This software integrates analytical components through the concepts of "plugins," and a plugin is available for the generation of Reactome FI networks from gene lists[7].

Based on all of the above, we propose a strategy to extract functionally connected modules from lists of differentially expressed coding genes by following one of the analytical approaches detailed under "Differential Expression Analysis." Our strategy involves application of the Reactome search for FI to selected lists of genes with their relative Log2 Fold Change values (up- or down-) in the neurodegenerative brain. Manual selection from Cytoscape of a particular FI network containing a subset of the input gene lists enables to plugin a request to globally evaluate pathway and GO (MF/BP/CC) enrichment within this network. Given the importance and relevance of transcript modules, their FI plugin identification in the main networks of Cytoscape or Reactome should be followed by repeated enrichment analysis on each module. An update to the Reactome FI interaction module has been recently added (in 2013); however, using a more regularly maintained annotation resource such as Ingenuity could be important in terms of the sensibility and specificity of network identification. Enriched pathway lists can then be compared and intersected between different comparisons and conditions, yielding a high-profile view of the main functional clusters mobilized under disease progression or, simply, in the healthy/diseased transition. **Figure 2** presents an example of such a functional module based on NGS differential expression analysis from LOAD compared to non-demented brain and generated from the main FI network. This module highlights a calculated enrichment in down-regulated major histocompatibility complex genes, supporting the recent report by Zhang et al. (2013).

INTERPRETING LONG ncRNAs THROUGH FUNCTIONAL ANNOTATION AND TRANSCRIPTIONAL NETWORKS; PRIMARY APPLICATION TO A NEURODEGENERATION STUDY

The ncRNA-oriented interpretation of NGS transcriptome datasets in disease (and often in neurodegeneration) studies involves innovative and promising emerging directions. These include integration of the information derived from the differential analysis of coding and ncRNAs based on biomedical annotations reported in specialized resources such as ncRNA databases, Pubmed and OMIM. In addition, interesting semi-supervised learning methods have recently been proposed for efficient classification of lncRNA and disease state based on lncRNA expression profiles and associated comparisons (Chen and Yan, 2013; Yang et al., 2014). A recently proposed global prediction method for functional annotation of lncRNAs (Guo et al., 2013) involves the construction of a so-called "bi-colored" biological network combining two type vertices (protein-coding and non-coding genes) as well as two type edges (co-expression and PPi's) in the network. A number of case studies, including brain-expressed lncRNAs with predicted neuronal functions, suggest an advantage of bi-colored networks as compared to, for instance, co-expression networks (Guo et al., 2013). Although this approach has only been applied to murine data and is not yet available as usable software, it is clearly a very promising and powerful predictive annotation method.

The rapidly growing list of ncRNA sequences annotated in public databases such as Noncode (Xie et al., 2014)[8] has reached the noticeable total number of 210,831 lncRNAs in its latest release (v.4). However, immediately usable and well-established methods for understanding the functional role of lncRNAs are still

[4] http://www.ingenuity.com/products/ipa

[5] http://www.reactome.org/

[6] http://www.cytoscape.org

[7] http://wiki.reactome.org/index.php/Reactome_FI_Cytoscape_Plugin

[8] http://www.noncode.org

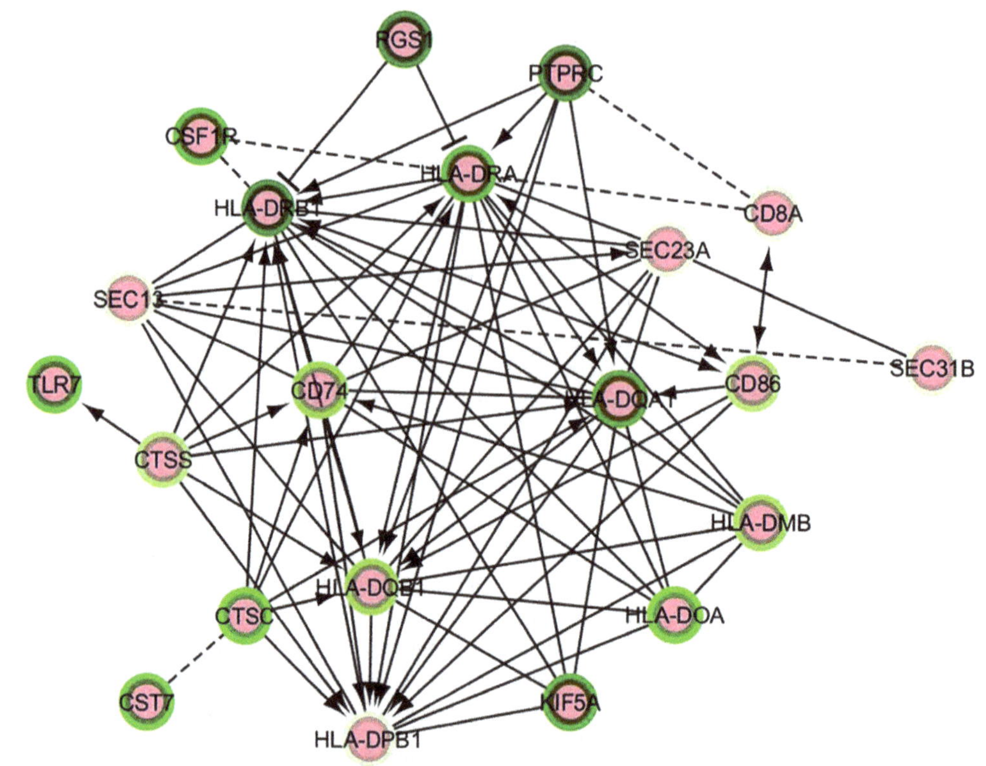

FIGURE 2 | A functional interaction network module from an AD vs. control NGS dataset analysis. The intensity of the green color in the border of the nodes represent the Log2FC – darker green corresponds to minor negative Log2FC, i.e., the most down-regulated genes. The edges represent functional interactions detected between the nodes; these can be non-directed, directed stimulatory (arrows), directed repressor (T-shaped edges) or inferred (discontinuous line edges).

lacking, even for those associated with the phenotype of interest. Likewise, it is still impossible to readily integrate the regulatory roles of differentially expressed lncRNAs with the gene networks of differentially regulated coding RNAs identified in the samples of interest. A simple strategy we propose to address this issue is to integrate the representation of regulatory relationships between coding and non-coding genes in terms of networks by combining the use of publicly available information resources (specialized ncRNA databases, PubMed etc.) and the Cytoscape software. The starting point is a table of regulatory links, e.g., literature search for ncRNAs/coding gene or PPi relationships in neurodegenerative diseases, starting from NGS transcriptome-based ncRNA gene list. **Table 1** presents an example for such a study based on datasets derived from AD vs. normal control brains.

This table can be suitably reformatted and elaborated in Cytoscape, generating one or more network representation. In **Figure 3**, every interaction type described in **Table 1** corresponds to a different edge line format; for instance, the "alternative splicing" relationship is represented by continuous line edges between the nodes; "repress_transcription" by a discontinuous point and segment line; "promotes_amyloid beta" by a double line edge and so on. Diamonds and ellipses represent ncRNA and coding genes, respectably. Directions of edges represent the direction of the FI, with arrow colors specifying positive (red), negative (green), or unknown (black) interactions. Such visual representation of literature-derived lncRNA/coding RNA interactions can be a useful starting point for integrating other functional information associated with the coding genes in these nodes.

A parallel strategy has recently been extended by another group (Xie et al., 2014), generating two distinct networks which can be integrated through a single bipartite lncRNA-disease network: a lncRNA-implicated disease network (lncDN), in which the nodes are disease and the links are lncRNAs; and a disease-associated lncRNA network (DlncN), in which the ncRNAs are nodes and the diseases are edges. Formal network analysis techniques, such as analysis of the network degree of distribution or topology and comparison with random networks highlighted the biological plausibility of this initial representation. The starting approach was the same as the one proposed here [data mining of specialized databases such as LncRNADisease (Chen et al., 2013) and manual paper scanning], and two tables were released: one linking diseases (including AD) with lncRNAs and another linking lncRNAs with other elements such as other RNAs, proteins, transcription factors and so on. These tables could be used to originate representations in Cytoscape with the method described above including also original information from the transcriptome NGS experiment under examination.

Current strategies for constructing databases of interaction networks primarily rely on the "heuristic" interactions derived

Table 1 | A selection of known coding/non-coding or coding/coding gene or protein–protein interactions involved in neurodegenerative diseases, derived from the current literature.

Gene_ID	ncRNA ?	TGT_ID	ncRNA ?	Interaction_type	Direction	Pos/Neg	Reference
A51	Y	SORL1	N	Alternative_splicing	>	?	Ma et al. (2009)
BACE1-AS	Y	BACE1	N	Post-transcriptionally_activate	>	+	Faghihi et al. (2008)
17A	Y	GABA B2	N	Alternative_splicing	>	?	Massone et al. (2011)
NMD29	Y	APP	N	Promotes_amyloid beta	>	+	Massone et al. (2012)
HAR1F	Y	REST	N	Repress_transcription	<	−	Johnson et al. (2010)
HAR1R	Y	REST	N	Repress_transcription	<	−	Johnson et al. (2010)
BDNFOS	Y	BDNF	N	Post-transcriptionally_repress	>	−	Ferrer et al. (2000)
UCHL1-AS	Y	UCHL1	N	Post-transcriptionally_activate	>	+	Carrieri et al. (2012)
HTTAS	Y	HTT	N	Post-transcriptionally_repress	>	−	Chung et al. (2011)
BACE1	N	APP	N	Promotes_amyloid beta	>	?	Goedert and Spillantini (2006)
HTT	N	BDNF	N	Promotes_transport	>	+	Gauthier et al. (2004)
UCHL1	N	APP	N	Unknown	?	?	Cottrell et al. (2005)
HTT	N	REST	N	Promotes_proper_localization	>	+	Zuccato et al. (2003)

The first and third columns report the source and target genes for a given interaction. The second and fourth column report whether the gene or the target is a non-coding RNA. The fifth column reports a range of classified interaction types which have been created "ad hoc" from what is available from the literature. The sixth column reports the direction of the interaction, the seventh column whether this is a positive or a negative interaction, and the last column reports the relevant reference.

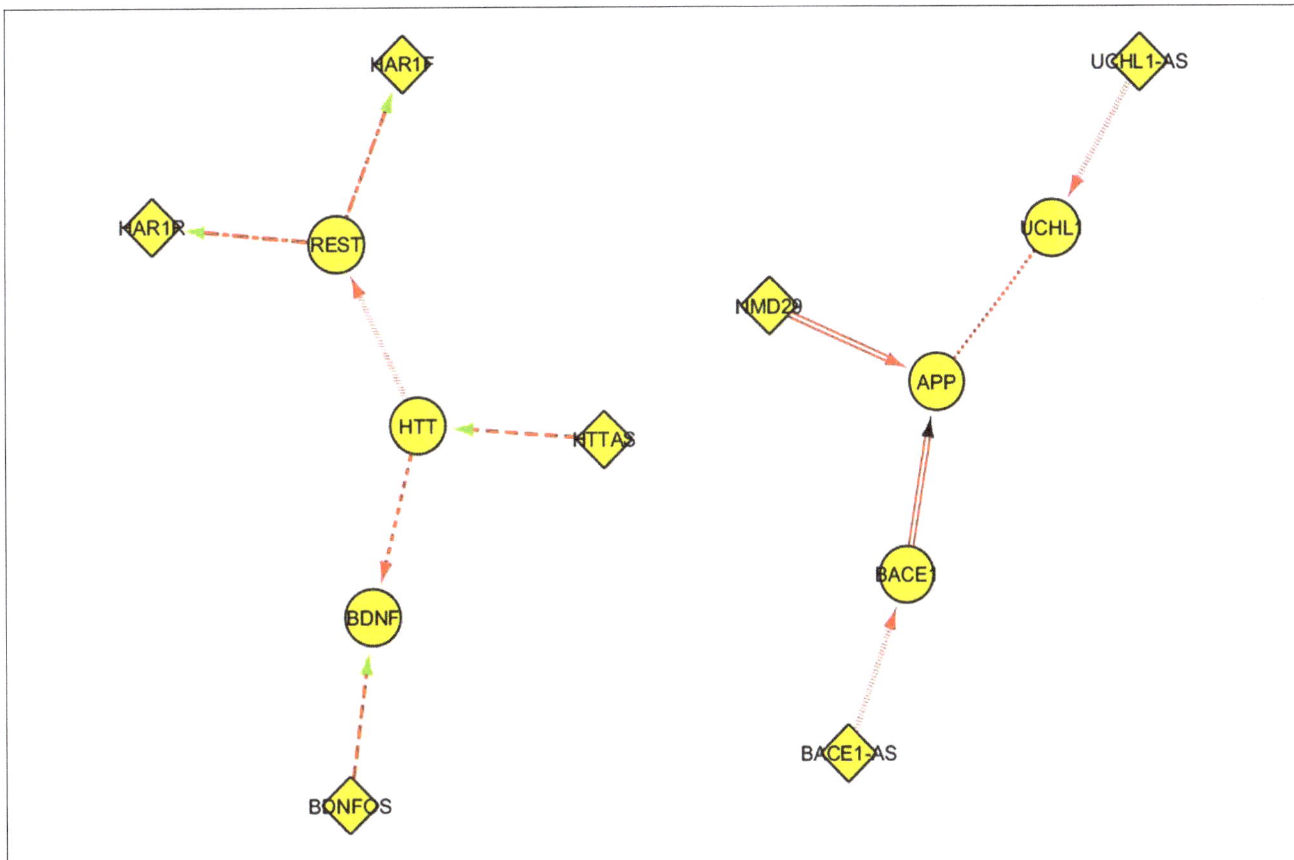

FIGURE 3 | A Cytoscape network representation of ncRNA/coding RNA and coding RNA/coding RNA manually annotated functional interactions described in Table 1. Diamonds represent ncRNA genes, ellipses represent coding genes. The functional meaning of the graphical format of the edges, including the color, is explained in the main text.

from careful database and literature scans. Yet more recently, a growing number of databases of RNA–RNA and protein-RNA interactions from CLIP-Seq experiments report annotated interaction networks between miRNA–circRNAs, miRNA–mRNA, and miRNA–lncRNAs (Li et al., 2014; Yuan et al., 2014). In particular, NPinter[9] is focused on interactions between ncRNAs (excluding tRNAs and rRNAs) and other biomolecules (proteins, RNAs and genomic DNA). These interactions are represented with the same Cytoscape web layout we propose here, are annotated as far as this is currently possible and their use may complement the procedure described above, providing a functional view of entire NGS transcriptome analyses, with focus on lncRNAs.

ACKNOWLEDGMENTS

We thank Mr Shahar Barbash, Jerusalem and Dr. Giulia Soldà of the University of Milan for fruitful discussions and useful insights on the construction of the ncRNA-coding RNA interaction table. This manuscript includes bioinformatics concepts, tools and strategies for whole transcriptome analysis derived from the FP7 Radiant project, in which Alessandro Guffanti is a PI for Genomnia srl (http://www.radiant-project.eu/).

REFERENCES

Altar, C. A., Cai, N., Bliven, T., Juhasz, M., Conner, J. M., Acheson, A. L., et al. (1997). Anterograde transport of brain-derived neurotrophic factor and its role in the brain. *Nature* 389, 856–860. doi: 10.1038/39885

Barbash, S., and Soreq, H. (2012). Threshold-independent meta-analysis of Alzheimer's disease transcriptomes shows progressive changes on hippocampal functions, epigenetics and microRNA regulation. *Curr. Alzheimer Res.* 9, 425–435. doi: 10.2174/156720512800492512

Berson, A., Barbash, S., Shaltiel, G., Goll, Y., Hanin, G., Greenberg, D. S., et al. (2012). Cholinergic-associated loss of hnRNP-A/B in Alzheimer's disease impairs cortical splicing and cognitive function in mice. *EMBO Mol. Med.* 4, 730–742. doi: 10.1002/emmm.201100995

Bi, Y., and Davuluri, R. V. (2013). NPEBseq: nonparametric empirical bayesian-based procedure for differential expression analysis of RNA-seq data. *BMC Bioinformatics* 14:262. doi: 10.1186/1471-2105-14-262

Bilguvar, K., Tyagi, N. K., Ozkara, C., Tuysuz, B., Bakircioglu, M., Choi, M., et al. (2013). Recessive loss of function of the neuronal ubiquitin hydrolase UCHL1 leads to early-onset progressive neurodegeneration. *Proc. Natl. Acad. Sci. U.S.A.* 110, 3489–3494. doi: 10.1073/pnas.1222732110

Carrieri, C., Cimatti, L., Biagioli, M., Beugnet, A., Zucchelli, S., Fedele, S., et al. (2012). Long non-coding antisense RNA controls Uchl1 translation through an embedded SINEB2 repeat. *Nature* 491, 454–457. doi: 10.1038/nature11508

Cesana, M., Cacchiarelli, D., Legnini, I., Santini, T., Sthandier, O., Chinappi, M., et al. (2011). A long noncoding RNA controls muscle differentiation by functioning as a competing endogenous RNA. *Cell* 147, 358–369. doi: 10.1016/j.cell.2011.09.028

Chen, G., Wang, Z., Wang, D., Qiu, C., Liu, M., Chen, X., et al. (2013). LncRNADisease: a database for long-non-coding RNA-associated diseases. *Nucleic Acids Res.* 41, D983–D986. doi: 10.1093/nar/gks1099

Chen, X., and Yan, G. Y. (2013). Novel human lncRNA-disease association inference based on lncRNA expression profiles. *Bioinformatics* 29, 2617–2624. doi: 10.1093/bioinformatics/btt426

Chung, D. W., Rudnicki, D. D., Yu, L., and Margolis, R. L. (2011). A natural antisense transcript at the Huntington's disease repeat locus regulates HTT expression. *Hum. Mol. Genet.* 20, 3467–3477. doi: 10.1093/hmg/ddr263

Ciarlo, E., Massone, S., Penna, I., Nizzari, M., Gigoni, A., Dieci, G., et al. (2013). An intronic ncRNA-dependent regulation of SORL1 expression affecting Aβ formation is upregulated in post-mortem Alzheimer's disease brain samples. *Dis. Model. Mech.* 6, 424–433. doi: 10.1242/dmm.009761

Cooper-Knock, J., Kirby, J., Ferraiuolo, L., Heath, P. R., Rattray, M., and Shaw, P. J. (2012). Gene expression profiling in human neurodegenerative disease. *Nat. Rev. Neurol.* 8, 518–530. doi: 10.1038/nrneurol.2012.156

Costa, V., Esposito, R., Aprile, M., and Ciccodicola, A. (2012). Non-coding RNA and pseudogenes in neurodegenerative diseases: "The (un)Usual Suspects." *Front. Genet.* 3:231. doi: 10.3389/fgene.2012.00231

Cottrell, B. A., Galvan, V., Banwait, S., Gorostiza, O., Lombardo, C. R., Williams, T., et al. (2005). A pilot proteomic study of amyloid precursor interactors in Alzheimer's disease. *Ann. Neurol.* 58, 277–289. doi: 10.1002/ana.20554

Faghihi, M. A., Modarresi, F., Khalil, A. M., Wood, D. E., Sahagan, B. G., Morgan, T. E., et al. (2008). Expression of a noncoding RNA is elevated in Alzheimer's disease and drives rapid feed-forward regulation of β-secretase. *Nat. Med.* 14, 723–730. doi: 10.1038/nm1784

Fatica, A., and Bozzoni, I. (2013). Long non-coding RNAs: new players in cell differentiation and development. *Nat. Rev. Genet.* 15, 7–21. doi: 10.1038/nrg3606

Ferrer, I., Goutan, E., Marın, C., Rey, M. J., and Ribalta, T. (2000). Brain-derived neurotrophic factor in Huntington disease. *Brain Res.* 866, 257–261. doi: 10.1016/S0006-8993(00)02237-X

Gauthier, L. R., Charrin, B. C., Borrell-Pagès, M., Dompierre, J. P., Rangone, H., Cordelières, F. P., et al. (2004). Huntingtin controls neurotrophic support and survival of neurons by enhancing BDNF vesicular transport along microtubules. *Cell* 118, 127–138. doi: 10.1016/j.cell.2004.06.018

Gharami, K., Xie, Y., An, J. J., Tonegawa, S., and Xu, B. (2008). Brain-derived neurotrophic factor over-expression in the forebrain ameliorates Huntington's disease phenotypes in mice. *J. Neurochem.* 105, 369–379. doi: 10.1111/j.1471-4159.2007.05137.x

Glaus, P., Honkela, A., and Rattray, M. (2012). Identifying differentially expressed transcripts from RNA-seq data with biological variation. *Bioinformatics* 28, 1721–1728. doi: 10.1093/bioinformatics/bts260

Goedert, M., and Spillantini, M. G. (2006). A century of Alzheimer's disease. *Science* 314, 777–781. doi: 10.1126/science.1132814

Guo, X., Gao, L., Liao, Q., Xiao, H., Ma, X., Yang, X., et al. (2013). Long non-coding RNAs function annotation: a global prediction method based on bi-colored networks. *Nucleic Acids Res.* 41, e35. doi: 10.1093/nar/gks967

Johnson, R., Richter, N., Jauch, R., Gaughwin, P. M., Zuccato, C., Cattaneo, E., et al. (2010). Human accelerated region 1 noncoding RNA is repressed by REST in Huntington's disease. *Physiol. Genomics* 41, 269–274. doi: 10.1152/physiolgenomics.00019.2010

Karni, S., Soreq, H., and Sharan, R. (2009). A network-based method for predicting disease-causing genes. *J. Comput. Biol.* 16, 181–189. doi: 10.1089/cmb.2008.05TT

Khanin, R., and Wit, E. (2006). How scale-free are biological networks. *J. Comput. Biol.* 13, 810–818. doi: 10.1089/cmb.2006.13.810

Leroy, E., Boyer, R., Auburger, G., Leube, B., Ulm, G., Mezey, E., et al. (1998). The ubiquitin pathway in Parkinson's disease. *Nature* 395, 451–452. doi: 10.1038/26652

Lesage, S., and Brice, A. (2009). Parkinson's disease: from monogenic forms to genetic susceptibility factors. *Hum. Mol. Genet.* 18, R48–R59. doi: 10.1093/hmg/ddp012

Li, J. H., Liu, S., Zhou, H., Qu, L. H., and Yang, J. H. (2014). starBase v2.0: decoding miRNA-ceRNA, miRNA-ncRNA and protein-RNA interaction networks from large-scale CLIP-Seq data. *Nucleic Acids Res.* 42, D92–D97. doi: 10.1093/nar/gkt1248

Ma, Q. L., Galasko, D. R., Ringman, J. M., Vinters, H. V., Edland, S. D., Pomakian, J., et al. (2009). Reduction of SorLA/LR11, a sorting protein limiting β-amyloid production, in Alzheimer disease cerebrospinal fluid. *Arch. Neurol.* 66, 448–457. doi: 10.1001/archneurol.2009.22

Massone, S., Ciarlo, E., Vella, S., Nizzari, M., Florio, T., Russo, C., et al. (2012). NDM29, a RNA polymerase III-dependent non coding RNA, promotes amyloidogenic processing of APP and amyloid β secretion. *Biochim. Biophys. Acta* 1823, 1170–1177. doi: 10.1016/j.bbamcr.2012.05.001

Massone, S., Vassallo, I., Fiorino, G., Castelnuovo, M., Barbieri, F., Borghi, R., et al. (2011). 17A, a novel non-coding RNA, regulates GABA B alternative splicing and signaling in response to inflammatory stimuli and in Alzheimer disease. *Neurobiol. Dis.* 41, 308–317. doi: 10.1016/j.nbd.2010.09.019

[9]http://www.bioinfo.org/NPInter

Matsui, M., Chu, Y., Zhang, H., Gagnon, K. T., Shaikh, S., Kuchimanchi, S., et al. (2013). Promoter RNA links transcriptional regulation of inflammatory pathway genes. *Nucleic Acids Res.* 41, 10086–100109. doi: 10.1093/nar/gkt777

Matthews, L., Gopinath, G., Gillespie, M., Caudy, M., Croft, D., de Bono, B., et al. (2009). Reactome knowledgebase of human biological pathways and processes. *Nucleic Acids Res.* 37(suppl. 1), D619–D622. doi: 10.1093/nar/gkn863

Mayburd, A., and Baranova, A. (2013). Knowledge-based compact disease models identify new molecular players contributing to early-stage Alzheimer's disease. *BMC Syst. Biol.* 7:121. doi: 10.1186/1752-0509-7-121

Mercer, T. R., Dinger, M. E., Sunkin, S. M., Mehler, M. F., and Mattick, J. S. (2008). Specific expression of long noncoding RNAs in the mouse brain. *Proc. Natl. Acad. Sci. U.S.A.* 105, 716–721. doi: 10.1073/pnas.0706729105

Modarresi, F., Faghihi, M. A., Lopez-Toledano, M. A., Fatemi, R. P., Magistri, M., Brothers, S. P., et al. (2012). Inhibition of natural antisense transcripts *in vivo* results in gene-specific transcriptional upregulation. *Nat. Biotech.* 30, 453–459. doi: 10.1038/nbt.2158

Poliseno, L., Salmena, L., Zhang, J., Carver, B., Haveman, W. J., and Pandolfi, P. P. (2010). A coding-independent function of gene and pseudogene mRNAs regulates tumour biology. *Nature* 465, 1033–1038. doi: 10.1038/nature09144

Robinson, M. D., McCarthy, D. J., and Smyth, G. K. (2010). edgeR: a Bioconductor package for differential expression analysis of digital gene expression data. *Bioinformatics* 26, 139–140. doi: 10.1093/bioinformatics/btp616

Rogaeva, E., Meng, Y., Lee, J. H., Gu, Y., Kawarai, T., Zou, F., et al. (2007). The neuronal sortilin-related receptor SORL1 is genetically associated with Alzheimer disease. *Nat. Genet.* 39, 168–177. doi: 10.1038/ng1943

Saito, R., Smoot, M. E., Ono, K., Ruscheinski, J., Wang, P. L., Lotia, S., et al. (2012). A travel guide to Cytoscape plugins. *Nat. Methods* 9, 1069–1076. doi: 10.1038/nmeth.2212

Soreq, L., Guffanti, A., Simchovitz, A., Salomonis, N., Bergman, H., Israel, Z., et al. (2014). Long non-coding RNA and alternative splicing modulations in Parkinson's leukocytes identified by RNA sequencing. *PLOS Comput. Biol.* (in press).

Subramanian, A., Tamayo, P., Mootha, V. K., Mukherjee, S., Ebert, B. L., Gillette, M. A., et al. (2005). Gene set enrichment analysis: a knowledge-based approach for interpreting genome-wide expression profiles. *Proc. Natl. Acad. Sci. U.S.A.* 102, 15545–15550. doi: 10.1073/pnas.0506580102

Trapnell, C., Williams, B. A., Pertea, G., Mortazavi, A. M., Kwan, G., van Baren, M. J., et al. (2010). Transcript assembly and quantification by RNA-Seq reveals unannotated transcripts and isoform switching during cell differentiation. *Nat. Biotechnol.* 28, 511–515. doi: 10.1038/nbt.1621

Wu, G., Feng, X., and Stein, L. (2010). A human functional protein interaction network and its application to cancer data analysis. *Genome Biol.* 11, R53. doi: 10.1186/gb-2010-11-5-r53

Xie, C., Yuan, J., Li, H., Li, M., Zhao, G., Bu, D., et al. (2014). NONCODEv4: exploring the world of long non-coding RNA genes. *Nucleic Acids Res.* 42, D98–D103. doi: 10.1093/nar/gkt1222

Yang, X., Gao, L., Guo, X., Shi, X., Wu, H., Song, F., et al. (2014). A network based method for analysis of lncRNA-disease associations and prediction of lncRNAs implicated in diseases. *PLoS ONE* 9:e87797. doi: 10.1371/journal.pone.0087797

Yuan, J., Wu, W., Xie, C., Zhao, G., Zhao, Y., and Chen, R. (2014). NPInter v2.0: an updated database of ncRNA interactions. *Nucleic Acids Res.* 42, D104–D108. doi: 10.1093/nar/gkt1057

Zeeberg, B. R., Qin, H., Narasimhan, S., Sunshine, M., Cao, H., Kane, D. W., et al. (2005). High-Throughput GoMiner, an 'industrial-strength' integrative gene ontology tool for interpretation of multiple-microarray experiments, with application to studies of Common Variable Immune Deficiency (CVID). *BMC Bioinformatics* 6:168. doi: 10.1186/1471-2105-6-168

Zhang, B., Gaiteri, C., Bodea, L. G., Wang, Z., McElwee, J., Podtelezhnikov, A. A., et al. (2013). Integrated systems approach identifies genetic nodes and networks in late-onset Alzheimer's disease. *Cell* 135, 707–720. doi: 10.1016/j.cell.2013.03.030

Zuccato, C., Tartari, M., Crotti, A., Goffredo, D., Valenza, M., Conti, L., et al. (2003). Huntingtin interacts with REST/NRSF to modulate the transcription of NRSE-controlled neuronal genes. *Nat. Genet.* 35, 76–83. doi: 10.1038/ng1219

6

Non-coding RNAs in chromatin disease involving neurological defects

Floriana Della Ragione[1,2], Miriam Gagliardi[1,2], Maurizio D'Esposito[1,2] and Maria R. Matarazzo[1,2]*

[1] *Functional Genomics and Epigenomics Laboratory, Institute of Genetics and Biophysics "ABT," Consiglio Nazionale delle Ricerche, Naples, Italy*
[2] *Laboratorio di Genomica e di Epigenomica, Istituto di Ricovero e Cura a Carattere Scientifico Neuromed, Pozzilli, Italy*

Novel classes of small and long non-coding RNAs (ncRNAs) are increasingly becoming apparent, being engaged in diverse structural, functional and regulatory activities. They take part in target gene silencing, play roles in transcriptional, post-transcriptional and epigenetic processes, such as chromatin remodeling, nuclear reorganization with the formation of silent compartments and fine-tuning of gene recruitment into them. Among their functions, non-coding RNAs are thought to act either as guide or scaffold for epigenetic modifiers that write, erase, and read the epigenetic signature over the genome. Studies on human disorders caused by defects in epigenetic modifiers and involving neurological phenotypes highlight the disruption of diverse classes of non-coding RNAs. Noteworthy, these molecules mediate a wide spectrum of neuronal functions, including brain development, and synaptic plasticity. These findings imply a significant contribution of ncRNAs in pathophysiology of the aforesaid diseases and provide new concepts for potential therapeutic applications.

Correspondence:
Maria R. Matarazzo, Institute of Genetics and Biophysics "ABT," Consiglio Nazionale delle Ricerche, Via Pietro Castellino 111, Naples 80131, Italy
e-mail: maria.matarazzo@igb.cnr.it

Keywords: Rett syndrome, ICF syndrome, non-coding RNA, chromatin, neurological desease, imprinting

INTRODUCTION

Our common view of the complexity of mammalian transcriptome has been revolutionized by the advent in the high-throughput sequencing highlighting that tens of thousands of sites produce transcripts with tiny protein-coding potential. Indeed, it is now increasingly clear that the vast majority of the genome is transcribed in both sense and antisense directions and this transcription is active in a cell context- and a developmental stage-specific way. Moreover, a rigorous distinction between protein-coding and non-coding transcripts is misleading, considering that some non-coding RNAs (ncRNAs) can be translated and other RNA transcripts may participate in regulatory and functional processes, rather than serving simply as intermediates for translation.

NcRNAs are commonly classified based on their size in two major groups: small ncRNA (sncRNAs, 20-30nt) which are involved in post-transcriptional regulation of target RNAs via RNAi, and/or modifying other RNAs, including microRNAs (miRNAs), Piwi-interacting RNAs (piRNAs) and small nucleolar RNAs (snoRNAs), and the heterogeneous group of long ncRNAs (lncRNAs, >200nt), such as transcribed ultraconserved regions (T-UCRs) and large intergenic ncRNAs (lincRNAs) (**Figure 1**).

MiRNAs are a class of small ncRNA with a role in post-transcriptional gene regulation through the base-pairing with the 3′-UTR of the target transcript. This interaction leads to degradation of the target or to inhibition of translation (Kim et al., 2009). siRNAs and piRNAs are small ncRNAs generated through the processing of LINE-1 and other retrotransposons, being involved in the silencing of repetitive elements (Saxena et al., 2012).

LncRNAs have roles in transcriptional and epigenetic regulation by recruiting transcription factors and chromatin-modifying complexes to specific nuclear and genomic sites (Khalil et al., 2009); in alternative splicing and other post-transcriptional RNA modifications through the assembly of nuclear domains containing RNA-processing factors (Wang and Chang, 2011; Caudron-Herger and Rippe, 2012). The emerging structural and functional activities of lncRNAs were categorized within a well-designed framework as molecules of signals, decoys, guides, and scaffolds (Wang and Chang, 2011).

NON-CODING RNAs IN NEURONAL FUNCTIONS

NcRNAs are involved in mediating a broad spectrum of biological processes especially those occurring in the central nervous system, where neural cells are highly expressing diverse classes of ncRNAs. Indeed, ncRNAs provide neural cells with the ability to precisely control the spatio-temporal expression of genes, which is a critical aspect for fulfilling complex neurobiological processes. The newest finding that in neural tissue mRNAs express significantly longer 3′UTRs, compared to other tissues, provides intriguing mechanisms for cell type-specific regulations that are governed by miRNAs, RNA-binding proteins and ribonucleoprotein aggregates (Wang and Yi, 2014).

For instance, various miRNAs show selective expression or are particularly abundant in brain (Kosik, 2006). Indeed, DICER ablation in mouse cerebral cortex, interrupting the biogenesis of all miRNAs, reduces the cortical size, by decreasing neural stem cell and neural progenitor pool, increasing apoptosis and affecting neuronal differentiation, whereas its ablation in postmitotic neurons in the cortex and hippocampus results in smaller cortex and increased cell death (Bian and Sun, 2011). Specific miRNAs have been implicated in neuronal differentiation and maintenance of neuronal phenotype (Im and Kenny, 2012), being integrated with the circuitry of CREB, repressor-element-1 (RE1)-silencing transcription factor REST and REST-corepressor 1 (CoREST), which

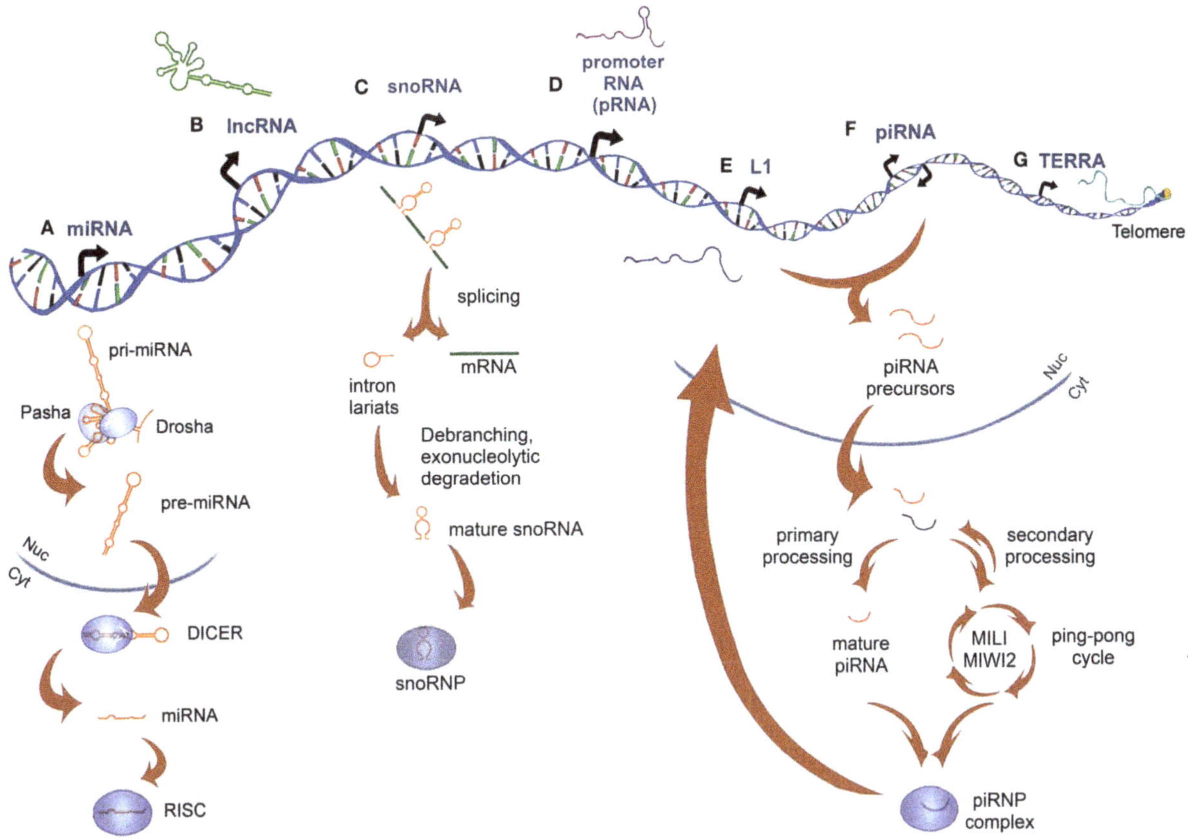

Syndrome	Non-coding RNA		References
Rett	miRNA	miR-30a/d; miR-381; miR-495; miR-29; miR-14a/b; miR-132; miR-212	Wang et al,2006; Im et al, 2010; Urdinguio et al, 2010
	lncRNA	AK081227; AK087060; Evf2; Gtl2/MEG3	Petazzi et al, 2013
	Repeats	LINE1; IAP; Major satellite	Muotri et al, 2010.
	piRNA	DQ541777	Saxena et al, 2012
ICF	miRNA	miR-338; miR-196a; miR-34b; miR-34c; miR-99b; let-7e; miR-125a	Aschrali et al, 2008; Gatto et al, 2010
	lncRNA	TERRA	Yehezkel et al, 2008
	Repeats	LINE1; Satellite-II; Satellite-α; NBL2	Heyn et al, 2012
	pRNA		Schmitz et al, 2010
Prader-Willy	lncRNA	Ube3a-ATS	Meng et al, 2012
Angelman	snoRNA	snord115; snord116	Sahoo et al, 2008
Beckwith-Wiedemann	miRNA	miR-483-5p	Han et al, 2013
	lncRNA	KCNQ1OT1	Choufani et al, 2013

FIGURE 1 | Non-coding RNAs: biogenesis and their relation to chromatin disorders. (A) MicroRNAs originate as primary miRNA (pri-miRNAs) that are processed by the DROSHA/PASHA complex in the nucleus. The resulting precursor miRNAs (pre-miRNAs) are exported into the cytoplasm, where they are processed by DICER1 to form mature miRNAs, which interact with RNA-induced silencing complex (RISC), acquiring a post-transcriptional silencing activity **(B)** Long non-coding RNA are heterogeneous transcripts, often longer than 2 kb, transcribed from intra- and intergenic regions by RNApol-II and, rarely, RNApol-III **(C)** Small nucleolar RNAs (snoRNAs) are codified primarily from introns. After the pre-mRNA generation, the transcript is spliced and the intron lariat is debranched and trimmed. The mature snoRNA interacts with ribonuclear proteins (RNPs), before being exported into the cytoplasm with a role in ribosomal RNA (rRNA) modification and processing, or retained into the nucleus, where it plays a role in alternative splicing and other unknown functions **(D)** In mouse, promoter-RNAs (pRNAs) are generated from intergenic regions located around 2 kb upstream to the pre-rRNA transcriptional start site. They are processed in molecules of 150–250 nucleotides and are thought to form a DNA:RNA triplex at the promoter, from which they are transcribed **(E)** Long interspersed nuclear elements-1 (LINE-1 or L1s) are retrotransposons dispersed throughout the genome that can be transcribed and inserted as extracopies of themselves **(F)** Piwi-interacting RNA (piRNA) originates as precursors from transposons and large piRNA clusters, then they are processed and exported into cytoplasm, where they undergo a primary or cyclic secondary processing (ping pong cycle, mediated by PIWI, MIWI, and MIWI2 proteins in mouse) and the assembly in piRNP complexes that modulate transposon activity and gene expression **(G)** Telomeric repeat-containing RNA (TERRA) is a large non-coding RNA transcribed from chromosome ends directly involved in the telomeric heterochromatin organization and preservation of telomere length. An up-to-date summary of the diverse class of ncRNAs, which have been functionally associated to Rett Syndrome and ICF Syndrome, as well as to the imprinting disease Prader-Willy/Angelman and Beckwith–Wiedemann syndromes, is reported in the table.

are master transcriptional and epigenetic regulators of neural genes and neural cell fate decisions (Qureshi and Mehler, 2012).

While most efforts have been devoted in identifying the neurobiological functions of miRNA, studies characterizing the expression and function of other classes of small and long ncRNAs in the central nervous system has begun to emerge. For instance, a specific set of piRNAs is highly expressed in the hippocampus, where they might play a role in spine morphogenesis (Lee et al., 2011). LncRNAs are also likely to have important roles in shaping brain development (Mercer et al., 2008; Ponjavic et al., 2009). A functional study examined the chromatin-state signature of neural progenitor cells (NPCs) identifying around one thousand lincRNAs, with some of them associated with hippocampal development, oligodendrocytes maturation and GABAergic-neuronal function (Guttman et al., 2009). A large percentage of these lincRNAs are involved in recruiting chromatin-modifying complexes to their genomic target sites, serving as scaffolds to specify the pattern of histone modifications (Tsai et al., 2010). Moreover, MeCP2 physically associates with RNCR3 (retinal non-coding RNA 3), unveiling new mechanisms of MeCP2/lncRNAs-mediated chromatin remodeling (Maxwell et al., 2013).

These observations provide insight into the complex interplay between ncRNAs and multifunctional epigenetic and transcriptional regulatory complexes coordinating neuronal lineage specification. In line with that, it is expected that if these ncRNAs regulate the development and maintenance of healthy neurons, their dysfunction may contribute to neurodevelopmental abnormalities (Qureshi and Mehler, 2012).

Here, we focused on the latest findings linking ncRNAs into the molecular and neural phenotypical defects of human disorders with deficiencies in (i) epigenetic modifiers, like MeCP2 (methyl-CpG-binding-protein-2) for the Rett syndrome (RTT) and DNMT3B (DNA-methyltrasferase-3B) for the Immumodeficiency, Centromeric instability, Facial anomalies (ICF) syndrome (Type1) or (ii) in the establishment of DNA methylation signature, as for the imprinting disorders (**Figure 1**).

Mutations in MeCP2 gene are linked to the severe postnatal neurodevelopmental disorder RTT syndrome, the second most common cause of mental retardation in females. It is characterized by developmental stagnation and regression, loss of purposeful hand movements and speech, stereotypic hand movements, deceleration of brain growth, autonomic dysfunction and seizures (Chahrour and Zoghbi, 2007). The ICF syndrome is caused by genetic defects in the catalytic activity of DNMT3B protein leading to genomic DNA hypomethylation and heterochromatin defects (Matarazzo et al., 2009). Beside immunological abnormalities, patients exhibit from mild to severe mental retardation and neurologic problems, including slow cognitive and motor development and psychomotor impairment (Ehrlich et al., 2006).

Defective inheritance of the imprinted signature is the main cause of the Prader–Willi (PWS) Angelman (AS) and Beckwith–Wiedemann syndromes (BWS). Both AS and PWS show learning dysfunctions and behavioral defects. Mutations or loss of the maternally-expressed gene UBE3A are responsible for AS, whereas loss of paternally-expressed genes, probably including SNRPN, causes PWS. BWS is caused by altered expression of imprinted genes belonging to a gene cluster at 11p15.5, and patients exhibits neurodevelopmental defects (Kent et al., 2008).

NON-CODING RNAs AS TRANSCRIPTIONAL AND POST-TRANSCRIPTIONAL REGULATORS

RTT is primarily caused by mutations in MECP2 gene, codifying a protein involved in both transcriptional repression and activation. Mecp2-null mice show many neurological symptoms recapitulating RTT (Della Ragione et al., 2012). Until recently, the classical approach to search for MeCP2 target genes involved in Rett pathogenesis was focused on protein-coding RNA transcripts. However, recent findings suggest a role of MeCP2 in transcriptional regulation of different classes of ncRNAs.

In 2010, two different large-scale analyses highlighted global dysregulation of miRNAs in MeCP2-null mice. Wu and colleagues identified several up- and down-regulated miRNAs in cerebella of Mecp2-deficient mice and, for many of them a direct promoter binding of MeCP2 was demonstrated. Interestingly, MeCP2 regulates the expression of a large cluster of miRNAs embedded within the Dlk1-Gtl2 imprinting domain, showing different levels of deregulation, suggesting the existence of miRNA-specific posttranscriptional regulation. Remarkably, MeCP2 silences miR-30a/d, miR-381 and miR-495, which in turn repress Brain-derived neurotrophic factor (BDNF), the down-regulated target gene in Mecp2-null mice (Wang et al., 2006); this suggests a multilayered MeCP2-mediated transcriptional regulation of BDNF (Wu et al., 2010).

Similarly, microarray expression analysis of Mecp2-null brains revealed alterations of several miRNAs. Noteworthy, deregulated miR-29 and miR-146 are known to have roles in neural and glial cells and its association with neurological disorders is reported (Urdinguio et al., 2007).

Although the classical form of RTT is associated with loss-of-function MECP2 mutations, duplication of this gene is responsible for RTT-like neurological phenotypes (Del Gaudio et al., 2006); therefore, a fine-tuning of MeCP2 level might be important for normal development.

In the last years, some reports highlighted a miRNAs contribution to maintain the correct levels of MeCP2. In rat neurons homeostatic mechanisms regulate MeCP2 levels through the stimulation of BDNF expression, which in turn induces miR132, thereby silencing MeCP2 expression (Klein et al., 2007). Later, it was shown that miR-212, located in the same cluster of miR-132, also targets MeCP2 and that MeCP2 silences the expression of both miRNAs, confirming the existence of a similar negative homeostatic feed-back loop between MeCP2 and mir-212, (Im et al., 2010).

Although several works highlighted a role of MeCP2 in transcriptional regulation of miRNAs, its involvement in the control of lncRNAs was poorly investigated. In Mecp2-deficient cerebella increased levels of Gtl2/MEG3, an imprinted ncRNA specifically expressed from maternal allele has been described. MeCP2-direct binding to the differentially methylated region controlling maternal specific expression was reported, suggesting a role of MeCP2 in the repression of paternal allele in the cerebellum (Jordan et al., 2007).

Very recently, the comparison of MeCP2-null and wt mouse brains transcriptome profiles highlighted 701 deregulated lncRNAs. Among lncRNAs with neuronal functions, the authors validated the up-regulation of AK081227 and AK087060, whose promoter is directly bound to MeCP2 in wt. Interestingly, the up-regulation of AK087060 is associated with an overexpression of the host gene, Arhgef26, codifying a Rho-guanin-nucleotide-exchange-factor (GEF) involved in neuronal functions, whereas the up-regulation of AK081227 is associated to a down-regulation of its host gene, the GABA-receptor-subunit-rho-2 (Gabrr2). Noteworthy, the GABAergic inhibitory neurotransmission is impaired in RTT (Coghlan et al., 2012). These findings indicate that lncRNAs deregulation in a MeCP2-deficient context may contribute to the RTT pathophysiology providing evidence for disrupted cis-regulated mechanisms in the disorder (Petazzi et al., 2013).

Recently, a functional link between ncRNAs, MeCP2 and GABAergic interneuron development has been found. Embryonic ventral forebrain-2 (Evf2) lncRNA is transcribed from the conserved Dlx-5/6 intergenic enhancer and regulates Dlx5 and Dlx6 expression during forebrain development by trans- and cis-acting mechanisms, respectively. It was shown that Evf2 recruits both DLX2 (activator) and MeCP2 (repressor) on the same ultraconserved Dlx5/6 enhancers in order to balance the correct expression of Dlx5 and Dlx6 during brain development. Remarkably, Evf2 loss causes GABAergic interneurons decrease in developing hippocampus. GABA-dependent inhibitory cortical activity is impaired in RTT-mice, thus MeCP2 and Evf2 loss may share common mechanisms (Bond et al., 2009). More recently, it is shown that MeCP2 represses Evf2 and Dlx5, whose expression is stimulated by DLX1/2 and that Evf2 prevents the DNA methylation of Dlx5/6 enhancer regardless MeCP2 (Berghoff et al., 2013). Altogether, these results suggest that ncRNAs deregulation may contribute to RTT pathoetiology.

While MECP2 reads and interprets the epigenetic signature, the *de novo* DNMT3B is the epigenetic factor establishing it during development.

Mutations interfering with its catalytic activity are known to affect the transcriptional profile of several hundred protein-coding genes in ICF patients' derived cells, with enriched functional classes including development and neurogenesis (Jin et al., 2008). Most of them do not exhibit promoter methylation defects, meaning that they are indirectly affected by DNMT3B deficiency (Matarazzo et al., 2004). Interestingly, a significant proportion of these genes are target of miRNAs, which are inversely deregulated in ICF-derived cells, suggesting that miRNAs are integrated in the DNMT3B-mediated regulatory circuitry modulating cell-specific gene expression program (Gatto et al., 2010). MiR-338 is the most up-regulated miRNAs with brain-specific functions, while among the down-regulated miRNAs, miR-196a is transcribed from intergenic regions within Hox genes clusters in vertebrates. As for the Hox genes, miR-196a acts as regulators of the nervous system development in embryos (Kosik, 2006). Intriguingly, LHX2, which is crucial for the proper development of cerebral cortex in mouse embryo is a miR-196a target gene, and results overexpressed in DNMT3B-deficient cells (Gatto et al., 2010).

Beyond the pivotal role of DNA methylation in miRNAs transcriptional control, there are examples describing the effect of ncRNAs on the epigenetic machinery and the DNMTs. The finding that a promoter-associated RNA recruits DNMT3B, inducing the methylation and the following repression of ribosomal RNA genes (rDNA) reveals a fascinating mechanism of RNA-dependent DNA methylation in mammals (Schmitz et al., 2010). Interestingly, DNMT3B exhibits binding specificity for a DNA:RNA-triplex, which are structures contributing to promoter-specific transcriptional repression by compromising transcription factor binding. That raises the exciting possibility that triplex-dependent recruitment of DNMT3B to specific genes might be a common function of regulatory ncRNAs.

Ribosomal RNAs are the target of another class of ncRNAs, the small nucleolar RNAs. These molecules are intermediate-sized ncRNAs (60–300 nt) predominantly intronic, which might be exported for processing the ribosomal RNA and/or remain in the nucleus for alternative splicing of mRNAs through yet unknown mechanisms.

They have been found playing an important role in imprinting disorders, specifically those with a neurodevelopmental component, such as PWS and AS. They are caused by several genetic and epigenetic mechanisms involving the 15q11–q13 imprinted locus, which contains a cluster of tandemly-arranged snoRNAs (Sahoo et al., 2008). Loss of the snoRNA HBII-52 has been associated to PWS, in which it regulates the alternative splicing of the serotonin receptor HTR2C precursor mRNA, resulting in a protein with reduced function. Additional snoRNAs at 15q11.2, including the Snord116 cluster, are even more likely candidates for causing PWS (Duker et al., 2010).

The PWS imprinting-control region contains multiple neuron-specific ncRNAs, including the antisense transcript to AS-causing ubiquitin-ligase Ube3a (Ube3a-ATS) (Meng et al., 2012). Neuron-specific transcriptional progression through Ube3a-ATS correlates with paternal Ube3a silencing. Intriguingly, topoisomerase inhibitors represses Ube3a-ATS inducing formation of DNA:RNA hybrids (R-loops), thus reverting the paternal allele silencing and providing a means to compensate for the loss of maternal Ube3a in AS patients (Powell et al., 2013).

Beckwith-Wiedemann (BWS) syndrome is also associated with altered expression of imprinted genes at 11p15.5. In particular, BWS results from increased expression of the paternally-expressed growth promoter IGF2 and/or reduced expression (or loss of function) of the maternal growth suppressor CDKN1C. An intragenic miRNA of the imprinted IGF2 (miR-483-5p) regulates MeCP2 levels through a human-specific binding site in the MECP2 long 3′-UTR. There is an inverse correlation of miR-483-5p and MeCP2 levels in developing human brains and fibroblasts from BWS patients. Importantly, the expression of miR-483-5p rescues abnormal dendritic spine phenotype of neurons overexpressing MeCP2.

LncRNA appear to play a key role in the BWS phenotype. KCNQ1OT1 is paternally transcribed from the imprinted-domain-2 of chromosome 11p15.5 (Weksberg et al., 2001). In the majority of BWS, loss of maternal methylation at IC2 is associated with bi-allelic transcription of the KCNQ1OT1 maternal allele (Choufani et al., 2013) and the bi-allelic silencing of the imprinted-domain genes, including the cell growth inhibitor CDKN1C (Diaz-Meyer et al., 2003). Notably, CDKN1C loss-of-function causes the typical overgrowth and increased risk to develop embryonic tumor in BWS patients.

NON-CODING RNAs AND TRANSCRIPTIONAL CONTROL OF REPEATS AND HETEROCHROMATIN

Recent reports highlighted a widespread misregulation of repeat-elements in Mecp2-deficient contexts. In rodents, MeCP2 loss is responsible for alteration of LINE1 neuronal transcription and retrotransposition (Muotri et al., 2010). An increased activity of L1 promoter in mouse Mecp2-null NPCs correlates to increased transcription. Noteworthy, increased L1 retrotransposition was also observed in NPCs generated from RTT patients induced pluripotent stem cells (iPSCs) and in postmortem brains from RTT patients. Therefore, MeCP2 seems to control L1 mobility in the nervous system and the absence of a functional protein may deregulate the retrotransposition with potential consequences for RTT (Muotri et al., 2010).

Further evidences on MeCP2-mediated regulation of repetitive elements showed that L1 retrotransposons, intracisternal-A-particles (IAP) and the major-satellite are up-regulated in Mecp2-null brains. These findings suggest that MeCP2 may act as a global regulator, probably by suppressing the spurious transcription of repetitive elements, thereby reducing the transcriptional noise (Skene et al., 2010).

LINE1 processing originates small ncRNAs including piRNAs, with a function related to the retrotransposons silencing. Therefore, it can be supposed that in a context of LINE1 excess, piRNAs may be also deregulated. The level of piRNAs in wt and Mecp2-null mouse cerebella by Wu et al. (2010) has been examined, finding 357 piRNAs expressed in wt cerebellum, the 59% of them showing a marked up-regulation in Mecp2-null mice. Intriguingly, the DQ541777 piRNA, important for the dendritic spine size that is impaired in Rett syndrome, is also overexpressed in Mecp2-null mice. In this light, it was proposed a model in which, in the absence of functional MeCP2 the overexpression of LINE-1 may lead to an increase in the piRNAs levels affecting the expression of specific genes deregulated in RTT (Saxena et al., 2012).

An important process in which the epigenetic players MeCP2 and DNMT3B interact with ncRNAs is the maintenance of the integrity at telomeric heterochromatin to prevent the telomere shortening (Deng et al., 2010). Telomeric-repeat-containing-RNAs (TERRAs) are lncRNAs transcribed from telomeres, involved in the formation of telomeric heterochromatin through a negative-feedback looping mechanism. TERRAs interact with several heterochromatin-associated proteins, including MeCP2, HP1, and H3K9 methyltrasferase. This interaction may be sufficient to nucleate heterochromatin complexes; the recruitment of DNMT3B and the establishment of CpG methylation at subtelomeres likely mediate this process. Indeed, in ICF-derived-cells TERRA levels are abnormally increased and telomeres are abnormally shortened (Yehezkel et al., 2008). The proposed mechanism implies that loss of CpG methylation at subtelomeres due to DNMT3B mutations results in a failure of TERRA-mediated feedback-looping. This allows for transcription factors to access to subtelomeres leading to a permissive chromatin state. Highly induced TERRA levels may contribute to telomere dysfunction in ICF cells either by inhibiting telomerase activity, forming RNA-DNAs hybrids with telomeres, or by interactions with telomere-binding proteins (Deng et al., 2010). The latest live imaging-based model, in which TERRA sequesters and delivers telomerase to the chromosome end from which the transcript originated, support the first mechanism (Cusanelli et al., 2013).

Genome-wide studies have reported an extensive reduction of DNA methylation at several repeat families, with satellite and transposons revealing the highest reduction. That implies the DNMT3B activity as crucial for centromere stability and transposon repression (Heyn et al., 2012). Overexpression of satellite II and satellite α DNA at pericentromeric and centromeric heterochromatin respectively has been indeed reported (Alexiadis et al., 2007), which might be functionally involved in the chromosomal aberrations in ICF syndrome.

CONCLUSIONS

Increasing reports highlighting aberrant regulation of different classes of ncRNAs in chromatin disorders characterized by neurological defects, open new perspectives for the comprehension of the pathogenetic mechanism of these disorders. These misregulated ncRNAs may be identified as responsible for specific subset of complex phenotypes, providing us with valuable means to the development of more effective therapeutic strategies based on RNA regulators.

Experimental approaches using high-throughput chemical screens are being proved to be suitable to find molecules that can both activate or inhibit the RNAi/miRNA pathway and, potentially correct some neurological defects (Li et al., 2010). Therapeutic strategies based on the design of specific oligonucleotides targeting ncRNAs, with the aim to specifically silence or replace the transcript, are being explored (Esteller, 2011) and appear very promising. However, their selective delivery into the CNS remains the most considerable challenge, and until now it has not been addressed effectively.

Noteworthy, recent reports indicated that miRNA expression profile in peripheral blood samples mirror the one present in the brain after cerebral ischaemia subsequent to stroke (Tan et al., 2009). In addition, neural cells can release ncRNAs in the blood and cerebrospinal fluid in membrane-bound exosomes (Skog et al., 2008). These evidences suggest that ncRNAs from body fluids might be used as biomarkers of neurological diseases. Further efforts are needed to decipher the intricate ncRNA world, and help to clarify how deregulation of ncRNAs may contribute to neuronal dysfunctions.

ACKNOWLEDGMENTS

The authors thank Anna Aliperti for the manuscript editing. Maria R. Matarazzo and Maurizio D'Esposito are supported by the UE Initial Training Network Project n. 238242 "DISCHROM" and the Epigenomics Flagship Project Epigen, MIUR-CNR.

REFERENCES

Alexiadis, V., Ballestas, M. E., Sanchez, C., Winokur, S., Vedanarayanan, V., Warren, M., et al. (2007). RNAPol-ChIP analysis of transcription from FSHD-linked tandem repeats and satellite DNA. *Biochim. Biophys. Acta* 1769, 29–40. doi: 10.1016/j.bbaexp.2006.11.006

Berghoff, E. G., Clark, M. F., Chen, S., Cajigas, I., Leib, D. E., and Kohtz, J. D. (2013). Evf2 (Dlx6as) lncRNA regulates ultraconserved enhancer methylation and the differential transcriptional control of adjacent genes. *Development* 140, 4407–4416. doi: 10.1242/dev.099390

Bian, S., and Sun, T. (2011). Functions of noncoding RNAs in neural development and neurological diseases. *Mol. Neurobiol.* 44, 359–373. doi: 10.1007/s12035-011-8211-3

Bond, A. M., Vangompel, M. J., Sametsky, E. A., Clark, M. F., Savage, J. C., Disterhoft, J. F., et al. (2009). Balanced gene regulation by an embryonic brain ncRNA is critical for adult hippocampal GABA circuitry. *Nat. Neurosci.* 12, 1020–1027. doi: 10.1038/nn.2371

Caudron-Herger, M., and Rippe, K. (2012). Nuclear architecture by RNA. *Curr. Opin. Genet. Dev.* 22, 179–187. doi: 10.1016/j.gde.2011.12.005

Chahrour, M., and Zoghbi, H. Y. (2007). The story of Rett syndrome: from clinic to neurobiology. *Neuron* 56, 422–437. doi: 10.1016/j.neuron.2007.10.001

Choufani, S., Shuman, C., and Weksberg, R. (2013). Molecular findings in Beckwith-Wiedemann syndrome. *Am. J. Med. Genet. C Semin. Med. Genet.* 163C, 131–140. doi: 10.1002/ajmg.c.31363

Coghlan, S., Horder, J., Inkster, B., Mendez, M. A., Murphy, D. G., and Nutt, D. J. (2012). GABA system dysfunction in autism and related disorders: from synapse to symptoms. *Neurosci. Biobehav. Rev.* 36, 2044–2055. doi: 10.1016/j.neubiorev.2012.07.005

Cusanelli, E., Romero, C. A., and Chartrand, P. (2013). Telomeric noncoding RNA TERRA is induced by telomere shortening to nucleate telomerase molecules at short telomeres. *Mol. Cell* 51, 780–791. doi: 10.1016/j.molcel.2013.08.029

Del Gaudio, D., Fang, P., Scaglia, F., Ward, P. A., Craigen, W. J., Glaze, D. G., et al. (2006). Increased MECP2 gene copy number as the result of genomic duplication in neurodevelopmentally delayed males. *Genet. Med.* 8, 784–792. doi: 10.109701.gim.0000250502.28516.3c

Della Ragione, F., Filosa, S., Scalabri, F., and D'esposito, M. (2012). MeCP2 as a genome-wide modulator: the renewal of an old story. *Front. Genet.* 3:181. doi: 10.3389/fgene.2012.00181

Deng, Z., Campbell, A. E., and Lieberman, P. M. (2010). TERRA, CpG methylation and telomere heterochromatin: lessons from ICF syndrome cells. *Cell Cycle* 9, 69–74. doi: 10.4161/cc.9.1.10358

Diaz-Meyer, N., Day, C. D., Khatod, K., Maher, E. R., Cooper, W., Reik, W., et al. (2003). Silencing of CDKN1C (p57KIP2) is associated with hypomethylation at KvDMR1 in Beckwith-Wiedemann syndrome. *J. Med. Genet.* 40, 797–801. doi: 10.1136/jmg.40.11.797

Duker, A. L., Ballif, B. C., Bawle, E. V., Person, R. E., Mahadevan, S., Alliman, S., et al. (2010). Paternally inherited microdeletion at 15q11.2 confirms a significant role for the SNORD116 C/D box snoRNA cluster in Prader-Willi syndrome. *Eur. J. Hum. Genet.* 18, 1196–1201. doi: 10.1038/ejhg.2010.102

Ehrlich, M., Jackson, K., and Weemaes, C. (2006). Immunodeficiency, centromeric region instability, facial anomalies syndrome (ICF). *Orphanet J. Rare Dis.* 1, 2. doi: 10.1186/1750-1172-1-2

Esteller, M. (2011). Non-coding RNAs in human disease. *Nat. Rev. Genet.* 12, 861–874. doi: 10.1038/nrg3074

Gatto, S., Della Ragione, F., Cimmino, A., Strazzullo, M., Fabbri, M., Mutarelli, M., et al. (2010). Epigenetic alteration of microRNAs in DNMT3B-mutated patients of ICF syndrome. *Epigenetics* 5, 427–443. doi: 10.4161/epi.5.5.11999

Guttman, M., Amit, I., Garber, M., French, C., Lin, M. F., Feldser, D., et al. (2009). Chromatin signature reveals over a thousand highly conserved large non-coding RNAs in mammals. *Nature* 458, 223–227. doi: 10.1038/nature07672

Heyn, H., Vidal, E., Sayols, S., Sanchez-Mut, J. V., Moran, S., Medina, I., et al. (2012). Whole-genome bisulfite DNA sequencing of a DNMT3B mutant patient. *Epigenetics* 7, 542–550. doi: 10.4161/epi.20523

Im, H. I., Hollander, J. A., Bali, P., and Kenny, P. J. (2010). MeCP2 controls BDNF expression and cocaine intake through homeostatic interactions with microRNA-212. *Nat. Neurosci.* 13, 1120–1127. doi: 10.1038/nn.2615

Im, H. I., and Kenny, P. J. (2012). MicroRNAs in neuronal function and dysfunction. *Trends Neurosci.* 35, 325–334. doi: 10.1016/j.tins.2012.01.004

Jin, B., Tao, Q., Peng, J., Soo, H. M., Wu, W., Ying, J., et al. (2008). DNA methyltransferase 3B (DNMT3B) mutations in ICF syndrome lead to altered epigenetic modifications and aberrant expression of genes regulating development, neurogenesis and immune function. *Hum. Mol. Genet.* 17, 690–709. doi: 10.1093/hmg/ddm341

Jordan, C., Li, H. H., Kwan, H. C., and Francke, U. (2007). Cerebellar gene expression profiles of mouse models for Rett syndrome reveal novel MeCP2 targets. *BMC Med. Genet.* 8:36. doi: 10.1186/1471-2350-8-36

Kent, L., Bowdin, S., Kirby, G. A., Cooper, W. N., and Maher, E. R. (2008). Beckwith Weidemann syndrome: a behavioral phenotype-genotype study. *Am. J. Med. Genet. B Neuropsychiatr. Genet.* 147B, 1295–1297. doi: 10.1002/ajmg.b.30729

Khalil, A. M., Guttman, M., Huarte, M., Garber, M., Raj, A., Rivea Morales, D., et al. (2009). Many human large intergenic noncoding RNAs associate with chromatin-modifying complexes and affect gene expression. *Proc. Natl. Acad. Sci. U.S.A.* 106, 11667–11672. doi: 10.1073/pnas.0904715106

Kim, V. N., Han, J., and Siomi, M. C. (2009). Biogenesis of small RNAs in animals. *Nat. Rev. Mol. Cell Biol.* 10, 126–139. doi: 10.1038/nrm2632

Klein, M. E., Lioy, D. T., Ma, L., Impey, S., Mandel, G., and Goodman, R. H. (2007). Homeostatic regulation of MeCP2 expression by a CREB-induced microRNA. *Nat. Neurosci.* 10, 1513–1514. doi: 10.1038/nn2010

Kosik, K. S. (2006). The neuronal microRNA system. *Nat. Rev. Neurosci.* 7, 911–920. doi: 10.1038/nrn2037

Lee, E. J., Banerjee, S., Zhou, H., Jammalamadaka, A., Arcila, M., Manjunath, B. S., et al. (2011). Identification of piRNAs in the central nervous system. *RNA* 17, 1090–1099. doi: 10.1261/rna.2565011

Li, Y., He, C., and Jin, P. (2010). Emergence of chemical biology approaches to the RNAi/miRNA pathway. *Chem. Biol.* 17, 584–589. doi: 10.1016/j.chembiol.2010.05.014

Matarazzo, M. R., De Bonis, M. L., Vacca, M., Della Ragione, F., and D'esposito, M. (2009). Lessons from two human chromatin diseases, ICF syndrome and Rett syndrome. *Int. J. Biochem. Cell Biol.* 41, 117–126. doi: 10.1016/j.biocel.2008.07.026

Matarazzo, M. R., Lembo, F., Angrisano, T., Ballestar, E., Ferraro, M., Pero, R., et al. (2004). *In vivo* analysis of DNA methylation patterns recognized by specific proteins: coupling CHIP and bisulfite analysis. *Biotechniques* 37, 666–668, 670, 672–663.

Maxwell, S. S., Pelka, G. J., Tam, P. P., and El-Osta, A. (2013). Chromatin context and ncRNA highlight targets of MeCP2 in brain. *RNA Biol.* 10, 1741–1757. doi: 10.4161/rna.26921

Meng, L., Person, R. E., and Beaudet, A. L. (2012). Ube3a-ATS is an atypical RNA polymerase II transcript that represses the paternal expression of Ube3a. *Hum. Mol. Genet.* 21, 3001–3012. doi: 10.1093/hmg/dds130

Mercer, T. R., Dinger, M. E., Sunkin, S. M., Mehler, M. F., and Mattick, J. S. (2008). Specific expression of long noncoding RNAs in the mouse brain. *Proc. Natl. Acad. Sci. U.S.A.* 105, 716–721. doi: 10.1073/pnas.0706729105

Muotri, A. R., Marchetto, M. C., Coufal, N. G., Oefner, R., Yeo, G., Nakashima, K., et al. (2010). L1 retrotransposition in neurons is modulated by MeCP2. *Nature* 468, 443–446. doi: 10.1038/nature09544

Petazzi, P., Sandoval, J., Szczesna, K., Jorge, O. C., Roa, L., Sayols, S., et al. (2013). Dysregulation of the long non-coding RNA transcriptome in a Rett syndrome mouse model. *RNA Biol.* 10, 1197–1203. doi: 10.4161/rna.24286

Ponjavic, J., Oliver, P. L., Lunter, G., and Ponting, C. P. (2009). Genomic and transcriptional co-localization of protein-coding and long non-coding RNA pairs in the developing brain. *PLoS Genet.* 5:e1000617. doi: 10.1371/journal.pgen.1000617

Powell, W. T., Coulson, R. L., Gonzales, M. L., Crary, F. K., Wong, S. S., Adams, S., et al. (2013). R-loop formation at Snord116 mediates topotecan inhibition of Ube3a-antisense and allele-specific chromatin decondensation. *Proc. Natl. Acad. Sci. U.S.A.* 110, 13938–13943. doi: 10.1073/pnas.1305426110

Qureshi, I. A., and Mehler, M. F. (2012). Emerging roles of non-coding RNAs in brain evolution, development, plasticity and disease. *Nat. Rev. Neurosci.* 13, 528–541. doi: 10.1038/nrn3234

Sahoo, T., Del Gaudio, D., German, J. R., Shinawi, M., Peters, S. U., Person, R. E., et al. (2008). Prader-Willi phenotype caused by paternal deficiency for the HBII-85 C/D box small nucleolar RNA cluster. *Nat. Genet.* 40, 719–721. doi: 10.1038/ng.158

Saxena, A., Tang, D., and Carninci, P. (2012). piRNAs warrant investigation in Rett Syndrome: an omics perspective. *Dis. Markers* 33, 261–275. doi: 10.3233/DMA-2012-0932

Schmitz, K. M., Mayer, C., Postepska, A., and Grummt, I. (2010). Interaction of noncoding RNA with the rDNA promoter mediates recruitment of DNMT3b and silencing of rRNA genes. *Genes Dev.* 24, 2264–2269. doi: 10.1101/gad.590910

Skene, P. J., Illingworth, R. S., Webb, S., Kerr, A. R., James, K. D., Turner, D. J., et al. (2010). Neuronal MeCP2 is expressed at near histone-octamer levels and globally alters the chromatin state. *Mol. Cell* 37, 457–468. doi: 10.1016/j.molcel.2010.01.030

Skog, J., Wurdinger, T., Van Rijn, S., Meijer, D. H., Gainche, L., Sena-Esteves, M., et al. (2008). Glioblastoma microvesicles transport RNA and proteins that promote tumour growth and provide diagnostic biomarkers. *Nat. Cell Biol.* 10, 1470–1476. doi: 10.1038/ncb1800

Tan, K. S., Armugam, A., Sepramaniam, S., Lim, K. Y., Setyowati, K. D., Wang, C. W., et al. (2009). Expression profile of MicroRNAs in young stroke patients. *PLoS ONE* 4:e7689. doi: 10.1371/journal.pone.0007689

Tsai, M. C., Manor, O., Wan, Y., Mosammaparast, N., Wang, J. K., Lan, F., et al. (2010). Long noncoding RNA as modular scaffold of histone modification complexes. *Science* 329, 689–693. doi: 10.1126/science.1192002

Urdinguio, R. G., Pino, I., Ropero, S., Fraga, M. F., and Esteller, M. (2007). Histone H3 and H4 modification profiles in a Rett syndrome mouse model. *Epigenetics* 2, 11–14. doi: 10.4161/epi.2.1.3698

Wang, H., Chan, S. A., Ogier, M., Hellard, D., Wang, Q., Smith, C., et al. (2006). Dysregulation of brain-derived neurotrophic factor expression and neurosecretory function in Mecp2 null mice. *J. Neurosci.* 26, 10911–10915. doi: 10.1523/JNEUROSCI.1810-06.2006

Wang, K. C., and Chang, H. Y. (2011). Molecular mechanisms of long noncoding RNAs. *Mol. Cell* 43, 904–914. doi: 10.1016/j.molcel.2011.08.018

Wang, L., and Yi, R. (2014). 3′UTRs take a long shot in the brain. *Bioessays* 36, 39–45. doi: 10.1002/bies.201300100

Weksberg, R., Nishikawa, J., Caluseriu, O., Fei, Y. L., Shuman, C., Wei, C., et al. (2001). Tumor development in the Beckwith-Wiedemann syndrome is associated with a variety of constitutional molecular 11p15 alterations including imprinting defects of KCNQ1OT1. *Hum. Mol. Genet.* 10, 2989–3000. doi: 10.1093/hmg/10.26.2989

Wu, H., Tao, J., Chen, P. J., Shahab, A., Ge, W., Hart, R. P., et al. (2010). Genome-wide analysis reveals methyl-CpG-binding protein 2-dependent regulation of microRNAs in a mouse model of Rett syndrome. *Proc. Natl. Acad. Sci. U.S.A.* 107, 18161–18166. doi: 10.1073/pnas.1005595107

Yehezkel, S., Segev, Y., Viegas-Pequignot, E., Skorecki, K., and Selig, S. (2008). Hypomethylation of subtelomeric regions in ICF syndrome is associated with abnormally short telomeres and enhanced transcription from telomeric regions. *Hum. Mol. Genet.* 17, 2776–2789. doi: 10.1093/hmg/ddn177

7

NMDA receptor-dependent regulation of miRNA expression and association with Argonaute during LTP *in vivo*

Balagopal Pai[1†], Taweeporn Siripornmongcolchai[1†], Birgitte Berentsen[1], Ashraf Pakzad[1], Christel Vieuille[1], Ståle Pallesen[2], Maciej Pajak[3], T. Ian Simpson[3,4], J. Douglas Armstrong[3], Karin Wibrand[1] and Clive R. Bramham[1]*

[1] Department of Biomedicine and K.G. Jebsen Centre for Research on Neuropsychiatric Disorders, University of Bergen, Bergen, Norway
[2] Department of Psychosocial Science, University of Bergen, Bergen, Norway
[3] Institute for Adaptive and Neural Computation, School of Informatics, University of Edinburgh, Edinburgh, UK
[4] Biomathematics and Statistics Scotland, JCMB, Edinburgh, UK

***Correspondence:**
Clive R. Bramham, Department of Biomedicine and K.G. Jebsen Centre for Research on Neuropsychiatric Disorders, University of Bergen, Jonas Lies vei 91, N-5009 Bergen, Norway e-mail: clive.bramham@biomed.uib.no
† Shared first authorship.

microRNAs (miRNAs) are major regulators of protein synthesis in the brain. A major goal is to identify changes in miRNA expression underlying protein synthesis-dependent forms of synaptic plasticity such as long-term potentiation (LTP). Previous analyses focused on changes in miRNA levels in total lysate samples. Here, we asked whether changes in total miRNA accurately reflect changes in the amount of miRNA bound to Argonaute protein within the miRNA-induced silencing complex (miRISC). Ago2 immunoprecipitation was used to isolate RISC-associated miRNAs following high-frequency stimulation (HFS)-induced LTP in the dentate gyrus of anesthetized rats. Using locked-nucleic acid-based PCR cards for high-throughput screening and independent validation by quantitative TaqMan RT-PCR, we identified differential regulation of Ago2-associated and total miRNA expression. The ratio of Ago2/total miRNA expression was regulated bidirectionally in a miRNA-specific manner and was largely dependent on N-methyl-D-aspartate receptor (NMDA) activation during LTP induction. The present results identify miRNA association with Ago2 as a potential control point in activity-dependent synaptic plasticity in the adult brain. Finally, novel computational analysis for targets of the Ago2-associated miRNAs identifies 21 pathways that are enriched and differentially targeted by the miRNAs including axon guidance, mTOR, MAPK, Ras, and LTP.

Keywords: synaptic plasticity, microRNA, RNA-induced silencing complex, Argonaute, microRNA target prediction, gene expression, protein synthesis, hippocampus

INTRODUCTION

Stable forms of activity-dependent synaptic plasticity require coordinated gene transcription and bursts of protein synthesis and degradation. Rapid regulation of local protein synthesis in dendrites is considered important for synaptic homeostasis and plasticity (Bramham and Wells, 2007; Martin and Ephrussi, 2009). In recent years miRNAs have emerged as key modulators of neuronal protein synthesis. miRNAs are short non-coding RNAs (~22 nucleotides) that bind to partially complementary sites on the 3′ UTR of target mRNAs where they act to inhibit protein synthesis (Filipowicz et al., 2008; Djuranovic et al., 2011; Huntzinger and Izaurralde, 2011). Many new brain-specific miRNAs have appeared with vertebrate and primate evolution and roles for specific miRNAs in neurogenesis, dendritic spine morphogenesis, synaptic regulation, plasticity, and memory storage have been demonstrated (Vo et al., 2005; Krichevsky et al., 2006; Rajasethupathy et al., 2009; Siegel et al., 2009; Mellios et al., 2011; Tognini et al., 2011). The target diversity, specificity, and activity-dependent regulation make miRNAs attractive as modulators of local protein synthesis and synaptic plasticity.

In the canonical biogenesis pathway, miRNAs are transcribed as long primary transcripts and processed in the nucleus by the RNase III enzyme Drosha to generate a stem-loop structured precursor. The precursor miRNA is then exported to the cytoplasm where a second RNase III enzyme, Dicer, generates a mature double-stranded miRNA intermediate. One of these strands, the guide strand, is recognized and bound by the protein Argonaute (Ago), which further functions in recruitment of the multi-protein, miRNA-induced silencing complex (miRISC) (Bartel, 2004). The passenger strand of the miRNA duplex is normally destroyed. Once assembled on target bound miRNA, the miRISC inhibits protein synthesis by repressing translation, promoting mRNA decay, or some combination of the two processes (Filipowicz et al., 2008; Huntzinger and Izaurralde, 2011; Béthune et al., 2012; Djuranovic et al., 2012).

MicroRNA activity is modulated through changes in miRNA biogenesis, miRNA turnover, and regulation of RISC effector proteins (Lugli et al., 2005; Ashraf et al., 2006; Kosik, 2006; Banerjee et al., 2009; Krol et al., 2010a,b; Wibrand et al., 2010) A previous study on miRNA expression in dentate gyrus long-term potentiation (LTP) provided evidence for rapid, activity-dependent decay of several mature miRNAs in addition to upregulation of miRNA by transcription (Wibrand et al., 2010). In that study and previous work on chemically induced LTP (Park and Tang, 2009), miRNA levels were measured in whole tissue lysate. The general assumption has been that guide-stranded mature miRNA is predominantly, if not exclusively, bound to Argonaute. However, mounting evidence suggest that miRNA binding to Argonaute is both reversible and regulated (Meister, 2013).

Using Ago2 immunoprecipitation, we demonstrate rapid, differential regulation of Ago2-associated and total miRNAs following LTP induction in the dentate gyrus *in vivo*. The ratio of Ago2/total miRNA expression was regulated bidirectionally in a miRNA-specific manner and was coupled to N-methyl-D-aspartate (NMDA) receptor-dependent LTP induction. Hence, these findings identify regulation of miRNA:Ago2 interactions as a potential control point in long-term synaptic plasticity of the adult dentate gyrus.

Finally we use an integrated miRNA target prediction approach to inform pathway enrichment analyses in which we find that many of the major pathways traditionally associated with the regulation of synaptic plasticity are targeted, including the mTOR, MAPK, and Ras pathways. Surprisingly, the axon guidance pathway is the most highly enriched, but includes many genes already known to play a role in synaptic plasticity.

MATERIALS AND METHODS

In vivo ELECTROPHYSIOLOGY

Experiments were carried out under ethical standards approved by the Norwegian Committee for Experiments on Animals. *In vivo* electrophysiological experiments were carried out on 30 adult male rats of the Sprague–Dawley outbred strain, weighing 250–350 g. The electrophysiological procedures have been detailed elsewhere (Messaoudi et al., 2002; Panja et al., 2009). Rats were anesthetized with urethane and electrodes were stereotactically placed for selective stimulation of the medial perforant pathway and recording of evoked field potentials in the hilar region of the dentate gyrus. A concentric bipolar stimulating electrode (input impedance ~40 MΩ; tip separation 500 μm; SNEX 100; Rhodes Medical Instruments, Woodland Hills, CA) was lowered into the dorsomedial aspect of the angular bundle for stimulation of the medial perforant path.

The recording electrode was slowly lowered into the dorsal hippocampus until a positive-going field EPSP (fEPSP) of maximum slope was obtained in the dentate hilus (7.9 mm posterior to bregma and 4.2 mm lateral from midline for stimulation; 3.9 mm posterior and 2.3 mm lateral for recording). Biphasic rectangular test pulses of 150 μs duration were applied every 30 s throughout the experiment (0.033 Hz) except during the period of high-frequency stimulation (HFS). Responses were allowed to stabilize, and 20 min of baseline recording was obtained. HFS consisted of 400-Hz, 8-pulse stimulus trains repeated 4 times with 10 s between each train. HFS was applied three times with 5 min between each session. The total number of pulses was 128. After HFS, evoked responses were collected for periods of 30 and 120 min. Signals from the dentate hilus were amplified, filtered (1 Hz and 10 Hz), and digitized (25 Hz). Acquisition and analysis of field potentials were accomplished using Data Wave Technologies Work Bench Software (Longmont, CO). The maximum slope of the fEPSP was measured and the averages of four consecutive responses were obtained.

INTRAHIPPOCAMPAL INFUSION

The recording electrode with an attached guide cannula was lowered into the dentate gyrus as described for the recording electrode above. An inner infusion cannula (31 gauge) was then inserted so it protruded 300 μm below the end of the guide. The tip of the infusion cannula was located in the deep stratum lacunosum-moleculare of field CA1, 700 μm above the hilar recording site and 300–400 μm above the medial perforant synapse (Messaoudi et al., 2007). The inner infusion cannula was connected via a polyethylene (PE50) tube to a 3 μl Hamilton syringe (Reno, NV) and infusion pump. 0.3 μl of 2-Amino-5-phosphonopentanoic acid (AP5, 50 mM prepared in 1× PBS; Tocris) was infused over 12 min at a rate of 0.085 μl/min, and test pulse stimulation was continued for a further 18 min prior to HFS.

DENTATE GYRUS DISSECTION AND SAMPLE PREPARATION

At the end of the electrophysiological recordings rats were decapitated, the brain was extracted and rinsed with ice-cold saline and both hippocampi were removed within less than 3 min. The dentate gyri were then rapidly dissected on ice and immediately frozen on dry ice.

ARGONAUTE 2 IMMUNOPRECIPITATION

Immunoprecipitation was performed according to Choe et al. (2010) with minor modifications. Forty microliters of protein G-sepharose (17061801, GE Health Care Bioscience AB) was incubated with 3 μg of mouse monoclonal Ago2 antibody (anti-EIF2C2) (H00027161-M01, Abnova) at room temperature in a rotary shaker (25 rpm) for 1.5 h. Immunoprecipitation using purified mouse IgG (558509, BD Pharmingen) served as a control for detection of non-specific protein binding. The sepharose beads were blocked with 2% yeast tRNA (R4018, Sigma-Aldrich) and 1% BSA (9048-46-8, Sigma-Aldrich) in 1× PBS at room temperature in a rotary shaker (25 rpm) for 30 min. Dentate gyri were homogenized (Dounce homogenizer) in ice cold lysis buffer containing 25 mM Tris (Ambion Life Sciences, Carlsbad, CA, USA), 150 mM NaCl, 2 mM MgCl2, 0.5% NP-40 (Ambion Life Sciences, Carlsbad, CA, USA), 0.5 mM DTT (Ambion Life Sciences, Carlsbad, CA, USA), 0.4 unit RNAse inhibitor (Ambion Life Sciences, Carlsbad, CA, USA), and protease inhibitor cocktail (Roche Diagnostics GmbH) 1 tablet/10 ml. The homogenate was centrifuged at 4°C (10,000 rpm, 15 min) and subjected to pre-clearing with 40 μl protein-G sepharose at 4°C for 30 min, and centrifuged at 3000 rpm for 3 min. The protein concentration of the pre-cleared supernatant was determined by the BCA Protein Assay (BCA Protein Assay kit 23227, Thermo Scientific). A small aliquot of the supernatant was separately stored at 4°C for analysis of total lysate (input). The antibody bound beads were incubated with 750 μg of pre-cleared protein at 4°C in a rotary shaker (25 rpm) for 2.5 h. Non-specifically bound proteins were removed from the sepharose beads by giving four washes: first wash using lysis buffer, second wash with lysis buffer containing

900 mM NaCl instead of 150 mM, a third wash in the standard lysis buffer, and a final wash in lysis buffer containing 0.05% NP-40.

RNA ISOLATION

The Ago2 immunoprecipitate (referred to as Ago2 IP or Ago2 pellet) and the input samples were treated with 250 μl DNAse solution containing 25 μl of 10× DNAse1 buffer, 1 unit DNAse1 (Ambion Life Sciences, Carlsbad, CA, USA) and 50 unit RNAse inhibitor (Ambion Life Sciences, Carlsbad, CA, USA) at 37°C for 20 min for genomic DNA removal. Both the input (containing total RNA including all miRNAs) and the Ago2 IP (containing all RNAs in Ago2 complex including Ago2-associated miRNAs) were then treated with 500 μl of Trizol (Ambion Life Sciences, Carlsbad, CA, USA) for 5 min and 200 μl of Chloroform (Sigma-Aldrich, St. Louis, MO, USA), and subjected to centrifugation at 4°C, 14,000 rpm for 15 min. The water phase containing RNA was collected. RNA was precipitated in a solution containing 500 μl isopropanol, 5 μg glycogen (Ambion Life Sciences, Carlsbad, CA, USA), and 10% v/v ammonium acetate (Ambion Life Sciences, Carlsbad, CA, USA) at –20°C for at least 16 h. The preparation was then centrifuged at 4°C, 14,000 rpm for 45–60 min. The pellet was washed once in 100% ethanol, and once in 80% ethanol prior to centrifugation at 4°C, 14,000 rpm for 20 min. The RNA pellet was air-dried for 15 min, and dissolved in 25 μl of nuclease-free water. The quantity and quality of the RNA were determined by absorbance measurement at 260/280 nm. The quality of the total RNA was assessed by PCR-Quality Control (PCR-QC) using TaqMan® Gene expression assays (Applied Biosystems, Life Sciences, Carlsbad, CA, USA) for amplification of miRNAs which are known to express in the brain: miR-347 (assay 1334) and miR-151 (assay 1330). Argonaute immunoprecipitation was validated by western blot analysis of Ago2 protein in cortex, cornu ammonis, dentate gyrus, and HEK293 cells transfected with GFP-Ago2 vector.

HIGH-THROUGHPUT PCR CARD ANALYSIS OF microRNA EXPRESSION

High-throughput PCR analysis was performed using the miRCURY LNA universal RT miRNA Ready-to-Use PCR Mouse and Rat panel 1, V2.R (PCR card 203706, Exiqon). Twenty nanograms total RNA was reverse-transcribed to cDNA according to the universal cDNA synthesis kit instructions (203300, Exiqon). The qPCR was performed according to the SYBR Green Master Mix Universal RT kit instructions (203400, Exiqon). The PCR reaction was performed on a Roche Light Cycler® 480 II (Roche Applied Science). Briefly, a poly-A tail is added to the mature miRNA template. The cDNA template is then amplified using miR-specific LNA™ enhanced forward and reverse primers that are pre-aliquoted in the PCR card. The reverse primers detect the poly-T tail and the 3′ part of the mature microRNA sequence, ensuring specific amplification of the mature microRNA.

Of 384 wells in the PCR card, 373 wells contain different primer sets for 373 miRNAs of known sequences present in mirBase version 16. In addition, 11 wells are used for the following controls: an empty well (blank), three interplate-calibrators, a primer pair specific to synthetic oligo-RNA template in the cDNA synthesis master mix (for quality control of cDNA synthesis), and wells for the six reference genes miR-423-3p, miR-103, miR-191, u6 (small nucleolar RNA), RNU-5G (small nucleolar RNA), and rnu-1A1 (small nucleolar RNA).

The data analysis was performed according to the manufacturer's instructions (Exiqon GenEx qPCR analysis software). For each of three rats, the Ct (threshold cycle) values from the input and Ago2 IP samples collected at 30 and 120 min post-HFS were normalized using global normalization, an appropriate approach for large scale analysis (>100 assays) in which most miRNAs are not regulated. The Ct value of each miRNA was normalized to the mean Ct of all the miRNAs represented on the PCR card. Differences in miRNA expression between the treated and contralateral control dentate gyrus were compared by a Student's *t*-test with Dunn–Bonferroni correction (GeneEx software). One-Way ANOVA and *post hoc* Fisher's LSD was additionally applied to the data analysis in order to allow detection of possible false-negative results from Dunn–Bonferroni correction.

TaqMan REAL-TIME RT-PCR ANALYSIS OF microRNA

Ten nanograms total RNA was reverse-transcribed to cDNA according to the TaqMan® miRNA reverse transcription Kit instructions (4366597, Applied Biosystems) provided along with the TaqMan® RT primer specific to miRNA of interest. TaqMan® RT primers (Applied Biosystems) RT00-2602 (miR-384-5p), RT00-0413 (miR-29b), RT00-0522 (miR-219), RT00-2017 (miR-592), RT00-0580 (miR-20a), RT00-0382 (let-7f), RT00-2230 (miR-330-5p), RT00-0548 (miR-338), RT00-0526 (miR-223), RT00-2551 (miR-212), RT00-0480 (miR-181a), RT000426 (miR-34a), RT000395 (miR-19a), RT001061 (miR-326), and RT00-0492 (miR-193a) were used.

To identify the most stable gene for normalization, multi-factor ANOVA for multiple comparisons was used to analyze the Ct (threshold cycle) values of 373 miRNAs in Ago IP at 30 and 120 min and in input at 30 and 120 min (from the PCR cards). Two genes (miR-345-3p and miR-214) with most stable expression across samples (with highest *P*-value and lowest SD in Multi-Factor ANOVA analysis) were tested by qPCR in Ago2 IP ($n = 6$) and input samples ($n = 6$) in both treated and control dentate gyrus obtained at 30 min post-HFS. Rno-miR-345-3p was found to be the most stably expressed with the lowest range of Ct values among all samples, and therefore was used as an optimal normalizer in qPCR validation of miRNA expression.

cDNA pre-amplification was performed to allow accurate and reliable qPCR analyses of low abundance miRNAs. Fourteen cycles of exponential phase cDNA pre-amplification was performed according to the TaqMan® PreAmp Master Mix instructions (4391128, Applied Biosystems). The pre-amplified cDNA was diluted 10 times and subjected to qPCR. The qPCR was performed on a Roche Light Cycler®480 II (Roche Applied Science) using diluted pre-amplified cDNA from the individual dentate gyrus input and Ago2 IP samples. After reverse transcription and pre-amplification, qPCR was analyzed in a 25 μl reaction volume using 2× TaqMan® Universal PCR Master Mix II with no uracil-N-glycosylase (Applied Biosystems). PCR quantification was performed in triplicate using the relative standard curve method to determine gene expression levels. TaqMan®Gene expression assays (Applied Biosystems) were used corresponding to the TaqMan® RT primers used in cDNA synthesis.

QUANTITATIVE PCR ANALYSIS OF *Arc* mRNA

For analysis of *Arc* mRNA, 2 μg total RNA was reverse-transcribed to cDNA according to the MMLV reverse transcriptase kit instructions (2043, Ambion). qPCR was performed on a Roche Light Cycler® 480 II (Roche Applied Science) using cDNA corresponding to 10 ng total RNA of individual homogenized dentate gyrus. The qPCR was analyzed in 25 μl reaction using 2×TaqMan® PCR mix (Applied Biosystems). The qPCR quantification was performed in triplicate using relative standard curve method to determine gene expression levels. Ubiquitin-B was used as a housekeeping gene to normalize and determine the expression level for *Arc*. TaqMan®Gene expression assays (Applied Biosystems): Rn00571208_g1 (*Arc*) and Rn03062801_g1 (ubiquitin-B) were used.

STATISTICAL ANALYSIS FOR qPCR VALIDATION

Statistical analyses were performed using SPSS (version 16). Two miRNAs (miR-181a and miR-193a) were undetectable in the control dentate gyrus because their Ct values were greater than 40, and were therefore excluded from the analyses. One-Way ANOVA was used to analyze relative expression differences between the treated and contralateral control dentate gyrus in both Ago2 IP and input for all miRNAs. The expression levels between different miRNAs, as well as the differences between treatment groups were analyzed using a One-Way ANOVA and Fisher's LSD *post hoc* test. Fold changes in treated dentate gyrus relative to the contralateral control dentate gyrus were calculated for Ago2 IP and input samples from the individual rats and averaged.

microRNA TARGET PREDICTION

To identify the putative target genes of each miRNA we first queried four of the most widely used target prediction sources; DIANA (Maragkakis et al., 2011), miRanda (Griffiths-Jones et al., 2008), TargetScan (Friedman et al., 2009), and PicTar (Lall et al., 2006). Both DIANA and PicTar report miRNA targets in *Mus musculus* which we projected into *Rattus norvegicus* using only direct orthologs extracted from the Ensembl Compara database (Vilella et al., 2009).

We next quantified the agreement between predicted target lists using Rank Product (RP) analysis (Breitling et al., 2004; Eisinga et al., 2013). Briefly, each gene was ordered by quality score and the geometric mean of the gene rank calculated across prediction sources. Missing ranks were imputed for target genes missing only one rank value, genes missing more source values were discarded. To assess the robustness of the computed ranks we performed a bootstrap analysis with 1000 permutations of rank order using the Bioconductor RankProd package (Hong et al., 2006). In order to minimize the elimination of true positive targets, genes with RP ($p > 0.5$) were used in subsequent pathway analysis.

PATHWAY ANALYSIS

Integrated miRNA target gene lists from the RP step were used as input to pathway enrichment analyses by hypergeometric testing using the Bioconductor KEGGprofile package (Zhao, 2012). Gene to KEGG pathway mappings were retrieved for every pathway in the KEGG database (Kanehisa et al., 2011) and used to identify pathways that were enriched in predicted miRNA target genes ($p \leq 0.05$).

RESULTS

VALIDATION OF ARGONAUTE-2 IMMUNOPRECIPITATION

Dentate gyrus lysates were immunoprecipitated with an Ago2-specific antibody or control, non-immune IgG, and expression of the brain-specific miRNAs, miR-151, and miR-347, was examined by qPCR. miR-151 and miR-347 levels were enriched more than 100-fold in the Ago2 IP (**Figure 1A**). Furthermore, western blot analysis detected Ago2 protein at 97 kDa in the Ago2 pellet from naïve rat dentate gyrus, but not in the non-immune IgG pellet (**Figure 1B**). As a positive control, ectopically expressed Ago2-GFP was detected in HEK293 cells (**Figure 1B**). The results confirm immunoprecipitation of Ago2 and Ago2-associated miRNAs.

HIGH-THROUGHPUT miRNA EXPRESSION PROFILING

Brief bursts of HFS applied to the medial perforant path of anesthetized rats induced stable LTP of the fEPSP slope (**Figure 2A**).

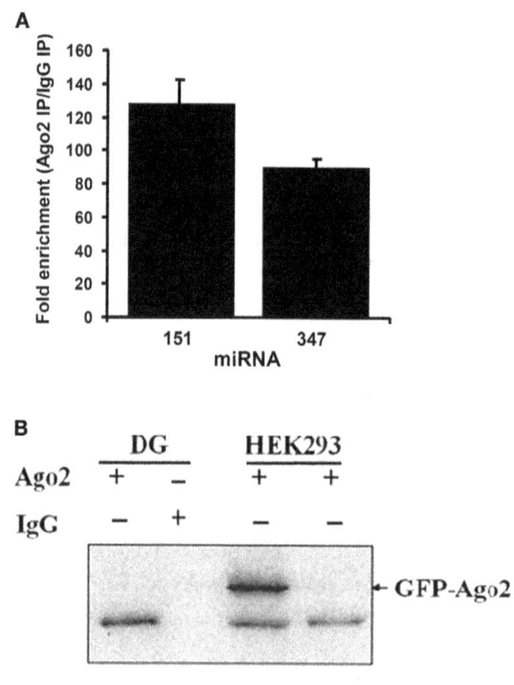

FIGURE 1 | Validation of Argonaute 2 immunoprecipitation. (A) Specific Ago2-immunoprecipitation of brain-enriched miRNAs. TaqMan qPCR for brain-enriched miR-347 and miR-151 was performed in Ago2 immunoprecipitated (IP) or non-immune mouse IgG immunoprecipitated samples from dentate gyrus. Values are means (+s.e.m.; $n = 3$) expressed as fold enrichment in the Ago2 IP relative to IgG IP. **(B)** Ago2 immunoblots following immunoprecipitation of dentate gyrus (DG) samples with Ago2 antibody or non-immune mouse IgG. A band at ~97 kDa corresponding to Ago2 was detected in Ago2, but not IgG, IP. As a positive control, HEK293 cells were transfected with GFP-Ago2. Endogenous Ago2 protein (lower band) and GFP-Ago2 fusion protein (arrow; band at ~127 kDa) were detected in transfected cells.

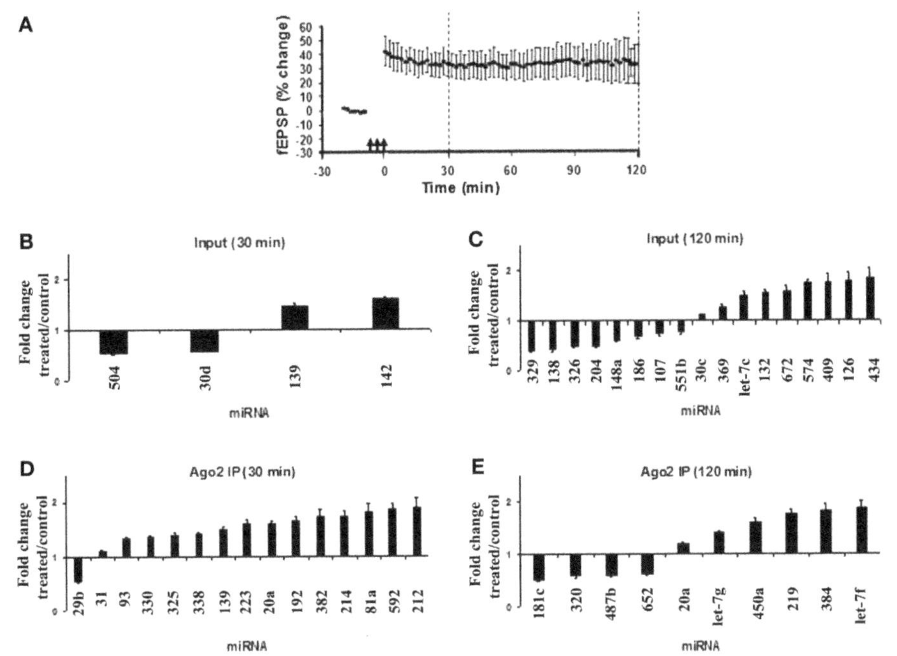

FIGURE 2 | Modulation of miRNA expression in total lysates and Ago2 immunoprecipitates following LTP induction. (A) Time course plot showing changes in the medial perforant path-evoked fEPSP slope expressed as a percentage of baseline. Values are mean ± s.e.m. ($n = 3$). Dentate gyrus tissue was obtained at 30 or 120 min post-HFS. **(B–E)** miRNA PCR cards from Exiqon were used to screen 373 miRNAs in total lysates (input) and Ago2 immunoprecipitates following high-frequency stimulation (HFS). Data for input and Ago2 IP samples for each time point were normalized to the respective global mean of all miRNAs expressed on the card. Values are mean (+s.e.m.) changes in HFS-treated dentate gyrus relative to the contralateral control ($n = 3$). Values are significantly different from control (Student's t-test with Dunn–Bonferroni correction, $p < 0.05$). **(B)** Fold change in miRNA expression in dentate gyrus input at 30 min post-HFS. **(C)** Fold change in miRNA expression in dentate gyrus input at 120 min post-HFS. **(D)** Fold change in miRNA expression in dentate gyrus Ago2 immunoprecipitate at 30 min post-HFS. **(E)** Fold change in miRNA expression in dentate gyrus Ago2 immunoprecipitates at 120 min post-HFS.

The dentate gyrus was rapidly micro-dissected at 30 or 120 min post-HFS. miRNA expression in the HFS-treated dentate gyrus was compared with the contralateral, unstimulated dentate gyrus which served as an internal control. High-throughput expression profiling of Ago2 IP and input samples was performed using pre-aliquoted, locked-nucleic acid based miRNA PCR primer sets in 384-well PCR plates. As there is no known reference gene stably expressed in both the Ago2 pellet and input, a global normalization was performed in which the Ct value of each miRNA was normalized to the mean Ct of all the miRNAs represented on the PCR card. Statistical differences in miRNA expression between the treated and control dentate gyrus were assessed by a Student's t-test with Dunn–Bonferroni correction.

In dentate gyrus lysates (inputs), at 30 min post-HFS, only 4 of 376 miRNAs represented on the panel exhibited significantly altered expression. Fold-changes ranged between a decrease of 0.49-fold (miR-504) and an increase of 1.55-fold (miR-142) relative to the contralateral control dentate gyrus (**Figure 2B**). At 120 min post-HFS, 17 miRNAs were significantly regulated, ranging between a maximum decrease of 0.65 fold (miR-329) and maximum increase of 1.79 fold (miR-434) (**Figure 2C**). In agreement with previous results (Wibrand et al., 2012), miR-132 was significantly upregulated at 120 min post-HFS in dentate gyrus lysates (**Figure 2C**). The high-throughput analysis of input samples indicate predominantly delayed (2 h), bidirectional changes in miRNA expression following HFS.

In Ago2 IP samples, 14 miRNAs were upregulated at 30 min post-HFS, and only miR-29b was downregulated (**Figure 2D**). At 120 min, 10 miRNAs were regulated (**Figure 2E**). None of the miRNAs exhibiting altered expression in the Ago2 pellet at 30 or 120 min post-HFS were also regulated in the input samples. Thus, the PCR card analysis revealed rapid, differential regulation of miRNAs in the Ago2-immunoprecipitated fraction relative to total miRNA.

LTP-SPECIFIC, DIFFERENTIAL REGULATION OF Ago2-ASSOCIATED AND TOTAL miRNA EXPRESSION: qPCR VALIDATION

TaqMan-based qPCR analysis of independent samples was used to validate changes in Ago2-immunoprecipitated miRNAs at 30 min post-HFS. In the qPCR validation, four experimental groups were used in order to identify miRNA regulation specific to LTP induction. The treatment groups were: (1) HFS + LFT; $n = 6$, (2) block of LTP induction by local intrahippocampal infusion of the NMDAR antagonist, AP5 (AP5 + HFS + LFT; $n = 4$). (3) LFT alone; $n = 5$, and (4) AP5 + LFT; $n = 5$. As shown in **Figure 3A**, LTP was blocked when HFS was applied in the presence of AP5. No changes in field potentials occurred in the LFT and AP5 + LFT treatment groups.

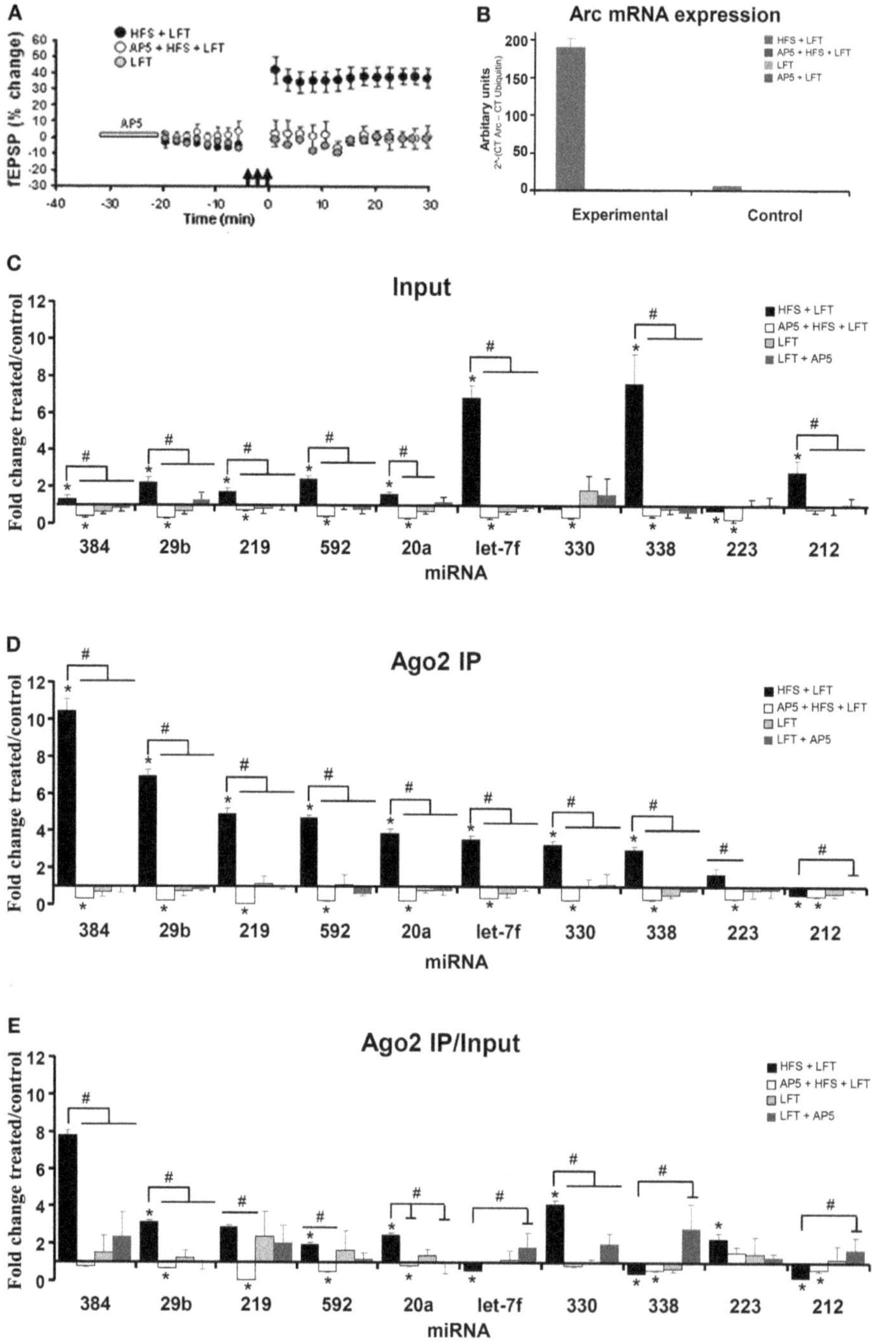

FIGURE 3 | Differential expression of Ago2-associated and total miRNAs linked to NMDA receptor-dependent LTP induction. (A) Time course plot showing changes in the medial perforant path-evoked fEPSP slope expressed as a percentage of baseline. Values are mean (±s.e.m.). HFS + LFT, $n = 6$; AP5 + HFS + LFT, $n = 4$; LFT, $n = 3$. Dentate gyrus tissue was obtained at 30 min. **(B)** Quantitative PCR was used to validate the expression of *Arc* mRNA. Changes in *Arc* mRNA levels in the treated and contralateral control dentate gyrus lysate samples were analyzed. The PCR data was normalized to the expression of *Ubiquitin-B* using the ΔCt method. Values are mean (+s.e.m.). HFS + LFT, $n = 6$; AP5 + HFS + LFT, $n = 4$; LFT, $n = 3$: AP5 + LFT, $n = 5$. **(C–E)** Quantitative TaqMan PCR was used for independent analysis of 10 selected miRNAs from the PCR card screen. The same set of miRNAs were analyzed in the input sample **(C)** and Ago2-immunoprecipitate **(D)**. qPCR data was normalized to expression of miR-345-3p. **(C)** Fold change in miRNA expression in dentate gyrus input samples at 30 min. Bar graph shows mean fold change (+s.e.m.) in treated dentate gyrus relative to control, contralateral dentate gyrus. Significant differences between the HFS group and other treatment groups are indicated (#; $p < 0.05$). Significant difference between the ispilateral (treated) and contralateral (control) dentate gyrus are indicated (*). HFS + LFT, $n = 6$; AP5 + HFS + LFT, $n = 4$; LFT alone, $n = 5$; AP5 + LFT, $n = 5$. **(D)** Fold change in miRNA expression in dentate gyrus Ago2 immunoprecipitates at 30 min post-HFS. Significant differences between the HFS group and other treatment groups are

(Continued)

FIGURE 3 | Continued
indicated (#; $p < 0.05$). Significant difference between the ispilateral (treated) and contralateral (control) dentate gyrus are indicated (*). **(E)** Relative fold change in miRNA expression in dentate gyrus Ago2 immunoprecipitates compared to dentate gyrus lysates (Ago2/input expression ratios) at 30 min post-HFS. Bar graph shows relative fold change in treated dentate gyrus relative to control, contralateral dentate gyrus. Significant differences between the HFS group and other treatment groups are indicated (#; $p < 0.05$). Significant difference between the ispilateral (treated) and contralateral (control) dentate gyrus are indicated (*).

As a functional validation of LTP-specific gene expression in the dentate gyrus, qPCR analysis of *Arc* mRNA was performed. *Arc* is an immediate early gene of importance for protein synthesis-dependent synaptic plasticity and memory storage (Bramham et al., 2010). NMDAR-dependent *Arc* expression is tightly linked to LTP induction in the dentate gyrus (Messaoudi et al., 2007; Panja et al., 2009). *Arc* mRNA expression was elevated 34-fold in the HFS + LFT treated dentate gyrus relative to contralateral dentate gyrus and this increase was blocked by AP5-infusion and was absent in groups receiving LFT only (**Figure 3B**).

Eleven miRNAs from the high-throughput screen were chosen for qPCR validation. These selected miRNAs included the seven most strongly upregulated miRNAs (miR-330, miR-338, miR-223, miR-20a, miR-181a, miR-592, miR-212) in the Ago2 IP at 30 min, the only downregulated miRNA (miR-29b) in the Ago2 IP at 30 min, and the three most strongly upregulated miRNAs (miR-219, miR-384, let-7f) in the Ago2 IP at 120 min post-HFS (significant by *t*-test with Dunn–Bonferroni correction and 1-Way ANOVA with LSD test). For normalization of the qPCR data, miR-345-3p was used as the most stably expressed miRNA across samples. miR-181a levels were detected in the HFS-treated dentate gyrus but were below the detection limit in the contralateral (unstimulated) dentate gyrus. miR-181a was therefore excluded from quantitative analysis.

The results of the qPCR analysis of the 10 miRNAs examined are shown in **Figures 3C–E**. The Ct values obtained in treated dentate gyrus were normalized to control Ct values in the contralateral dentate gyrus for each rat. This was done separately for the input (**Figure 3C**) and Ago2 IP (**Figure 3D**) samples. Eight of the 10 miRNAs with altered expression in the Ago2 IP on the PCR card were similarly regulated by qPCR (**Table A1**). Overall, larger increases were obtained by TaqMan qPCR, which may reflect a wider dynamic range of Ct values obtained by cDNA amplification in the TaqMan analysis. Robust quantitative differences in miRNA expression were observed between input samples and Ago2 IP samples. Five miRNAs (miR-384, miR-29b, miR-219, miR-592, and miR-20a) exhibited 2 to 5-fold greater increases in expression in the Ago2 immunoprecipitate than in the input samples, relative to contralateral control values (**Figures 3C,D**). miR-330 and miR-223 expression was unchanged or slightly decreased in input samples at 30 min post-HFS but enhanced in the Ago2 IP. In contrast, miR-let7f and miR-338 exhibited 2-fold greater increases in the input sample compared to the Ago2 pellet. Finally, miR-212 was elevated in the input sample, but was significantly decreased in abundance in the Ago2 pellet.

Next we examined the role of NMDA receptor activation in regulation of miRNA expression. Local infusion of AP5 blocked LTP induction and prevented the increase in miRNA expression in input samples and Ago2 IP samples. Remarkably, all 10 miRNAs, including those that were not regulated or decreased in the HFS group, exhibited a significant decrease in expression when HFS was applied in the presence of AP5. No significant changes in miRNA expression were observed in Ago2 IP or input samples of the LFT or LFT + AP5 treatment groups. An analysis of the Ago2/input ratios revealed two distinct patterns of miRNA expression (**Figure 3E**). Seven miRNAs (miR-384, miR-29b, miR-219, miR-592, miR-20a, miR-330, and miR-223) showed enhanced, NMDAR-dependent association with Ago2. In contrast, 3 miRNAs (miR-let7f, miR-338, and miR-212) exhibited decreased expression in the Ago2 IP relative to input.

REGULATION OF *Arc*-TARGETING miRNAs

Recently, Wibrand et al. (2012) identified a set of miRNAs which bind to the *Arc* 3′ UTR and inhibit Arc protein expression in HEK293 cells and primary hippocampal neuronal cultures. Given the central role of Arc mRNA expression and translation in dentate gyrus LTP (Messaoudi et al., 2007; Panja et al., 2009), we were interested in determining the Ago2/IP expression pattern of Arc-targeting miRNAs. In input samples, all three miRNAs examined (miR-34a, miR-19a, miR-326) showed enhanced expression 30 min post-HFS and decreased expression below the contralateral control level when HFS was given in the presence of AP5 (**Figure 4A**). Analysis of the Ago2 IP and Ago2 IP/input expression ratios revealed enhanced NMDAR-dependent association of miR-34a with Ago2 make this (**Figures 4B,C**). In contrast, miR-19a showed no change and miR-326 had a significantly decreased Ago2/IP expression ratio following HFS. When AP5 was infused prior to HFS, the Ago2/IP expression ratio of miR-19a and miR-326 was increased, indicating NMDAR-dependent dissociation of these miRNA from Ago2 (**Figure 4C**).

STABLE EXPRESSION OF ARGONAUTE 2 PROTEIN DURING LTP

Levels of Argonaute protein are known to influence the stability of miRNA (Winter and Diederichs, 2011). We therefore examined the expression of Argonaute protein as a potential mechanism for the differential regulation of total and Ago2-immunoprecipitated miRNAs. As shown in **Figure 5**, immunoblot analysis showed no change in Ago2 expression in input and Ago2-immunoprecipated samples at 30 and 120 min post-HFS (**Figure 5**).

miRNA TARGET GENE PREDICTION AND PATHWAY ANALYSIS

In order to better understand the potential downstream effects of the activity-dependent enhanced and depleted Ago2-associated miRNAs we integrated predictions from four of the most commonly used miRNA target prediction resources; DIANA (Maragkakis et al., 2011), miRanda (Griffiths-Jones et al., 2008), TargetScan (Friedman et al., 2009), and PicTar (Lall et al., 2006) using the RP method (Breitling et al., 2004). This allowed us to mitigate for the poor agreement normally found between

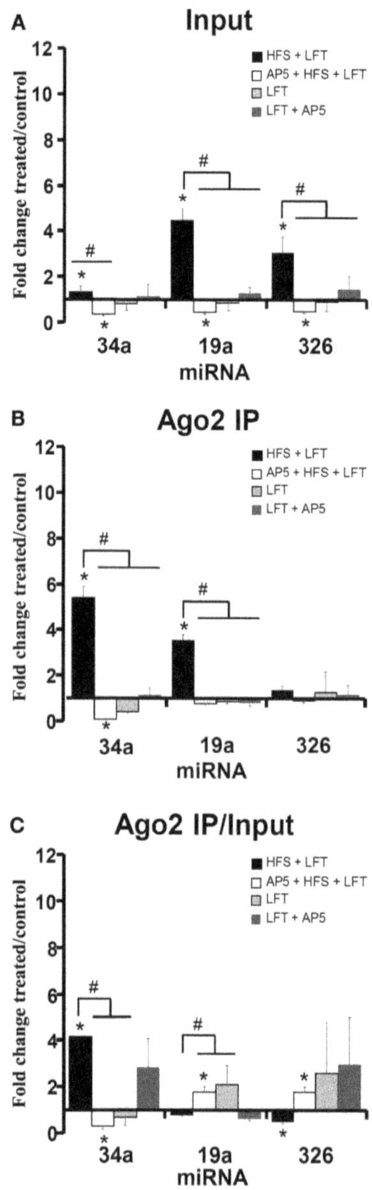

FIGURE 4 | Regulation of *Arc*-targeting miRNAs in LTP. Quantitative PCR was used to examine the expression of a set of 3 *Arc*-associated miRNAs at 30 min. The same set of miRNAs were analyzed in the input sample **(A)** and Ago2 immunoprecipitate **(B)**. The qPCR data was normalized to the expression of miR-345-3p. **(A)** Fold change in *Arc*-associated miRNA expression in dentate gyrus lysates at 30 min post-HFS. Bar graph shows mean fold change (+s.e.m.) in treated dentate gyrus relative to control, contralateral dentate gyrus. HFS + LFT, $n = 6$; AP5 + HFS + LFT, $n = 4$; LFT alone, $n = 5$; AP5 + LFT, $n = 5$. Significant differences between the HFS group and other treatment groups are indicated (#; $p < 0.05$). Significant difference between the ispilateral (treated) and contralateral (control) dentate gyrus are indicated (*). **(B)** Fold change in *Arc*-associated miRNA expression in dentate gyrus Ago2 immunoprecipitates at 30 min post-HFS. Significant differences between the HFS group and other treatment groups are indicated (#; $p < 0.05$). Significant difference between the ispilateral (treated) and contralateral (control) dentate gyrus are indicated (*). **(C)** Relative fold change in *Arc*-associated miRNA expression in dentate gyrus Ago2 immunoprecipitates compared to dentate gyrus lysates (Ago2/input

(Continued)

FIGURE 4 | Continued

expression ratios) at 30 min post-HFS. Significant differences between the HFS group and other treatment groups are indicated (#; $p < 0.05$). Significant difference between the ispilateral (treated) and contralateral (control) dentate gyrus are indicated (*).

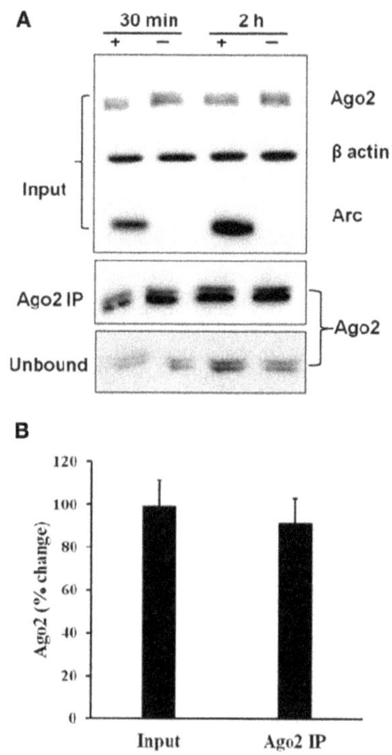

FIGURE 5 | Stable expression of Argonaute 2 protein during LTP. (A) Immunoprecipitation of Ago2 30 and 120 min post-HFS. Representative immunoblot of Ago2 expression levels in input, Ago2 immunoprecipitate (Ago2 IP), and unbound fraction. **(B)** Bar graph shows mean % change (+s.e.m.) in Ago2 levels in input and Ago2-IP samples of treated dentate gyrus relative to the contralateral citation(untreated) dentate gyrus ($n = 17$).

different target gene prediction algorithms (Reyes-Herrera and Ficarra, 2012). Target gene list sizes for miRNAs with activity-dependent association with Ago2 for the 8 enhanced miRNAs were 97 (miR-20a), 156 (miR-219), 58 (miR-223), 114 (miR-29b), 30 (miR-330), 91 (miR-34a), 156 (miR-384), and 53 (miR-592) and for the 5 depleted miRNAs were 52 (let-7f), 55 (miR-338), 47 (miR-212), 255 (miR-19a), 32 (miR-326).

We next created three union target gene sets of 684 (enhanced), 418 (depleted), and 1019 (combined) predicted miRNA target genes to use as input for pathway enrichment analysis using the Bioconductor KEGGprofile package (Zhao, 2012). The combined list miRNA targets are strongly enriched in a number of key biological pathways relevant to activity-dependent synaptic plasticity (**Table 1**) including MAPK, mTOR, and Ras signaling pathways.

Of particular note is the greater than 4-fold over-representation ($p = 4.73 \times 10^{-11}$) of genes traditionally involved in the mediation of axon guidance. **Figure 6** shows a schematic of the axon navigation pathway annotated to show

Table 1 | KEGG pathways targeted by the 13 activity-dependent miRNAs.

KEGG	Pathway	*N*	*FC*	*p*
4360	Axon guidance	25	4.32	4.72E-11
4510	Focal adhesion	30	3.23	1.37E-09
4151	PI3K-Akt signaling pathway	35	2.28	5.02E-07
4320	Dorso-ventral axis formation	7	7.15	2.58E-06
4014	Ras signaling pathway	24	2.29	2.68E-05
4010	MAPK signaling pathway	25	2.15	5.46E-05
4150	mTOR signaling pathway	10	3.51	9.65E-05
4070	Phosphatidylinositol signaling system	11	3.01	2.27E-04
4350	TGF-beta signaling pathway	10	2.74	8.76E-04
4720	Long-term potentiation	8	2.77	2.06E-03
4144	Endocytosis	19	1.82	2.87E-03
4725	Cholinergic synapse	11	2.19	3.86E-03
4810	Regulation of actin cytoskeleton	17	1.74	6.99E-03
4722	Neurotrophin signaling pathway	11	2.01	7.52E-03
562	Inositol phosphate metabolism	7	2.35	8.92E-03
3018	RNA degradation	8	2.22	8.97E-03
4310	Wnt signaling pathway	12	1.90	9.12E-03
4120	Ubiquitin mediated proteolysis	11	1.82	1.58E-02
4340	Hedgehog signaling pathway	5	2.34	1.84E-02
3060	Protein export	3	2.81	2.00E-02
4728	Dopaminergic synapse	10	1.72	2.83E-02

KEGG, KEGG accession number; N, number of target genes in pathway; FC, fold enrichment over expected.

the targeting of enhanced and depleted miRNAs. The enhanced miRNA pool remarkably targets receptors of all four signaling families of the pathway; ephrins, netrins, semaphorins, and Slits as well as MAPK1 and GSK3β which have well-established roles in the regulation of activity-dependent synaptic plasticity. Both enhanced and depleted microRNAs appear to heavily target genes involved in ephrin signal transduction especially the cascade directly upstream of MAPK1. The only place where enhanced and depleted targets directly oppose each other is in differential targeting of the Robo1 and Robo2 receptors for Slit1/2.

Pathway enrichment analyses with the individual enhanced and depleted lists produce very similar pathway enrichment profiles to the combined lists (see **Tables A2, A3**).

DISCUSSION

microRNA levels are dictated by a multistep biogenesis pathway and probably multiple mechanisms for miRNA decay (Kai and Pasquinelli, 2010; Meister, 2013). Knowledge of miRNA expression during synaptic plasticity has so far relied on measurements in lysates from whole tissue or subcellular fractions. In the canonical biogenesis pathway, the guide strand of the mature miRNAs is bound by Ago to form the miRISC. Mature miRNA is considered to be present predominantly in tight complex with Argonaute. The present analysis of LTP in the dentate gyrus of anesthetized rats demonstrates differential regulation of mature miRNA expression in whole lysates and the Ago2 immunoprecipitated fraction. Both quantitatively and qualitatively, miRNA expression in tissue lysates does not accurately reflect changes in the miRNA content of the Ago2-RISC. The ratio of Ago2/total miRNA expression was regulated bidirectionally in a miRNA-specific manner and was largely dependent on NMDA receptor activation during LTP induction. The present results identify miRNA association with Ago2 as a potential control point in activity-dependent synaptic plasticity in the adult brain.

The high-throughput screen comparing HFS-treated and contralateral dentate gyrus indicated dynamic and differential regulation of total and Ago2-immunoprecipated miRNAs. A systemic validation using TaqMan qPCR demonstrated differential regulation at 30 min post-HFS. When comparing miRNA Ago2/input expression ratios, eight miRNAs (miR-384, miR-29b, miR-219, miR-592, miR-20a, miR-330 miR-223, and miR-34a) exhibited increases relative to the contralateral dentate gyrus, whereas five miRNAs (miR-let7f, miR-338, miR-212, miR-19a, and miR-326) showed decreases in this ratio. The results demonstrate activity-dependent, miRNA-specific regulation of miRNA abundance in the Ago2-RISC relative to total miRNA. The enhanced expression of miRNA and enhanced associated with Ago2 was specific to NMDA receptor-dependent LTP induction, as was the decrease in the Ago2/input ratio for miR-let7f and miR-326. These changes in miRNA expression were blocked when HFS was applied in the presence of NMDAR antagonist, AP5, and were absent when low-frequency test stimulation was applied alone or in combination with AP5 infusion. We therefore conclude that LTP induction is coupled to NMDAR-dependent regulation of miRNA expression and miRNA-specific interactions with Ago2. In addition, those miRNAs upregulated following HFS exhibited significant downregulation upon LTP block by AP5, which was not seen in the low-frequency test stimulation control groups. This indicates that HFS also acts through an unknown, NMDAR-independent mechanism to downregulate miRNA expression and its association with Ago2. Finally, this work does not exclude the possibility of small changes in miRNA expression in the contralateral dentate gyrus, although we have demonstrated LTP-specific regulation of miRNAs in the HFS-treated dentate gyrus.

Consistent with our previous work (Wibrand et al., 2010), expression of miR-212 and miR-132 was increased in dentate gyrus lysates at 120 min post-HFS. Wibrand and colleagues observed NMDAR-dependent decreases in mature miR-212 and miR-132 in the absence of NMDAR-dependent effects on precursor miRNA levels, suggesting that NMDAR signaling promotes decay of the mature miRNAs. Consistent with increased turnover, decreased expression was observed for ~50% of the miRNAs that were regulated in the input samples at 30 and 120 min post-HFS. However, the present work focused on qPCR validation of miRNAs that were upregulated in the Ago2 IP.

Park and Tang (2009) used miRNA arrays to determine the temporal expression profiles of 62 miRNAs in adult mouse hippocampal slices following induction of chemical LTP (C-LTP) and metabotropic glutamate receptor-dependent LTD (mGluR-LTD). The study demonstrated regulation of total (lysate) miRNA expression for the majority of miRNAs (50/61) by both C-LTP and mGluR-LTD. Most regulated miRNAs exhibited rapid upregulation at 15 min and declined thereafter but were still upregulated 2 h after LTP or LTD induction. In the present *in vivo* study, LTP was induced by patterned HFS of the medial perforant path

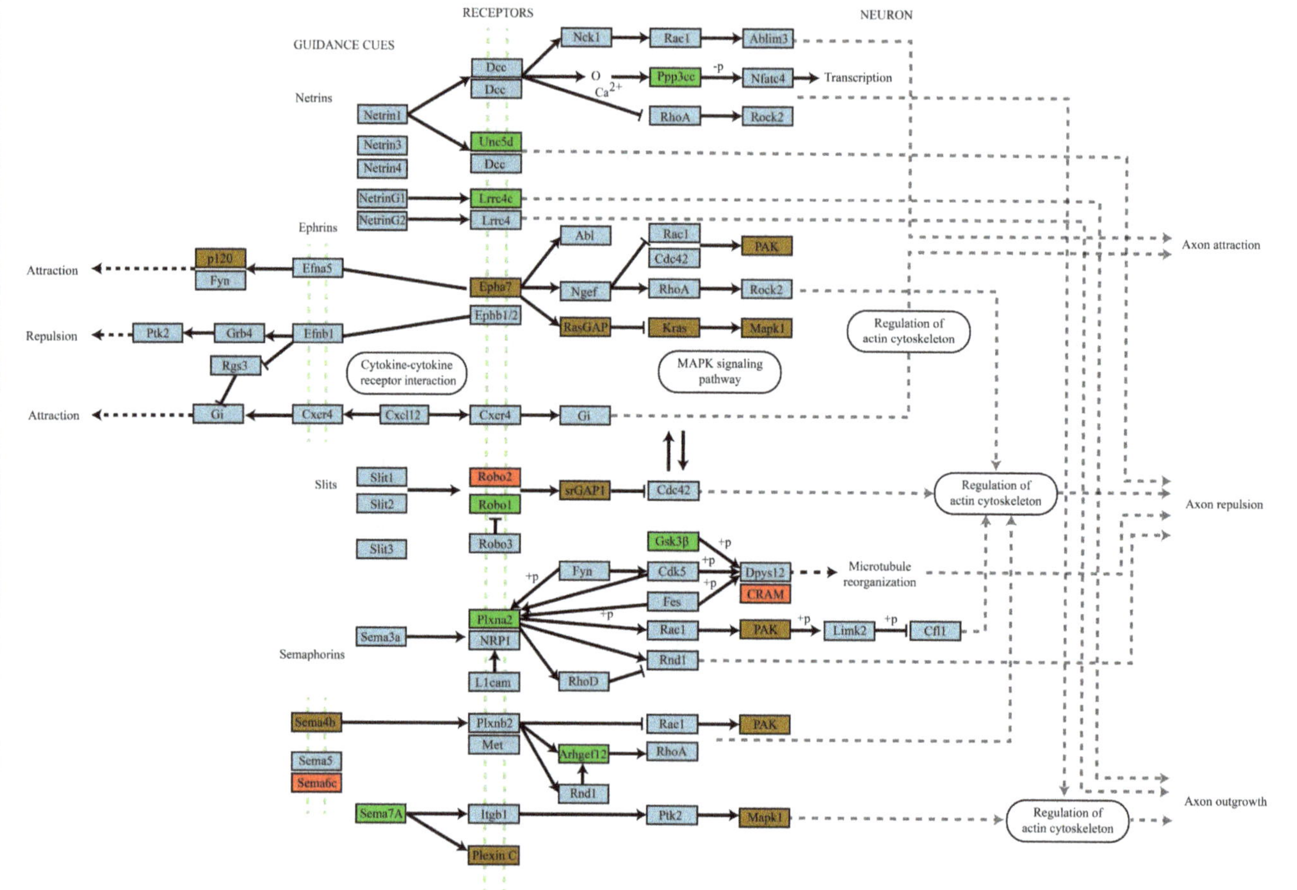

FIGURE 6 | Axon navigation pathway targeting by miRNAs that differentially associate with Ago2 in an activity-dependent manner. Genes targeted by miRNAs that differentially associate with Ago2 in an activity-dependent manner are color coded by whether they are targeted by enhanced (green box), depleted (red box), or by both enhanced and depleted miRNAs (brown box). The involvement of all four guidance molecule families and their convergence on signal transduction systems classically associated with activity-dependent synaptic plasticity suggests an important role for these receptor mediated signaling pathways in plasticity.

input to the dentate gyrus. Rapid regulation at 30 min post-HFS was also observed in the present study, particularly in the Ago2 IP samples. However, the high-throughput screen shows delayed (2 h) bidirectional changes in miRNA expression in both Ago2 immunoprecipitates and lysates.

REGULATON OF Ago2-microRNA INTERACTIONS

The differential regulation of Ago2 immunoprecipitated and total miRNA expression indicates the existence of a substantial non-Ago2-bound or "free" miRNA fraction. A key issue to be resolved is the nature of the non-Ago2-bound pool. This pool may consist of (1) mature miRNAs in the RISC loading complex ready to be loaded onto Ago, (2) miRNAs discharged from Ago following degradation of the target mRNA, (3) miRNAs weakly bound to Ago2 which dissociate during sample preparation, and (4) miRNAs bound to other members of the Argonaute family.

Co-expression of Argonaute family proteins (Ago1, 2, 3, and 4) occurs in many animal cell types including neurons. The four Ago proteins appear to play overlapping roles in mammals (Juvvuna et al., 2012; Meister, 2013). All mammalian Ago proteins contain PAZ, MID, and PIWI domains. The PAZ domain anchors the 3′-end of the miRNA, while the MID domain harbors a binding pocket for the 5′-end of the miRNA. The PIWI domain of Ago2, but not of other mammalian Ago proteins, has endonucleolytic activity capable of cleaving perfectly complementary sites. In mammals, however, miRNAs bind predominantly to partially complementary mRNA and Ago2-mediated "slicing" of target mRNA is uncommon. Rather, the mammalian Ago-RISC inhibits translation and promotes deadenylation-induced mRNA decay. Recent work suggests a sequential mechanism whereby rapid translation inhibition is followed by slow mRNA degradation (Béthune et al., 2012; Djuranovic et al., 2012).

Mammalian miRNAs are thought to be randomly sorted onto the four Argonaute proteins rather than targeted to specific Ago proteins (Dueck et al., 2012; Wang et al., 2012). If this is true for the brain, then analysis of Ago2 immunoprecipitated miRNAs can be considered representative of miRNA regulation as a whole. Wang et al. (2012) immunoprecipitated Ago1–3 from mouse keratinocytes and human melanoma cells and performed qPCR analysis to quantify the levels of miRNAs that interact with each

Ago species. Ago2 interacted with a majority of miRNAs (60%), compared with Ago1 (30%) and Ago3 (<10%) in a proportion that matched the abundance of each Ago. However, processing of some miRNA precursors is mediated by Ago2 rather than Dicer. Dueck et al. (2012) demonstrated that ectopically expressed miR-451 in HEK293 cells is not only processed by Ago2 but also loaded exclusively onto Ago2-associated RISC. Once associated with Ago2, the mature miRNA is not exchanged with other Ago family proteins. In medium spiny neurons of the striatum, Ago2 (but not other Agos) contributes to the expression of some 25% of mature miRNAs (Schaefer et al., 2010). Therefore, it is possible that the Ago2 immunoprecipitated miRNAs identified in the present study are skewed toward Ago2 processing-dependent miRNAs. Immunoprecipitation of other Ago family proteins is needed to address the issue.

Recent work suggests that miRNA loading onto Ago is a regulated process. The minimal RISC loading complex consists of Dicer, the double-stranded RNA-binding protein, TRBP, heat-shock protein 90, and Ago. The current view is that miRNA loading onto Ago occurs in two-steps (Meister, 2013). The mature microRNA duplex is first bound by TRBP, which repositions the duplex on Dicer in an orientation that affords correct strand selection. The actual transfer of the miRNA duplex to Ago is mediated by heat shock protein 90 (HSP90), which binds Ago and keeps it in an open state capable of capturing the miRNA. Additional mechanisms likely exist for sequestering miRNA from Ago. For example, the RNA-binding protein, hnRNP E2, has been shown to reversibly sequester miR-328 away from Ago, Dicer, and other proteins of the RISC loading complex (Eiring et al., 2010).

A set of positive-charged arginine amino acids concentrated in the nucleotide-binding channel in Ago stabilizes the interaction of the protein with miRNA (Wang et al., 2010). However, molecular dynamic simulations and thermodynamic analysis indicate that conformational changes within the flexible PAZ domain could affect the recognition and release of miRNA (Wang et al., 2010). Recent evidence suggests that Ago2 is also extensively regulated by phosphorylation. A highly conserved tyrosine (Y529) located in the 5′-end-binding pocket of Ago2's MID domain can be phosphorylated (Rüdel et al., 2011). This phosphorylation inhibits small RNA binding to Ago2, suggesting that it may serve as a reversible molecular switch on miRNA binding. If Ago2 conformation is so regulated during LTP, this could provide a basis for the reversible modulation of Ago2:miRNA binding.

By stabilizing guide-stranded mature miRNA, Ago vastly extends the half-life of miRNA. Downregulation or ectopic expression of Ago results in decreased or enhanced miRNA levels, respectively (Winter and Diederichs, 2011). Hence, changes in Ago2 abundance would be expected to influence miRNA levels. However, modulation of Ago2 levels does not appear to be a contributing mechanism in LTP, as there was no change in the amount of total or immunoprecipitated Ago2 at 30 or 120 min after LTP induction.

Work in *C. elegans* suggests that target mRNA availability is a key factor in determining the release of miRNA from Argonaute and subsequent degradation of the miRNA (Chatterjee and Grosshans, 2009). miRNA binding to target stabilizes the miRNA:Ago interaction. miRNAs bound to abundant and stable mRNA will themselves be stable. Upon degradation of the target mRNA, miRNAs are released from Ago and degraded. Accordingly, changes in the mRNA expression profile during LTP are likely to influence the ratio of Ago2-bound to free miRNA in an miRNA-specific manner.

Circular RNAs (circRNAs) are a major class of regulatory RNAs which function to sponge endogenous miRNAs (Hansen et al., 2013; Memczak et al., 2013). CircRNAs are diverse (at least 2000 in human and mouse), abundantly expressed in brain, and contain numerous miRNA binding sites. miR-7 binding to a specific circRNA (csRS-7) results in robust derepression of miR-7 mRNA targets in neurons. Although miRNAs remain bound to Ago on circRNAs, circRNAs are resistant to miRISC-mediated destabilization. As a result, any movement or exchange of miRNAs between their binding sites on circRNA and mRNA is likely to shift the balance between free and Ago2-associated miRNA. Regulation of circRNAs in LTP is hypothetical at present, but could potentially contribute to rapid changes in the Ago2-miRNA pool.

A recent study in cortical synaptosomes suggests that axon terminals accumulate, store, and secrete miRNAs (Xu et al., 2013). Synaptosomes are biochemical fractions containing axon terminals that are pinched-off and released, often together with components of the postsynaptic membrane. The authors characterized miRNA profiles in synaptosomes using microarrays and qPCR. Endogenous Ago2-bound miRNAs were enriched in the synaptic vesicle fraction. Synthetic miR-125 was also taken up by the synaptosomes through a non-specific endocytic mechanism. Interestingly, the proportion of Ago2/total miRNAs in the synaptosome varied considerably among the 21 miRNAs, indicating that a miRNA-specific, non-Ago2-bound pool exists. Upon KCL-evoked depolarization, endogenous miRNAs are secreted from synaptosomes still attached to Ago2. It is therefore possible that secretion of Ago2 bound miRNAs, from postsynaptic or presynaptic compartments, alters the equilibrium between free and Ago2-bound miRNAs.

miRNA TARGET PREDICTION AND PATHWAY ANALYSIS

Central to our understanding of miRNA function is the identification of their direct molecular targets. To date, no direct binding screens have taken place in experimental systems relevant to activity-dependent synaptic plasticity although techniques now exist to do so (Helwak et al., 2013). In the absence of such data we rely on miRNA target prediction algorithms that use structural, sequence and evolutionary based features of known miRNA-binding sites (Reyes-Herrera and Ficarra, 2012). Despite their widespread adoption, however, there is poor agreement between predictions made by different algorithms for the same miRNA. We adopted the RP approach to identify the most consistently predicted target genes from four of the most widely used miRNA target prediction algorithms. This produced mutually supportive target gene lists of on average 100 genes per miRNA that had lost 94.9% of predicted targets during the cross-comparison analysis by RP (**Table A4**).

Comparison of the biological pathways targeted by miRNAs with enhanced and depleted activity-dependent Ago2 association revealed 21 significantly enriched pathways ($p \leq 0.05$). Among these were many previously reported to play roles in the regulation of activity-dependent synaptic plasticity in four broad categories including *remodeling and turnover pathways:* cell-cell adhesion (Gerrow and El-Husseini, 2006), actin cytoskeletal rearrangement (Bosch and Hayashi, 2012), endocytosis (Huganir and Nicoll, 2013; Jiang and Ehlers, 2013) proteolysis and protein export (Bingol and Sheng, 2011), *signal transduction pathways*: ERK/MAPK (English and Sweatt, 1997; Rosenblum et al., 2002; Ying et al., 2002; Kelleher et al., 2004), PI3K-Akt, mTOR (Hoeffer and Klann, 2010), Ras (Stornetta and Zhu, 2011), TGFβ, neurotrophin, and Wnt (Poon et al., 2013), *process pathways*: LTP, cholinergic and dopaminergic synapse activity and *developmental pathways*: axon guidance and dorso-ventral axis formation. This latter group show the highest and most significant enrichment in our miRNA targets and emerging evidence supports a central role for classical developmental pathways such as axon guidance in the regulation of synaptic plasticity (Wibrand et al., 2006; Knafo and Esteban, 2012). Indeed the intracellular signaling pathways through which netrins (Bayat et al., 2012; Horn et al., 2013), ephrins (Lim et al., 2008; Klein, 2009), Slits (Soderling et al., 2007), and semaphorins (Pasterkamp and Giger, 2009) operate are the same pathways found to be functional during activity-dependent synaptic plasticity.

CLOSING COMMENTS

In sum, the present work provides evidence for bidirectional changes in miRNA expression compatible with regulated shuttling of miRNA to and from Ago2 in the adult dentate gyrus. As recent work has succeeded in cell-specific expression profiling of Ago2-associated miRNAs in brain (He et al., 2012), it will be important to elucidate the signaling pathways and cell biological mechanisms that dictate time-dependent interactions of miRNA with Argonautes. In addition, the bioinformatic predictions for biological processes modulated by Ago2-regulated miRNAs strongly point to regulation of mechanisms classically involved in axon guidance.

ACKNOWLEDGMENTS

Funded by the University of Bergen, the Lundbeck Foundation, The Research Council of Norway, and European Research Area Networks in systems biology (ERA-SysBio+). Karin Wibrand was supported by a grant from Bergen Medical Research Foundation (BMFS). Maciej Pajak was funded by grants EP/F500385/1 and BB/F529254/1.

REFERENCES

Ashraf, S. I., McLoon, A. L., Sclarsic, S. M., and Kunes, S. (2006). Synaptic protein synthesis associated with memory is regulated by the RISC pathway in Drosophila. *Cell* 124, 191–205. doi: 10.1016/j.cell.2005.12.017

Banerjee, S., Neveu, P., and Kosik, K. S. (2009). A coordinated local translational control point at the synapse involving relief from silencing and MOV10 degradation. *Neuron* 64, 871–884. doi: 10.1016/j.neuron.2009.11.023

Bartel, D. P. (2004). MicroRNAs: genomics, biogenesis, mechanism, and function. *Cell* 116, 281–297. doi: 10.1016/S0092-8674(04)00045-5

Bayat, M., Baluchnejadmojarad, T., Roghani, M., Goshadrou, F., Ronaghi, A., and Mehdizadeh, M. (2012). Netrin-1 improves spatial memory and synaptic plasticity impairment following global ischemia in the rat. *Brain Res.* 1452, 185–194. doi: 10.1016/j.brainres.2012.03.008

Béthune, J., Artus-Revel, C. G., and Filipowicz, W. (2012). Kinetic analysis reveals successive steps leading to miRNA-mediated silencing in mammalian cells. *EMBO Rep.* 13, 716–723. doi: 10.1038/embor.2012.82

Bingol, B., and Sheng, M. (2011). Deconstruction for reconstruction: the role of proteolysis in neural plasticity and disease. *Neuron* 69, 22–32. doi: 10.1016/j.neuron.2010.11.006

Bosch, M., and Hayashi, Y. (2012). Structural plasticity of dendritic spines. *Curr. Opin. Neurobiol.* 22, 383–388. doi: 10.1016/j.conb.2011.09.002

Bramham, C. R., Alme, M. N., Bittins, M., Kuipers, S. D., Nair, R. R., Pai, B., et al. (2010). The Arc of synaptic memory. *Exp. Brain Res.* 200, 125–140. doi: 10.1007/s00221-009-1959-2

Bramham, C. R., and Wells, D. G. (2007). Dendritic mRNA: transport, translation and function. *Nat. Rev. Neurosci.* 8, 776–789. doi: 10.1038/nrn2150

Breitling, R., Armengaud, P., Amtmann, A., and Herzyk, P. (2004). Rank products: a simple, yet powerful, new method to detect differentially regulated genes in replicated microarray experiments. *FEBS Lett.* 573, 83–92. doi: 10.1016/j.febslet.2004.07.055

Chatterjee, S., and Grosshans, H. (2009). Active turnover modulates mature microRNA activity in *Caenorhabditis elegans*. *Nature* 461, 546–549. doi: 10.1038/nature08349

Choe, J., Cho, H., Lee, H. C., and Kim, Y. K. (2010). microRNA/Argonaute 2 regulates nonsense-mediated messenger RNA decay. *EMBO Rep.* 11, 380–386. doi: 10.1038/embor.2010.44

Djuranovic, S., Nahvi, A., and Green, R. (2011). A parsimonious model for gene regulation by miRNAs. *Science* 331, 550–553. doi: 10.1126/science.1191138

Djuranovic, S., Nahvi, A., and Green, R. (2012). miRNA-mediated gene silencing by translational repression followed by mRNA deadenylation and decay. *Science* 336, 237–240. doi: 10.1126/science.1215691

Dueck, A., Ziegler, C., Eichner, A., Berezikov, E., and Meister, G. (2012). microRNAs associated with the different human Argonaute proteins. *Nucleic Acids Res.* 40, 9850–9862. doi: 10.1093/nar/gks70

Eiring, A. M., Harb, J. G., Neviani, P., Garton, C., Oaks, J. J., Spizzo, R., et al. (2010). miR-328 functions as an RNA decoy to modulate hnRNP E2 regulation of mRNA translation in leukemic blasts. *Cell* 140, 652–665. doi: 10.1016/j.cell.2010.01.007

Eisinga, R., Breitling, R., and Heskes, T. (2013). The exact probability distribution of the rank product statistics for replicated experiments. *FEBS Lett.* 587, 677–682. doi: 10.1016/j.febslet.2013.01.037

English, J. D., and Sweatt, J. D. (1997). A requirement for the mitogen-activated protein kinase cascade in hippocampal long term potentiation. *J. Biol. Chem.* 272, 19103–19106. doi: 10.1074/jbc.272.31.19103

Filipowicz, W., Bhattacharyya, S. N., and Sonenberg, N. (2008). Mechanisms of post-transcriptional regulation by microRNAs: are the answers in sight? *Nat. Rev. Genet.* 9, 102–14. doi: 10.1038/nrg2290

Friedman, R. C., Farh, K. K.-H., Burge, C. B., and Bartel, D. P. (2009). Most mammalian mRNAs are conserved targets of microRNAs. *Genome Res.* 19, 92–105. doi: 10.1101/gr.082701.108

Gerrow, K., and El-Husseini, A. (2006). Cell adhesion molecules at the synapse. *Front. Biosci.* 11, 2400–2419. doi: 10.2741/1978

Griffiths-Jones, S., Saini, H. K., van Dongen, S., and Enright, A. J. (2008). miRBase: tools for microRNA genomics. *Nucleic Acids Res.* 36, D154–D158. doi: 10.1093/nar/gkm952

Hansen, T. B., Jensen, T. I., Clausen, B. H., Bramsen, J. B., Finsen, B., Damgaard, C. K., et al. (2013). Natural RNA circles function as efficient microRNA sponges. *Nature* 495, 384–388. doi: 10.1038/nature11993

He, M., Liu, Y., Wang, X., and Zhang, M. (2012). Cell-type-based analysis of microRNA profiles in the mouse brain. *Neuron* 73, 35–48. doi: 10.1016/j.neuron.2011.11.010

Helwak, A., Kudla, G., Dudnakova, T., and Tollervey, D. (2013). Mapping the human miRNA interactome by CLASH reveals frequent noncanonical binding. *Cell* 153, 654–665. doi: 10.1016/j.cell.2013.03.043

Hoeffer, C. A., and Klann, E. (2010). mTOR signaling: at the crossroads of plasticity, memory and disease. *Trends Neurosci.* 33, 67–75. doi: 10.1016/j.tins.2009.11.003

Hong, F., Breitling, R., McEntee, C. W., Wittner, B. S., Nemhauser, J. L., and Chory, J. (2006). RankProd: a bioconductor package for detecting differentially expressed genes in meta-analysis. *Bioinformatics* 22, 2825–2827. doi: 10.1093/bioinformatics/btl476

Horn, K. E., Glasgow, S. D., Gobert, D., Bull, S.-J., Luk, T., Girgis, J., et al. (2013). DCC expression by neurons regulates synaptic plasticity in the adult brain. *Cell Rep.* 3, 173–185. doi: 10.1016/j.celrep.2012.12.005

Huganir, R. L., and Nicoll, R. A. (2013). AMPARs and synaptic plasticity: the last 25 years. *Neuron* 80, 704–717. doi: 10.1016/j.neuron.2013.10.025

Huntzinger, E., and Izaurralde, E. (2011). Gene silencing by microRNAs: contributions of translational repression and mRNA decay. *Nat. Rev. Genet.* 12, 99–110. doi: 10.1038/nrg2936

Jiang, Y., and Ehlers, M. D. (2013). Review modeling autism by SHANK gene mutations in mice. *Neuron* 78, 8–27. doi: 10.1016/j.neuron.2013.03.016

Juvvuna, P. K., Khandelia, P., Lee, L. M., and Makeyev, E. V. (2012). Argonaute identity defines the length of mature mammalian microRNAs. *Nucleic Acids Res.* 40, 6808–6820. doi: 10.1093/nar/gks293

Kai, Z. S., and Pasquinelli, A. E. (2010). MicroRNA assassins: factors that regulate the disappearance of miRNAs. *Nat. Struct. Mol. Biol.* 17, 5–10. doi: 10.1038/nsmb.1762

Kanehisa, M., Goto, S., Sato, Y., Furumichi, M., and Tanabe, M. (2011). KEGG for integration and interpretation of large-scale molecular data sets. *Nucleic Acids Res.* 40, D109–D114. doi: 10.1093/nar/gkr988

Kelleher, R. J., Govindarajan, A., Jung, H.-Y., Kang, H., and Tonegawa, S. (2004). Translational control by MAPK signaling in long-term synaptic plasticity and memory. *Cell* 116, 467–479. doi: 10.1016/S0092-8674(04)00115-1

Klein, R. (2009). Bidirectional modulation of synaptic functions by Eph/ephrin signaling. *Nat. Neurosci.* 12, 15–20. doi: 10.1038/nn.2231

Knafo, S., and Esteban, J. A. (2012). Common pathways for growth and for plasticity. *Curr. Opin. Neurobiol.* 22, 405–411. doi: 10.1016/j.conb.2012.02.008

Kosik, K. S. (2006). The neuronal microRNA system. *Nat. Rev. Neurosci.* 7, 911–920. doi: 10.1038/nrn2037

Krichevsky, A. M., Sonntag, K.-C., Isacson, O., and Kosik, K. S. (2006). Specific microRNAs modulate embryonic stem cell-derived neurogenesis. *Stem Cells* 24, 857–864. doi: 10.1634/stemcells.2005-0441

Krol, J., Busskamp, V., Markiewicz, I., Stadler, M. B., Ribi, S., Richter, J., et al. (2010a). Characterizing light-regulated retinal microRNAs reveals rapid turnover as a common property of neuronal microRNAs. *Cell* 141, 618–631. doi: 10.1016/j.cell.2010.03.039

Krol, J., Loedige, I., and Filipowicz, W. (2010b). The widespread regulation of microRNA biogenesis, function and decay. *Nat. Rev. Genet.* 11, 597–610. doi: 10.1038/nrg2843

Lall, S., Grün, D., Krek, A., Chen, K., Wang, Y.-L., Dewey, C. N., et al. (2006). A genome-wide map of conserved microRNA targets in *C. elegans*. *Curr. Biol.* 16, 460–471. doi: 10.1016/j.cub.2006.01.050

Lim, B. K., Matsuda, N., and Poo, M. (2008). Ephrin-B reverse signaling promotes structural and functional synaptic maturation *in vivo*. *Nat. Neurosci.* 11, 160–169. doi: 10.1038/nn2033

Lugli, G., Larson, J., Martone, M. E., Jones, Y., and Smalheiser, N. R. (2005). Dicer and eIF2c are enriched at postsynaptic densities in adult mouse brain and are modified by neuronal activity in a calpain-dependent manner. *J. Neurochem.* 94, 896–905. doi: 10.1111/j.1471-4159.2005.03224.x

Maragkakis, M., Vergoulis, T., Alexiou, P., Reczko, M., Plomaritou, K., Gousis, M., et al. (2011). DIANA-microT Web server upgrade supports Fly and Worm miRNA target prediction and bibliographic miRNA to disease association. *Nucleic Acids Res.* 39, W145–W148. doi: 10.1093/nar/gkr294

Martin, K. C., and Ephrussi, A. (2009). mRNA localization: gene expression in the spatial dimension. *Cell* 136, 719–730. doi: 10.1016/j.cell.2009.01.044

Meister, G. (2013). Argonaute proteins: functional insights and emerging roles. *Nat. Rev. Genet.* 14, 447–459. doi: 10.1038/nrg3462

Mellios, N., Sugihara, H., Castro, J., Banerjee, A., Le, C., Kumar, A., et al. (2011). miR-132, an experience-dependent microRNA, is essential for visual cortex plasticity. *Nat. Neurosci.* 14, 1240–1242. doi: 10.1038/nn.2909

Memczak, S., Jens, M., Elefsinioti, A., Torti, F., Krueger, J., Rybak, A., et al. (2013). Circular RNAs are a large class of animal RNAs with regulatory potency. *Nature* 495, 333–338. doi: 10.1038/nature11928

Messaoudi, E., Kanhema, T., Soulé, J., Tiron, A., Dagyte, G., da Silva, B., et al. (2007). Sustained Arc/Arg3.1 synthesis controls long-term potentiation consolidation through regulation of local actin polymerization in the dentate gyrus *in vivo*. *J. Neurosci.* 27, 10445–10455. doi: 10.1523/JNEUROSCI.2883-07.2007

Messaoudi, E., Ying, S.-W., Kanhema, T., Croll, S. D., and Bramham, C. R. (2002). Brain-derived neurotrophic factor triggers transcription-dependent, late phase long-term potentiation *in vivo*. *J. Neurosci.* 22, 7453–7461.

Panja, D., Dagyte, G., Bidinosti, M., Wibrand, K., Kristiansen, A.-M., Sonenberg, N., et al. (2009). Novel translational control in Arc-dependent long term potentiation consolidation *in vivo*. *J. Biol. Chem.* 284, 31498–31511. doi: 10.1074/jbc.M109.056077

Park, C. S., and Tang, S. J. (2009). Regulation of microRNA expression by induction of bidirectional synaptic plasticity. *J. Mol. Neurosci.* 38, 50–56. doi: 10.1007/s12031-008-9158-3

Pasterkamp, R. J., and Giger, R. J. (2009). Semaphorin function in neural plasticity and disease. *Curr. Opin. Neurobiol.* 19, 263–274. doi: 10.1016/j.conb.2009.06.001

Poon, V. Y., Choi, S., and Park, M. (2013). Growth factors in synaptic function. *Front. Synaptic Neurosci.* 5:6. doi: 10.3389/fnsyn.2013.00006

Rajasethupathy, P., Fiumara, F., Sheridan, R., Betel, D., Puthanveettil, S. V., Russo, J. J., et al. (2009). Characterization of small RNAs in aplysia reveals a role for miR-124 in constraining synaptic plasticity through CREB. *Neuron* 63, 803–817. doi: 10.1016/j.neuron.2009.05.029

Reyes-Herrera, P. H., and Ficarra, E. (2012). One decade of development and evolution of microRNA target prediction algorithms. *Genomics Proteomics Bioinformatics* 10, 254–263. doi: 10.1016/j.gpb.2012.10.001

Rosenblum, K., Futter, M., Voss, K., Erent, M., Skehel, P. A., French, P., et al. (2002). The role of extracellular regulated kinases I/II in late-phase long-term potentiation. *J. Neurosci.* 22, 5432–5441.

Rüdel, S., Wang, Y., Lenobel, R., Körner, R., Hsiao, H.-H., Urlaub, H., et al. (2011). Phosphorylation of human Argonaute proteins affects small RNA binding. *Nucleic Acids Res.* 39, 2330–2343. doi: 10.1093/nar/gkq1032

Schaefer, A., Im, H.-I., Venø, M. T., Fowler, C. D., Min, A., Intrator, A., et al. (2010). Argonaute 2 in dopamine 2 receptor-expressing neurons regulates cocaine addiction. *J. Exp. Med.* 207, 1843–1851. doi: 10.1084/jem.20100451

Siegel, G., Obernosterer, G., Fiore, R., Oehmen, M., Bicker, S., Christensen, M., et al. (2009). A functional screen implicates microRNA-138-dependent regulation of the depalmitoylation enzyme APT1 in dendritic spine morphogenesis. *Nat. Cell Biol.* 11, 705–716. doi: 10.1038/ncb1876

Soderling, S. H., Guire, E. S., Kaech, S., White, J., Zhang, F., Schutz, K., et al. (2007). A WAVE-1 and WRP signaling complex regulates spine density, synaptic plasticity, and memory. *J. Neurosci.* 27, 355–365. doi: 10.1523/JNEUROSCI.3209-06.2006

Stornetta, R. L., and Zhu, J. J. (2011). Ras and rap signaling in synaptic plasticity and mental disorders. *Neuroscientist* 17, 54–78. doi: 10.1177/1073858410365562

Tognini, P., Putignano, E., Coatti, A., and Pizzorusso, T. (2011). Experience-dependent expression of miR-132 regulates ocular dominance plasticity. *Nat. Neurosci.* 14, 1237–1239. doi: 10.1038/nn.2920

Vilella, A. J., Severin, J., Ureta-Vidal, A., Heng, L., Durbin, R., and Birney, E. (2009). EnsemblCompara GeneTrees: complete, duplication-aware phylogenetic trees in vertebrates. *Genome Res.* 19, 327–335. doi: 10.1101/gr.073585.107

Vo, N., Klein, M. E., Varlamova, O., Keller, D. M., Yamamoto, T., Goodman, R. H., et al. (2005). A cAMP-response element binding protein-induced microRNA regulates neuronal morphogenesis. *Proc. Natl. Acad. Sci. U.S.A.* 102, 16426–16431. doi: 10.1073/pnas.0508448102

Wang, D., Zhang, Z., O'Loughlin, E., Lee, T., Houel, S., O'Carroll, D., et al. (2012). Quantitative functions of argonaute proteins in mammalian development. *Genes Dev.* 26, 693–704. doi: 10.1101/gad.182758.111

Wang, Y., Li, Y., Ma, Z., Yang, W., and Ai, C. (2010). Mechanism of microRNA-target interaction: molecular dynamics simulations and thermodynamics analysis. *PLoS Comput. Biol.* 6:e1000866. doi: 10.1371/journal.pcbi.1000866

Wibrand, K., Messaoudi, E., Håvik, B., Steenslid, V., Løvlie, R., Steen, V. M., et al. (2006). Identification of genes co-upregulated with Arc during BDNF-induced long-term potentiation in adult rat dentate gyrus *in vivo*. *Eur. J. Neurosci.* 23, 1501–1511. doi: 10.1111/j.1460-9568.2006.04687.x

Wibrand, K., Pai, B., Siripornmongcolchai, T., Bittins, M., Berentsen, B., Ofte, M. L., et al. (2012). MicroRNA regulation of the synaptic plasticity-related gene Arc. *PLoS ONE* 7:e41688. doi: 10.1371/journal.pone.0041688

Wibrand, K., Panja, D., Tiron, A., Ofte, M. L., Skaftnesmo, K.-O., Lee, C. S., et al. (2010). Differential regulation of mature and precursor microRNA expression by NMDA and metabotropic glutamate receptor activation during LTP in the adult dentate gyrus *in vivo*. *Eur. J. Neurosci.* 31, 636–645. doi: 10.1111/j.1460-9568.2010.07112.x

Winter, J., and Diederichs, S. (2011). Argonaute proteins regulate microRNA stability. *RNA Biol.* 8, 1149–1157. doi: 10.4161/rna.8.6.17665

Xu, J., Chen, Q., Zen, K., Zhang, C., and Zhang, Q. (2013). Synaptosomes secrete and uptake functionally active microRNAs via exocytosis and endocytosis pathways. *J. Neurochem.* 124, 15–25. doi: 10.1111/jnc.12057

Ying, S.-W., Futter, M., Rosenblum, K., Webber, M. J., Hunt, S. P., Bliss, T. V. P., et al. (2002). Brain-derived neurotrophic factor induces long-term potentiation in intact adult hippocampus: requirement for ERK activation coupled to CREB and upregulation of Arc synthesis. *J. Neurosci.* 22, 1532–1540.

Zhao, S. (2012). *KEGGprofile: an Annotation and Visualization Package for Multi-Types and Multi-Groups Expression Data in KEGG Pathway*. R package version 1.2.0. R/Bioconductor.

APPENDIX

Table A1 | Comparison of PCR card screening to Taqman qPCR validation results.

miRNA	miRNA levels in Ago2 IP following LTP induction	
	PCR card	qPCR
384	↑	↑
29b	↓	↑
219	↑	↑
592	↑	↑
20a	↑	↑
let-7f	↑	↑
330	↑	↑
338	↑	↑
223	↑	↑
212	↑	↓
34a	–	↑
19a	–	↑
326	–	–

Significantly increased expression (↑); significantly decreased expression (↓); no change (–).

Table A2 | Neural related pathways enriched in targets with decreased activity-dependent Ago2 association.

KEGG	Pathway name	*N*	*FC*	*P*
4360	Axon guidance	19	4.71	1.93E-09
4510	Focal adhesion	24	3.70	3.23E-09
4151	PI3K-Akt signaling pathway	28	2.62	3.46E-07
4512	ECM-receptor interaction	11	4.07	1.23E-05
4150	mTOR signaling pathway	8	4.03	1.35E-04
4070	Phosphatidylinositol signaling system	9	3.54	1.91E-04
4010	MAPK signaling pathway	18	2.22	3.11E-04
4320	Dorso-ventral axis formation	4	5.86	4.66E-04
4014	Ras signaling pathway	16	2.19	7.16E-04
562	Inositol phosphate metabolism	7	3.37	9.74E-04
4728	Dopaminergic synapse	10	2.46	2.15E-03
3018	RNA degradation	7	2.78	3.29E-03
4350	TGF-beta signaling pathway	7	2.75	3.55E-03
4310	Wnt signaling pathway	9	2.04	1.14E-02
4720	Long-term potentiation	5	2.48	1.45E-02
5031	Amphetamine addiction	5	2.48	1.45E-02
4810	Regulation of actin cytoskeleton	12	1.76	1.57E-02
4330	Notch signaling pathway	4	2.53	1.98E-02
5034	Alcoholism	10	1.77	2.25E-02
4722	Neurotrophin signaling pathway	7	1.83	3.44E-02
4730	Long-term depression	4	2.08	4.15E-02

Table A3 | Neural related pathways enriched in targets with increased activity-dependent Ago2 association.

KEGG	Pathway name	*N*	*FC*	*P*
4360	Axon guidance	13	6.01	2.13E-08
4320	Dorso-ventral axis formation	5	13.66	1.11E-06
4010	MAPK signaling pathway	14	3.22	1.77E-05
4540	Gap junction	7	4.73	9.98E-05
4014	Ras signaling pathway	12	3.07	1.01E-04
4725	Cholinergic synapse	7	3.72	5.10E-04
4720	Long-term potentiation	5	4.62	6.69E-04
4120	Ubiquitin mediated proteolysis	7	3.09	1.68E-03
4350	TGF-beta signaling pathway	5	3.66	2.23E-03
4722	Neurotrophin signaling pathway	6	2.93	3.96E-03
4530	Tight junction	6	2.61	7.31E-03
4730	Long-term depression	3	2.91	1.89E-02
4721	Synaptic vesicle cycle	3	2.86	1.99E-02
4510	Focal adhesion	7	2.01	2.00E-02
4150	mTOR signaling pathway	3	2.82	2.10E-02
4810	Regulation of actin cytoskeleton	7	1.91	2.60E-02
4310	Wnt signaling pathway	5	2.12	2.86E-02
4668	TNF signaling pathway	4	2.23	3.21E-02
4020	Calcium signaling pathway	6	1.91	3.40E-02
4340	Hedgehog signaling pathway	2	2.50	4.46E-02
4151	PI3K-Akt signaling pathway	9	1.57	4.82E-02
5034	Alcoholism	5	1.65	7.58E-02

Table A4 | Reduction in target gene list size resulting from rank product analysis.

miRNA	UTn	RPn
let-7f	2195	52
miR-19a	1806	255
miR-20a	2244	97
miR-212	1365	47
miR-219	2205	156
miR-223	1274	58
miR-29b	2684	114
miR-326	1455	32
miR-330	2005	30
miR-338	2055	55
miR-34a	1588	91
miR-384	2064	156
miR-592	437	53
Total	23377	1196 (5.1%)

UTn, Unique targets; RPn, Rank products.

8

Regulation of microRNA expression in the neuronal stem cell niches during aging of the short-lived annual fish *Nothobranchius furzeri*

Eva Terzibasi Tozzini[1‡], Aurora Savino[1‡], Roberto Ripa[1], Giorgia Battistoni[1†], Mario Baumgart[2] and Alessandro Cellerino[1,2]*

[1] *Laboratorio di Biologia, Scuola Normale Superiore, Pisa, Italy*
[2] *Fritz Lipmann Institute for Age Research, Leibniz Institute, Jena, Germany*

In the last decade, our group has intensively studied the annual fish *Nothobranchius furzeri* as a new experimental model in Biology specifically applied to aging research. We previously studied adult neuronal stem cells of *N. furzeri in vivo* and we demonstrated an age-dependent decay in adult neurogenesis. More recently we identified and quantified the expression of miRNAs in the brain of *N. furzeri* and we detected 165 conserved miRNAs and found that brain aging in this fish is associated with coherent up-regulation of well-known tumor suppressor miRNAs, as well as down-regulation of well-known onco miRNAs – In the present work we characterized the expression of miR-15a, miR-20a, and microRNA cluster 17–92 in the principal neurogenic niches of the brain of young and old subjects of *N. furzeri*, by using *in situ* hybridization techniques, together with proliferating-cell nuclear antigen immuno-staining for a simultaneous visualization of the neuronal progenitors. We found that: (1) the expression of miR-15a is higher in the brain of old subjects and concentrates mainly in the principal neurogenic niches of telencephalon and optic tectum, (2) the expression of miR-20a is higher in the brain of young subjects, but more widespread to the areas surrounding the neurogenic niches, (3) finally, the expression of the microRNA cluster 17–92 is higher in the brain of young subjects, concentrated mainly in the principal neurogenic niches of telencephalon and cerebellum, and with reduced intensity in the optic tectum. Taken together, our data show that these microRNAs, originally identified in whole-brain analysis, are specifically regulated in the stem cell niche during aging.

Keywords: microRNA regulation, *Nothobranchius furzeri*, adult neurogenesis, aging, neuronal stem cells, maturation, *in situ* hybridization

Correspondence:
Alessandro Cellerino, Laboratorio di Biologia, Scuola Normale Superiore di Pisa, Via Moruzzi 1, 56124 Pisa, Italy
e-mail: a.cellerino@sns.it

[†]*Present address:*
Giorgia Battistoni, Cold Spring Harbour Laboratory, Watson School of Biological Sciences, Huntington, NY, USA

[‡] *Eva Terzibasi Tozzini and Aurora Savino have contributed equally to this work.*

INTRODUCTION

MicroRNAs (miRNAs) are abundant non-coding RNAs around 20–22 nucleotides in length, which are emerging as important key players in the regulation of gene expression. miRNAs are transcribed by RNA Polymerase II (i.e., the same Polymerase which transcribes protein-coding RNAs) as long transcripts called primary transcripts and undergo a complex processing before being included in a ribonucleic complex. Several miRNAs can be grouped in a genomic cluster and co-transcribed, and may be hosted within an intron of a protein-coding gene. MiRNAs bind, due to sequence complementarity, to specific sites in the 3′ untranslated region of their target mRNAs, thereby silencing expression of the gene product via translational repression and/or mRNA degradation. Indeed, they represent a new level of gene regulation acting at the post-transcriptional level. Up to now, several thousands of miRNAs have been predicted and identified in animals, plants and viruses (www.mirbase.org).

A feature of miRNAs is their combinatorial regulation: a given miRNA can target a multitude of different mRNAs and a given target might similarly be targeted by multiple miRNAs; for this reason, they frequently represent the central nodes of several regulatory networks and may act as rheostat to provide stability and fine-tuning to gene expression networks (Osella et al., 2011; Siciliano et al., 2013). Moreover, they are promising candidates for functional studies by genome-wide transcriptional analysis, thanks to some specific features: (i) miRNAs are highly conserved in vertebrates (cases of 100% identity between fish and mammals are not uncommon) and are thought to be an evolutionarily ancient component of genetic regulation; (ii) in a single tissue, relatively few miRNAs are expressed (hundreds vs. tenths of thousands mRNAs); (iii) they represent in their context the biologically active molecule, since they directly bind and control the target mRNAs: measurements of miRNA concentrations allow a more direct inference of a biological function.

In the last decade, our group has intensively studied the annual fish *Nothobranchius furzeri* as a new experimental model in Biology. This fish inhabits ephemeral pools in semi-arid *bushveld* of Southern Mozambique characterized by scarce and erratic precipitations and have adapted to the seasonal drying of their environment by producing desiccation-resistant eggs which can remain dormant in the dry mud for one and maybe more years by entering into diapause (Genade et al., 2005). Due to very short duration of the rain season, the natural lifespan of these animals is limited to a few months (Terzibasi Tozzini et al., 2013). They represent the vertebrate species with the shortest captive lifespan and also the fastest maturation (Genade et al., 2005; Blazek et al., 2013). In addition, they express a series of conserved aging markers and are amenable to genetic manipulations, making them an attractive model system for aging research (Valenzano et al., 2006; Hartmann et al., 2009, 2011; Terzibasi et al., 2009; Di Cicco et al., 2011; Valenzano et al., 2011; Hartmann and Englert, 2012; Allard et al., 2013). Fish brains are characterized by a very active adult neurogenesis with stem cell niches distributed along the entire rostro–caudal extent of the ventricular surface (Zupanc and Horschke, 1995; Adolf et al., 2006; Grandel et al., 2006; Kuroyanagi et al., 2010). Adult neurogenesis in mammals is known to decrease dramatically with age (Kuhn et al., 1996; Pekcec et al., 2008; Ben Abdallah et al., 2010; Knoth et al., 2010). Adult neurogenesis in mammals is restricted to two neurogenic niches in the telencephalon (TEL). Adult neurogenesis in teleosts, on the other hand, is widespread along the entire rostro–caudal axis and it is therefore unclear whether the same age-dependent decay is observed as in mammals. We therefore studied adult neuronal stem cells of *N. furzeri in vivo* and demonstrated an age-dependent decay in adult neurogenesis in terms both of incorporation of nucleotide analogs and expression of specific markers. In addition, RNA-seq experiments revealed age-dependent down-regulation of cell cycle genes during aging of *N. furzeri* brain (Petzold et al., 2013). We also observed a dramatic up-regulation of GFAP protein in the radial (neurogenic) glia of aged *N. furzeri* brains. All these data indicate a drastic reduction of neuronal stem cell activity during *N. furzeri* aging (Terzibasi Tozzini et al., 2012).

In the present paper, we use *N. furzeri* to model age-dependent decay of neurogenesis. We specifically analyzed the telencephalic neurogeneic niches that share the same embryonic origin with the mammalian adult niches (Adolf et al., 2006) and in particular the ventral niche that is homologous to the subventricular (subpallial) zone and the dorsal region that is homologous to pallial zone. For comparisons, we also analyzed the germinal zone of the optic tectum (OT), that is specific to teleosts and its stem cells do not show a glial phenotype (Terzibasi Tozzini et al., 2012). This would allow us to differentiate between conserved expression patterns in the telencephalic niches from possible teleost-specific expression pattern detectable only in the OT.

We previously used small RNA sequencing to identify and quantify expression of miRNAs in the brain of *N. furzeri* using miRBase as reference. We could detect 165 conserved miRNAs and found that brain aging in *N. furzeri* is associated with coherent up-regulation of well-known tumor suppressor miRNAs (such as miR-15a) that show positive interactions with TP53 and negative interactions with MYC, while the opposite is true for down-regulated miRNAs, such as miR-20a and other miRNAs belonging to the miRNA cluster 17–92 (Baumgart et al., 2012). Further, several of these miRNAs are regulated in the primate brain as well (Somel et al., 2010). This regulation is probably linked to the age-dependent reduction in adult neurogenesis observed in *Nothobranchius* species, as it would be suggested also by down-regulation of miR-9, a miRNA enriched in adult neuronal precursors (Terzibasi Tozzini et al., 2012).

The prototypic miRNA let-7 was originally shown to regulate the timing of developmental events in *Caenorhabditis elegans* (Reinhart et al., 2000) and later to regulate the age-dependent loss of regeneration in *C. elegans* (Zou et al., 2013). Studies in Vertebrates have indicated that the timing of miRNAs expression can regulate the timely generation of neurons with different cell-fates (Cremisi, 2013). Aim of the present work was to characterize the expression pattern for some miRNAs which are regulated during aging of *N. furzeri* brain, focusing on miRNAs known to be regulators of the cell cycle, since it has been previously demonstrated (Terzibasi Tozzini et al., 2012) that neuronal stem cells (NSCs) decrease with age. The miRNA cluster 17–92 is the prototypical oncogenic miRNA *locus* and it is up-regulated in a variety of cancers. It codes for six miRNAs: miR-17a, miR-18a, miR-19a, miR-20a, miR-19b, and miR-92a (Mogilyansky and Rigoutsos, 2013) and this organization is conserved in teleost fish (Guo et al., 2013). Its expression is controlled by the prototypical oncogene MYC and it targets known oncosuppressors such as PTEN and CDKN1A and pro-apoptotic genes such as BCL2L11 thereby contributing to oncogenic transformation (Mogilyansky and Rigoutsos, 2013). The miRNA cluster 17–92 is also associated to aging, as it is down-regulated during senescence of human cells both *in vitro* and *in vivo* (Hackl et al., 2010), cardiac aging in mice (van Almen et al., 2011) and aging of *N. furzeri* brain (Baumgart et al., 2012). Recent studies have shown that miR-17–92 cluster also regulates neuronal stem cell expansion and axonal elongation of embryonic neuronal precursors via targeting of PTEN (Bian et al., 2013; Zhang et al., 2013). On the other side, miR-15a is a known oncosuppressor that is regulated by TP53 and targets cell-cycle and anti-apoptotic proteins (Finnerty et al., 2010). Action of miR-15a in the nervous system is unknown, but during normal development of the heart miR-15a induces mitotic cycle exit of postnatal cardiomyocytes (Porrello et al., 2011). Expression of miR-15a increases during aging of *N. furzeri* (Baumgart et al., 2012) and may contribute to reduced activity of neuronal stem cells. We therefore decided to analyze miR-15a and, on the other side, miR-20a and cluster 17–92, for more in-depth investigations and analyzed their expression at the cellular level in the neurogenic niches of young- and old-fish.

RESULTS

We analyzed the expression of miR-15a, miR-20a and miRNA cluster 17–92 in the brain of young and old subjects of *N. furzeri*, by using *in situ* hybridization techniques, together with proliferating-cell nuclear antigen (PCNA) immuno-staining for a simultaneous visualization of the neurogenetic niches.

CLONING OF THE GENOMIC microRNA CLUSTER 17–92 From *N. furzeri*

In order to isolate the miRNA cluster 17–92 from *N. furzeri,* we designed primers covering the sequences of miR-17-5p and miR-92a-3p (**Figure 1**). The primers amplified a fragment of 857 bp. Alignment of this fragment with the corresponding genomic regions of *Oryzias latipes, Tetraodon nigrovirids* and *Danio rerio* revealed the expected conservation in the regions of all the pre-miRNA of the cluster. Alignment of the

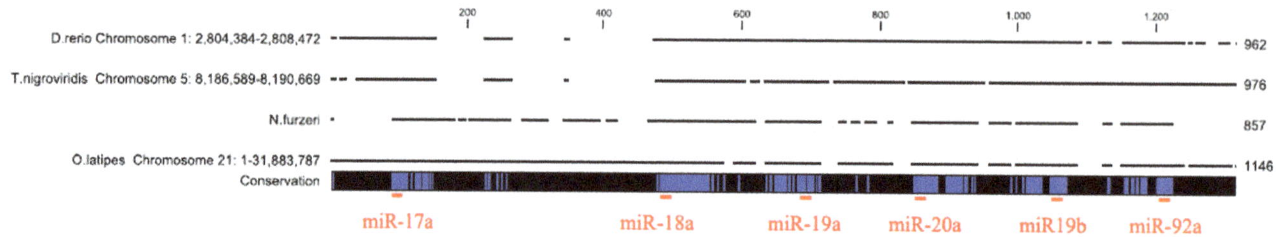

FIGURE 1 | Alignment of the microRNA cluster 17–92 from the four teleost species. The genomic regions of *D. rerio*, *T. nigroviridis*, and *O. latipes* were aligned to the fragment amplified in *N. furzeri*. The blue vertical bars indicate identical nucleotides. The localization of the mature miRNA sequences is indicated by a red horizontal bar.

sequences corresponding to the mature miRNAs of the cluster revealed 100% conservation in teleosts of miR-17, miR-18a, miR-20a, miR-19b, and miR-92a. The sequence of miR-19a showed a single position variation both in *N. furzeri* compared with the other three species (13 T > C, **Figure 2**) and in *O. latipes* compared with the other three species (19 A > G, **Figure 2**).

Species/Abbrv	* * * * * * * * * * * * * * * * * * * * *
1. D. rerio	TGTGCAAATCTATGCAAAACTGA
2. N. furzeri	TGTGCAAATCTACGCAAAACTGA
3. O. latipes	TGTGCAAATCTATGCAAAGCTGA
4. T. nigroviri	TGTGCAAATCTATGCAAAACTGA

FIGURE 2 | Alignment of the miR-19a-3p from the four teleost species. The non-conserved sites are indicated in color.

EXPRESSION OF miR-15a IS HIGHER IN THE BRAIN OF OLD SUBJECTS AND CONCENTRATES MAINLY IN THE PRINCIPAL NEUROGENETIC NICHES OF TEL AND OT

To visualize expression of miR-15a in *N. furzeri* brain we used a probe for fru-miR-15a whose sequence is identical to that of *N. furzeri*. **Figures 3A,B** show an overview of miR-15a distribution in young- and old-subjects, respectively, in a low-power overview and double labeling. The neurogenic activity is detected by immunohistochemistry for PCNA and visualized as a green fluorescence staining and labeling for the miRNA obtained using and LNA probe is shown as red fluorescence. Three regions of interest are indicated in the hemi-brains horizontal section, and represent areas were some of the most active neurogenetic niches are located (Terzibasi Tozzini et al., 2012): TEL and relative sub-regions (acTEL, antero-central TEL; lpTEL, latero-posterior TEL), OT and Cerebellum (CRB). As expected from previous results (Terzibasi Tozzini et al., 2012), PCNA positive cells (green) are more numerous in all neurogenic areas of the young brains (**Figures 3A,C,E**) as compared to the old ones (**Figures 3B,D,F**). Expression of miR-15a is overlapping with the neurogenic niches but is weaker in the young-subject (**Figure 3A**) as compared to the old-subject (**Figure 3B**). This is in line with the up-regulation of miR-15 detected by qPCR and miRNA-seq (Baumgart et al., 2012). The distribution of miR-15a can be appreciated more in detail in the magnifications of the different regions (**Figures 4–6**): in the TEL, miR-15a expression is primarily concentrated in the acTEL (**Figures 4Bi,ii**) and in the lpTEL (**Figures 5Bi,ii**) neurogenetic niches, and staining is clearly more prominent in the old, as compared to the young subject (**Figures 4Ai,ii** and **5Ai,ii** for acTEL and lpTEL, respectively). In the old OT, miR-15a expression is concentrated in the posterior margin (**Figures 6Bi,ii**, red), co-localizing with the proliferative niche of PCNA positive cells (**Figures 6Bi,ii**, green). Notably, the young subject presents a weaker miR15a expression in the same area.

EXPRESSION OF miR-20a IS HIGHER IN THE BRAIN OF YOUNG SUBJECTS, BUT MORE WIDESPREAD TO THE AREAS SURROUNDING THE NEUROGENIC NICHES

To visualize expression of miR-20a in *N. furzeri* a LNA probe designed against dre-miR-20a was used. An overview of miR-20 expression into young and old brain is shown in **Figures 3C,D**, respectively, and its presence is clearly higher in the young tissue with respect to the old one, in line with previous results of qPCR and miRNA-seq (Baumgart et al., 2012). Unlike miR-15a, which results highly concentrated into the neurogenic niches, miR-20a shows a more widespread distribution through acTEL, CRB, and OT regions of young subjects. MiR-20a expression can be appreciated more in detail in the magnification panels (**Figures 4–6**): in the acTEL region of the young brain (**Figures 4Ci,ii**) red fluorescence indicates a strong expression of miR-20a into the centro-ventricular neurogenetic niche (evidenced by the green fluorescence of PCNA positive cells) and, at a lower level, in the surrounding areas. Its expression is radically reduced in the same regions of the old brain (**Figures 4Di,ii**). A similar situation can be observed for the lpTEL region (**Figures 5C,D** rows) and the OT (**Figures 6C,D** rows), where the young tissue shows in both cases a stronger and more diffuse miR-20a expression (**Figures 5** and **6C** rows), compared to the old one (**Figures 5** and **6D** rows).

EXPRESSION OF THE microRNA CLUSTER 17–92 IS HIGHER IN THE BRAIN OF YOUNG SUBJECTS, CONCENTRATED MAINLY IN THE PRINCIPAL NEUROGENIC NICHES OF TELENCEPHALON AND CEREBELLUM, AND WITH REDUCED INTENSITY IN THE OPTIC TECTUM

Finally, we performed an ISH in young- versus old-brains to evaluate the expression of the primary transcript (pri-miRNA)

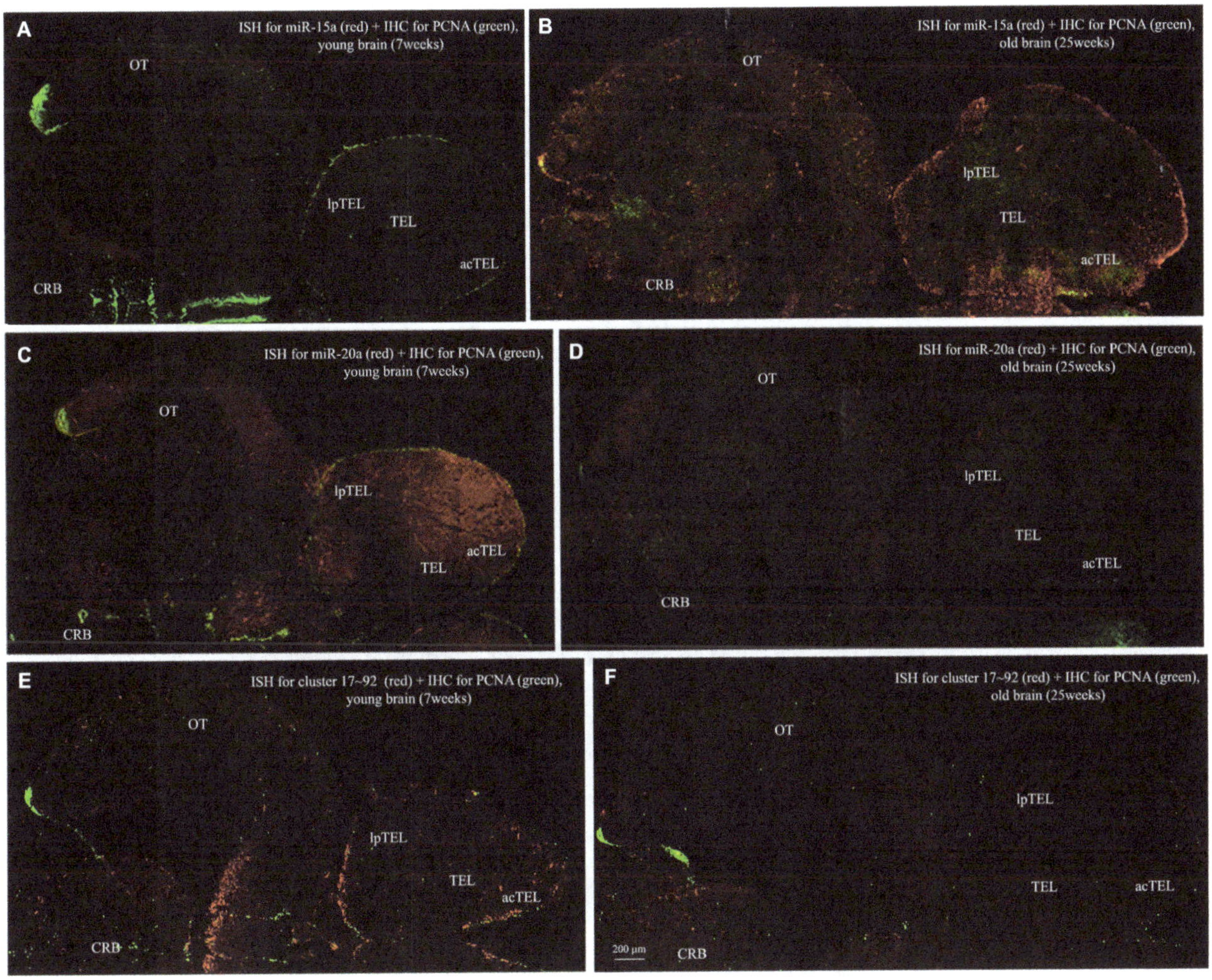

FIGURE 3 | Overviews of *Nothobranchius furzeri* hemi-brain. In situ Hybridization (ISH, in red) for miR15 **(A,B)**, miR20 **(C,D)** and Cluster17–92 **(E,F)**, double stained with PCNA (in green) by immunohistochemistry (IHC), in young (**A,C,E**, 7 weeks old**)** versus old (**B,D,F**, 25 weeks old) subjects. TEL, telencephalon; acTEL, antero-central telencephalon; lpTEL, latero-posterior telencephalon; OT, optic tectum; CRB, cerebellum.

for the miRNA cluster 17–92 during aging. The overview of its expression in young and old hemi-brains is represented in **Figures 3E,F**, respectively. Similarly to miR-20a, the pri-miRNA is more expressed in the young brain as compared to the old one, but in this case its distribution results mainly concentrated into the neurogenic niches of the TEL (better appreciated in the magnifications of the acTEL and lpTEL of **Figures 4** and **5**, respectively, **E** and **F** rows) and CRB (magnifications not shown). Compared to these regions, the young OT is characterized by a weaker, but still present, expression of miRNA cluster 17–92 (magnifications of **Figures 6E,F** rows) partially extended to the region adjacent to the proliferative niche of the posterior margin (**Figure 6E**), and expression is undetectable in the old OT.

DISCUSSION

The action of miRNA was widely investigated in the context of tumor biology. The role of miRNAs on the context of brain aging and neurogenesis until recently concentrated on miR-9 and miR-124 (Leucht et al., 2008; Cheng et al., 2009; Maiorano and Mallamaci, 2010; Coolen et al., 2012). Here, we used in situ hybridization to localize the cells expressing one prototypical oncogenic miRNA cluster (miR-17–92) and one prototypical oncosuppressor miRNA (miR-15a) in the brain of *N. furzeri* during aging. Both miRNAs were detected preferentially in the neurogenic niches and the sites of expression did not change during aging. However, at a qualitative level, opposing temporal patterns were apparent: during aging, the intensity of labeling for miR-17–92 primary transcripts and miR-20a decreases while the intensity of labeling for miR-15a increases. This is consistent with previous quantitative analysis of miRNA-seq and qPCR of whole brain extracts showing that, during aging, the expression of the miR-17–92 miRNA cluster decreases and the expression of miR-15a increases (Baumgart et al., 2012). The brain of *N. furzeri* contains widespread neuronal stem cells and is characterized by a drastic age-dependent reduction of neurogenesis (Terzibasi Tozzini et al., 2012). It is therefore likely that

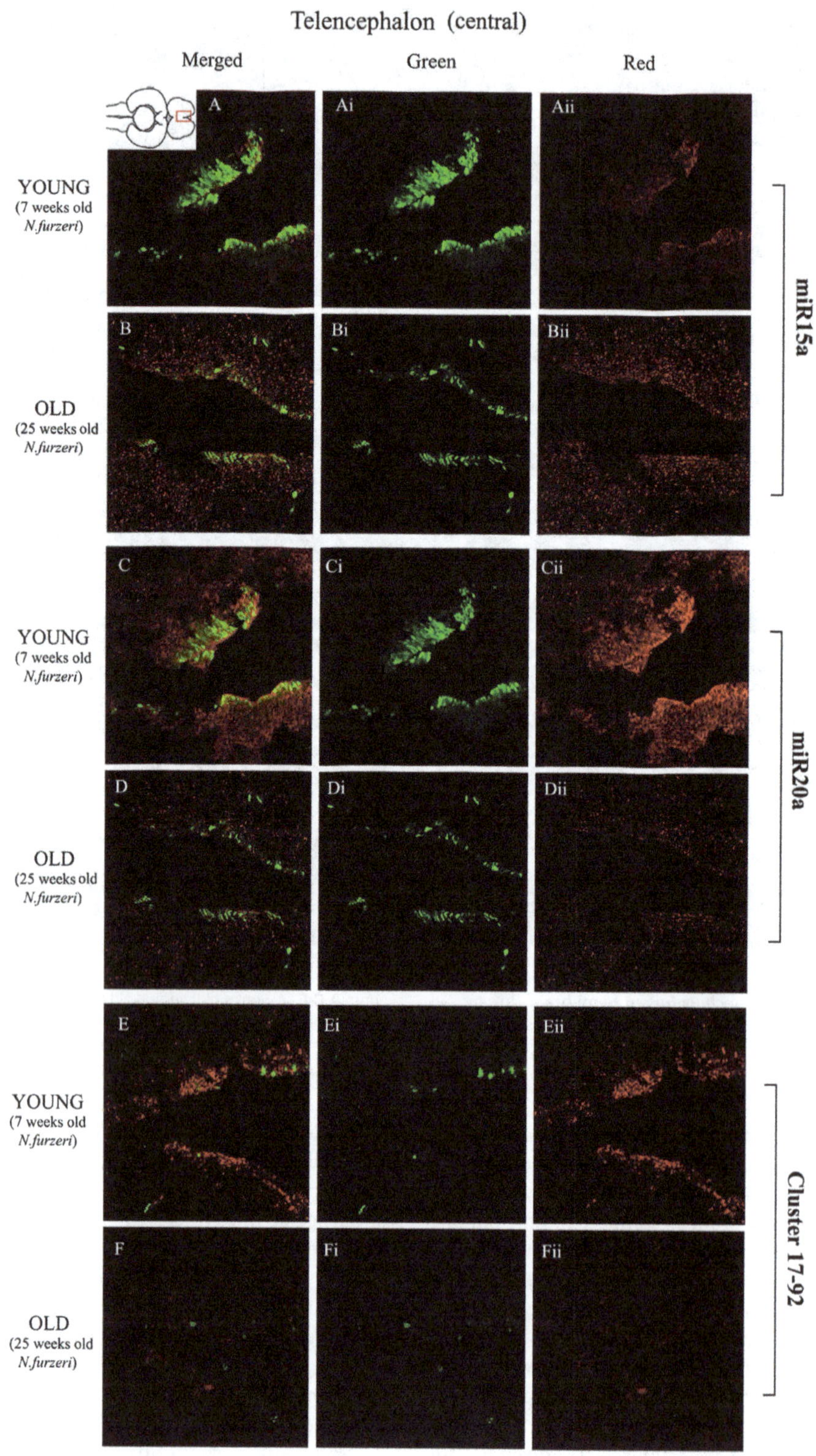

FIGURE 4 | Magnification of the central region of the telencephalon (cTEL) stained in green for PCNA by IHC, and in red for miR15 (A,B strips), miR20 (C,D strips) and Cluster17-92 (E,F strips) by ISH. The upper inset on **A** shows an overview of a horizontal brain section: the location of the cTEL is indicated by the red rectangle. The left column of the panel **(A–F)** shows the merged channels for the double staining; **A,B** refer to ISH for miR15a, respectively, in a young versus an old representative subject. **C,D** refer to ISH for miR20a, respectively, in a young versus an old representative subject. **E,F** refer to ISH for Cluster17–92, respectively, in a young versus an old representative subject. Central **(Ai–Fi)** and right **(Aii–Fii)** columns show the green and red single channel of the respective image on the left.

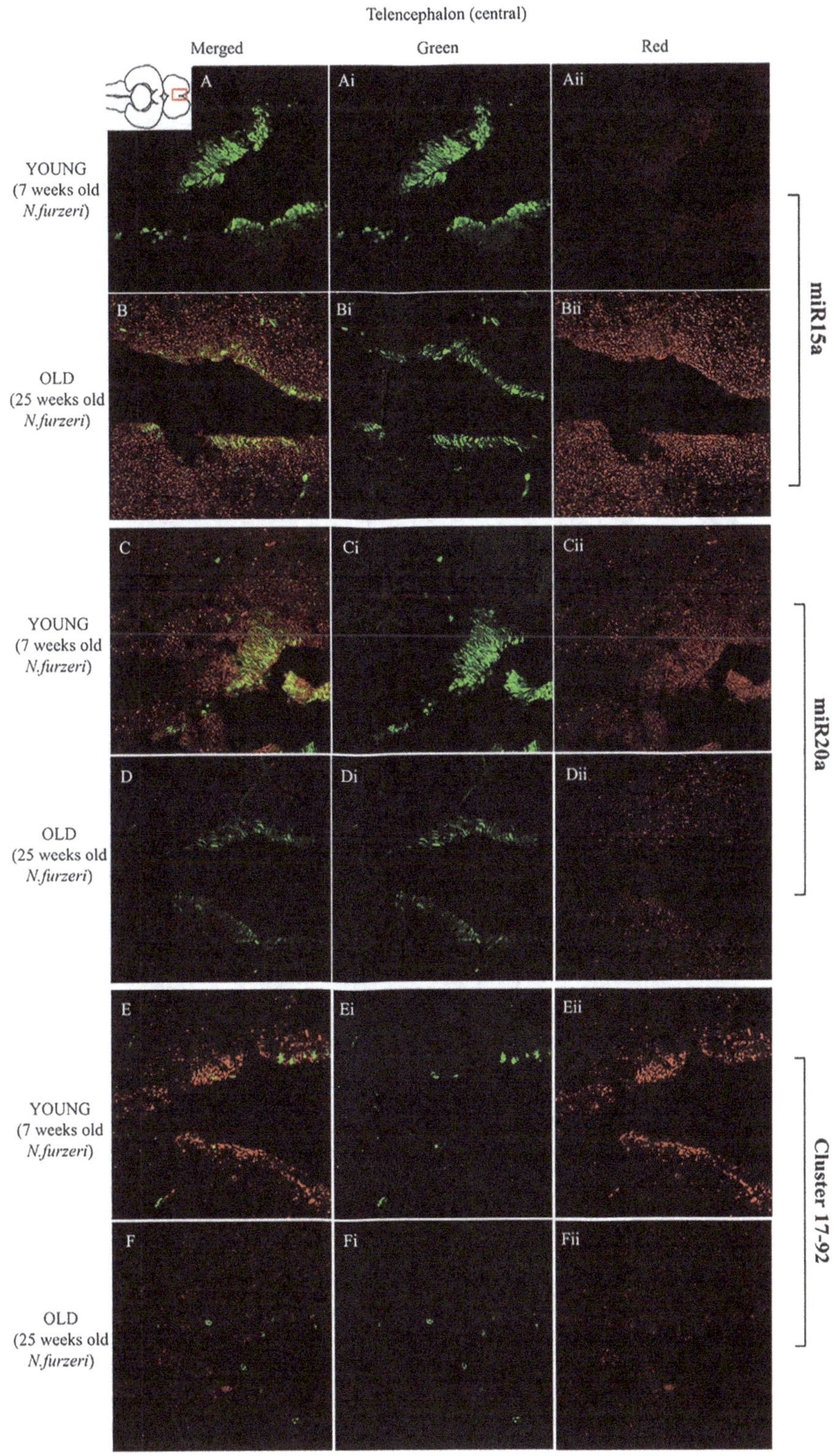

FIGURE 5 | Magnification of the latero-posterior region of the telencephalon (lpTEL) stained in green for PCNA by IHC, and in red for miR15 (A,B strips), miR20 (C,D strips), and Cluster17–92 (E,F strips) by ISH. The lower inset on **Aii** shows an overview of a horizontal brain section: the location of the lpTEL is indicated by the red rectangle. The left column of the panel (**A–F**) shows the merged channels for the double staining; **A,B** refer to ISH for miR15a, respectively, in a young versus an old representative subject. **C,D** refer to ISH for miR20a, respectively, in a young versus an old representative subject. **E,F** refer to ISH for Cluster17–92, respectively, in a young versus an old representative subject. Central (**Ai–Fi**) and right (**Aii–Fii**) columns show the green and red single channel of the respective image on the left.

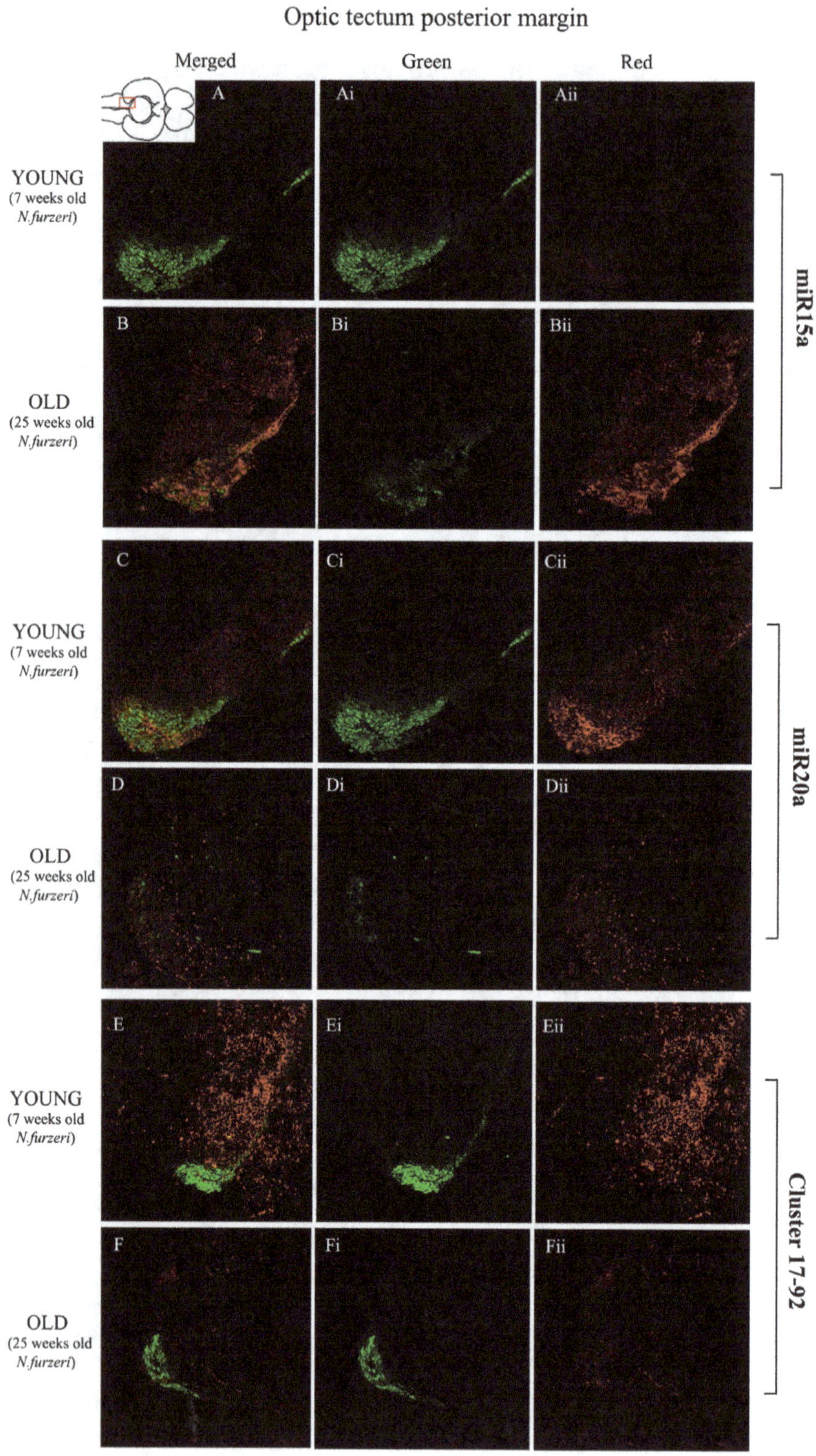

FIGURE 6 | Magnification of the posterior margin of the optic tectum (pOT) stained in green for PCNA by IHC, and in red for miR15 (A,B strips), miR20 (C,D strips) and Cluster17–92 (E,F strips) by ISH. The upper inset on **A** shows an overview of a horizontal brain section: the location of the pOT is indicated by the red rectangle. The left column of the panel (**A–F**) shows the merged channels for the double staining; **A,B** refer to ISH for miR15a, respectively, in a young versus an old representative subject. **C,D** refer to ISH for miR20a, respectively, in a young versus an old representative subject. **E,F** refer to ISH for cluster17–92, respectively, in a young versus an old representative subject. Central (**Ai–Fi**) and right (**Aii–Fii**) columns show the green and red single channel of the respective image on the left.

regulation of these miRNAs in the stem cell niche generates a signal that is detected by quantitative techniques in whole-brain extracts.

The miRNA cluster 17–92 is down-regulated during aging in a variety of models (Hackl et al., 2010; van Almen et al., 2011; Baumgart et al., 2012), but no data are present as to the site of expression of miRNA cluster 17–92 in the brain. We could specifically show that this gene is expressed in the neurogenic nice but also cells surrounding it. This indicates that miRNA cluster 17–92 is important for adult neuronal stem cell function, but remains activates also in newborn neurons. Indeed recent studies have shown that miR-17–92 cluster regulates neuronal stem cell expansion and axonal elongation of embryonic neuronal precursors via targeting of PTEN (Bian et al., 2013; Zhang et al., 2013). In young animals, the expression of miR-20a (one of the members of the cluster) is more widespread that the expression of the primary transcript. This is expected, since primary transcripts have very short half-life while mature miRNAs are thought to be long-lived.

miRNA-15a act as a general negative regulator of the cell cycle (Finnerty et al., 2010) and induces mitotic cycle exit of postnatal cardiomyocytes (Porrello et al., 2011). Therefore, increased expression of miR-15a in the aged neuronal stem cells is consistent with reduced cell cycle activity.

Our data suggest that miR-17–92 cluster and miR-15a play opposing roles in the regulation of stem cell activity and that their age-dependent imbalance is part of the mechanisms responsible for age-dependent reduction of adult neurogenesis.

MATERIALS AND METHODS

FISH BREEDING AND HOUSING CONDITIONS

All experiments were performed on group-house *N. furzeri* of the MZM-04/10 strain. The protocols of fish maintenance were carried out in accordance with all animal use practices established by the Italian Ministry of Health (Number 96/2003a).

Eggs were maintained on wet peat moss at room temperature in sealed Petri dishes. When embryos had developed, eggs were hatched by flushing the peat with tap water at 16–18°C. Embryos were scooped with a cut plastic pipette and transferred to a clean vessel. Fry were fed with newly hatched *Artemia nauplii* for the first 2 weeks and then weaned with finely chopped *Chironomus* larvae. Starting at the fourth week of life, fish were moved to 40-l tanks at a maximum density of 20 fish per tank equipped with air-driven sponge filters. The aquarium room's temperature was set at a constant 26°C. Twice a week the bottom of the tanks was siphoned and 50% of the water was exchanged with tempered tap water.

TISSUE COLLECTION AND PREPARATION

Fish were euthanized with MS-222 and cooled on crushed ice for 5 min before dissection. Whole brains from young (7 weeks) and old (25 weeks) animals were dissected and fixed by immersion in 4% paraformaldehyde/0.1 M phosphate buffer (pH 7.4), and then cryoprotected with a two-step immersion at 20% and then 30% sucrose solution for at least 12 h each. Finally the tissues were embedded at −20°C in Neg50 crio-embedding medium (Thermo Scientific); series of 16 μm thick sections were cut with a Leica cryostat and collected on Superfrost plus slides® (Thermo Scientific).

CLONING OF miR-17–92 Locus of *N. furzeri* AND PROBE PREPARATION

PCR was performed on cDNA using GoTaq polymerase (Promega), 56 degrees for annealing temperature, and 60 s elongation time using the following primers:

Forward: CAAAGTGCTTACAGTGCAGGT

T7-Reverse: GTAATACGACTCACTATAGGG-GGCCGGGACA AGTGCAATACC

0.5 μg of PCR products that contain T7 RNA polymerase promoter at the 3′ ends were used as templates for in vitro transcription. Probes were transcribed using DIG RNA labeling kit (SP6/T7) (Roche), according to the manufacturer's protocol.

The sequence of the *N. furzeri* miR-17–92 locus was deposited in GeneBank (Accession Number: KF986732). LNA probes for the mature form of fru-miR-15a (MI0003469) and dre-miR-20a (MI0001907) were directly ordered from Exiqon (Denmark)

IN SITU HYBRIDIZATION

We performed *in situ* Hybridization using two different probes: classical RNA probes, to detect transduction products expression of specific genes, and LNA probes, to detect the expression of several mature miRNAs (functional form) of our interest.

All *in situ* Hybridization protocols has been performed on 16 μm thick cryo-sections of fish brain. Slides were dried for 2 h at 37°C, washed in PBS twice for 3 min, and then treated for 8 min with Proteinase K (diluted 1:80000 starting from stocks of 20 mg/mL). After that, slides were washed in Glycine (2 mg/mL in PBT) twice for 5 min, to stop the reaction. Then, sections were fixed with PFA 4% for 20 min at room temperature, and washed in PBT (three times for 3 min). Pre-hybridization were performed covering the slides with 200 μl of hybridization buffer under parafilm coverslips (to avoid evaporation) at hybridization temperature (60°C for classic RNA probes; 37°C for LNA probes) for 30 min. Hybridization was performed covering each slide with a solution of the specific antisense probe, or LNA 3′ DIG labeled exiqon probe diluted in both cases in 200 μl of hybridization buffer to a final concentration of 1 μg/mL. Parafilm coverslips were used and slides incubated at hybridization temperature overnight. Before using them, diluted RNA probes (not LNA) have been denatured for 5 min at 80°C. In order to avoid drying out the slides the whole process has been carried out in wet chamber with PBS.

After hybridization, 2× SSC has been used to remove the coverslip. Slides were first washed in 1× SSC, twice for 20 min, and then in 0.2× SSC twice for 20 min, always at hybridization temperature. A final washing step was done in PBT three times for 5 min at room temperature.

For the probe revelation slides were incubated with blocking solution for 30 min at room temperature and then with Anti-Dig-AP Fab Fragments Ab [1/2000] in blocking solution overnight at 4°C.

Washings in PBT, 3 times for 5 min, and in NMNT, 3 times for 5 min at room temperature, have been conducted before adding Fast Red solution (Roche Tablets; 1 in 2 mL Tris-HCl 0.1 M, pH = 8.2). To avoid the formation of precipitate, Fast Red tablets have been vortexed for 5 min in Tris-HCl and then filtered. Observation has been conducted every 20 min with a Zeiss fluorescence microscope until the signal detection (1–10 h depending on the probe used). The staining has been stopped washing well in PBS (at least 3 times for 5 min) at room temperature.

HISTOLOGY: PCNA STAINING

After ISH procedure, slides were processed to stain the population of proliferating cells in the neurogenetic niches, following the standard procedures of immunohistochemistry: we used the primary antibody against PCNA commercially available from DAKO (mouse monoclonal, clone PC10, code: M0879) diluted 1:500. Visualization of the primary antibody was performed with the secondary antibody Alexa Fluor® 488 (goat anti-mouse, Life Technologies, code: A10680) diluted 1:400. The staining has been stopped washing well in PBS (at least 3 times for 5 min) at room temperature. Then slides were closed with a specific mounting (Fluoroshield, Sigma) and analyzed with a confocal microscope (Leica TCS).

AUTHOR CONTRIBUTIONS

Eva Terzibasi Tozzini designed the study, performed *in situ* hybridization, confocal acquisition and imaging, and wrote the paper. Aurora Savino performed most part of the *in situ* hybridization experiments and part of the confocal acquisition for this reason she should be considered co-first author together with Eva Terzibasi Tozzini. Giorgia Battistoni performed *in situ* hybridization. Roberto Ripa and Mario Baumgart performed the cloning of the standard and LNA probes. Alessandro Cellerino designed and supervised the study and wrote the paper. All authors read and approved the final manuscript.

ACKNOWLEDGMENTS

This work was partially supported by the DFG Grant CE 46/5-1 to Alessandro Cellerino and by the MFAG 11511 (AIRC Association) to Eva Terzibasi Tozzini and by an internal grant of the Scuola Normale Superiore.

REFERENCES

Adolf, B., Chapouton, P., Lam, C. S., Topp, S., Tannhauser, B., Strahle, U., et al. (2006). Conserved and acquired features of adult neurogenesis in the zebrafish telencephalon. *Dev. Biol.* 295, 278–293. doi: 10.1016/j.ydbio.2006.03.023

Allard, J. B., Kamei, H., and Duan, C. (2013). Inducible transgenic expression in the short-lived fish *Nothobranchius furzeri*. *J. Fish Biol.* 82, 1733–1738. doi: 10.1111/jfb.12099

Baumgart, M., Groth, M., Priebe, S., Appelt, J., Guthke, R., Platzer, M., et al. (2012). Age-dependent regulation of tumor-related microRNAs in the brain of the annual fish *Nothobranchius furzeri*. *Mech. Ageing Dev.* 133, 226–233. doi: 10.1016/j.mad.2012.03.015

Ben Abdallah, N. M., Slomianka, L., Vyssotski, A. L., and Lipp, H. P. (2010). Early age-related changes in adult hippocampal neurogenesis in C57 mice. *Neurobiol. Aging* 31, 151–161. doi: 10.1016/j.neurobiolaging.2008.03.002

Bian, S., Hong, J., Li, Q., Schebelle, L., Pollock, A., Knauss, J. L., et al. (2013). MicroRNA cluster miR-17-92 regulates neural stem cell expansion and transition to intermediate progenitors in the developing mouse neocortex. *Cell Rep.* 3, 1398–1406. doi: 10.1016/j.celrep.2013.03.037

Blazek, R., Polacik, M. J., and Reichard, M. (2013). Rapid growth, early maturation and short generation time in African annual fishes. *Evodevo* 4, 24. doi: 10.1186/2041-9139-4-24

Cheng, L. C., Pastrana, E., Tavazoie, M., and Doetsch, F. (2009). miR-124 regulates adult neurogenesis in the subventricular zone stem cell niche. *Nat. Neurosci.* 12, 399–408. doi: 10.1038/nn.2294

Coolen, M., Thieffry, D., Drivenes, O., Becker, T. S., and Bally-Cuif, L. (2012). miR-9 controls the timing of neurogenesis through the direct inhibition of antagonistic factors. *Dev. Cell* 22, 1052–1064. doi: 10.1016/j.devcel.2012.03.003

Cremisi, F. (2013). MicroRNAs and cell fate in cortical and retinal development. *Front. Cell Neurosci.* 7:141. doi: 10.3389/fncel.2013.00141

Di Cicco, E., Tozzini, E. T., Rossi, G., and Cellerino, A. (2011). The short-lived annual fish *Nothobranchius furzeri* shows a typical teleost aging process reinforced by high incidence of age-dependent neoplasias. *Exp. Gerontol.* 46, 249–256. doi: 10.1016/j.exger.2010.10.011

Finnerty, J. R., Wang, W. X., Hebert, S. S., Wilfred, B. R., Mao, G., and Nelson, P. T. (2010). The miR-15/107 group of microRNA genes: evolutionary biology, cellular functions, and roles in human diseases. *J. Mol. Biol.* 402, 491–509. doi: 10.1016/j.jmb.2010.07.051

Genade, T., Benedetti, M., Terzibasi, E., Roncaglia, P., Valenzano, D. R., Cattaneo, A., et al. (2005). Annual fishes of the genus *Nothobranchius* as a model system for aging research. *Aging Cell* 4, 223–233. doi: 10.1111/j.1474-9726.2005.00165.x

Grandel, H., Kaslin, J., Ganz, J., Wenzel, I., and Brand, M. (2006). Neural stem cells and neurogenesis in the adult zebrafish brain: origin, proliferation dynamics, migration and cell fate. *Dev. Biol.* 295, 263–277. doi: 10.1016/j.ydbio.2006.03.040

Guo, L., Yang, S., Zhao, Y., Wu, Q., and Chen, F. (2013). Dynamic evolution of mir-17-92 gene cluster and related miRNA gene families in vertebrates. *Mol. Biol. Rep.* 40, 3147–3153. doi: 10.1007/s11033-012-2388-z

Hackl, M., Brunner, S., Fortschegger, K., Schreiner, C., Micutkova, L., Muck, C., et al. (2010). miR-17, miR-19b, miR-20a, and miR-106a are down-regulated in human aging. *Aging Cell* 9, 291–296. doi: 10.1111/j.1474-9726.2010.00549.x

Hartmann, N., and Englert, C. (2012). A microinjection protocol for the generation of transgenic killifish (Species: *Nothobranchius furzeri*). *Dev. Dyn.* 241, 1133–1141. doi: 10.1002/dvdy.23789

Hartmann, N., Reichwald, K., Lechel, A., Graf, M., Kirschner, J., Dorn, A., et al. (2009). Telomeres shorten while Tert expression increases during ageing of the short-lived fish *Nothobranchius furzeri*. *Mech. Ageing Dev.* 130, 290–296. doi: 10.1016/j.mad.2009.01.003

Hartmann, N., Reichwald, K., Wittig, I., Drose, S., Schmeisser, S., Luck, C., et al. (2011). Mitochondrial DNA copy number and function decrease with age in the short-lived fish *Nothobranchius furzeri*. *Aging Cell* 10, 824–831. doi: 10.1111/j.1474-9726.2011.00723.x

Knoth, R., Singec, I., Ditter, M., Pantazis, G., Capetian, P., Meyer, R. P., et al. (2010). Murine features of neurogenesis in the human hippocampus across the lifespan from 0 to 100 years. *PLoS ONE* 5:e8809. doi: 10.1371/journal.pone.0008809

Kuhn, H. G., Dickinson-Anson, H., and Gage, F. H. (1996). Neurogenesis in the dentate gyrus of the adult rat: age-related decrease of neuronal progenitor proliferation. *J. Neurosci.* 16, 2027–2033.

Kuroyanagi, Y., Okuyama, T., Suehiro, Y., Imada, H., Shimada, A., Naruse, K., et al. (2010). Proliferation zones in adult medaka (*Oryzias latipes*) brain. *Brain Res.* 1323, 33–40. doi: 10.1016/j.brainres.2010.01.045

Leucht, C., Stigloher, C., Wizenmann, A., Klafke, R., Folchert, A., and Bally-Cuif, L. (2008). MicroRNA-9 directs late organizer activity of the midbrain-hindbrain boundary. *Nat. Neurosci.* 11, 641–648. doi: 10.1038/nn.2115

Maiorano, N. A., and Mallamaci, A. (2010). The pro-differentiating role of miR-124: indicating the road to become a neuron. *RNA Biol.* 7, 528–533. doi: 10.4161/rna.7.5.12262

Mogilyansky, E., and Rigoutsos, I. (2013). The miR-17/92 cluster: a comprehensive update on its genomics, genetics, functions and increasingly important and numerous roles in health and disease. *Cell Death Differ.* 20, 1603–1614. doi: 10.1038/cdd.2013.125

Osella, M., Bosia, C., Cora, D., and Caselle, M. (2011). The role of incoherent microRNA-mediated feedforward loops in noise buffering. *PLoS Comput. Biol.* 7:e1001101. doi: 10.1371/journal.pcbi.1001101

Pekcec, A., Baumgartner, W., Bankstahl, J. P., Stein, V. M., and Potschka, H. (2008). Effect of aging on neurogenesis in the canine brain. *Aging Cell* 7, 368–374. doi: 10.1111/j.1474-9726.2008.00392.x

Petzold, A., Reichwald, K., Groth, M., Taudien, S., Hartmann, N., Priebe, S., et al. (2013). The transcript catalogue of the short-lived fish *Nothobranchius furzeri* provides insights into age-dependent changes of mRNA levels. *BMC Genomics* 14:185. doi: 10.1186/1471-2164-14-185

Porrello, E. R., Johnson, B. A., Aurora, A. B., Simpson, E., Nam, Y. J., Matkovich, S. J., et al. (2011). MiR-15 family regulates postnatal mitotic arrest of cardiomyocytes. *Circ. Res.* 109, 670–679. doi: 10.1161/CIRCRESAHA.111.248880

Reinhart, B. J., Slack, F. J., Basson, M., Pasquinelli, A. E., Bettinger, J. C., Rougvie, A. E., et al. (2000). The 21-nucleotide let-7 RNA regulates developmental timing in *Caenorhabditis elegans. Nature* 403, 901–906. doi: 10.1038/35002607

Siciliano, V., Garzilli, I., Fracassi, C., Criscuolo, S., Ventre, S., and Di Bernardo, D. (2013). MiRNAs confer phenotypic robustness to gene networks by suppressing biological noise. *Nat. Commun.* 4, 2364. doi: 10.1038/ncomms3364

Somel, M., Guo, S., Fu, N., Yan, Z., Hu, H. Y., Xu, Y., et al. (2010). MicroRNA, mRNA, and protein expression link development and aging in human and macaque brain. *Genome Res.* 20, 1207–1218. doi: 10.1101/gr.106849.110

Terzibasi, E., Lefrancois, C., Domenici, P., Hartmann, N., Graf, M., and Cellerino, A. (2009). Effects of dietary restriction on mortality and age-related phenotypes in the short-lived fish *Nothobranchius furzeri. Aging Cell* 8, 88–99. doi: 10.1111/j.1474-9726.2009.00455.x

Terzibasi Tozzini, E., Baumgart, M., Battistoni, G., and Cellerino, A. (2012). Adult neurogenesis in the short-lived teleost *Nothobranchius furzeri*: localization of neurogenic niches, molecular characterization and effects of aging. *Aging Cell* 11, 241–251. doi: 10.1111/j.1474-9726.2011.00781.x

Terzibasi Tozzini, E., Dorn, A., Ng'oma, E., Polacik, M., Blazek, R., Reichwald, K., et al. (2013). Parallel evolution of senescence in annual fishes in response to extrinsic mortality. *BMC Evol. Biol.* 13:77. doi: 10.1186/1471–2148-13–77

Valenzano, D. R., Sharp, S., and Brunet, A. (2011). Transposon-mediated transgenesis in the short-lived African killifish *Nothobranchius furzeri*, a vertebrate model for aging. *G3 (Bethesda)* 1, 531–538. doi: 10.1534/g3.111.001271

Valenzano, D. R., Terzibasi, E., Cattaneo, A., Domenici, L., and Cellerino, A. (2006). Temperature affects longevity and age-related locomotor and cognitive decay in the short-lived fish *Nothobranchius furzeri. Aging Cell* 5, 275–278. doi: 10.1111/j.1474-9726.2006.00212.x

van Almen, G. C., Verhesen, W., Van Leeuwen, R. E., Van De Vrie, M., Eurlings, C., Schellings, M. W., et al. (2011). MicroRNA-18 and microRNA-19 regulate CTGF and TSP-1 expression in age-related heart failure. *Aging Cell* 10, 769–779. doi: 10.1111/j.1474-9726.2011.00714.x

Zhang, Y., Ueno, Y., Liu, X. S., Buller, B., Wang, X., Chopp, M., et al. (2013). The MicroRNA-17-92 cluster enhances axonal outgrowth in embryonic cortical neurons. *J. Neurosci.* 33, 6885–6894. doi: 10.1523/JNEUROSCI.5180-12.2013

Zou, Y., Chiu, H., Zinovyeva, A., Ambros, V., Chuang, C. F., and Chang, C. (2013). Developmental decline in neuronal regeneration by the progressive change of two intrinsic timers. *Science* 340, 372–376. doi: 10.1126/science.1231321

Zupanc, G. K., and Horschke, I. (1995). Proliferation zones in the brain of adult gymnotiform fish: a quantitative mapping study. *J. Comp. Neurol.* 353, 213–233. doi: 10.1002/cne.903530205

9

MicroRNAs regulate neuronal plasticity and are involved in pain mechanisms

Sara Elramah[1,2], Marc Landry[1,2] and Alexandre Favereaux[1,2] *

[1] Interdisciplinary Institute for Neuroscience, UMR 5297, University of Bordeaux, Bordeaux, France
[2] Interdisciplinary Institute for Neuroscience, UMR 5297, Centre National de la Recherche Scientifique, Bordeaux, France

***Correspondence:**
Alexandre Favereaux, Interdisciplinary Institute for Neuroscience, UMR 5297, University of Bordeaux, 146, rue Léo Saignat, 33 077 Bordeaux Cedex, France
e-mail: alexandre.favereaux@u-bordeaux2.fr

MicroRNAs (miRNAs) are emerging as master regulators of gene expression in the nervous system where they contribute not only to brain development but also to neuronal network homeostasis and plasticity. Their function is the result of a cascade of events including miRNA biogenesis, target recognition, and translation inhibition. It has been suggested that miRNAs are major switches of the genome owing to their ability to regulate multiple genes at the same time. This regulation is essential for normal neuronal activity and, when affected, can lead to drastic pathological conditions. As an example, we illustrate how deregulation of miRNAs can affect neuronal plasticity leading to chronic pain. The origin of pain and its dual role as a key physiological function and a debilitating disease has been highly debated until now. The incidence of chronic pain is estimated to be 20–25% worldwide, thus making it a public health problem. Chronic pain can be considered as a form of maladaptive plasticity. Long-lasting modifications develop as a result of global changes in gene expression, and are thus likely to be controlled by miRNAs. Here, we review the literature on miRNAs and their targets responsible for maladaptive plasticity in chronic pain conditions. In addition, we conduct a retrospective analysis of miRNA expression data published for different pain models, taking into account recent progress in our understanding of the role of miRNAs in neuronal plasticity.

Keywords: microRNA, gene expression, neuron, plasticity, pain

INTRODUCTION

MicroRNAs (miRNAs) are non-coding, endogenous ~23 nucleotide (nt) RNAs that regulate target-gene expression by either translation inhibition or mRNA degradation (Bartel, 2009). They were first discovered in *C. elegans* where *lin-4* plays a critical role in the developmental orchestration (Lee et al., 1993). Since then, the number of identified miRNAs has reached a thousand in many species. Owing to their uncommon targeting properties, a single miRNA species can bind and regulate multiple targets, and it is now thought that the expression of most, if not all, genes involves modulation by miRNAs. Thus, the "macro switch" function of miRNAs in neuronal development is now well documented (Li and Jin, 2010). More recently, accruing evidence established miRNAs as essential regulators of proper neuronal function. In particular, it was demonstrated that miRNAs regulate many proteins involved in neuronal adaptation to network activity. miRNAs take part in the morphological and functional changes sustaining neuronal plasticity. For instance, miR-134 is expressed in hippocampal neurons where it regulates the LIM-domain kinase 1, which represses cofilin, an actin depolymerization factor, thus modifying spine morphology (Schratt et al., 2006). Another example is miR-284, which regulates the expression of the glutamate receptor GluA2 at the neuromuscular junction in *Drosophila* (Karr et al., 2009).

As an actor in neuronal plasticity, miRNAs are likely to play a role in the onset and maintenance of neurological diseases. Indeed screening strategies have identified altered expression of specific miRNAs in Alzheimer's, Parkinson's, Huntington's disease, and Tourette syndrome patients (Johnson et al., 2012; Salta and De Strooper, 2012). While these results raise hope for new treatments, more work is needed to fully differentiate the miRNA changes that trigger pathological mechanisms from those resulting from the disease. A tempting hypothesis is that long-term alteration of miRNA pathways normally regulating basal neuron function could lead to disease. Long-lasting modifications of gene expression are thought to result in chronic disease such as neuropathic pain. Therefore, miRNA deregulation could play a key role in chronic pain.

Here, we briefly examine current knowledge on miRNA biogenesis, target recognition, and regulation. Then, we review the literature to highlight miRNAs that are involved in neuronal plasticity, with a special focus on chronic pain pathologies.

miRNA BIOGENESIS

To date, miRbase, a specialized miRNA database, comprises 1872 entries for the human genome (Griffiths-Jones et al., 2006; Kozomara and Griffiths-Jones, 2011). miRNA genes are present on all chromosomes, with the exception of the human Y chromosome. Nearly 50% of miRNA-coding genes are situated within the intergenic space and possess their own regulatory elements (Lagos-Quintana et al., 2001; Corcoran et al., 2009). In contrast, 40% of miRNAs genes are positioned within introns (Rodriguez et al., 2004; Smalheiser et al., 2008), and 10% are located within exon terminals. As a consequence, the expression of half of the miRNA genes depends on the regulation of their host gene, so they may be involved in the control of genetic networks related to the expected function of the host gene product (O'Carroll and Schaefer, 2013). An interesting feature is that many miRNA genes are grouped within clusters, with an intergenic distance ranging from 0.1 to 50 kb, and exhibit a similar expression pattern (Baskerville and Bartel, 2005). In addition, miRNAs within clusters are often, but not always, related to each other, while miRNAs from the same family are occasionally clustered (Lagos-Quintana et al., 2001; Lau et al., 2001).

Transcription of miRNAs is performed by either RNA Polymerase II or RNA Polymerase III, producing primary miRNA (pri-miRNA), a large stem-loop structure (3–4 kb in length) with a 5′ cap and a poly(A) tail (Cai et al., 2004; Lee et al., 2004). Then, this pri-miRNA structure is recognized and processed by the microprocessor complex which is composed of the ribonuclease Drosha (RNase III enzyme), the RNA-binding protein (RBP) DGCR8 (DiGeorge syndrome critical region gene 8; Lee et al., 2003; Denli et al., 2004; Gregory et al., 2004) and other auxiliary factors (Han et al., 2004), generating ~60- to 70-nt-long stem-loop precursor miRNAs (pre-miRNA; Morlando et al., 2008). Processing of pri-miRNAs into pre-miRNAs occurs concomitantly with transcriptional events, thus rapidly constituting a nuclear pool of pre-miRNAs (Morlando et al., 2008). The next step to functional miRNAs is the export of pre-miRNAs from the nucleus to the cytoplasm by the karyopherin protein family member, Exportin-5, in a GTP-dependent manner (Yi et al., 2003; Bohnsack et al., 2004; Lund et al., 2004). Once in the cytoplasm, the pre-miRNA is loaded into the RNA-induced silencing complex (RISC) loading complex, where it is further processed into a ~21-nt-long miRNA duplex by Dicer, a type-III ribonuclease (Bernstein et al., 2001; Hutvágner et al., 2001; Ketting et al., 2001; Knight and Bass, 2001). At this stage, only one strand is finally incorporated into the RISC, the "guide" strand, whereas the other strand called "the passenger" is likely degraded. The criteria defining which of the two strands is loaded into the RISC still need to be clarified but it appears that, in most of the cases, it is the one whose 5′ end is less tightly paired (Khvorova et al., 2003; Schwarz et al., 2003).

Another processing pathway independent of the Drosha/DGCR8 microprocessor machinery and previously discovered in *Drosophila* and *C. elegans* (Okamura et al., 2007; Ruby et al., 2007a) has been recently identified in mammals. The so-called mirtons are directly spliced from the introns of mRNA coding genes, directly exported to the cytoplasm and processed by Dicer (Okamura et al., 2007; Ruby et al., 2007a).

TARGET RECOGNITION AND TRANSLATION INHIBITION

BASICS OF miRNA:mRNA INTERACTIONS

Loading of the "guide" strand into the Argonaute protein of the RISC makes it functional and ready to generate mRNA inhibition (Hutvágner and Zamore, 2002; Mourelatos et al., 2002). The mechanisms and the consequent magnitude of this regulation are dependent on the characteristics of the miRNA:target mRNA binding. Thus, in metazoans, extensive base pairing has been demonstrated to induce mRNA cleavage (Hutvágner and Zamore, 2002; Rhoades et al., 2002; Yekta et al., 2004), whereas imperfect binding leads to target repression through translational inhibition and/or mRNA destabilization (Lee et al., 1993; Wightman et al., 1993; Lim et al., 2005). In addition, the location of miRNA binding sites in the target mRNA plays a predominant role on the efficacy of the regulation. Although binding of miRNA has been demonstrated in the 5′ untranslated region (UTR) and the open reading frame (ORF) of mRNA (Easow et al., 2007; Lytle et al., 2007; Chi et al., 2009; Leung et al., 2011), these sites are less effective than those located in the 3′UTR (Kloosterman et al., 2004; Farh et al., 2005; Lewis et al., 2005; Lim et al., 2005; Grimson et al., 2007; Ruby et al., 2007b; Baek et al., 2008). This might reflect the fact that in 5′UTR and ORF, the translation machinery has a higher affinity than the RISC, thus displacing the silencing complex (Bartel, 2009).

The nucleotide sequence in the target mRNA that is engaged in miRNA binding is called the miRNA recognition element (MRE; Shukla et al., 2011) or "seed region" (Bartel, 2004). miRNA target recognition and seed region classification have been extensively reviewed previously (see Bartel, 2009). The composition of this seed region varies but always involves a sequence with conserved Watson–Crick pairing (i.e., the hydrogen bonding that pairs guanine–cytosine and adenine–thymine) to the 5′ region of the miRNA centered on nucleotides 2–7 (Bartel, 2009). Several types of seed regions exist depending on the length and composition of the sequence involved in miRNA:mRNA binding, resulting in different affinities and inhibition properties. These include canonical sites with a 6- to 8-nt match between miRNA and mRNA, and non-canonical sites that include additional pairing at the 3′ end of the miRNA. Additional factors have been shown to affect miRNA seed efficacy such as AU-rich sites, which have been shown to be more effective (Lewis et al., 2005; Grimson et al., 2007; Nielsen et al., 2007; Pasquinelli, 2012).

Other factors include the position of the seed within the 3′UTR of the target-mRNA (Grimson et al., 2007), with sites at the extremities of the 3′UTR being more accessible than those in the middle because long UTRs may form occlusive interactions, thus greatly reducing miRNA site accessibility.

Another important feature is site multiplicity, where the presence of multiple sites for the same or different miRNAs on the target-mRNA increases the repression response. Multiple sites might contribute to target mRNA inhibition in either a non-cooperative manner or cooperatively. miRNA cooperation results in a stronger repression than the sum of the individual and independent sites. Cooperative regulation implies that seed sequences are within a 40-nt region but with a minimum 8 nt gap between them (Doench et al., 2003; Grimson et al., 2007; Nielsen et al., 2007; Saetrom et al., 2007).

Given the large and growing number of miRNA species, the enormous number of putative target mRNAs and the length of their 3′UTR sequences, the manual prediction of miRNA:mRNA interactions would be impossible. Therefore, computational analysis using algorithms and prediction databases is the usual method to identify miRNA targets. Hence, target prediction programs are based on seed region recognition tools that basically list all the sites with miRNA-binding properties and rank them accordingly to the kind of seed, conservation across evolution and some of the above-mentioned factors known to modulate site efficiency (for review, see Reyes-Herrera and Ficarra, 2012).

However, despite refinements of prediction tools, the percentage of predicted targets that pass the experimental validation stage is still sub-optimal. Therefore, it often constitutes a time-consuming bottleneck in miRNA studies that involve complex experimental paradigms. In line with this, recent data suggest that miRNA:mRNA interactions sometimes involve the 3′ end of miRNAs with little evidence for 5′ contacts, and some of these interactions have been shown to be functional (Helwak et al., 2013). In addition, other parameters not taken into account in these algorithms could affect the accuracy of target prediction tools. For instance, there is the importance of the secondary structure of RNA and its association with RBPs, which influence target site accessibility, and thereby its regulation (Brodersen and Voinnet, 2009).

MECHANISMS OF miRNA-MEDIATED INHIBITION OF TRANSLATION

miRNA binding to its target mRNA is the starting point of a post-transcriptional regulation of gene expression occurring in the cytoplasm, mostly by translational repression or mRNA degradation (Valencia-Sanchez et al., 2006; Jackson and Standart, 2007; Nilsen, 2007; Pillai et al., 2007; Standart and Jackson, 2007). In fact, microRNA-induced silencing complex (miRISC)-mediated gene inhibition has been demonstrated to arise from three putative mechanisms: (i) site-specific cleavage, (ii) enhanced mRNA decay, and (iii) translational inhibition. Thanks to recent studies combining cutting-edge transcriptomic and proteomic analyses, a genome-wide view of the changes elicited by miRNA down or up-regulation on the protein output is now available (Baek et al., 2008; Selbach et al., 2008; Hendrickson et al., 2009; Guo et al., 2010). These experimental data are critical for validating the prediction tools for miRNA targeting as well as for comparing the respective roles of the different modes of action driven by miRNAs.

Site-specific cleavage

This Ago2-mediated process requires full complementarity between miRNA and its target (Hammond et al., 2001; Hutvágner and Zamore, 2002), which seems to be very limited in mammals (Yekta et al., 2004; Hornstein et al., 2005). Loading of the miRNA into the Ago2 protein involves conformational changes which should enhance Watson–Crick pairing to the target mRNA. In contrast to this rare event, translational inhibition or mRNA degradation, which both result from partial binding of miRNA to mRNA, seem to be the most widely occurring mechanisms in mammals (for review, see Fabian et al., 2010).

Translational repression

Protein translation repression by miRNAs may result from various mechanisms: inhibition of translation initiation, inhibition of translation elongation; protein degradation while translation is being processed, premature termination of the translation (also known as ribosome drop-off); or a combination of some of these mechanisms (Bagga et al., 2005; Pillai et al., 2005; Nottrott et al., 2006; Petersen et al., 2006).

At the translation initiation step, miRNAs can inhibit protein production by disrupting the interaction between the 5′-cap and the 3′-poly(A) tail of the mRNA. The mechanisms involved are not fully understood but it is thought that Ago could compete with eukaryotic translation initiation factor 4 for mRNA-cap binding (Humphreys et al., 2005; Kiriakidou et al., 2007). Furthermore, miRNAs could prevent translation by inhibiting the association of the ribosomal subunits (Chendrimada et al., 2007; Thermann and Hentze, 2007).

At the post-initiation stage, translation inhibition by miRNAs could be mediated by premature termination and ribosome drop-off (Petersen et al., 2006), stalling of the elongation by slowing down the ribosome process (Rüegsegger et al., 2001; Mootz et al., 2004), or co-translational degradation of nascent polypeptides (Nottrott et al., 2006). However, experimental evidence for these mechanisms and explaining their interdependence is still only partial. As summarized by Filipowicz et al. (2008), the inhibition of translation at the initiation or elongation phase is perhaps not exclusive and it is likely that initiation is always inhibited. However, ribosomes queuing on the mRNA when elongation is also inhibited may hide this obligate mechanism (Filipowicz et al., 2008).

Enhanced mRNA decay

Large-scale analyses of the expression of miRNAs and their predicted mRNA targets have shown an inverse correlation, strongly suggesting that mRNA degradation is a hallmark of miRNA-mediated inhibition of transcripts (Chekulaeva and Filipowicz, 2009). A likely scenario relies on the deadenylation of the mRNA target, which would prevent circularization of the transcript. Circularization is an essential mechanism for mRNA translation that also prevents mRNA degradation, since linear transcripts are more prone to degradation (Wakiyama et al., 2007). Nevertheless, whether deadenylation precedes (Wakiyama et al., 2007; Iwasaki et al., 2009) or follows (Fabian et al., 2009; Zdanowicz et al., 2009) translational inhibition is still an unresolved issue.

Beyond the question of the mechanisms responsible for mRNA translation inhibition, there is the issue of the sub-cellular localization of this regulation. The most popular hypothesis posits that mRNAs under miRNA-mediated inhibition are stored (Brengues et al., 2005; Bhattacharyya et al., 2006) and degraded (Eulalio et al., 2007; Parker and Sheth, 2007) into cytoplasmic particles called processing bodies or glycine-tryptophan (GW) bodies. These cytoplasmic foci are free of translational machinery but are enriched in proteins that are required for efficient mRNA inhibition (Jakymiw et al., 2005; Liu et al., 2005; Rehwinkel et al., 2005; Behm-Ansmant et al., 2006).

miRNAs ARE REGULATORS OF NEURONAL ACTIVITY

Although the way miRNAs regulate their targets is still imperfectly understood, it is widely accepted that they play a major role in gene expression regulation. As such, miRNA have a crucial function in neuronal development where they seem to act as a master switch of the genome (for review, see Sun et al., 2013). In the mature nervous system, increasing evidence suggests that miRNA are important for normal neuronal function (Rajasethupathy et al., 2009; Edbauer et al., 2010; Cohen et al., 2011; Tognini et al., 2011; Dorval et al., 2012; Hsu et al., 2012; Lee et al., 2012; Saba et al., 2012).

The role of miRNA in neuronal function intermingles (i) miRNA that regulates neuronal activity with (ii) neuronal activity that modulates miRNA expression, which could in turn regulate targets with an impact on neuronal activity (feed-forward loop). In addition, neuronal activity should not be considered as a whole but as the output of thousands of synaptic inputs. Upon stimulation, single synapses or sets of synapses can go through intense and selective modifications in an independent manner for long periods of time (Martin and Kosik, 2002; Nelson and Turrigiano, 2008; Wibrand et al., 2010). Although short-term modifications of synapses could mainly be the result of post-translational events, long-term changes require regulation of gene expression at the transcriptional and post-transcriptional levels (Martin and Kosik, 2002; Wibrand et al., 2010). Thus, local post-transcriptional regulation regulated by activity is certainly a key element for the maintenance and plasticity of neural connections (Ashraf and Kunes, 2006; Sutton and Schuman, 2006; Bramham and Wells, 2007). Indeed, it has been demonstrated that specific mRNAs and components of the translational machinery, including ribosomes and other non-coding RNAs, are localized to dendritic regions of neurons, where they are likely to serve local translation (Steward and Levy, 1982; Davis et al., 1987; Torre and Steward, 1992; Trembleau et al., 1994; Landry and Hökfelt, 1998; Steward and Schuman, 2001). Localization of mRNAs into dendrites is an active phenomenon involving the 3′UTR sequence of messenger where RBPs bind to initiate transport (for review, see Doyle and Kiebler, 2011; Goldie and Cairns, 2012). In particular, some mRNAs are located at the post-synaptic density (PSD) as polyribosome structures (Wells, 2012). Some of these mRNAs encode proteins such as kinases and translational control factors, which are attractive candidates to mediate synaptic changes (Eberwine et al., 2001; Steward and Schuman, 2001). Interestingly, the number of polyribosome-containing spines increases in response to the long-term potentialization (LTP) protocol (Ostroff et al., 2002), and their PSD area enlarges when compared to polyribosome-free spines. This indicates that the presence of polyribosomes produces these structural changes, which were previously ascribed to changes in synaptic strength (Martin and Kosik, 2002). It has been suggested that this local translation mechanism could play a major role in synaptic plasticity and therefore contribute to the molecular basis of learning and memory (Kang and Schuman, 1996; Campbell and Holt, 2001; Kim et al., 2004).

Recently, miRNAs have been proposed as mediators regulating local protein synthesis at the synaptic level. miRNAs are enriched in the brain (Lagos-Quintana et al., 2002; Krichevsky et al., 2003; Kim et al., 2004; Sempere et al., 2004; Kosik and Krichevsky, 2005), where they have been shown to be differently expressed not only in distinct areas (Landgraf et al., 2007; Bak et al., 2008; Olsen et al., 2009), but also at the synaptic level (Pichardo-Casas et al., 2012). Moreover, studies on synaptoneurosomes revealed the abundance of several components of the miRNAs biogenesis pathway and their silencing complex machinery at PSDs (Lugli et al., 2005; Pichardo-Casas et al., 2012). Thus, dendritic mRNA translation can be modulated by miRNAs which have been selectively transported as mature or pre-miRNAs. In response to synaptic activity, this miRNA-driven regulation can either increase or decrease local mRNA translation through different mechanisms (**Figure 1**). Interestingly, not all miRNAs have the same regulation upon stimulus. However, it is not clear whether the involvement of these different types of regulation depends on the type of synaptic activity or on the type of stimulus.

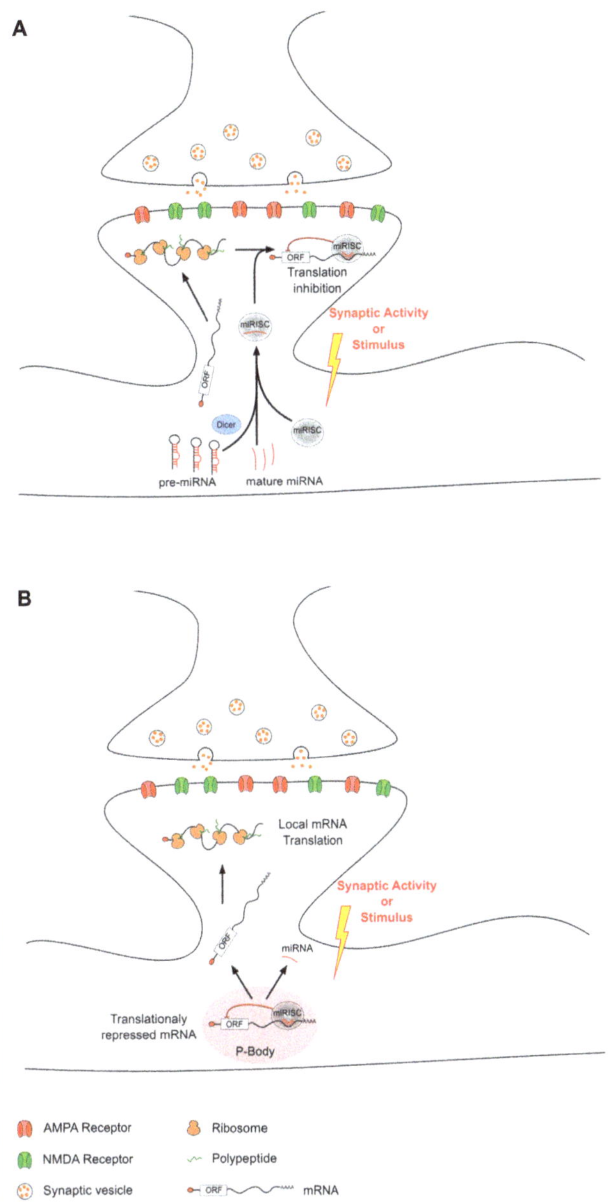

FIGURE 1 | MicroRNAs can modulate local translation in response to changes in synaptic activity. After transport from the soma to the dendrites, some mRNAs are locally translated into proteins. This local translation mechanism can be modulated in response to synaptic activity changes by dendritic miRNAs that have also been transported from the soma. This miRNA-driven mechanism can either decrease **(A)** or increase **(B)** local translation. **(A)** Decrease of local translation could be the result of an activity-related miRNA loading into miRISC and specific binding to target mRNAs. **(B)** Increase of translation may be the consequence of an unbinding of miRNA from target-mRNAs which could then escape P-body and undergo local translation.

In addition to their role in physiological conditions, accruing evidence suggests that miRNAs play an important role in the pathological mechanisms of neurodegenerative diseases (reviewed in Johnson et al., 2012; Salta and De Strooper, 2012). Hence, alterations of specific miRNAs have been associated with Alzheimer's, Parkinson's, Huntington's disease, and Tourette syndrome. Furthermore, in other debilitating diseases of the nervous system, miRNA deregulation has been correlated with altered neuronal activity, as in chronic pain, which is characterized by increased excitability within the pain circuitry. One of the first demonstrations of the role of miRNAs in chronic pain came from a study by Zhao et al. (2010) where a conditional knockout of Dicer was targeted to sodium channel Nav1.8-positive nociceptor neurons in the dorsal root ganglia (DRG). This impairment of miRNA function induced a strong attenuation of inflammatory pain, suggesting that miRNAs are necessary to enhance excitability of this subpopulation of neurons in response to inflammation mediators. Here, we review specific miRNAs that have been shown to play a role in the regulation of neuronal activity and highlight their possible association with pain processes (summarized in **Table 1**). In some cases, the causal role of miRNA in pain mechanisms is strongly suggested by targeted-mRNAs identification and functional studies. On the other hand, we conducted a retrospective analysis of miRNA expression data published for different pain models and speculated about their potential implication based on their known targets in normal neuronal activity.

FUNCTIONAL IMPLICATION OF miRNA IN NEURONAL PLASTICITY AND PAIN SENSITIZATION

One of the first studies reporting the control of local translation by miRNA at the synapse upon synaptic activity showed that miR-134 negatively regulates LIMK1 in an activity-dependent manner (Schratt et al., 2006). LIMK1 is a protein kinase that controls actin filament dynamics through inhibition of actin depolymerizing factor (ADF)/cofilin (Bamburg, 1999). This regulation could be critical for synaptic transmission, synaptic integration, and plasticity since the majority of the excitatory synapses are formed on dendritic spines, which are actin-rich protrusions from the dendritic shaft (Hering and Sheng, 2001; Bonhoeffer and Yuste, 2002; Spruston, 2008). The study demonstrated the compartmentalization of miR-134 and its target LIMK1 mRNA at the synapto-dendritic area. It has been proposed that the miR-134 association with LIMK1 mRNA keeps the LIMK1 mRNA in a dormant state while it is being transported within dendrites to synaptic sites. Over-expression of miR-134 inhibits LIMK1 mRNA local translation, resulting in a negative regulation of the size of the dendritic spines. Exposure of neurons to external stimuli like the neurotrophic factor brain-derived neurotrophic factor (BDNF) reduces miR-134 inhibition on LIMK1 mRNA translation (Schratt et al., 2006). Recently, the same group reported

Table 1 | MicroRNAs involved in plasticity and pain mechanisms.

miRNA	Involvement in plasticity mechanisms			Involvement in pain mechanisms		
	Plasticity protocols	**Identified targets**	**Reference**	**Pain models**	**Identified targets**	**Reference**
miR-134	BDNF exposure	LIMK1	Schratt et al. (2006)	Inflammation/CCI	ND	Bai et al. (2007), Genda et al. (2013)
miR-132	Bicuculline/KCl/monocular deprivation	P250GAP /MeCP2	Vo et al. (2005), Klein et al. (2007), Wayman et al. (2008), Mellios et al. (2011), Tognini et al. (2011)	CRPS/CCI	ND	Orlova et al. (2011), Arai et al. (2013)
miR-188	Long-term-potentiation	Nrp-2	Lee et al. (2012)	CCI	ND	Arai et al. (2013)
miR-29a/b	Psychoactive drugs	Arpc3	Lippi et al. (2011)	Inflammation/CRPS/ CCI	ND	Bai et al. (2007), Orlova et al. (2011), Genda et al. (2013)
miR-181a	Psychoactive drugs	GluA2	Schaefer et al. (2010), Chandrasekar and Dreyer (2011), Saba et al. (2012)	Neuropathic/ zymosan-induced pelvic pain	$GABA_{A\alpha-1}$	Li et al. (2013), Sengupta et al. (2013)
miR-219	Disturbance of NMDA signaling	CaMKIIγ	Kocerha et al. (2009)	Traumatic spinal cord injury/CCI	ND	Liu et al. (2009), Genda et al. (2013)
miR-125	Fragile X syndrome	NR2A	Edbauer et al. (2010)	CCI	ND	Arai et al. (2013)
miR-124	Neuronal differentiation/axon guidance	Sema3A/RhoG/ Zif268	Baudet et al. (2012), Franke et al. (2012), Yang et al. (2012)	Inflammation/nerve injury	MeCP2	Bai et al. (2007), Wu et al. (2011), Willemen et al. (2012), Kynast et al. (2013)

CCI, chronic constriction injury; CRPS, complex regional pain syndrome; ND, not determined.

another mechanism by which pre-miR-134 is transported to dendritic sites. Replacing the loop sequence of pre-miR-134 with the loop of a non-dendritic pre-miRNA abolished dendritic accumulation of pre-miR-134. Mutagenesis analysis revealed that the five central loop nucleotides are critical because of an interaction with the Asp-Glu-Ala-His-box (DEAH-box) helicase DEAH box protein 36 (DHX36). DHX36 is known to compete with Dicer *in vitro*, and Argonaute complexes that contain DHX36 are devoid of Dicer activity (Höck et al., 2007). Indeed, knockdown of DHX36 displayed a significant reduction in the percentage of dendritic pre-miR-134, without affecting the global levels of pre-miR-134 or mature miR-134. Consistently with the role of miR-134 on spine morphology, functional experiments revealed that DHX36 negatively regulates dendritic spine morphogenesis in hippocampal neurons (Bicker et al., 2013).

One of the first studies on a possible role of miRNAs in pain showed that miR-134 is modulated in the trigeminal ganglion in response to inflammatory pain (Bai et al., 2007). These authors induced inflammatory pain by injecting complete Freund's adjuvant (CFA) into the rat masseter muscle, a paradigm known to produce transient inflammation accompanied by allodynia. Interestingly, miR-134 was down-regulated at the onset of pain, 30 min after CFA injection, returned to control level 1 day later, showed an over-expression rebound at day 4 and finally returned to control level at day 12. This phasic deregulation of miR-134 expression suggests that it could be an adaptive response to the early phase of inflammation. Another study in the chronic constriction injury (CCI) model showed that miR-134 was up-regulated in the dorsal horn of the spinal cord at day 14 after surgery (Genda et al., 2013). In this case, miR-134 deregulation occurred later after the onset of the painful behavior and could have been a consequence of the pain mechanisms. In contrast, our own results show that miR-134 was down-regulated 7 days after injury in the dorsal horn of a rat model of sciatic nerve ligation. This was accompanied by an up-regulation of LIMK1, the miR-134 target (A. Salam et al., unpublished data). Therefore, it will be important to undertake functional studies to elucidate the role of miR-134 in chronic pain.

miR-132 is another example of activity-modulated miRNA. Experiments where neuronal activity is increased through a bicuculline-mediated blockade of $GABA_A$ inhibitory tone showed a rapid increase in the expression of miR-132 precursor and mature miR-132 (Wayman et al., 2008). Interestingly, this regulation was attenuated by pretreatment with the selective *N*-methyl-D-aspartate receptor (NMDAR) antagonist amino-5-phosphonovaleric acid (APV). In addition, KCl treatment increased transcription of the miR-132 precursor, suggesting that different modalities of neuronal activity stimulation also trigger a similar miR-132 increase. The explanation lies in the pathway leading to miR-132 over-expression. Indeed, inhibitors for CaM kinase, MEK–ERK (mitogen-activated protein kinase kinase–extracellular signal-regulated kinase) or CREB (cAMP response element-binding protein), all prevent miR-132 up-regulation upon activity enhancement, suggesting that miR-132 is regulated predominantly by the CREB pathway. miR-132 directly targets p250GAP, a protein known to inhibit Rho family GTPases (Taniguchi et al., 2003; Zhao et al., 2003). The final outcome of miR-132 over-expression is an increase in dendrite morphogenesis, presumably as a response to Rac activity. Indeed, the same group recently proposed that miR-132 regulates dendritic spinogenesis through the Rac1-Pak actin remodeling pathway (Impey et al., 2010). Another target of miR-132 is methyl CpG-binding protein 2 (MeCP2), which is involved in dendritic development and synaptogenesis and whose modulation can affect synaptic plasticity (Klein et al., 2007). Additional evidence of miR-132 having an impact on neuronal morphology came from transgenic experiments where the genomic locus containing miR-132 (and miR-212 as well) was deleted, leading to a dramatic decrease in dendritic length, arborization, and spine density (Magill et al., 2010). The impact of miR-132 regulation on spinogenesis is revealed in synaptic plasticity paradigms. For instance, *in vitro* short-term plasticity is affected by miR-132 over-expression without altering basal synaptic transmission (Lambert et al., 2010). *In vivo*, short-term recognition memory is impaired by miR-132 over-expression in the perirhinal cortex. This results from a deficit in both long-term depression and potentiation (Scott et al., 2012). In the visual cortex, two recent studies demonstrated that miR-132 is a key component of experience-dependent plasticity. Tognini et al. (2011) showed that monocular deprivation decreased miR-132 expression in the cortex contralateral to the deprived eye. Counterbalancing this miR-132 decrease with miR-132 mimic supplementation completely blocked ocular dominance plasticity. At the same time, Mellios et al. (2011) identified miR-132 as the miRNA whose expression is the most affected by dark rearing and/or monocular deprivation. In addition, miR-132 inhibition occluded ocular dominance plasticity after monocular deprivation, which is associated with an altered maturation of dendritic spines. Finally, a recent study on olfactory bulb neurons born in the neonatal subventricular zone revealed that miR-132 is essential for normal dendritic complexity and spine morphology (Pathania et al., 2012). In conclusion, and as previously proposed (Tognini and Pizzorusso, 2012), finely regulated miR-132 expression seems to be essential for plasticity. Thus, too high an expression would make dendritic spines too stable. Too low an expression would lead to very unstable spines, thus impeding synaptic plasticity.

Vo et al. (2005) demonstrated that BDNF triggered miR-132 up-regulation in cortical neurons. Interestingly, BDNF was recently identified as a modulator of nociception. BDNF is up-regulated in the DRG and the spinal cord in inflammatory and neuropathic pain models (reviewed in Merighi et al., 2008 and Vanelderen et al., 2010, respectively), where it is associated with an increased excitatory synaptic drive. In addition, in most cases, intrathecal BDNF injections exhibit pro-nociceptive effects (Merighi et al., 2008). Thus, one could hypothesize that the effect of BDNF on nociceptive behavior could partially be the result of a BDNF-driven miR-132 over-expression. Thus, BDNF would induce an up-regulation of miR-132, which in turn would increase dendrite morphogenesis and arborization in the nociceptive pathway, resulting in an increased transmission of the pain signal. In patients with complex regional pain syndrome (CRPS), a disabling chronic neuropathic pain affecting one or more extremities, miR-132 blood levels were significantly altered (Orlova et al., 2011). Apart from the direct nociceptive pathway, other nervous structures like the limbic system may influence pain perception. Indeed, the hippocampus is thought to be part of the descending anti-nociceptive system, potentially exerting an inhibitory role in neuropathic pain (Basbaum and Fields, 1979). Arai et al. (2013) screened miRNA expression in the hippocampus of animals submitted to the CCI paradigm of neuropathic pain. miR-132 was down-regulated early after the onset of the neuropathic behavior and stayed under-expressed until the latest time-point analyzed. Thus, it is tempting to hypothesize that this modulation of miR-132 could lower the excitatory drive of the hippocampus and therefore lower the anti-nociceptive effect on the spinal pain pathway.

miR-188 is another activity-regulated miRNA with a proven synaptic plasticity tuning function. Lee et al. (2012) found that miR-188 was up-regulated in hippocampal slices in response to the LTP protocol. Neuropilin-2 (Nrp-2), one of the predicted targets of miR-188, is down-regulated after the LTP procedure and luciferase experiments confirmed the interaction. Nrp-2 is a receptor of semaphorin 3F, which induces the repulsion of neuronal growth cones expressing Nrp-2 (Kolodkin and Ginty, 1997; Kruger et al., 2005). In addition, miR-188 treatment can rescue the decreased miniature excitatory postsynaptic current (mEPSC) frequency and reduction of spine density induced by Nrp-2 over-expression, suggesting that miR-188 plays a role in synaptic plasticity by buffering Nrp-2 expression.

Despite its potentially crucial role in neuronal function, evidence for the involvement of miR-188 in pain mechanisms is very scarce. However, one study reported an altered expression under pain conditions. Arai et al. (2013) quantified a down-regulation of miR-188 in the hippocampus of CCI animals but the significance of this modification remains to be elucidated.

The role of miRNAs in dendritic spine remodeling as a substrate for synaptic plasticity has also been evidenced *in vivo*. Lippi et al. (2011) exposed adult mice to psychoactive drugs like nicotine, cocaine, or amphetamine and quantified miRNA expression in different brain regions. Many miRNAs were regulated in response to these neuroadaptation paradigms, and especially the miR-29a/b locus was consistently over-expressed. *In vitro* experiments confirmed that these miRNAs were up-regulated in an activity-dependent manner. Arpc3 was identified as a target of miR-29a/b. This protein is part of the ARP2/3 actin nucleation complex which plays a critical role in actin branching, a mechanism involved in dendritic spine maturation. Therefore, this work strongly suggests that miR-29a/b regulates the activity-dependent structural plasticity associated with psycho-stimulant exposure.

Several studies identified a deregulation of miR-29a/b in pain conditions. The first evidence came from Bai et al. (2007) who reported a down-regulation of this miRNA in the trigeminal ganglion neurons after inflammatory muscle pain. It was later confirmed in two other pain conditions, the CRPS (Orlova et al., 2011) and the CCI model (Genda et al., 2013). Nevertheless, these studies did not investigate the subsequent regulation of Arpc3 or any other target of miR-29a/b, so the role of miR-29a/b in pain processing still needs to be elucidated.

In the context of chronic exposure to drugs of abuse, Saba et al. (2012) focused their attention on the regulation of miRNAs in the nucleus accumbens. This is one of the most important brain regions in behavioral responses to drugs of abuse and is elicited by dopamine release. Synaptoneurosome preparations revealed a strong enrichment of miR-181a in response to treatment. A previous study showed that miR-181a expression in the striatum was regulated by Ago2 in cocaine addiction (Schaefer et al., 2010). This miRNA was predicted to target GluA2 and was confirmed in luciferase experiments (Saba et al., 2012). In addition, miR-181a over-expression in hippocampal cultures reduced AMPA (α-amino-3-hydroxy-5-methyl-4-isoxazolepropionic acid) receptor surface clusters, spine volume, and mEPSC frequency. Finally, the association between miR-181a and drugs of abuse has been highlighted (Chandrasekar and Dreyer, 2011). In that study, lentiviral over-expression of miR-181a in the nucleus accumbens enhanced cocaine-induced conditioned place preference. Two studies performed on the miRNA expression in the dorsal horn of spinal cord in neuropathic pain models quantified a down-regulation of miR-181a (Li et al., 2013) or other members of the miR-181 family, namely miR-181b/c/d (von Schack et al., 2011). Thus, this miR-181 down-regulation could lead to an up-regulation of the excitatory receptor GluA2 in the nociceptive pathway.

Involvement of AMPA receptors in neuropathic pain mechanisms has already been suggested (for review, see Garry and Fleetwood-Walker, 2004). Unfortunately, the expression of GluA2 was not assessed in these two miRNA studies. Interestingly, another study on a different model, chronic pelvic pain, revealed a role of miR-181a through the regulation of a different target, the inhibitory receptor $GABA_{A\alpha-1}$ (Sengupta et al., 2013). Pelvic pain was experimentally elicited by intra-vesicular injections of zymosan (a carbohydrate extracted from yeast and known to induce inflammation) into the bladder at postnatal day 14. This induced long-lasting neuroanatomical and neurophysiological changes in the nociceptive system still present at postnatal day 60. At that stage, zymosan-treated animals were characterized by visceral hypersensitivity, an up-regulation of miR-181a and a down-regulation of $GABA_{A\alpha-1}$ expression in the lombo-sacral segment of the spinal cord. Bioinformatics analyses identified multiple sites for miR-181a/b in the 3′UTR of $GABA_{A\alpha-1}$ and luciferase experiments proved the inhibitory effect of miR-181a on $GABA_{A\alpha-1}$ translation. These results strongly suggest that this miR-181a-induced down-regulation of $GABA_A$ receptors results in a loss of inhibition in the spinal cord sustaining long-lasting visceral hypersensitivity. They highlight the importance of target identification in miRNA studies.

N-methyl-D-aspartate receptors are another kind of glutamate receptor known to play a crucial role in synaptic transmission and plasticity. Altered NMDA-mediated signaling is associated with behavioral impairments in psychiatric disorders. Kocerha et al. (2009) demonstrated that miR-219 is down-regulated in the prefrontal cortex in response to pharmacological or genetic disturbances of NMDA signaling. In addition, they showed that miR-219 targets calcium/calmodulin-dependent protein kinase II (CaMKII) subunit γ, a downstream component of the NMDA signaling cascade. Thus, miR-219 down-regulation upon NMDA inhibition appears to be a compensatory mechanism that attenuates behavioral disorders associated with acute receptor antagonism.

Two miRNA screening studies suggest that miR-219 may be involved in pain mechanisms. The first evidence came from a model of traumatic spinal cord injury where miR-219 was significantly down-regulated 7 days after contusion (Liu et al., 2009). On the contrary, sciatic nerve ligation (CCI model) was demonstrated to induce an up-regulation of this miRNA (Genda et al., 2013). However, in both cases the investigation of targeted mRNA still needs to be conducted to shed light on the pathological role of miR-219 in pain pathways. In addition, the group of M. Sheng demonstrated that the expression of the NR2A subunit of NMDARs was regulated by miR-125b in hippocampal neurons (Edbauer et al., 2010). Indeed, endogenous miR-125b affected NMDAR composition and therefore induced functional changes in channel kinetics. As a consequence, miR-125b expression is likely to be critical for synaptic plasticity. Interestingly, a CCI pain model induced the down-regulation of miR-125b in the hippocampus (Arai et al., 2013), a structure that is part of the descending anti-nociceptive system.

miR-124 is one of the most abundant miRNAs in the brain and its role in the development of the mammalian brain is now well established. Thus, miR-124 is a neuronal differentiation promoter that also acts as an inhibitor of neuronal stem cells (Cheng et al., 2009; Yoo et al., 2009; Åkerblom et al., 2012). During *X. laevis* development, miR-124 plays a crucial role in timing the axon pathfinding of retinal ganglion cells (RGCs; Baudet et al., 2012). Thus, a key event in the correct navigation of RGC axons is a change in growth cone sensitivity to guidance cues. Baudet et al. (2012) demonstrated that miR-124 regulates the initiation of growth cone responsiveness to semaphorin Sema3A. In addition, miR-124 was shown to regulate neuronal process complexity by modulating the small GTPase RhoG (Franke et al., 2012). Indeed, RhoG is a critical modulator of the actin cytoskeleton. Consequently, RhoG inhibits axonal branching so miR-124-mediated inhibition of RhoG stimulates axonal and dendritic complexity. Yang et al. (2012) demonstrated that miR-124 is a direct regulator of the transcription factor Zif268, which is essential for activity-related modulation of synaptic transmission and cognition.

In the context of chronic pain, miR-124 down-regulation in DRG neurons was reported in inflammatory muscle pain (Bai et al., 2007), as well as in sciatic nerve after peripheral nerve crush (Wu et al., 2011). Moreover, intrathecal injection of miR-124 had an anti-nociceptive effect in both inflammatory and nerve injury-induced chronic pain models (Willemen et al., 2012). Finally, Niederberger's group showed that intravenous injection of miR-124 alleviates the nociceptive response to the formalin test and identified the target involved as MeCP2 (Kynast et al., 2013). Thus, in addition to miR-132 (Klein et al., 2007), miR-124a also regulates MeCP2 translation. MeCP2 is an epigenetic modulator of BDNF, one of the major players in inflammatory pain mechanisms (Merighi et al., 2008).

One of the interesting characteristics of miRNAs that has been conserved through evolution is that a given miRNA has the potential to regulate multiple targets owing to the permissive hybridization to target mRNAs. This mechanism of action is now well accepted and it can have an important impact on gene expression regulation. Thus, one or few miRNAs could regulate the expression of multiple genes that participate in the same function or which constitute the different subunits of a macromolecular complex (Ferretti et al., 2008; Harraz et al., 2012).

In the context of chronic pain, we demonstrated such a multiple targeting by one miRNA. Indeed, we showed that a single miRNA, miR-103, simultaneously regulates the expression of the three subunits of the Cav1.2-comprising L-type calcium channel (Cav1.2-LTC) in an integrative regulation. Sensitization to pain involves the activation of various types of voltage-gated calcium channels. Some control synaptic transmission (Matthews and Dickenson, 2001; Bourinet et al., 2005; Altier et al., 2007) while others regulate intrinsic membrane properties. Among the latter, Cav1.2-LTC regulates gene expression underlying long-term plastic changes (Dolmetsch et al., 2001; Fossat et al., 2010). miR-103-mediated modulation of Cav1.2 function is bidirectional since knocking-down or over-expressing miR-103 respectively up- or down-regulate the level of Cav1.2-LTC translation. Functionally, we showed that miR-103 knockdown in naive rats results in hypersensitivity to pain. Moreover, miR-103 was down-regulated in neuropathic animals and miR-103 intrathecal applications successfully relieved pain, thus identifying miR-103 as a possible novel therapeutic target in neuropathic chronic pain (Favereaux et al., 2011).

ACTIVITY-INDUCED MODULATION OF miRNA LEVELS

A set of evidence is growing to suggest that miRNAs can regulate neuronal activity by modulating the expression of ion channels, the morphology of dendritic spines and the molecular pathways downstream from receptor activation. However, the mechanisms that induce an activity-related modulation of miRNA-mediated inhibition of target genes remain poorly understood. Recent reports mostly in non-neuronal cells showed that it involves regulation of both the metabolism and function of miRNAs, and some of these mechanisms were also found to play a crucial role in neurons (for review, see Krol et al., 2010b). Below, we summarize the known mechanisms that modulate miRNA levels as a result of activity variations in neurons.

First, modulation of miRNA levels in response to activity could result from transcription regulation as for mRNAs. Indeed, Nomura et al. (2008) found that the transcription of miR-184, a brain-specific miRNA, is repressed by the binding of MeCP2. miR-184 is an imprinted gene exclusively expressed from the paternal allele. Interestingly, enhancement of neuronal activity by high-KCl treatment induced MeCP2 phosphorylation and the consequent release of phosphorylated MeCP2 from the miR-184 promoter region. Thus, the increase in miR-184 levels in response to neuronal activity involves at least an augmented transcription of miR-184.

CREB is a transcription factor that plays a crucial role in nervous system development and plasticity (reviewed in Lonze and Ginty, 2002). A genome-wide screen for CREB-binding sites identified hundreds of locations that are associated with non-coding RNAs and miRNAs, including miR-132 (Vo et al., 2005). DNase I footprinting assay confirmed the CREB binding at two consensus cAMP regulatory elements (CREs) in the close 5′ region of the miR-212/-132 locus. CREB is known to be activated by neurotrophins such as BDNF, and the authors demonstrated that miR-132 transcription was enhanced in response to BDNF. In addition, CREB inhibition partially blocked the BDNF-induced increase of miR-132, strongly suggesting that this mechanism involved the CREB pathway. Wayman et al. (2008) demonstrated that miR-132 is regulated by CREB in an activity-dependent manner. Hence, in hippocampal neuronal cultures, inhibition of $GABA_A$ inhibitory tone with bicuculline increased synaptic activity and the levels of miR-132 precursor and mature forms. Interestingly, blockade of CREB-dependent transcription abolished the miR-132 up-regulation in response to synaptic activity.

Second, the function of miRNA can be modulated by regulating miRISC components. Hence, MOV10, the mammalian ortholog of the SDE3 helicase Armitage in *Drosophila* (Ashraf et al., 2006), is present at synapses and undergoes rapid proteolysis in response to NMDAR-mediated activity (Banerjee et al., 2009). As a consequence, it relieves miRNA-mediated translation inhibition of key proteins at the synapse like CaMKII or LIMK1 (Ashraf et al., 2006; Banerjee et al., 2009).

Another possible mechanism could be the activity-dependent regulation of dendritic P-bodies. Cougot et al. (2008) demonstrated that ribonucleoprotein particles (RNPs) with a P-body-like structure are present in dendrites and that they exhibit motorized movements upon synaptic activation to relocate to distant sites (Cougot et al., 2008). In addition, neuronal activation induced a loss of AGO2 from these P-body-like structures, suggesting that it may regulate local translation. Thus, inhibited messenger RNPs (mRNPs) may be stored in these particles at resting state and then be released in response to synaptic activity in order to be translated.

Besides regulation of miRISC components, recent evidence suggests that synergistic pathways may contribute to miRNA function and could therefore be activity-regulated. Hence, FMRP (fragile X mental retardation protein) is a protein with multiple RNA-binding domains that acts as a translational suppressor of particular mRNAs (Bassell and Warren, 2008). Interestingly, FMRP interacts with RISC proteins and miRNAs, although it is not necessary for miRNA-mediated inhibition (Caudy et al., 2002; Ishizuka et al., 2002; Jin et al., 2004). Edbauer et al. (2010) recently showed that both FMRP and miR-125b bound NR2A NMDAR subunit mRNA, thus leading to translation inhibition. Moreover, the inhibition of NR2A by FMRP is enhanced by miR-125b and FMRP depletion reversed miR-125b effects, strongly suggesting a synergistic effect.

Finally, obtaining a net change in miRNA levels without affecting miRNA transcription could be the result of miRNA decay alterations. Indeed, recent evidence suggests that miRNA turnover is fast in neuronal cells owing to rapid decay (Krol et al., 2010a). In addition, the authors demonstrated that the rate of miRNA decay is activity-dependent. Thus, blocking neuronal activity with either tetrodotoxin (TTX; inhibiting action potentials) or 6-nitro-sulfamoyl-benzo-quinoxaline-dione/3-carboxy-piperazin-propyl phosphonic acid (NBQX/CPP; inhibiting glutamate transmission) reduced miRNA decay. Some elements of the enzymatic machinery involved in miRNA degradation have recently been discovered (Ramachandran and Chen, 2008; Chatterjee and Grosshans, 2009). However, the factors responsible for the rapid and activity-dependent miRNA decay in neurons are still unknown and constitute a new challenge. The most recent breakthrough in our understanding of miRNA regulation in neurons came from an underestimated RNA class, circular RNAs (circRNAs). circRNAs were first discovered in plants (Sanger et al., 1976) and then in unicellular organisms (Grabowski et al., 1981), but the best-known circRNA is the sex-determining region Y RNA (Sry) which is highly expressed in testes (Capel et al., 1993). Recently, two groups identified a brain-expressed circRNA [(named CDR1as (cerebellar degeneration-related protein 1 antisense) or circular RNA sponge for miR-7 (ciRS-7)] that contains roughly 70 target sites for miR-7 (Hansen et al., 2013; Memczak et al., 2013). This circRNA acts as a natural miRNA sponge since it binds several miR-7 copies at a time, thus reducing miR-7 inhibition on mRNA targets. Interestingly, a very recent study identified miR-7 as a regulator of neuronal activity in chronic pain conditions. Hence, Sakai et al. (2013) showed that miR-7a was strongly down-regulated in the DRG of neuropathic pain models in animals. They demonstrated that miR-7a targets the β2-subunit of voltage-gated sodium channel, thus increasing the excitability of nociceptive neurons. In addition, miR-7a exogenous over-expression in DRG of injured animals alleviated neuropathic pain.

CONCLUSION

How miRNAs regulate neuronal function in response to activity and whether deregulation of these mechanisms triggers pathological states are still poorly understood. For instance, are the miRNA pathways that control neuronal fate during development also involved in brain homeostasis? What are the mechanisms that could modulate miRNA expression in response to neuronal activity? Do the pathways involved in miRNA regulation depend on the kind of stimulus or on the miRNA species? What is the spatial resolution of miRNA control on local translation? What is the therapeutic potential of targeting activity-regulated miRNA?

The analysis of miRNA regulation in challenging pathological conditions such as chronic pain may help to highlight crucial miRNA mechanisms that are discreet in basal conditions. In the past few years, many studies have screened for miRNA expression in various animal models and in cohorts of patients with diverse neurodegenerative diseases. Although highlighting biomarker miRNAs with a possible value for therapeutic approaches, this kind of approach does not improve our understanding of miRNA targeting and function in pathological mechanisms. Indeed, it would be risky to evaluate targets of candidate miRNAs on algorithm-based prediction databases only, since the number of putative targets is very large and confirmation of targeting sometimes difficult to achieve. Therefore, it will be important to improve miRNA target prediction tools maybe by considering recent experimental data suggesting that "seed" region may not be the only signature of miRNA targeting (Helwak et al., 2013). Moreover, it would be interesting to compare miRNA and mRNA expression data as often as possible in the light of experimentally confirmed miRNA:mRNA interactions.

Nevertheless, the various experimental paradigms with their sometimes conflicting data could hinder progress toward a better understanding of miRNA function. Therefore, the use of unified experimental parameters could further clarify the role of miRNA in neuronal plasticity. The large body of pre-existing data provides solid evidence for the involvement of miRNA regulation in both physiological and pathological conditions. Thus, miRNA is an attractive potential therapeutic target.

ACKNOWLEDGMENTS

This work received funding from the Centre National de la Recherche Scientifique, Agence Nationale pour la Recherche (grant MirPAIN), Association pour la Recherche sur le Cancer (ARC), Conseil Régional Aquitaine. We acknowledge Y. Le Feuvre and C. Baudet for helpful comments on the manuscript.

REFERENCES

Åkerblom, M., Sachdeva, R., Barde, I., Verp, S., Gentner, B., Trono, D., et al. (2012). MicroRNA-124 is a subventricular zone neuronal fate determinant. *J. Neurosci.* 32, 8879–8889. doi: 10.1523/JNEUROSCI.0558-12.2012

Altier, C., Dale, C. S., Kisilevsky, A. E., Chapman, K., Castiglioni, A. J., Matthews, E. A., et al. (2007). Differential role of N-type calcium channel splice isoforms in pain. *J. Neurosci.* 27, 6363–6373. doi: 10.1523/JNEUROSCI.0307-07.2007

Arai, M., Genda, Y., Ishikawa, M., Shunsuke, T., Okabe, T., and Sakamoto, A. (2013). The miRNA and mRNA changes in rat hippocampi after chronic constriction injury. *Pain Med.* 14, 720–729. doi: 10.1111/pme.12066

Ashraf, S. I., and Kunes, S. (2006). A trace of silence: memory and microRNA at the synapse. *Curr. Opin. Neurobiol.* 16, 535–539. doi: 10.1016/j.conb.2006.08.007

Ashraf, S. I., McLoon, A. L., Sclarsic, S. M., and Kunes, S. (2006). Synaptic protein synthesis associated with memory is regulated by the RISC pathway in *Drosophila*. *Cell* 124, 191–205. doi: 10.1016/j.cell.2005.12.017

Baek, D., Villén, J., Shin, C., Camargo, F. D., Gygi, S. P., and Bartel, D. P. (2008). The impact of microRNAs on protein output. *Nature* 455, 64–71. doi: 10.1038/nature07242

Bagga, S., Bracht, J., Hunter, S., Massirer, K., Holtz, J., Eachus, R., et al. (2005). Regulation by let-7 and lin-4 miRNAs results in target mRNA degradation. *Cell* 122, 553–563. doi: 10.1016/j.cell.2005.07.031

Bai, G., Ambalavanar, R., Wei, D., and Dessem, D. (2007). Downregulation of selective microRNAs in trigeminal ganglion neurons following inflammatory muscle pain. *Mol. Pain* 3, 15. doi: 10.1186/1744-8069-3-15

Bak, M., Silahtaroglu, A., Møller, M., Christensen, M., Rath, M. F., Skryabin, B., et al. (2008). MicroRNA expression in the adult mouse central nervous system. *RNA* 14, 432–444. doi: 10.1261/rna.783108

Bamburg, J. R. (1999). Proteins of the ADF/cofilin family: essential regulators of actin dynamics. *Annu. Rev. Cell Dev. Biol.* 15, 185–230. doi: 10.1146/annurev.cellbio.15.1.185

Banerjee, S., Neveu, P., and Kosik, K. S. (2009). A coordinated local translational control point at the synapse involving relief from silencing and MOV10 degradation. *Neuron* 64, 871–884. doi: 10.1016/j.neuron.2009.11.023

Bartel, D. P. (2004). MicroRNAs: genomics, biogenesis, mechanism, and function. *Cell* 116, 281–297. doi: 10.1016/S0092-8674(04)00045-5

Bartel, D. P. (2009). MicroRNAs: target recognition and regulatory functions. *Cell* 136, 215–233. doi: 10.1016/j.cell.2009.01.002

Basbaum, A. I., and Fields, H. L. (1979). The origin of descending pathways in the dorsolateral funiculus of the spinal cord of the cat and rat: further studies on the anatomy of pain modulation. *J. Comp. Neurol.* 187, 513–531. doi: 10.1002/cne.901870304

Baskerville, S., and Bartel, D. P. (2005). Microarray profiling of microRNAs reveals frequent coexpression with neighboring miRNAs and host genes. *RNA* 11, 241–247. doi: 10.1261/rna.7240905

Bassell, G. J., and Warren, S. T. (2008). Fragile X syndrome: loss of local mRNA regulation alters synaptic development and function. *Neuron* 60, 201–214. doi: 10.1016/j.neuron.2008.10.004

Baudet, M., Zivraj, K. H., Abreu-Goodger, C., Muldal, A., Armisen, J., Blenkiron, C., et al. (2012). miR-124 acts through CoREST to control onset of Sema3A sensitivity in navigating retinal growth cones. *Nat. Neurosci.* 15, 29–38. doi: 10.1038/nn.2979

Behm-Ansmant, I., Rehwinkel, J., Doerks, T., Stark, A., Bork, P., and Izaurralde, E. (2006). mRNA degradation by miRNAs and GW182 requires both CCR4:NOT deadenylase and DCP1:DCP2 decapping complexes. *Genes Dev.* 20, 1885–1898. doi: 10.1101/gad.1424106

Bernstein, E., Caudy, A. A., Hammond, S. M., and Hannon, G. J. (2001). Role for a bidentate ribonuclease in the initiation step of RNA interference. *Nature* 409, 363–366. doi: 10.1038/35053110

Bhattacharyya, S. N., Habermacher, R., Martine, U., Closs, E. I., and Filipowicz, W. (2006). Relief of microRNA-mediated translational repression in human cells subjected to stress. *Cell* 125, 1111–1124. doi: 10.1016/j.cell.2006.04.031

Bicker, S., Khudayberdiev, S., Weiß, K., Zocher, K., Baumeister, S., and Schratt, G. (2013). The DEAH-box helicase DHX36 mediates dendritic localization of the neuronal precursor-microRNA-134. *Genes Dev.* 27, 991–996. doi: 10.1101/gad.211243.112

Bohnsack, M. T., Czaplinski, K., and Gorlich, D. (2004). Exportin 5 is a RanGTP-dependent dsRNA-binding protein that mediates nuclear export of pre-miRNAs. *RNA* 10, 185–191. doi: 10.1261/rna.5167604

Bonhoeffer, T., and Yuste, R. (2002). Spine motility. Phenomenology, mechanisms, and function. *Neuron* 35, 1019–1027. doi: 10.1016/S0896-6273(02)00906-6

Bourinet, E., Alloui, A., Monteil, A., Barrere, C., Couette, B., Poirot, O., et al. (2005). Silencing of the Cav3.2 T-type calcium channel gene in sensory neurons demonstrates its major role in nociception. *EMBO J.* 24, 315–324. doi: 10.1038/sj.emboj.7600515

Bramham, C. R., and Wells, D. G. (2007). Dendritic mRNA: transport, translation and function. *Nat. Rev. Neurosci.* 8, 776–789. doi: 10.1038/nrn2150

Brengues, M., Teixeira, D., and Parker, R. (2005). Movement of eukaryotic mRNAs between polysomes and cytoplasmic processing bodies. *Science* 310, 486–489. doi: 10.1126/science.1115791

Brodersen, P., and Voinnet, O. (2009). Revisiting the principles of microRNA target recognition and mode of action. *Nat. Rev. Mol. Cell Biol.* 10, 141–148. doi: 10.1038/nrm2619

Cai, X., Hagedorn, C. H., and Cullen, B. R. (2004). Human microRNAs are processed from capped, polyadenylated transcripts that can also function as mRNAs. *RNA* 10, 1957–1966. doi: 10.1261/rna.7135204

Campbell, D. S., and Holt, C. E. (2001). Chemotropic responses of retinal growth cones mediated by rapid local protein synthesis and degradation. *Neuron* 32, 1013–1026. doi: 10.1016/S0896-6273(01)00551-7

Capel, B., Swain, A., Nicolis, S., Hacker, A., Walter, M., Koopman, P., et al. (1993). Circular transcripts of the testis-determining gene Sry in adult mouse testis. *Cell* 73, 1019–1030. doi: 10.1016/0092-8674(93)90279-Y

Caudy, A. A., Myers, M., Hannon, G. J., and Hammond, S. M. (2002). Fragile X-related protein and VIG associate with the RNA interference machinery. *Genes Dev.* 16, 2491–2496. doi: 10.1101/gad.1025202

Chandrasekar, V., and Dreyer, J. (2011). Regulation of miR-124, Let-7d, and miR-181a in the accumbens affects the expression, extinction, and reinstatement of cocaine-induced conditioned place preference. *Neuropsychopharmacology* 36, 1149–1164. doi: 10.1038/npp.2010.250

Chatterjee, S., and Grosshans, H. (2009). Active turnover modulates mature microRNA activity in *Caenorhabditis elegans*. *Nature* 461, 546–549. doi: 10.1038/nature08349

Chekulaeva, M., and Filipowicz, W. (2009). Mechanisms of miRNA-mediated post-transcriptional regulation in animal cells. *Curr. Opin. Cell Biol.* 21, 452–460. doi: 10.1016/j.ceb.2009.04.009

Chendrimada, T. P., Finn, K. J., Ji, X., Baillat, D., Gregory, R. I., Liebhaber, S. A., et al. (2007). MicroRNA silencing through RISC recruitment of eIF6. *Nature* 447, 823–828. doi: 10.1038/nature05841

Cheng, L., Pastrana, E., Tavazoie, M., and Doetsch, F. (2009). miR-124 regulates adult neurogenesis in the subventricular zone stem cell niche. *Nat. Neurosci.* 12, 399–408. doi: 10.1038/nn.2294

Chi, S. W., Zang, J. B., Mele, A., and Darnell, R. B. (2009). Argonaute HITS-CLIP decodes microRNA-mRNA interaction maps. *Nature* 460, 479–486. doi: 10.1038/nature08170

Cohen, J. E., Lee, P. R., Chen, S., Li, W., and Fields, R. D. (2011). MicroRNA regulation of homeostatic synaptic plasticity. *Proc. Natl. Acad. Sci. U.S.A.* 108, 11650–11655. doi: 10.1073/pnas.1017576108

Corcoran, D. L., Pandit, K. V., Gordon, B., Bhattacharjee, A., Kaminski, N., and Benos, P. V. (2009). Features of mammalian microRNA promoters emerge from polymerase II chromatin immunoprecipitation data. *PLoS ONE* 4:e5279. doi: 10.1371/journal.pone.0005279

Cougot, N., Bhattacharyya, S. N., Tapia-Arancibia, L., Bordonné, R., Filipowicz, W., Bertrand, E., et al. (2008). Dendrites of mammalian neurons contain specialized P-body-like structures that respond to neuronal activation. *J. Neurosci.* 28, 13793–13804. doi: 10.1523/JNEUROSCI.4155-08.2008

Davis, L., Banker, G. A., and Steward, O. (1987). Selective dendritic transport of RNA in hippocampal neurons in culture. *Nature* 330, 477–479. doi: 10.1038/330477a0

Denli, A. M., Tops, B. B. J., Plasterk, R. H. A., Ketting, R. F., and Hannon, G. J. (2004). Processing of primary microRNAs by the Microprocessor complex. *Nature* 432, 231–235. doi: 10.1038/nature03049

Doench, J. G., Petersen, C. P., and Sharp, P. A. (2003). siRNAs can function as miRNAs. *Genes Dev.* 17, 438–442. doi: 10.1101/gad.1064703

Dolmetsch, R. E., Pajvani, U., Fife, K., Spotts, J. M., and Greenberg, M. E. (2001). Signaling to the nucleus by an L-type calcium channel-calmodulin complex through the MAP kinase pathway. *Science* 294, 333–339. doi: 10.1126/science.1063395

Dorval, V., Smith, P. Y., Delay, C., Calvo, E., Planel, E., Zommer, N., et al. (2012). Gene network and pathway analysis of mice with conditional ablation of Dicer in post-mitotic neurons. *PLoS ONE* 7:e44060. doi: 10.1371/journal.pone.0044060

Doyle, M., and Kiebler, M. A. (2011). Mechanisms of dendritic mRNA transport and its role in synaptic tagging. *EMBO J.* 30, 3540–3552. doi: 10.1038/emboj.2011.278

Easow, G., Teleman, A. A., and Cohen, S. M. (2007). Isolation of microRNA targets by miRNP immunopurification. *RNA* 13, 1198–1204. doi: 10.1261/rna.563707

Eberwine, J., Miyashiro, K., Kacharmina, J. E., and Job, C. (2001). Local translation of classes of mRNAs that are targeted to neuronal dendrites. *Proc. Natl. Acad. Sci. U.S.A.* 98, 7080–7085. doi: 10.1073/pnas.121146698

Edbauer, D., Neilson, J. R., Foster, K. A., Wang, C. F., Seeburg, D. P., Batterton, M. N., et al. (2010). Regulation of synaptic structure and function by FMRP-associated microRNAs miR-125b and miR-132. *Neuron* 65, 373–384. doi: 10.1016/j.neuron.2010.01.005

Eulalio, A., Behm-Ansmant, I., and Izaurralde, E. (2007). P bodies: at the crossroads of post-transcriptional pathways. *Nat. Rev. Mol. Cell Biol.* 8, 9–22. doi: 10.1038/nrm2080

Fabian, M. R., Mathonnet, G., Sundermeier, T., Mathys, H., Zipprich, J. T., Svitkin, Y. V., et al. (2009). Mammalian miRNA RISC recruits CAF1 and PABP to affect PABP-dependent deadenylation. *Mol. Cell* 35, 868–880. doi: 10.1016/j.molcel.2009.08.004

Fabian, M. R., Sonenberg, N., and Filipowicz, W. (2010). Regulation of mRNA translation and stability by microRNAs. *Annu. Rev. Biochem.* 79, 351–379. doi: 10.1146/annurev-biochem-060308-103103

Farh, K. K., Grimson, A., Jan, C., Lewis, B. P., Johnston, W. K., Lim, L. P., et al. (2005). The widespread impact of mammalian microRNAs on mRNA repression and evolution. *Science* 310, 1817–1821. doi: 10.1126/science.1121158

Favereaux, A., Thoumine, O., Bouali-Benazzouz, R., Roques, V., Papon, M., Salam, S. A., et al. (2011). Bidirectional integrative regulation of Cav1.2 calcium channel by microRNA miR-103: role in pain. *EMBO J.* 30, 3830–3841. doi: 10.1038/emboj.2011.249

Ferretti, E., De Smaele, E., Miele, E., Laneve, P., Po, A., Pelloni, M., et al. (2008). Concerted microRNA control of Hedgehog signalling in cerebellar neuronal progenitor and tumour cells. *EMBO J.* 27, 2616–2627. doi: 10.1038/emboj.2008.172

Filipowicz, W., Bhattacharyya, S. N., and Sonenberg, N. (2008). Mechanisms of post-transcriptional regulation by microRNAs: are the answers in sight? *Nat. Rev. Genet.* 9, 102–114. doi: 10.1038/nrg2290

Fossat, P., Dobremez, E., Bouali-Benazzouz, R., Favereaux, A., Bertrand, S. S., Kilk, K., et al. (2010). Knockdown of L calcium channel subtypes: differential effects in neuropathic pain. *J. Neurosci.* 30, 1073–1085. doi: 10.1523/JNEUROSCI.3145-09.2010

Franke, K., Otto, W., Johannes, S., Baumgart, J., Nitsch, R., and Schumacher, S. (2012). miR-124-regulated RhoG reduces neuronal process complexity via ELMO/Dock180/Rac1 and Cdc42 signalling. *EMBO J.* 31, 2908–2921. doi: 10.1038/emboj.2012.130

Garry, E. M., and Fleetwood-Walker, S. M. (2004). A new view on how AMPA receptors and their interacting proteins mediate neuropathic pain. *Pain* 109, 210–213. doi: 10.1016/j.pain.2004.04.002

Genda, Y., Arai, M., Ishikawa, M., Tanaka, S., Okabe, T., and Sakamoto, A. (2013). microRNA changes in the dorsal horn of the spinal cord of rats with chronic constriction injury: a TaqMan® Low Density Array study. *Int. J. Mol. Med.* 31, 129–137. doi: 10.3892/ijmm.2012.1163

Goldie, B. J., and Cairns, M. J. (2012). Post-transcriptional trafficking and regulation of neuronal gene expression. *Mol. Neurobiol.* 45, 99–108. doi: 10.1007/s12035-011-8222-0

Grabowski, P. J., Zaug, A. J., and Cech, T. R. (1981). The intervening sequence of the ribosomal RNA precursor is converted to a circular RNA in isolated nuclei of Tetrahymena. *Cell* 23, 467–476. doi: 10.1016/0092-8674(81)90142-2

Gregory, R. I., Yan, K., Amuthan, G., Chendrimada, T., Doratotaj, B., Cooch, N., et al. (2004). The microprocessor complex mediates the genesis of microRNAs. *Nature* 432, 235–240. doi: 10.1038/nature03120

Griffiths-Jones, S., Grocock, R. J., van Dongen, S., Bateman, A., and Enright, A. J. (2006). miRBase: microRNA sequences, targets and gene nomenclature. *Nucleic Acids Res.* 34, D140–D144. doi: 10.1093/nar/gkj112

Grimson, A., Farh, K. K., Johnston, W. K., Garrett-Engele, P., Lim, L. P., and Bartel, D. P. (2007). MicroRNA targeting specificity in mammals: determinants beyond seed pairing. *Mol. Cell* 27, 91–105. doi: 10.1016/j.molcel.2007.06.017

Guo, H., Ingolia, N. T., Weissman, J. S., and Bartel, D. P. (2010). Mammalian microRNAs predominantly act to decrease target mRNA levels. *Nature* 466, 835–840. doi: 10.1038/nature09267

Hammond, S. M., Boettcher, S., Caudy, A. A., Kobayashi, R., and Hannon, G. J. (2001). Argonaute2, a link between genetic and biochemical analyses of RNAi. *Science* 293, 1146–1150. doi: 10.1126/science.1064023

Han, J., Lee, Y., Yeom, K., Kim, Y., Jin, H., and Kim, V. N. (2004). The Drosha-DGCR8 complex in primary microRNA processing. *Genes Dev.* 18, 3016–3027. doi: 10.1101/gad.1262504

Hansen, T. B., Jensen, T. I., Clausen, B. H., Bramsen, J. B., Finsen, B., Damgaard, C. K., et al. (2013). Natural RNA circles function as efficient microRNA sponges. *Nature* 495, 384–388. doi: 10.1038/nature11993

Harraz, M. M., Eacker, S. M., Wang, X., Dawson, T. M., and Dawson, V. L. (2012). MicroRNA-223 is neuroprotective by targeting glutamate receptors. *Proc. Natl. Acad. Sci. U.S.A.* 109, 18962–18967. doi: 10.1073/pnas.1121288109

Helwak, A., Kudla, G., Dudnakova, T., and Tollervey, D. (2013). Mapping the human miRNA interactome by CLASH reveals frequent noncanonical binding. *Cell* 153, 654–665. doi: 10.1016/j.cell.2013.03.043

Hendrickson, D. G., Hogan, D. J., McCullough, H. L., Myers, J. W., Herschlag, D., Ferrell, J. E., et al. (2009). Concordant regulation of translation and mRNA abundance for hundreds of targets of a human microRNA. *PLoS Biol.* 7:e1000238. doi: 10.1371/journal.pbio.1000238

Hering, H., and Sheng, M. (2001). Dendritic spines: structure, dynamics and regulation. *Nat. Rev. Neurosci.* 2, 880–888. doi: 10.1038/35104061

Höck, J., Weinmann, L., Ender, C., Rüdel, S., Kremmer, E., Raabe, M., et al. (2007). Proteomic and functional analysis of Argonaute-containing mRNA-protein complexes in human cells. *EMBO Rep.* 8, 1052–1060. doi: 10.1038/sj.embor.7401088

Hornstein, E., Mansfield, J. H., Yekta, S., Hu, J. K., Harfe, B. D., McManus, M. T., et al. (2005). The microRNA miR-196 acts upstream of Hoxb8 and Shh in limb development. *Nature* 438, 671–674. doi: 10.1038/nature04138

Hsu, R., Schofield, C. M., Dela Cruz, C. G., Jones-Davis, D. M., Blelloch, R., and Ullian, E. M. (2012). Loss of microRNAs in pyramidal neurons leads to specific changes in inhibitory synaptic transmission in the prefrontal cortex. *Mol. Cell. Neurosci.* 50, 283–292. doi: 10.1016/j.mcn.2012.06.002

Humphreys, D. T., Westman, B. J., Martin, D. I. K., and Preiss, T. (2005). MicroRNAs control translation initiation by inhibiting eukaryotic initiation factor 4E/cap and poly(A) tail function. *Proc. Natl. Acad. Sci. U.S.A.* 102, 16961–16966. doi: 10.1073/pnas.0506482102

Hutvágner, G., McLachlan, J., Pasquinelli, A. E., Bálint, E., Tuschl, T., and Zamore, P. D. (2001). A cellular function for the RNA-interference enzyme Dicer in the maturation of the let-7 small temporal RNA. *Science* 293, 834–838. doi: 10.1126/science.1062961

Hutvágner, G., and Zamore, P. D. (2002). A microRNA in a multiple-turnover RNAi enzyme complex. *Science* 297, 2056–2060. doi: 10.1126/science.1073827

Impey, S., Davare, M., Lesiak, A., Fortin, D., Ando, H., Varlamova, O., et al. (2010). An activity-induced microRNA controls dendritic spine formation by regulating Rac1-PAK signaling. *Mol. Cell. Neurosci.* 43, 146–156. doi: 10.1016/j.mcn.2009.10.005

Ishizuka, A., Siomi, M. C., and Siomi, H. (2002). A *Drosophila* fragile X protein interacts with components of RNAi and ribosomal proteins. *Genes Dev.* 16, 2497–2508. doi: 10.1101/gad.1022002

Iwasaki, S., Kawamata, T., and Tomari, Y. (2009). *Drosophila* argonaute1 and argonaute2 employ distinct mechanisms for translational repression. *Mol. Cell* 34, 58–67. doi: 10.1016/j.molcel.2009.02.010

Jackson, R. J., and Standart, N. (2007). How do microRNAs regulate gene expression? *Sci. STKE* 2007, re1. doi: 10.1126/stke.3672007re1

Jakymiw, A., Lian, S., Eystathioy, T., Li, S., Satoh, M., Hamel, J. C., et al. (2005). Disruption of GW bodies impairs mammalian RNA interference. *Nat. Cell Biol.* 7, 1267–1274. doi: 10.1038/ncb1334

Jin, P., Zarnescu, D. C., Ceman, S., Nakamoto, M., Mowrey, J., Jongens, T. A., et al. (2004). Biochemical and genetic interaction between the fragile X mental retardation protein and the microRNA pathway. *Nat. Neurosci.* 7, 113–117. doi: 10.1038/nn1174

Johnson, R., Noble, W., Tartaglia, G. G., and Buckley, N. J. (2012). Neurodegeneration as an RNA disorder. *Prog. Neurobiol.* 99, 293–315. doi: 10.1016/j.pneurobio.2012.09.006

Kang, H., and Schuman, E. M. (1996). A requirement for local protein synthesis in neurotrophin-induced hippocampal synaptic plasticity. *Science* 273, 1402–1406. doi: 10.1126/science.273.5280.1402

Karr, J., Vagin, V., Chen, K., Ganesan, S., Olenkina, O., Gvozdev, V., et al. (2009). Regulation of glutamate receptor subunit availability by microRNAs. *J. Cell Biol.* 185, 685–697. doi: 10.1083/jcb.200902062

Ketting, R. F., Fischer, S. E., Bernstein, E., Sijen, T., Hannon, G. J., and Plasterk, R. H. (2001). Dicer functions in RNA interference and in synthesis of small RNA involved in developmental timing in *C. elegans*. *Genes Dev.* 15, 2654–2659. doi: 10.1101/gad.927801

Khvorova, A., Reynolds, A., and Jayasena, S. D. (2003). Functional siRNAs and miRNAs exhibit strand bias. *Cell* 115, 209–216. doi: 10.1016/S0092-8674(03)00801-8

Kim, J., Krichevsky, A., Grad, Y., Hayes, G. D., Kosik, K. S., Church, G. M., et al. (2004). Identification of many microRNAs that copurify with polyribosomes in mammalian neurons. *Proc. Natl. Acad. Sci. U.S.A.* 101, 360–365. doi: 10.1073/pnas.2333854100

Kiriakidou, M., Tan, G. S., Lamprinaki, S., De Planell-Saguer, M., Nelson, P. T., and Mourelatos, Z. (2007). An mRNA m7G cap binding-like motif within human Ago2 represses translation. *Cell* 129, 1141–1151. doi: 10.1016/j.cell.2007.05.016

Klein, M. E., Lioy, D. T., Ma, L., Impey, S., Mandel, G., and Goodman, R. H. (2007). Homeostatic regulation of MeCP2 expression by a CREB-induced microRNA. *Nat. Neurosci.* 10, 1513–1514. doi: 10.1038/nn2010

Kloosterman, W. P., Wienholds, E., Ketting, R. F., and Plasterk, R. H. A. (2004). Substrate requirements for let-7 function in the developing zebrafish embryo. *Nucleic Acids Res.* 32, 6284–6291. doi: 10.1093/nar/gkh968

Knight, S. W., and Bass, B. L. (2001). A role for the RNase III enzyme DCR-1 in RNA interference and germ line development in *Caenorhabditis elegans*. *Science* 293, 2269–2271. doi: 10.1126/science.1062039

Kocerha, J., Faghihi, M. A., Lopez-Toledano, M. A., Huang, J., Ramsey, A. J., Caron, M. G., et al. (2009). MicroRNA-219 modulates NMDA receptor-mediated neurobehavioral dysfunction. *Proc. Natl. Acad. Sci. U.S.A.* 106, 3507–3512. doi: 10.1073/pnas.0805854106

Kolodkin, A. L., and Ginty, D. D. (1997). Steering clear of semaphorins: neuropilins sound the retreat. *Neuron* 19, 1159–1162. doi: 10.1016/S0896-6273(00)80408-0

Kosik, K. S., and Krichevsky, A. M. (2005). The elegance of the microRNAs: a neuronal perspective. *Neuron* 47, 779–782. doi: 10.1016/j.neuron.2005.08.019

Kozomara, A., and Griffiths-Jones, S. (2011). miRBase: integrating microRNA annotation and deep-sequencing data. *Nucleic Acids Res.* 39, D152–D157. doi: 10.1093/nar/gkq1027

Krichevsky, A. M., King, K. S., Donahue, C. P., Khrapko, K., and Kosik, K. S. (2003). A microRNA array reveals extensive regulation of microRNAs during brain development. *RNA* 9, 1274–1281. doi: 10.1261/rna.5980303

Krol, J., Busskamp, V., Markiewicz, I., Stadler, M. B., Ribi, S., Richter, J., et al. (2010a). Characterizing light-regulated retinal microRNAs reveals rapid turnover as a common property of neuronal microRNAs. *Cell* 141, 618–631. doi: 10.1016/j.cell.2010.03.039

Krol, J., Loedige, I., and Filipowicz, W. (2010b). The widespread regulation of microRNA biogenesis, function and decay. *Nat. Rev. Genet.* 11, 597–610. doi: 10.1038/nrg2843

Kruger, R. P., Aurandt, J., and Guan, K. (2005). Semaphorins command cells to move. *Nat. Rev. Mol. Cell Biol.* 6, 789–800. doi: 10.1038/nrm1740

Kynast, K. L., Russe, O. Q., Möser, C. V., Geisslinger, G., and Niederberger, E. (2013). Modulation of central nervous system-specific microRNA-124a alters the inflammatory response in the formalin test in mice. *Pain* 154, 368–376. doi: 10.1016/j.pain.2012.11.010

Lagos-Quintana, M., Rauhut, R., Lendeckel, W., and Tuschl, T. (2001). Identification of novel genes coding for small expressed RNAs. *Science* 294, 853–858. doi: 10.1126/science.1064921

Lagos-Quintana, M., Rauhut, R., Yalcin, A., Meyer, J., Lendeckel, W., and Tuschl, T. (2002). Identification of tissue-specific microRNAs from mouse. *Curr. Biol.* 12, 735–739. doi: 10.1016/S0960-9822(02)00809-6

Lambert, T. J., Storm, D. R., and Sullivan, J. M. (2010). MicroRNA132 modulates short-term synaptic plasticity but not basal release probability in hippocampal neurons. *PLoS ONE* 5:e15182. doi: 10.1371/journal.pone.0015182

Landgraf, P., Rusu, M., Sheridan, R., Sewer, A., Iovino, N., Aravin, A., et al. (2007). A mammalian microRNA expression atlas based on small RNA library sequencing. *Cell* 129, 1401–1414. doi: 10.1016/j.cell.2007.04.040

Landry, M., and Hökfelt, T. (1998). Subcellular localization of preprogalanin messenger RNA in perikarya and axons of hypothalamo-posthypophyseal magnocellular neurons: an in situ hybridization study. *Neuroscience* 84, 897–912. doi: 10.1016/S0306-4522(97)00567-8

Lau, N. C., Lim, L. P., Weinstein, E. G., and Bartel, D. P. (2001). An abundant class of tiny RNAs with probable regulatory roles in *Caenorhabditis elegans*. *Science* 294, 858–862. doi: 10.1126/science.1065062

Lee, K., Kim, J., Kwon, O., An, K., Ryu, J., Cho, K., et al. (2012). An activity-regulated microRNA, miR-188, controls dendritic plasticity and synaptic transmission by downregulating neuropilin-2. *J. Neurosci.* 32, 5678–5687. doi: 10.1523/JNEUROSCI.6471-11.2012

Lee, R. C., Feinbaum, R. L., and Ambros, V. (1993). The *C. elegans* heterochronic gene lin-4 encodes small RNAs with antisense complementarity to lin-14. *Cell* 75, 843–854. doi: 10.1016/0092-8674(93)90529-Y

Lee, Y., Ahn, C., Han, J., Choi, H., Kim, J., Yim, J., et al. (2003). The nuclear RNase III Drosha initiates microRNA processing. *Nature* 425, 415–419. doi: 10.1038/nature01957

Lee, Y., Kim, M., Han, J., Yeom, K., Lee, S., Baek, S. H., et al. (2004). MicroRNA genes are transcribed by RNA polymerase II. *EMBO J.* 23, 4051–4060. doi: 10.1038/sj.emboj.7600385

Leung, A. K. L., Young, A. G., Bhutkar, A., Zheng, G. X., Bosson, A. D., Nielsen, C. B., et al. (2011). Genome-wide identification of Ago2 binding sites from mouse embryonic stem cells with and without mature microRNAs. *Nat. Struct. Mol. Biol.* 18, 237–244. doi: 10.1038/nsmb.1991

Lewis, B. P., Burge, C. B., and Bartel, D. P. (2005). Conserved seed pairing, often flanked by adenosines, indicates that thousands of human genes are microRNA targets. *Cell* 120, 15–20. doi: 10.1016/j.cell.2004.12.035

Li, H., Shen, L., Ma, C., and Huang, Y. (2013). Differential expression of miRNAs in the nervous system of a rat model of bilateral sciatic nerve chronic constriction injury. *Int. J. Mol. Med.* 32, 219–226. doi: 10.3892/ijmm.2013.1381

Li, X., and Jin, P. (2010). Roles of small regulatory RNAs in determining neuronal identity. *Nat. Rev. Neurosci.* 11, 329–338. doi: 10.1038/nrn2739

Lim, L. P., Lau, N. C., Garrett-Engele, P., Grimson, A., Schelter, J. M., Castle, J., et al. (2005). Microarray analysis shows that some microRNAs downregulate large numbers of target mRNAs. *Nature* 433, 769–773. doi: 10.1038/nature03315

Lippi, G., Steinert, J. R., Marczylo, E. L., D'Oro, S., Fiore, R., Forsythe, I. D., et al. (2011). Targeting of the Arpc3 actin nucleation factor by miR-29a/b regulates dendritic spine morphology. *J. Cell Biol.* 194, 889–904. doi: 10.1083/jcb.201103006

Liu, J., Rivas, F. V., Wohlschlegel, J., Yates JR3, Parker, R., and Hannon, G. J. (2005). A role for the P-body component GW182 in microRNA function. *Nat. Cell Biol.* 7, 1261–1266. doi: 10.1038/ncb1333

Liu, N., Wang, X., Lu, Q., and Xu, X. (2009). Altered microRNA expression following traumatic spinal cord injury. *Exp. Neurol.* 219, 424–429. doi: 10.1016/j.expneurol.2009.06.015

Lonze, B. E., and Ginty, D. D. (2002). Function and regulation of CREB family transcription factors in the nervous system. *Neuron* 35, 605–623. doi: 10.1016/S0896-6273(02)00828-0

Lugli, G., Larson, J., Martone, M. E., Jones, Y., and Smalheiser, N. R. (2005). Dicer and eIF2c are enriched at postsynaptic densities in adult mouse brain and are modified by neuronal activity in a calpain-dependent manner. *J. Neurochem.* 94, 896–905. doi: 10.1111/j.1471-4159.2005.03224.x

Lund, E., Güttinger, S., Calado, A., Dahlberg, J. E., and Kutay, U. (2004). Nuclear export of microRNA precursors. *Science* 303, 95–98. doi: 10.1126/science.1090599

Lytle, J. R., Yario, T. A., and Steitz, J. A. (2007). Target mRNAs are repressed as efficiently by microRNA-binding sites in the 5′ UTR as in the 3′ UTR. *Proc. Natl. Acad. Sci. U.S.A.* 104, 9667–9672. doi: 10.1073/pnas.0703820104

Magill, S. T., Cambronne, X. A., Luikart, B. W., Lioy, D. T., Leighton, B. H., Westbrook, G. L., et al. (2010). microRNA-132 regulates dendritic growth and arborization of newborn neurons in the adult hippocampus. *Proc. Natl. Acad. Sci. U.S.A.* 107, 20382–20387. doi: 10.1073/pnas.1015691107

Martin, K. C., and Kosik, K. S. (2002). Synaptic tagging – who's it? *Nat. Rev. Neurosci.* 3, 813–820. doi: 10.1038/nrn942

Matthews, E. A., and Dickenson, A. H. (2001). Effects of ethosuximide, a T-type Ca(2+) channel blocker, on dorsal horn neuronal responses in rats. *Eur. J. Pharmacol.* 415, 141–149. doi: 10.1016/S0014-2999(01)00812-3

Mellios, N., Sugihara, H., Castro, J., Banerjee, A., Le, C., Kumar, A., et al. (2011). miR-132, an experience-dependent microRNA, is essential for visual cortex plasticity. *Nat. Neurosci.* 14, 1240–1242. doi: 10.1038/nn.2909

Memczak, S., Jens, M., Elefsinioti, A., Torti, F., Krueger, J., Rybak, A., et al. (2013). Circular RNAs are a large class of animal RNAs with regulatory potency. *Nature* 495, 333–338. doi: 10.1038/nature11928

Merighi, A., Salio, C., Ghirri, A., Lossi, L., Ferrini, F., Betelli, C., et al. (2008). BDNF as a pain modulator. *Prog. Neurobiol.* 85, 297–317. doi: 10.1016/j.pneurobio.2008.04.004

Mootz, D., Ho, D. M., and Hunter, C. P. (2004). The STAR/Maxi-KH domain protein GLD-1 mediates a developmental switch in the translational control of *C. elegans* PAL-1. *Development* 131, 3263–3272. doi: 10.1242/dev.01196

Morlando, M., Ballarino, M., Gromak, N., Pagano, F., Bozzoni, I., and Proudfoot, N. J. (2008). Primary microRNA transcripts are processed co-transcriptionally. *Nat. Struct. Mol. Biol.* 15, 902–909. doi: 10.1038/nsmb.1475

Mourelatos, Z., Dostie, J., Paushkin, S., Sharma, A., Charroux, B., Abel, L., et al. (2002). miRNPs: a novel class of ribonucleoproteins containing numerous microRNAs. *Genes Dev.* 16, 720–728. doi: 10.1101/gad.974702

Nelson, S. B., and Turrigiano, G. G. (2008). Strength through diversity. *Neuron* 60, 477–482. doi: 10.1016/j.neuron.2008.10.020

Nielsen, C. B., Shomron, N., Sandberg, R., Hornstein, E., Kitzman, J., and Burge, C. B. (2007). Determinants of targeting by endogenous and exogenous microRNAs and siRNAs. *RNA* 13, 1894–1910. doi: 10.1261/rna.768207

Nilsen, T. W. (2007). Mechanisms of microRNA-mediated gene regulation in animal cells. *Trends Genet.* 23, 243–249. doi: 10.1016/j.tig.2007.02.011

Nomura, T., Kimura, M., Horii, T., Morita, S., Soejima, H., Kudo, S., et al. (2008). MeCP2-dependent repression of an imprinted miR-184 released by depolarization. *Hum. Mol. Genet.* 17, 1192–1199. doi: 10.1093/hmg/ddn011

Nottrott, S., Simard, M. J., and Richter, J. D. (2006). Human let-7a miRNA blocks protein production on actively translating polyribosomes. *Nat. Struct. Mol. Biol.* 13, 1108–1114. doi: 10.1038/nsmb1173

O'Carroll, D., and Schaefer, A. (2013). General principals of miRNA biogenesis and regulation in the brain. *Neuropsychopharmacology* 38, 39–54. doi: 10.1038/npp.2012.87

Okamura, K., Hagen, J. W., Duan, H., Tyler, D. M., and Lai, E. C. (2007). The mirtron pathway generates microRNA-class regulatory RNAs in *Drosophila*. *Cell* 130, 89–100. doi: 10.1016/j.cell.2007.06.028

Olsen, L., Klausen, M., Helboe, L., Nielsen, F. C., and Werge, T. (2009). MicroRNAs show mutually exclusive expression patterns in the brain of adult male rats. *PLoS ONE* 4:e7225. doi: 10.1371/journal.pone.0007225

Orlova, I. A., Alexander, G. M., Qureshi, R. A., Sacan, A., Graziano, A., Barrett, J. E., et al. (2011). MicroRNA modulation in complex regional pain syndrome. *J. Transl. Med.* 9, 195. doi: 10.1186/1479-5876-9-195

Ostroff, L. E., Fiala, J. C., Allwardt, B., and Harris, K. M. (2002). Polyribosomes redistribute from dendritic shafts into spines with enlarged synapses during LTP in developing rat hippocampal slices. *Neuron* 35, 535–545. doi: 10.1016/S0896-6273(02)00785-7

Parker, R., and Sheth, U. (2007). P bodies and the control of mRNA translation and degradation. *Mol. Cell* 25, 635–646. doi: 10.1016/j.molcel.2007.02.011

Pasquinelli, A. E. (2012). MicroRNAs and their targets: recognition, regulation and an emerging reciprocal relationship. *Nat. Rev. Genet.* 13, 271–282. doi: 10.1038/nrg3162.

Pathania, M., Torres-Reveron, J., Yan, L., Kimura, T., Lin, T. V., Gordon, V., et al. (2012). miR-132 enhances dendritic morphogenesis, spine density, synaptic integration, and survival of newborn olfactory bulb neurons. *PLoS ONE* 7:e38174. doi: 10.1371/journal.pone.0038174

Petersen, C. P., Bordeleau, M., Pelletier, J., and Sharp, P. A. (2006). Short RNAs repress translation after initiation in mammalian cells. *Mol. Cell* 21, 533–542. doi: 10.1016/j.molcel.2006.01.031

Pichardo-Casas, I., Goff, L. A., Swerdel, M. R., Athie, A., Davila, J., Ramos-Brossier, M., et al. (2012). Expression profiling of synaptic microRNAs from the adult rat brain identifies regional differences and seizure-induced dynamic modulation. *Brain Res.* 1436, 20–33. doi: 10.1016/j.brainres.2011.12.001

Pillai, R. S., Bhattacharyya, S. N., Artus, C. G., Zoller, T., Cougot, N., Basyuk, E., et al. (2005). Inhibition of translational initiation by Let-7 MicroRNA in human cells. *Science* 309, 1573–1576. doi: 10.1126/science.1115079

Pillai, R. S., Bhattacharyya, S. N., and Filipowicz, W. (2007). Repression of protein synthesis by miRNAs: how many mechanisms? *Trends Cell Biol.* 17, 118–126. doi: 10.1016/j.tcb.2006.12.007

Rajasethupathy, P., Fiumara, F., Sheridan, R., Betel, D., Puthanveettil, S. V., Russo, J. J., et al. (2009). Characterization of small RNAs in *Aplysia* reveals a role for miR-124 in constraining synaptic plasticity through CREB. *Neuron* 63, 803–817. doi: 10.1016/j.neuron.2009.05.029

Ramachandran, V., and Chen, X. (2008). Degradation of microRNAs by a family of exoribonucleases in *Arabidopsis*. *Science* 321, 1490–1492. doi: 10.1126/science.1163728

Rehwinkel, J., Behm-Ansmant, I., Gatfield, D., and Izaurralde, E. (2005). A crucial role for GW182 and the DCP1:DCP2 decapping complex in miRNA-mediated gene silencing. *RNA* 11, 1640–1647. doi: 10.1261/rna.2191905

Reyes-Herrera, P. H., and Ficarra, E. (2012). One decade of development and evolution of microRNA target prediction algorithms. *Genomics Proteomics Bioinformatics* 10, 254–263. doi: 10.1016/j.gpb.2012.10.001

Rhoades, M. W., Reinhart, B. J., Lim, L. P., Burge, C. B., Bartel, B., and Bartel, D. P. (2002). Prediction of plant microRNA targets. *Cell* 110, 513–520. doi: 10.1016/S0092-8674(02)00863-2

Rodriguez, A., Griffiths-Jones, S., Ashurst, J. L., and Bradley, A. (2004). Identification of mammalian microRNA host genes and transcription units. *Genome Res.* 14, 1902–1910. doi: 10.1101/gr.2722704

Ruby, J. G., Jan, C. H., and Bartel, D. P. (2007a). Intronic microRNA precursors that bypass Drosha processing. *Nature* 448, 83–86. doi: 10.1038/nature05983

Ruby, J. G., Stark, A., Johnston, W. K., Kellis, M., Bartel, D. P., and Lai, E. C. (2007b). Evolution, biogenesis, expression, and target predictions of a substantially expanded set of *Drosophila* microRNAs. *Genome Res.* 17, 1850–1864. doi: 10.1101/gr.6597907

Rüegsegger, U., Leber, J. H., and Walter, P. (2001). Block of HAC1 mRNA translation by long-range base pairing is released by cytoplasmic splicing upon induction of the unfolded protein response. *Cell* 107, 103–114. doi: 10.1016/S0092-8674(01)00505-0

Saba, R., Störchel, P. H., Aksoy-Aksel, A., Kepura, F., Lippi, G., Plant, T. D., et al. (2012). Dopamine-regulated microRNA miR-181a controls GluA2 surface expression in hippocampal neurons. *Mol. Cell. Biol.* 32, 619–632. doi: 10.1128/MCB.05896-11

Saetrom, P., Heale, B. S. E., Snøve, O. J., Aagaard, L., Alluin, J., and Rossi, J. J. (2007). Distance constraints between microRNA target sites dictate efficacy and cooperativity. *Nucleic Acids Res.* 35, 2333–2342. doi: 10.1093/nar/gkm133

Sakai, A., Saitow, F., Miyake, N., Miyake, K., Shimada, T., and Suzuki, H. (2013). miR-7a alleviates the maintenance of neuropathic pain through regulation of neuronal excitability. *Brain* 136(Pt 9), 2738–2750. doi: 10.1093/brain/awt191

Salta, E., and De Strooper, B. (2012). Non-coding RNAs with essential roles in neurodegenerative disorders. *Lancet Neurol.* 11, 189–200. doi: 10.1016/S1474-4422(11)70286-1

Sanger, H. L., Klotz, G., Riesner, D., Gross, H. J., and Kleinschmidt, A. K. (1976). Viroids are single-stranded covalently closed circular RNA molecules existing as highly base-paired rod-like structures. *Proc. Natl. Acad. Sci. U.S.A.* 73, 3852–3856. doi: 10.1073/pnas.73.11.3852

Schaefer, A., Im, H., Venø, M. T., Fowler, C. D., Min, A., Intrator, A., et al. (2010). Argonaute 2 in dopamine 2 receptor-expressing neurons regulates cocaine addiction. *J. Exp. Med.* 207, 1843–1851. doi: 10.1084/jem.20100451

Schratt, G. M., Tuebing, F., Nigh, E. A., Kane, C. G., Sabatini, M. E., Kiebler, M., et al. (2006). A brain-specific microRNA regulates dendritic spine development. *Nature* 439, 283–289. doi: 10.1038/nature04367

Schwarz, D. S., Hutvágner, G., Du, T., Xu, Z., Aronin, N., and Zamore, P. D. (2003). Asymmetry in the assembly of the RNAi enzyme complex. *Cell* 115, 199–208. doi: 10.1016/S0092-8674(03)00759-1

Scott, H. L., Tamagnini, F., Narduzzo, K. E., Howarth, J. L., Lee, Y., Wong, L., et al. (2012). MicroRNA-132 regulates recognition memory and synaptic plasticity in the perirhinal cortex. *Eur. J. Neurosci.* 36, 2941–2948. doi: 10.1111/j.1460-9568.2012.08220.x

Selbach, M., Schwanhäusser, B., Thierfelder, N., Fang, Z., Khanin, R., and Rajewsky, N. (2008). Widespread changes in protein synthesis induced by microRNAs. *Nature* 455, 58–63. doi: 10.1038/nature07228

Sempere, L. F., Freemantle, S., Pitha-Rowe, I., Moss, E., Dmitrovsky, E., and Ambros, V. (2004). Expression profiling of mammalian microRNAs uncovers a subset of brain-expressed microRNAs with possible roles in murine and human neuronal differentiation. *Genome Biol.* 5, R13. doi: 10.1186/gb-2004-5-3-r13

Sengupta, J. N., Pochiraju, S., Kannampalli, P., Bruckert, M., Addya, S., Yadav, P., et al. (2013). MicroRNA-mediated $GABA_{A\alpha-1}$ receptor subunit down-regulation in adult spinal cord following neonatal cystitis-induced chronic visceral pain in rats. *Pain* 154, 59–70. doi: 10.1016/j.pain.2012.09.002

Shukla, G. C., Singh, J., and Barik, S. (2011). MicroRNAs: processing, maturation, target recognition and regulatory functions. *Mol. Cell. Pharmacol.* 3, 83–92.

Smalheiser, N. R., Lugli, G., Torvik, V. I., Mise, N., Ikeda, R., and Abe, K. (2008). Natural antisense transcripts are co-expressed with sense mRNAs in synaptoneurosomes of adult mouse forebrain. *Neurosci. Res.* 62, 236–239. doi: 10.1016/j.neures.2008.08.010

Spruston, N. (2008). Pyramidal neurons: dendritic structure and synaptic integration. *Nat. Rev. Neurosci.* 9, 206–221. doi: 10.1038/nrn2286

Standart, N., and Jackson, R. J. (2007). MicroRNAs repress translation of m7Gppp-capped target mRNAs in vitro by inhibiting initiation and promoting deadenylation. *Genes Dev.* 21, 1975–1982. doi: 10.1101/gad.1591507

Steward, O., and Levy, W. B. (1982). Preferential localization of polyribosomes under the base of dendritic spines in granule cells of the dentate gyrus. *J. Neurosci.* 2, 284–291.

Steward, O., and Schuman, E. M. (2001). Protein synthesis at synaptic sites on dendrites. *Annu. Rev. Neurosci.* 24, 299–325. doi: 10.1146/annurev.neuro.24.1.299

Sun, A. X., Crabtree, G. R., and Yoo, A. S. (2013). MicroRNAs: regulators of neuronal fate. *Curr. Opin. Cell Biol.* 25, 215–221. doi: 10.1016/j.ceb.2012.12.007

Sutton, M. A., and Schuman, E. M. (2006). Dendritic protein synthesis, synaptic plasticity, and memory. *Cell* 127, 49–58. doi: 10.1016/j.cell.2006.09.014

Taniguchi, S., Liu, H., Nakazawa, T., Yokoyama, K., Tezuka, T., and Yamamoto, T. (2003). p250GAP, a neural RhoGAP protein, is associated with and phosphorylated by Fyn. *Biochem. Biophys. Res. Commun.* 306, 151–155. doi: 10.1016/S0006-291X(03)00923-9

Thermann, R., and Hentze, M. W. (2007). *Drosophila* miR2 induces pseudo-polysomes and inhibits translation initiation. *Nature* 447, 875–878. doi: 10.1038/nature05878

Tognini, P., and Pizzorusso, T. (2012). MicroRNA212/132 family: molecular transducer of neuronal function and plasticity. *Int. J. Biochem. Cell Biol.* 44, 6–10. doi: 10.1016/j.biocel.2011.10.015

Tognini, P., Putignano, E., Coatti, A., and Pizzorusso, T. (2011). Experience-dependent expression of miR-132 regulates ocular dominance plasticity. *Nat. Neurosci.* 14, 1237–1239. doi: 10.1038/nn.2920

Torre, E. R., and Steward, O. (1992). Demonstration of local protein synthesis within dendrites using a new cell culture system that permits the isolation of living axons and dendrites from their cell bodies. *J. Neurosci.* 12, 762–772.

Trembleau, A., Morales, M., and Bloom, F. E. (1994). Aggregation of vasopressin mRNA in a subset of axonal swellings of the median eminence and posterior pituitary: light and electron microscopic evidence. *J. Neurosci.* 14, 39–53.

Valencia-Sanchez, M. A., Liu, J., Hannon, G. J., and Parker, R. (2006). Control of translation and mRNA degradation by miRNAs and siRNAs. *Genes Dev.* 20, 515–524. doi: 10.1101/gad.1399806

Vanelderen, P., Rouwette, T., Kozicz, T., Roubos, E., Van Zundert, J., Heylen, R., et al. (2010). The role of brain-derived neurotrophic factor in different animal models of neuropathic pain. *Eur. J. Pain* 14, 473.e1–e9. doi: 10.1016/j.ejpain.2009.09.006

Vo, N., Klein, M. E., Varlamova, O., Keller, D. M., Yamamoto, T., Goodman, R. H., et al. (2005). A cAMP-response element binding protein-induced microRNA regulates neuronal morphogenesis. *Proc. Natl. Acad. Sci. U.S.A.* 102, 16426–16431. doi: 10.1073/pnas.0508448102

von Schack, D., Agostino, M. J., Murray, B. S., Li, Y., Reddy, P. S., Chen, J., et al. (2011). Dynamic changes in the microRNA expression profile reveal multiple regulatory mechanisms in the spinal nerve ligation model of neuropathic pain. *PLoS ONE* 6:e17670. doi: 10.1371/journal.pone.0017670

Wakiyama, M., Takimoto, K., Ohara, O., and Yokoyama, S. (2007). Let-7 microRNA-mediated mRNA deadenylation and translational repression in a mammalian cell-free system. *Genes Dev.* 21, 1857–1862. doi: 10.1101/gad.1566707

Wayman, G. A., Davare, M., Ando, H., Fortin, D., Varlamova, O., Cheng, H. M., et al. (2008). An activity-regulated microRNA controls dendritic plasticity by down-regulating p250GAP. *Proc. Natl. Acad. Sci. U.S.A.* 105, 9093–9098. doi: 10.1073/pnas.0803072105

Wells, D. G. (2012). mRNA translation: regulating an out of soma experience. *Curr. Opin. Cell Biol.* 24, 554–557. doi: 10.1016/j.ceb.2012.06.005

Wibrand, K., Panja, D., Tiron, A., Ofte, M. L., Skaftnesmo, K. O., Lee, C. S., et al. (2010). Differential regulation of mature and precursor microRNA expression by NMDA and metabotropic glutamate receptor activation during LTP in the adult dentate gyrus in vivo. *Eur. J. Neurosci.* 31, 636–645. doi: 10.1111/j.1460-9568.2010.07112.x

Wightman, B., Ha, I., and Ruvkun, G. (1993). Posttranscriptional regulation of the heterochronic gene lin-14 by lin-4 mediates temporal pattern formation in *C. elegans*. *Cell* 75, 855–862. doi: 10.1016/0092-8674(93)90530-4

Willemen, H. L. D. M., Huo, X., Mao-Ying, Q., Zijlstra, J., Heijnen, C. J., and Kavelaars, A. (2012). MicroRNA-124 as a novel treatment for persistent hyperalgesia. *J. Neuroinflammation* 9, 143. doi: 10.1186/1742-2094-9-143

Wu, D., Raafat, M., Pak, E., Hammond, S., and Murashov, A. K. (2011). MicroRNA machinery responds to peripheral nerve lesion in an injury-regulated pattern. *Neuroscience* 190, 386–397. doi: 10.1016/j.neuroscience.2011.06.017

Yang, Y., Shu, X., Liu, D., Shang, Y., Wu, Y., Pei, L., et al. (2012). EPAC null mutation impairs learning and social interactions via aberrant regulation of miR-124 and Zif268 translation. *Neuron* 73, 774–788. doi: 10.1016/j.neuron.2012.02.003

Yekta, S., Shih, I., and Bartel, D. P. (2004). MicroRNA-directed cleavage of HOXB8 mRNA. *Science* 304, 594–596. doi: 10.1126/science.1097434

Yi, R., Qin, Y., Macara, I. G., and Cullen, B. R. (2003). Exportin-5 mediates the nuclear export of pre-microRNAs and short hairpin RNAs. *Genes Dev.* 17, 3011–3016. doi: 10.1101/gad.1158803

Yoo, A. S., Staahl, B. T., Chen, L., and Crabtree, G. R. (2009). MicroRNA-mediated switching of chromatin-remodelling complexes in neural development. *Nature* 460, 642–646. doi: 10.1038/nature08139

Zdanowicz, A., Thermann, R., Kowalska, J., Jemielity, J., Duncan, K., Preiss, T., et al. (2009). *Drosophila* miR2 primarily targets the m7GpppN cap structure for translational repression. *Mol. Cell* 35, 881–888. doi: 10.1016/j.molcel.2009.09.009

Zhao, C., Ma, H., Bossy-Wetzel, E., Lipton, S. A., Zhang, Z., and Feng, G. (2003). GC-GAP, a Rho family GTPase-activating protein that interacts with signaling adapters Gab1 and Gab2. *J. Biol. Chem.* 278, 34641–34653. doi: 10.1074/jbc.M304594200

Zhao, J., Lee, M. C., Momin, A., Cendan, C. M., Shepherd, S. T., Baker, M. D., et al. (2010). Small RNAs control sodium channel expression, nociceptor excitability, and pain thresholds. *J. Neurosci.* 30, 10860–10871. doi: 10.1523/JNEUROSCI.1980-10.2010

10

MicroRNA dysregulation in spinal cord injury: causes, consequences and therapeutics

Manuel Nieto-Diaz[1], Francisco J. Esteban[2], David Reigada[1], Teresa Muñoz-Galdeano[1], Mónica Yunta[1,3], Marcos Caballero-López[1], Rosa Navarro-Ruiz[1], Ángela del Águila[1] and Rodrigo M. Maza[1]*

[1] *Molecular Neuroprotection Group, Experimental Neurology Unit, Hospital Nacional de Parapléjicos (Servicio de Salud de Castilla-La Mancha), Toledo, Spain*
[2] *Departamento de Biología Experimental, Facultad de Ciencias Experimentales y de la Salud, Universidad de Jaén, Jaén, Spain*
[3] *Unidad de Patología Mitocondrial, Unidad Funcional de Investigación en Enfermedades Crónicas, Instituto de Salud Carlos III, Madrid, Spain*

Correspondence:
Rodrigo M. Maza, Molecular Neuroprotection Group, Experimental Neurology Unit, Hospital Nacional de Parapléjicos (Servicio de Salud de Castilla-La Mancha), Finca de la Peraleda, s/n, Toledo 45071, Spain
e-mail: rodrigom@sescam.jccm.es

Trauma to the spinal cord causes permanent disability to more than 180,000 people every year worldwide. The initial mechanical damage triggers a complex set of secondary events involving the neural, vascular, and immune systems that largely determine the functional outcome of the spinal cord injury (SCI). Cellular and biochemical mechanisms responsible for this secondary injury largely depend on activation and inactivation of specific gene programs. Recent studies indicate that microRNAs function as gene expression switches in key processes of the SCI. Microarray data from rodent contusion models reveal that SCI induces changes in the global microRNA expression patterns. Variations in microRNA abundance largely result from alterations in the expression of the cells at the damaged spinal cord. However, microRNA expression levels after SCI are also influenced by the infiltration of immune cells to the injury site and the death and migration of specific neural cells after injury. Evidences on the role of microRNAs in the SCI pathophysiology have come from different sources. Bioinformatic analysis of microarray data has been used to identify specific variations in microRNA expression underlying transcriptional changes in target genes, which are involved in key processes in the SCI. Direct evidences on the role of microRNAs in SCI are scarcer, although recent studies have identified several microRNAs (miR-21, miR-486, miR-20) involved in key mechanisms of the SCI such as cell death or astrogliosis, among others. From a clinical perspective, different evidences make clear that microRNAs can be potent therapeutic tools to manipulate cell state and molecular processes in order to enhance functional recovery. The present article reviews the actual knowledge on how injury affects microRNA expression and the meaning of these changes in the SCI pathophysiology, to finally explore the clinical potential of microRNAs in the SCI.

Keywords: spinal cord injury, microRNA, nervous system, cell death, inflammation, astrogliosis, therapeutics

INTRODUCTION

Spinal cord injury (SCI) is a dyscapacitating pathology with a global-incident rate estimated at 23 new traumatic SCI cases per million in 2007 (180,000 new cases/year; Lee et al., 2013). Recovery, even partial, from SCI was considered unachievable until the early 1980s when David and Aguayo (1981) demonstrated that spinal axons could regenerate under appropriate conditions. This seminal work initiated a burst of research aimed to understand the pathophysiology of the SCI and the development of therapeutic tools. The capacity of microRNAs to regulate cell state and function through post-transcriptionally silencing hundreds of genes are being acknowledged as an important actor in the pathophysiology of SCI. In this article, we review the known and potential roles of microRNAs in SCI and their possible therapeutic application. The article begins with an overview of the pathophysiology of SCI and the gene programs involved, followed by a general picture of microRNA biogenesis, function, and regulation, particularly in the central nervous system (CNS). Afterward, we discuss the observed global changes in microRNA expression following SCI and the role of mechanisms regulating microRNA biogenesis on SCI. We next explore the contribution of microRNA in the regulation of key processes of SCI such as inflammation, cell death, regeneration, or gliosis. The review ends with a brief perspective on the feasibility of microRNA-based therapeutics in the treatment of SCI.

AN OVERVIEW OF THE PATHOPHYSIOLOGY OF THE SPINAL CORD INJURY

The term spinal cord injury refers to the damage to the spinal cord caused by trauma or disease but also to the physiological response that develops after injury and that largely determines the functional deficits that will face the injured person. Although most SCI are traumatic, inflicted by mechanical causes due to accidents or violence, there are also a number of non-traumatic SCIs, mainly due to discopathies and tumors (Biering-Sorensen et al., 1990). The pathophysiology of the SCI is a complex intermingled set of events, responses, mechanisms, and processes, affecting the nervous, vascular, and immune systems, that develop during the months following the initial damage. Most participating cells reside in the spinal cord, but others are summoned to the injury site from the circulatory system. A brief description of the pathophysiology is provided in the following paragraphs. Detailed descriptions can be obtained in different reviews (Mautes et al., 2000; Dumont et al., 2001; Profyris et al., 2004; Liverman et al., 2005; Rowland et al., 2008; Oyinbo, 2011).

In the traumatic SCI, the mechanical trauma causes the compression, stretching, laceration, or transection of the spinal cord. The most common form of SCI is a compressive–contusive-type injury in which displaced components of the vertebral column, exert force on the cord causing both immediate traumatic injury and often sustained compression (Rowland et al., 2008). Once compression and contusion surpass structural thresholds, physical and biochemical alterations of the cells induce a cascade of systemic and local events that constitute the primary damage (Oyinbo, 2011). Local events include axon severing, membrane rupture and death of neurons, glia and endothelial cells. Surviving neurons at the injury site respond firing action potentials that shift the local levels of ions together with the ions released due to membrane shear. The resulting ion concentration reaches toxic levels that kill the nearby neurons. The barrage of action potentials also causes the release and accumulation of neurotransmitters that will cause further neuron and glial cell death by excitotoxicity. Mechanical trauma causes intraparenchymal hemorrhage (mainly in the small vessels of the gray substance) and, consequently, the disruption of the blood–spinal cord barrier together with edema and swelling at the spinal cord (Mautes et al., 2000). Vasospasm and thrombosis in the superficial vessels accompany hemorrhage causing hypoxia, ischemia, and increasing neural cell death. At a systemic level, primary damage causes a transient increase in systemic blood pressure that is followed by a prolonged hypotension (either hemorrhagic or neurogenic) causing further oxygen deprival to the spinal cord. Hypoxia – together with ion shifts inside and outside the neuron – seems to cause a temporal switch off of the spinal cord function at and below the injury site known as spinal shock.

In the minutes to months that follow the initial damage, the secondary phase of the SCI takes place. This secondary phase comprises several interrelated damage processes including vascular alterations, biochemical disturbances and cellular responses that lead to an inflammatory response and cell death that significantly expand the area of damage. Vascular alterations resulting from hemorrhage and ischemia are central constituents of the secondary injury cascade. Reduced perfusion of the spinal cord due to vasospasm and hypotension is followed by a period of reperfusion, which increases the production of oxygen- and nitrogen-derived free radicals [superoxide, hydroxyl radicals, nitric oxide (NO), peroxynitrite] already being produced during the period of ischemia (Dumont et al., 2001). All these species contribute to oxidative stress and exacerbates damage and cell death. Alterations in the vascular system also include the disruption of the blood–spinal cord barrier that extends far beyond the injury site for days and even weeks after injury. Release of cytokines [interleukin (IL)-1β, tumor necrosis factor-α (TNF-α)], matrix metalloproteinases, reactive oxygen species (ROS), etc., contribute to enhance vascular permeability (Mautes et al., 2000; Donnelly and Popovich, 2008) and – together with upregulation of cell adhesion molecules (CAMs and selectins) by endothelial cells (Mautes et al., 2000; Profyris et al., 2004; Donnelly and Popovich, 2008) – participate in the recruitment and infiltration of immune cells to the injured spinal cord.

Immune cells develop a key role in the pathophysiology of SCI. Neutrophils arrive to the injury site in the first hours after injury [peaking at 1 day post-injury (dpi) in rats and 1–3 dpi in humans, see Fleming et al., 2006] and disappear during the first week, although some evidences indicate a continued presence for long times (180 dpi in rats, according to Beck et al., 2010). Neutrophils remove debris, but mainly release assortments of proteins, including proteolytic and oxidative enzymes that "sterilize" the area but also contribute to extend tissue damage (Taoka et al., 1997). Neutrophils also release signaling proteins that attract macrophages. Macrophages resulting from the activation of spinal cord microglia or from blood monocytes infiltrate the injury in the first days after the injury, presenting a peak during the first week and persisting for months (Fleming et al., 2006). Microglial activation is triggered early after injury and induces a morphological and functional change in the phenotype of this cell, from a resting, ramified phenotype to a phagocytosis-capable, "macrophage-like" phenotype (Byrnes et al., 2006). Macrophages remove debris and dead cells, present antigens, and release pro-inflammatory and protective cytokines, ROS, NO, and proteases (Fleming et al., 2006). T lymphocytes enter the injured spinal cord mainly 1 week after injury. T cells are responsible for cell-mediated adaptive immunity, although their role in SCI remains controversial (Fleming et al., 2006). In rat models, it seems that immune cells tend to maintain or reduce their presence after this first burst of immune response following SCI. However, a recent study in rats demonstrates that immune cells present a time-dependent multiphasic response, with a late phase that mainly involves a peak of macrophages at 60 dpi (Beck et al., 2010). Contrary to the mixed beneficial and detrimental effects on the immune response in the initial phase, this late phase seems to be mainly beneficial and its blocking causes further functional deficits (Beck et al., 2010).

All previous events have strong effects on neural cells. Necrotic cell death initiated by the mechanical trauma spreads during the secondary phase due to excitotoxicity and the accumulation of free radicals (ROS and RNS) released by immune cells or during reperfusion. Free radicals cause lipid peroxidation as well as oxidative and nitrative damage to lipids, proteins, and nucleic acids, inducing the lysis of the cell membrane, altering the cytoskeleton and the organelles, and ultimately causing the death of neural cells (Oyinbo, 2011). Apoptosis and other forms of programed cell death are also important actors in secondary damage after SCI. Programed cell death seems to occur in at least two phases: an initial phase, in which apoptosis accompanies necrosis and a later phase, which is predominantly confined to white matter and that affects oligodendrocytes and microglia (Profyris et al., 2004). Calcium influx and possibly signaling through Fas/CD95 pathway are among the triggers proposed for programed cell death although other mechanisms may be also acting, including lost of trophic support (Liverman et al., 2005; Rowland et al., 2008).

Apoptosis of oligodendrocytes results in extended demyelination, the loss of the oligodendrocyte myelin sheath that insulate nerve axons and permit effective nervous signal conduction. As a consequence, axons crossing the injured segment/s but deprived from myelin sheath and experiencing alterations in the ion channels become unable to transmit signals to the brain and the body, even though they remain intact. Axotomy (axon sectioning) is also a major factor in SCI. Depending on aspects such as distance of axotomy to cell body, trophic support or neuronal type, the fate of axotomized neurons will differ strongly. A significant proportion of neurons, being severed close to the cell body or lacking enough tropic support, die after axotomy. Others retract the severed axon and develop a terminal retraction bulb. Conversely, some surviving neurons develop a regenerating response. These neurons experience hypertrophy of the cell body due to the increased synthesis of proteins that will be used in an attempt to regenerate the severed axon. Within this pro-regenerative response, intact neurons can also develop sprouts (collateral axonal branches) that may rewire unconnected targets (sometimes with undesired side effects). However, axon growth is strongly if not completely inhibited due to several inhibitors present at the injured spinal cord. Much of this inhibition is due to molecules associated to the oligodendrocyte myelin, such as NOGO, and other are consequence of the changes experienced by the astrocytes following injury. Astrocyte reactivity after SCI involves cellular changes characterized by an initial hypertrophic and a late hyperplasic response (Fawcett and Asher, 1999; Sahni et al., 2010). During the hypertrophic response, reactive astrocytes present a characteristic enlarged somata with thickened processes and upregulation of intermediate filament proteins, such as glial fibrillary acidic protein (GFAP) and vimentin (Pekny and Pekna, 2004). This initial hypertrophic response protects neural cells by up-taking the potentially excitotoxic glutamate, producing oxidative stress scavengers and repairing the blood–spinal cord barrier (Faulkner et al., 2004; Sofroniew, 2005). In the following hyperplastic phase during the subacute and chronic phases of the SCI, newly proliferated astrocytes with thinner processes forms a dense scar in the damaged area that inhibits of axon regeneration (Fawcett and Asher, 1999; Silver and Miller, 2004).

In the months and years that follow the damage, the SCI becomes chronic. Cell death, scarring, gliosis, and other local alterations of the tissue lead to the formation of cavities filled of fluid and surrounded by glial scar that can extend for several segments above and below the injury site (Liverman et al., 2005). Myelin loss and alterations in the functioning of the ion channels can lead to changes in the surviving neurons and dependent networks leading to chronic neuropathic pain and/or spasticity.

GENE EXPRESSION CHANGES AFTER SPINAL CORD INJURY

Most cell functions, responses, and phenotypic changes depend on the activation and/or suppression of a large number of transcriptional pathways (Di Giovanni et al., 2003). Microarray analyses in SCI models have identified gene expression changes that, to some extent, can be observed across different studies and even across different strains or species (Di Giovanni et al., 2003; Velardo et al., 2004). Prominent expression changes in the spinal cord following injury comprise clustered expression changes in genes associated to:

TRANSCRIPTION AND STRESS RESPONSE

Clusters including factors such as *NF-κB* (nuclear factor kappa-light-chain-enhancer of activated B cells), *c-fos*, *HSP-70* (70 kD heat shock protein) become upregulated early after injury and continue for at least 24 h (Song et al., 2001). Activation of transcription factors such as NF-κB or interferon regulatory factor (IRF)-1 mediates the increased expression of pro-inflammatory genes and modulates pivotal processes such as apoptosis or regeneration (Song et al., 2001). On the other hand, there is an early increase in chaperone expression (*HSP-70*) together with metallothioneins 1 and 2 (Aimone et al., 2004) that may protect cells from protein damage or oxidative stress. Further anti-oxidative stress genes become upregulated at much later times, including superoxide dismutases (SODs) 1 and 2, *catalase*, and *glutathione peroxidase* (GPX; Aimone et al., 2004).

INFLAMMATORY RESPONSE

Upregulation of pro-inflammatory genes, including cyclooxygenase (COX)-2, interleukins *IL-1β* and *IL-6*, TNF-α, is observed early after injury and persists during the first weeks to go back to normal levels at 14 days (Carmel et al., 2001; Song et al., 2001; Di Giovanni et al., 2003; Zhang et al., 2004). Chemokines involved in immune cell attraction [monocyte chemotactic protein (MCP)-1, macrophage inflammatory protein (MIP)-1β] and adhesion molecules participating in cell infiltration (integrins, intercellular and vascular CAMs, cadherins, and selectins) are also upregulated during the first hours after injury (Aimone et al., 2004). Changes in the expression of inflammatory genes take place in different spinal cord cells but has been particularly studied in microglia. According to a profiling study developed by Byrnes et al. (2006), activated microglia first express (peak at 4–24 h) pro-inflammatory molecules, including IL-1β, IL-6, CCL2 [chemokine (C–C motif) ligand 2]/MCP-1, CXCL2 [chemokine (C–X–C motif) ligand 2]/M1P2α, involved in the recruitment of immune cells to the damaged area. A second pulse of change in microglial gene expression occurs later (3–7 dpi in rats) and involves genes coding for cytochrome b-245 light chain protein (*CYBa*), cathepsin Y, Galectin-3, microglial response factor (MRF)-1, P38, cyclin D1, caspase 1, and leukocyte surface antigen CD53/OX44, that participate in the regulation of the immune response, phagocytosis, production of ROS, proliferation, and cell death. Other immune response genes related to phagocytosis including the classical complement pathway and the FC receptors show a persistent upregulation after injury (Aimone et al., 2004).

NEURON-ASSOCIATED GENES

A large cluster of genes coding for proteins involved in the potassium, calcium, and sodium pumps and channels as well as in synapsis, cell excitability, and neurotransmission show a significant decrease during the first week (Carmel et al., 2001; Velardo et al., 2004; De Biase et al., 2005; Wu et al., 2005). This decrease can reflect changes in the gene profile of the neurons but it may also reflect the advance of neuronal cell death that takes place after injury (Carmel et al., 2001; De Biase et al., 2005). Attempts of axonal regeneration in the weeks following injury are also accompanied by expression changes in a large group of genes that includes the overexpression of several plasticity and regeneration-associated proteins (*Ninjurin, Coronin 1b, Rab13, Growth Associated Protein-43, Neuritin, Ankyrin, Myelin oligodendrocyte glycoprotein*, and *cAMP*-related genes; Carmel et al., 2001; Song et al., 2001; Di Giovanni et al., 2003, 2005b).

CELL CYCLE AND CELL DEATH

Changes in the expression of cell cycle genes has been detected 24 h after injury, including upregulation of *c-myc, pcdna, gadd45a*, and cyclins (Di Giovanni et al., 2003). Activation of cell cycle genes may induce apoptosis in post-mitotic cells and, thus underlie post-SCI apoptosis of neurons. They may also be involved in astrocytic proliferation during the glial scar formation (Di Giovanni et al., 2003). Pro-apoptotic and anti-apoptotic genes also show significant expression changes, including upregulation of caspase-3, *Bax, Bak-1* in the first week after SCI and the later upregulation of protective *PI3K* and *Stat3* and downregulation of pro-apoptotic *GSK-3* (Carmel et al., 2001; Aimone et al., 2004). In addition, it has been observed the upregulation at 24 h of genes coding for different growth factors [transforming growth factor-β (TGF-β), platelet-derived growth factor, vascular endothelial growth factor] and anti-apoptotic proteins (survival of motor neurons proteins), which may contribute to prevent neural cell death (Song et al., 2001).

VASCULAR SYSTEM REGULATION AND ANGIOGENESIS

Hemorrhage and other early vascular events are reflected in the expression profile. Blood coagulation genes – platelet factor 4 (CXCL4), coagulation factors VIII, protein C, etc., – appear overexpressed in the first 24 h after injury and some remain for several weeks (Chamankhah et al., 2013). Genes such as angiopoietin are increased in the injury area in the week that follows the damage (Aimone et al., 2004). Other dysregulated genes related to vascular events include HIG (hypoxia-induced gene), which is downregulated late after injury (Aimone et al., 2004).

CHANGES IN GLIAL CELLS

Although less explored in global profile studies, there are important changes in gene expression in the glial cells related to astrocyte reactivity and the formation of the glial scar, as well as to the proliferation and remyelination attempts of oligodendrocytes. Among the best-characterized genes related to astrocyte reactivity and glial scar formation are those coding for GFAP, vimentin, and nestin, intermediate filaments highly overexpressed in reactive astrocytes. These genes are markedly upregulated during the first week after injury (Carmel et al., 2001; Wu et al., 2005). On the other hand, oligodendrocyte profiles are characterized by a decrease in cell specific genes due to the advance of oligodendrocyte death during the first weeks followed by an increase in proliferation and myelination genes (Wu et al., 2005).

MicroRNA BIOGENESIS, FUNCTION, AND REGULATION

As we have shown in the previous sections, SCI causes profound cellular changes that result from dysregulation of signaling pathways and structural proteins. Alteration of gene expression following SCI is likely accompanied by the post-transcriptional regulation of these modified gene networks. Among the known post-transcriptional regulators, microRNAs have recently attracted much attention due to their ability to inhibit mRNA translation.

MicroRNAs were first identified in *C. elegans* in 1993 (Lee et al., 1993). A small non-coding RNA (lin-4) was shown to regulate translation of lin-14 through RNA–RNA interaction. MicroRNAs constitute an abundant class of highly conserved small non-coding RNA molecules composed of 20–24 nucleotides in length, that post-transcriptional regulate gene expression. More than 2500 mature forms of microRNA sequences have been identified in humans (miRBase; Kozomara and Griffiths-Jones, 2011). MicroRNAs are transcribed from genomic DNA by RNA polymerase II or III in the form of large primary transcripts (pri-miRNAs) with functional secondary structures of stem-loop hairpins. The stem-loops structures are recognized and cleaved by the complex formed by the RNase III Drosha and the RNA-binding protein DGCR8, which leads to liberation of a precursor microRNA (pre-miRNA). Once processed, exportin 5 transports the pre-miRNAs from the nucleus to the cytosol, where an enzymatic complex containing Dicer process them to yield the 20- to 25-nucleotide duplex mature miRNAs. One strand (passenger) of the duplex is degraded and the other strand (guide) is integrated into a RNA-induced silencing complex (RISC), which facilitates the binding of the microRNAs to their target mRNA.

The predominant role of microRNAs in RISCs is to regulate post-transcriptional the expression of their target genes by translational repression, mRNA cleavage, or mRNA decay. The employed mechanism depends on the degree of complementarity between the microRNAs and their target mRNAs. When microRNAs perfectly or near-perfectly pairs the targeted mRNAs, as occurs in plants, cleavage of the mRNA takes place. On the contrary, when microRNAs imperfectly pair to their target mRNAs, as usually occurs in animals, translational repression or decay (due to microRNA-driven deadenylation) become the mechanisms mediating gene regulation. In animals, microRNAs have been proposed to downregulate gene expression mostly through the translational repression (Krichevsky, 2007), although a recent study showed that destabilization (and degradation) of target mRNAs is the major mechanism of miRNA gene repression in mammals (Guo et al., 2010).

Since microRNAs do not require perfect complementarity for target recognition in animals, a single microRNA can regulate multiple, even hundreds mRNAs (Lim et al., 2005; Baek et al., 2008; Selbach et al., 2008). At the same time, each mRNA can be regulated by many microRNAs (Krek et al., 2005; Krichevsky, 2007) and a given microRNA may have multiple binding sites in the same mRNA, thereby enhancing its overall effect (Bhalala et al., 2013). Computational predictions suggest that the more than 2000 known human microRNAs are able to repress the expression of at least a 20–30% of all protein-coding genes (Krichevsky, 2007) and up to the 60% according to Friedman et al. (2009) and Sayed and Abdellatif (2011). Besides a single miRNA can tune protein synthesis from thousands of genes, quantitative proteomics studies have found that the magnitude of the change is small under physiological conditions (less than fourfold; Guo et al., 2010). In fact, blocking microRNA biogenesis through DICER inhibition has modest effects on cell differentiation and organism patterning, although opposite results have also been reported (Kosik, 2010).

MicroRNAs are common components of regulatory pathways, and in many cases constitute molecular on–off switches in establishing cell fate and identity both under physiological and pathological conditions. The power of this regulatory mechanism lies in the unique ability of microRNAs to guide processes and cellular functions through precise titration of gene dosage, and the ability of a single microRNA to control the levels of a large cohort of gene products. Because microRNAs target multiple mRNAs, they can exert distributed control over broad target fields of functionally related mRNAs as opposed to focusing their control on a small number of genes in a "final common pathway." The action of an individual microRNA can lead to a cumulative reduction in expression of multiple components of one specific functional network, and several microRNAs may cooperatively target various mRNAs whose protein products are part of the same molecular pathway (Krek et al., 2005; Krol et al., 2010; Sluijter, 2013). MicroRNAs are often physically clustered in the genome, and these sets of microRNAs may target mRNAs with related biological functions at short distances in their protein–protein interaction map (Kim et al., 2009). Coordinated microRNA targeting of closely connected genes seems to be prevalent across pathways (Tsang et al., 2010). Thus, microRNAs provide broad and robust transcriptional regulation that can be governed either by individual microRNAs or by the combined action of multiple microRNAs.

MicroRNA networks are often specialized for specific cell types and there is a strong correlation between cell identity and patterns of microRNA expression (Kosik, 2010). The anticorrelated expression of microRNAs and their target mRNAs in developmental transitions and the mutually exclusive expression of target genes and microRNAs in neighboring tissues argues that microRNAs confer accuracy to developmental gene expression programs, thus ensuring tissue identity and supporting cell-lineage decisions, and reflect the basic role of miRNAs in establishing cell identity during development (Ebert and Sharp, 2012). MicroRNAs also serve as a buffer to assist cells in coping with environmental contingencies (Kosik, 2010). As markers of cell identity, miRNAs encode a representation of multiple cell states that all correspond to a single identity. That is, many different states comprise a single identity because cells must retain their identities in the face of both environmental changes and internal noise that can result in large variations in molecular composition. MicroRNAs are good candidates for setting boundary conditions upon coding transcripts to restrict protein levels within a range of values that maintain cell identity in the face of homeostatic compensatory changes. The RISC allows both the constitutive maintenance of cell identity by silencing mRNAs that are not part of the specialized cell's repertoire as well as the holding of mRNAs of an alternative identity in reserve (Lim et al., 2005). The environment that cells face is many times more complex than the biological adaptations available within the genome. Among the adaptive responses of cells to an environmental contingency is the up- or downregulation of proteins. The properties of miRNAs to adjust protein levels, their dispensability under basal conditions, their conservation, as well as the ease with which new miRNAs appear over evolutionary time all suggest that they are suited for environmental contingencies (Kosik, 2010). Wu et al. (2009) have proposed that miRNAs keep the system close to the mean and set expression boundaries of transcription factors, which are otherwise noisy.

MicroRNA IN THE NORMAL AND PATHOLOGICAL CENTRAL NERVOUS SYSTEM

MicroRNAs are highly expressed in the mammalian CNS, including the spinal cord (Miska et al., 2004; Kosik, 2006; Krichevsky, 2007; Bak et al., 2008). Their expression in the spinal cord seems to be specific and preserved through vertebrate evolution (Yunta et al., 2012). Moreover, experimental data reveal that some miRNAs are cell-type specific, such as miR-124 and miR-128, which are preferentially expressed in neurons, or miR-23 or miR-219, which are restricted to astrocytes and oligodendrocytes, respectively (Sempere et al., 2004; Smirnova et al., 2005; Lau et al., 2008). MicroRNAs serve essential roles in virtually every aspect of CNS function, including neurogenesis, neural development, and cellular responses leading to changes in synaptic plasticity (Krichevsky et al., 2003; Miska et al., 2004; Sempere et al., 2004; Stefani and Slack, 2008; Gangaraju and Lin, 2009; Li and Jin, 2010; Smith et al., 2010; Cochella and Hobert, 2012; Goldie and Cairns, 2012). For example, experimental overexpression or inhibition of miR-124 have demonstrated its key role in neuronal differentiation (Krichevsky et al., 2006; Makeyev et al., 2007; Visvanathan et al., 2007), whereas let-7b regulates neural stem cell proliferation and differentiation by targeting the stem cell regulator TLX and the cell cycle regulator cyclin D1 (Zhao et al., 2010a). MicroRNAs are also involved in the specification of glia. They have been shown to be critical regulators of oligodendrocyte differentiation and myelination in the vertebrate CNS, in particular miR-219 and miR-338 (Zhao et al., 2010b).

In addition to their role in the development and the functioning in the normal CNS, numerous evidences indicate that microRNA dysregulation is implicated in a wide range of neurological diseases. Several studies indicate that microRNA dysregulation can be associated to neurodegeneration, as in Alzheimer's disease where the downregulation of the miR-29 cluster has been proposed to contribute to increase BACE1 and amyloid-beta levels and thus to the development of the disease (see Saugstad, 2010). The role of microRNAs in neurodegeneration extends to other pathologies, such as Huntington and Parkinson diseases, or even to prion diseases (Saugstad, 2010). The evidences also suggest that microRNAs participate in psychiatric disorders, such as Schizophrenia, Tourette's syndrome, and bipolar disorder, as well as in developmental disorders, such as the Rett and fragile X syndromes (Kosik, 2006; Meza-Sosa et al., 2012). MicroRNAs also participate in the profound cellular changes that occur in the damaged CNS, where they play an active role in the regulation of typical features of CNS injuries, such as inflammation, apoptosis, cell proliferation, and differentiation (see this review for SCI or Bhalala et al., 2013 for a more general approach).

GLOBAL CHANGES IN microRNA EXPRESSION AND REGULATION OF microRNA BIOGENESIS IN SPINAL CORD INJURY

Several studies have analyzed microRNA expression and function in SCI (34 published paper in August, 2013 according to PubMed).

Seven of these studies include global analyses of microRNA expression based on microarrays. As shown in **Table 1**, the results from these studies strongly vary in the resulting overall patterns, both in the number (from as few as 10 significant expression changes to more than 250) and profile of changing microRNAs. Much of this variability can be ascribed to differences in SCI model, from ischemia-reperfusion to transection, compression, or contusion, to differences in the sampling time after injury, from 4 h to 14 days after injury, or to differences in the animal model (rats and mice of different strains). Besides, some results from comparable injury models and times still show strong differences. Technical differences among platforms, laboratories, sampling and analytical procedures, etc., may account for variability in microarray data (Git et al., 2010; Callari et al., 2012; Saugstad, 2013). In agreement, we have observed that the number of significant changes identified at 7 dpi vary from 257 to 2 depending on whether parametric (Student's *t*-test) or non-parametric (rank product test) tests are used (Yunta et al., 2012). However, discrepancies may also reveal variability in microRNA expression associated to differences in injury features. Injury severity is one of such factors. It is well known that severity determines several aspects of the SCI pathophysiology such as the inflammatory response or the nerve fiber preservation/destruction (Fehlings and Tator, 1995; Yang et al., 2005). In agreement, the expression of specific microRNAs (miR-129-2 and miR-146a) has been observed to correlate with functional score after injury, an accepted proximate to SCI severity (Strickland et al., 2011). Additional support for a severity effect on transcription comes from mRNA data. De Biase et al. (2005) observed strong differences in gene expression in contusive injuries of different severities, with a dramatic increase in

Table 1 | Global analyses of microRNA expression after SCI.

Study	SCI model	miRNA expression changes
Liu et al. (2009)	Animal: Sprague Dawley rats	4 hpo: 18 down, 23 up
	Contusion, NYU impactor (10 g, 12.5 mm)	1 dpo: 30 down, 27 up
	Level: T10	7 dpo: 30 down, 30 up
	Sampling: 4 h, 1 and 7 days	
Nakanishi et al. (2010)	Animal: C57BL/6 mice	12 hpo: 5 down, 5 up
	Compression, forceps (10 s).	
	Level: T11–T12	
	Sampling: 12 h	
Strickland et al. (2011)	Animal: Sprague Dawley rats	4 and 14 dpo: 32 down, 4 up
	Contusion, MASCIS impactor (10 g, 12.5 mm)	
	Level: T12–T13	
	Sampling: 4 and 14 days	
Jee et al. (2012a,b), Im et al. (2012)	Animal: ICR mice	265 exp. changes
	Transection	
	Level: T9–T10	
	Sampling: ?	
Yunta et al. (2012)	Animal: Wistar rats	1 dpo: 0 down, 0 up
	IH spinal cord impactor (200 kdynes)	3 dpo: 46 down, 5 up
	Level: T8	7 dpo: 192 down, 11 up
	Sampling: 1, 3, and 7 days	
Hu et al. (2013b)	Animal: Sprague Dawley rats	1 dpo: 5 down, 9 up
	Contusion, mod. Allen Weight Drop (8 g, 40 mm)	3 dpo: 5 down, 3 up
	Level: T10	
	Sampling: 1 and 3 days	
Hu et al. (2013a)	Animals: Rats	2 dpo: 10 down, 38 up
	Ischemic-Reperfusion	
	Level: lumbo-sacral segments	
	Sampling: 2 days	

Summary of models and results employed in published microarray analyses of miRNA expression in spinal cord injury. In all cases, data from injured animals was compared to data from Sham injured animals. Information from several studies was very limited and we would encourage authors to submit microarray data to public repositories as part of the process of publication, as suggested by the Microarray Gene Expression Data Society (http://www.mged.org). T, thoracic level; hpo, hours post-operation; dpo, days post-operation; up and down indicate up- and down-regulated microRNAs.

the number of genes with altered expression in moderate injuries relative to mild and severe ones. Thus, injury severity could be an important and interesting source of variation of microRNA expression that would merit further studies. Other injury features contribute to condition the microRNA profile of the spinal cord. Recently, Ziu et al. (2013) have compared the expression of six microRNAs after SCI with variable compression times showing that the duration of compression significantly alter the expression of different microRNAs.

Besides general variability in the microRNA expression patterns, Strickland et al. (2011) and our group (Yunta et al., 2012) observed a global downregulation of miRNA expression after a moderate contusive injury. Interestingly, studies by De Biase et al. (2005) and Byrnes et al. (2006) showed that moderate contusive injuries present a significant bias toward gene upregulation with a maximum at 7 days after injury, that contrast with the more balanced numbers of up- and downregulated genes observed in severe and mild injuries. Thus, the increase in the number of upregulated mRNA correlates with the general decrease of miRNA expression, which becomes particularly evident 1 week after injury (Yunta et al., 2012). Bioinformatic analyses based on miRNA target prediction data allowed us to show that almost one-third of the upregulated mRNAs in De Biase et al.'s (2005) study where targets of the downregulated microRNAs (Yunta et al., 2012). It is tempting to hypothesize that a generalized decrease in miRNA abundance reduces post-transcriptional regulation and thus causes an increase in mRNA levels after moderate SCI. Two questions immediately arise: why in moderate injuries? and, how do injuries regulate microRNA expression or biogenesis? Although we have no information to approach the first question, some is available to explore the effects of injuries on microRNA biogenesis. MicroRNA biogenesis can be regulated at different stages. The first layer governing miRNA abundance is the regulation of pri-miRNA transcription by binding of transcription factors (Treiber et al., 2012). C-Myc is one of such transcription factors, which is known to directly upregulate miR-17-92 cluster and, at the same time, to cause a widespread repression of microRNA expression (Chang et al., 2008). Interestingly, this transcription factor is significantly overexpressed at 4 and 24 h following a SCI (Di Giovanni et al., 2003). In agreement, the levels of several microRNAs repressed by c-Myc in Chang et al. (2008) experiments – miR-26a, miR-26b, miR-29a-c, miR-34a, miR-146a, miR-30a-e, let-7a, let-7d, let-7g, miR-99b, and miR-125 – become significantly decreased after SCI in our analysis whereas two members of the miR-17-92 cluster (miR-20a and miR-17) appear upregulated (Yunta et al., 2012). In addition to transcriptional regulation, processing of the pri- and pre-miRNA transcripts can be also regulated (Treiber et al., 2012). Blockage or downregulation of key proteins in the biogenesis pathway such Dicer, Drosha, DGCR8, or Exportin 5 leads to a reduction in the abundance of mature microRNAs and a accumulation of pri- and pre-microRNAs (Lee et al., 2008). Examples of this regulatory pathway are common in cancer (Lu et al., 2005) but also in other processes, such as liver regeneration after damage (Shu et al., 2011). Little is known about the variation in the expression and function of the microRNA biogenic machinery after SCI, however, Jee et al. (2012a) have recently described a downregulation of Dicer 7 days after contusive spinal cord. Dicer downregulation is consistent with the observed general depletion in miRNA abundance observed by Strickland et al. (2011) and Yunta et al. (2012). Additionally, growth factors such as bone morphogenetic proteins (BMPs) and TGF-β – overexpressed after SCI (McTigue et al., 2000; Xiao et al., 2010) – can contribute to regulate the microRNA biogenesis through activation of Smad proteins, which bind to pri-miRNA and enhance their Drosha-mediated processing to pre-miRNA (Davis et al., 2010). To what extent all these mechanisms contribute to the different patters of microRNA expression following SCI remains to be elucidated.

Microarray data allows identifying consistent changes in microRNA abundance following SCI. Considering those changes observed in at least two different studies, 36 microRNAs show consistent patterns of change (see **Table 2**). These changes illustrate the complexity of interpreting the microRNA expression changes from microarray data in the SCI due to the cellular heterogeneity of the spinal cord and the multiple changes that take place after injury. Expression changes in heterogeneous samples such as the spinal cord actually correspond to the weighted mean of the transcription programs of all cell types present in the sample (Lu et al., 2003). Thus, the observed expression changes may result either from changes in gene expression within a given cell type or to changes in the relative abundance of the expressing cell types, which severely constraints the conclusion that can be derived from the expression data (Wang et al., 2006; Gosink et al., 2007). In fact, heterogeneity could be a major reason why many gene expression analyses fail a rigorous validation (Clarke et al., 2010). After injury, the spinal cord experiences changes in the relative proportions of different cell types due to the necrotic and apoptotic death of neurons and oligodendrocytes (Grossman et al., 2001; Rowland et al., 2008) and the infiltration of immune cells (Grossman et al., 2001; Profyris et al., 2004). The death of specific cell types explains the downregulation of microRNAs associated with neurons, such as miR-124 and oligodendrocytes, miR-219 (Smirnova et al., 2005; Lau et al., 2008). Both microRNA show a sustained decrease in their levels that follows the progression of cell death in these neural cells. Interestingly, Liu et al. (2009) observed an increase in miR-124 abundance during the first 4 h. A similar upregulation was previously described in brain ischemia-reperfusion by Jeyaseelan et al. (2008), which proposed that such increase "indicates that injured brain cells could be actively involved in regeneration during the first 24 h of reperfusion." In parallel, the infiltration of immune and vascular cells explains the overexpression of specific microRNAs. The best characterized is miR-223, a neutrophil microRNA (Lindsay, 2008; Sonkoly and Pivarcsi, 2009; Izumi et al., 2011), whose upregulation reflects the infiltration of these immune cells during the acute phase of the spinal cord (Izumi et al., 2011; Yunta et al., 2012). Similarly, miR-451 – a red blood cell marker (Merkerova et al., 2008) – appears clearly increased in the first hours after injury to be later repressed or returned to control condition probably reflects the entrance of erythrocytes in the damaged area during the acute phase and their clearance later on.

MicroRNAs IN THE REGULATION OF INFLAMMATION FOLLOWING SCI

Spinal cord injury activates an inflammatory response that is initiated by the alteration of the blood–spinal cord barrier, followed by

Table 2 | Prominent changes in microRNA expression in murine models of spinal cord injury.

MicroRNA	Time after injury						
	4 h	**12 h**	**1 days**	**3 days**	**4 days**	**7 days**	**14 days**
miR-1		Up[2]	Up[1]	Down[4]	Down[3]	Up[1]/Down[4]	Down[3]
miR-100	Up[1]		Down[1]			Down[1,4]	
miR-103	Up[1]		Down[1]			Down[1,4]	
miR-107	Up[1]		Down[1]			Down[1,4]	
miR-124	Up[1]	Down[2]	Down[1]	Down[4]	Down[3]	Down[1,4]	Down[3]
miR-125b-3p			Down[5]			Down[4]	
miR-126			Down[5]	Down[5]		Down[4]	
miR-127	Up[1]		Down[1]	Down[4]		Down[1,4]	
miR-128	Up[1]		Down[1]	Down[4]		Down[1,4]	
miR-129-1					Down[3]		Down[3]
miR-129-2					Down[3]		Down[3]
miR-129-3p		Down[2]				Down[4]	
miR-129*	Down[1]		Down[1]			Down[1,4]	
miR-133a	Up[1]	Up[2]	Down[1]	Down[4]		Down[1,4]	
miR-133b	Up[1]	Up[2]	Down[1]	Down[4]		Down[1,4]	
miR-138	Down[1]		Down[1]	Down[4]		Down[1,4]	
miR-146a			Up[1]			Up[1,4]	
miR-17			Up[1]	Up[4]		Up[1]	
miR-181a	Up[1]		Down[1]			Down[1,4]	
miR-21			Up[1]	Up[4,5]	Up[3]	Up[1,4]	Down[3]
miR-219-2-3p	Down[1]		Down[1]			Down[1,4]	
miR-219-5p	Down[1]		Down[1]			Down[1,4]	
miR-223	Up[1]	Up[2]	Up[1,4]	Up[4]	Up[3]	Up[1,4]	Up[3]
miR-30b-5p	Down[1]		Down[1]			Down[1,4]	
miR-30c	Down[1]		Down[1]			Down[1,4]	
miR-30d	Down[1]		Down[1]			Down[1,4]	
miR-338*	Down[1]		Down[1]			Down[1,4]	
miR-342		Down[2]				Down[4]	
miR-34a	Down[1]		Down[1]	Down[4]		Down[1,4]	
miR-379*	Down[1]		Down[1]	Down[4]		Down[1,4]	
miR-451	Up[1]	Up[2]	Down[1]/Up vs 7 dpo[4]			Down[1]	
miR-487b	Up[1]		Down[1]			Down[1,4]	
miR-495	Down[1]	Down[2]	Down[1]	Down[4]		Down[1,4]	
miR-708			Down[5]	Down[4]		Down[4]	
miR-99a	Up[1]		Down[1]	Down[5]		Down[1,4]	
miR-let-7b			Down[5]	Down[5]		Down[4]	

The table details the changes in microRNA expression following spinal cord injury of dysregulated microRNAs according to, at least, two different studies. Data derived from the following microarray analyses: [1] Liu et al. (2009); [2] Nakanishi et al. (2010); [3] Strickland et al. (2011); [4] Yunta et al. (2012); [5] Hu et al. (2013a,b). Unless stated, Up and Down correspond to upregulated and downregulated respect to Sham control individuals respectively.

the sequential infiltration of peripheral immune cells, the activation of the microglia and the induction of inflammatory signaling pathways. MicroRNAs play important roles in controlling signaling pathways and the dynamics of the immune response during pathogenic immunological conditions (Lindsay, 2008; Sonkoly and Pivarcsi, 2009; Chen et al., 2013). Following SCI, several microRNAs undergo expression changes that can be related to the immune response, either associated with the invading immune cells or participating in the modulation of inflammatory pathways (**Figure 1**).

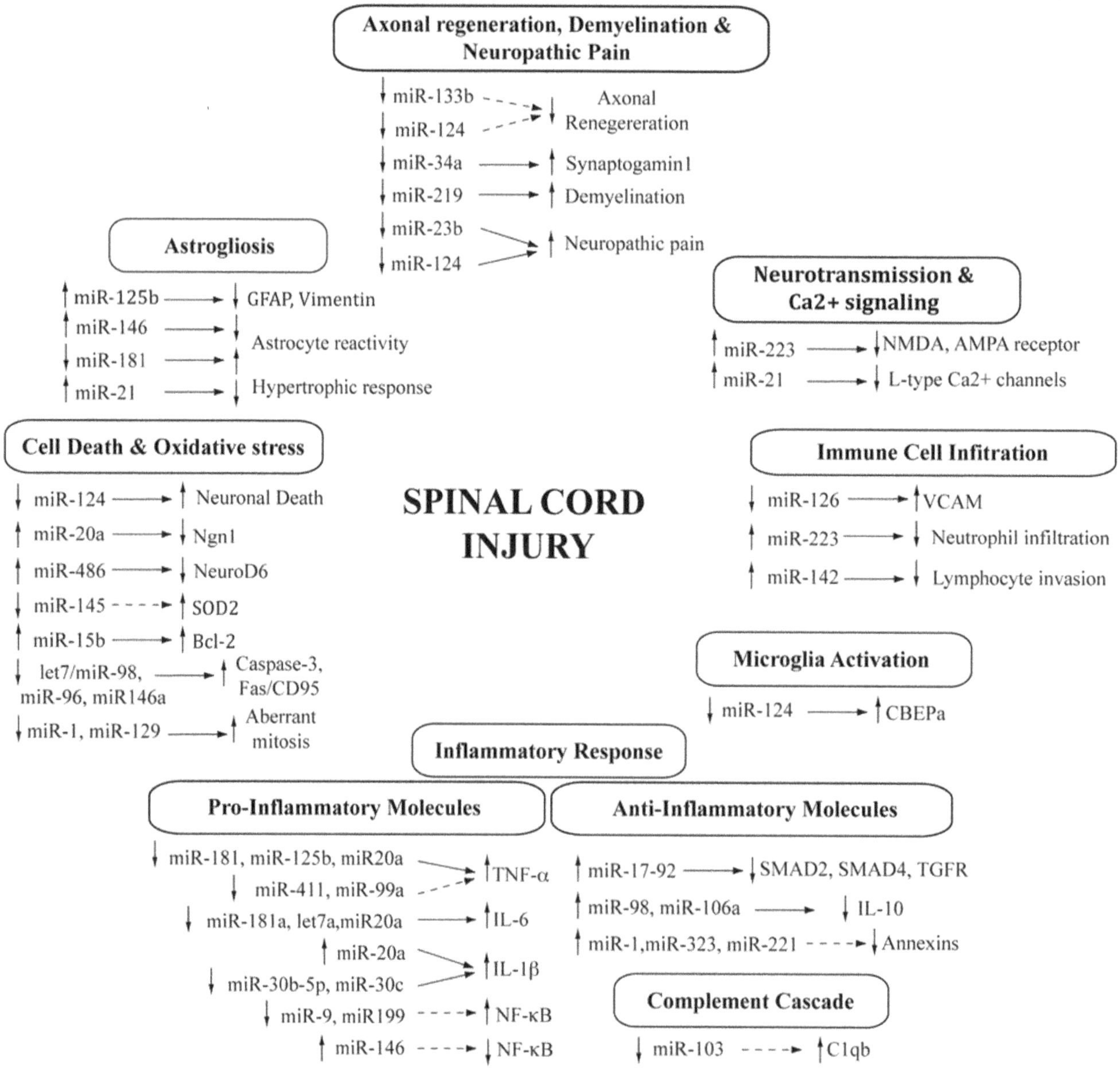

FIGURE 1 | MicroRNAs in the spinal cord injury pathophysiology. Diagram showing the cascade of processes triggered after SCI and the contribution of differentially expressed microRNAs. Changes in microRNA expression is indicated either as increased (up arrow) or decreased (down arrow) after SCI. Target genes are also shown (confirmed, direct regulation are indicated with a solid arrow, whereas those indirect or predicted are represented with a dashed arrow).

Immediately after the injury, the blood–spinal cord barrier becomes disturbed and the blood immune cells infiltrate the damaged area (Profyris et al., 2004; Jones et al., 2005). Early increases in the expression of CAMs play a key role in the process of immune cells recruitment and extravasation into the nervous tissue. Some of these expression changes can be controlled by microRNAs. In particular, the upregulation of *VCAM1* mRNA (Aimone et al., 2004) occurs in parallel to the downregulation of its regulator miR-126 (Harris et al., 2008) during the first week after injury (Yunta et al., 2012; Hu et al., 2013b). The subsequent immune cell infiltration is responsible for several changes in the microRNA profile of the spinal cord, as previously commented. Neutrophil infiltration explains the upregulation of miR-223 (Lindsay, 2008; Sonkoly and Pivarcsi, 2009; Izumi et al., 2011), whereas increased expression of the lymphocyte specific miR-142 (Wu et al., 2007) correlates with the access of these immune cells to the injury site during the first week (Yunta et al., 2012). MicroRNAs are also involved in the activation of microglia and macrophages. Particularly, the downregulation of miR-124 contributes to resting phenotype of microglia by targeting CEBPα, a master transcription factor important for the development of myeloid cells (Ponomarev et al., 2011; Guedes et al., 2013). miR-124 shows a sustained downregulation after injury (Deo et al., 2006; Liu et al., 2009; Nakanishi et al., 2010; Yunta et al., 2012) that may underlie microglial activation. However, miR-124 is a well-characterized neuronal microRNA and its downregulation likely reflects the extension of neuronal death that characterizes the secondary damage of SCI.

The inflammatory response is modulated by a number of key molecular immune mediators, such as cytokines, chemokines (TNF-α, IL-6, IL-1β) or the complement cascade (C1qb; Hausmann, 2003; Profyris et al., 2004; Jones et al., 2005), which are known targets of microRNAs. Particularly, overexpression of three key pro-inflammatory cytokines that modulate the inflammatory response in the SCI is likely regulated by microRNA experiencing expression changes after injury. Different SCI studies (Liu et al., 2009; Yunta et al., 2012) have suggested that increasing levels of the pro-inflammatory and pro-apoptotic factor TNF-α after injury (Tyor et al., 2002) may result from downregulation of its regulators miR-181 (Hutchison et al., 2013) and miR-125b (Tili et al., 2007) after SCI (Liu et al., 2009; Yunta et al., 2012; Hu et al., 2013b). Other microRNAs, such as miR-411, miR-99a, that appear downregulated after SCI (Liu et al., 2009; Yunta et al., 2012; Hu et al., 2013b) have been also predicted to target TNF-α by bioinformatics analysis. On the other hand, the increased levels of cytokine IL-6 during the first days after injury correlate with a reduced expression of its regulators let-7a (Iliopoulos et al., 2009) or miR-181a (Tili et al., 2007; Iliopoulos et al., 2009). Finally, the observed downregulation of miR-30b-5p and miR-30c during the first week after injury (Liu et al., 2009; Yunta et al., 2012) could be related to the overexpression of their target IL-1β. Additionally, it has been recently described that upregulation of miR-20a induces a cytotoxic environment with increased IL-6, TNF-α, IL-1-β, and COX-2 expression in the spinal cord (Jee et al., 2012b) due to miR-20a-mediated inhibition of neurogenin 1 (*NGN-1*). Inhibition of this microRNA – which is upregulated after injury (Liu et al., 2009; Jee et al., 2012b) – lead to a significant improvement in functional recovery associated to a reduced inflammation and the increased survival of motor neurons (Jee et al., 2012b).

Interestingly, pro-inflammatory cytokines lead to the activation of the NF-κB signaling pathway, which is also under microRNAs regulation (Ma et al., 2010). In particular, downregulation of miR-9 and miR-199 (Yunta et al., 2012) may induce the overexpression of the NF-κB pathway genes *p50NFkB* and *ikkb* (Chen et al., 2008; Bazzoni et al., 2009; Wang et al., 2011). The increased expression of miR-21 may also contribute to the regulation of this pathway but its role is less clear, as it exhibits both pro- and anti-inflammatory effects. miR-21 targets PTEN, a negative regulator of NF-κB (Iliopoulos et al., 2010), but also PDCD4, which promotes NF-κB activation and inhibits the expression of IL-10 (Frankel et al., 2008; Sheedy et al., 2010; Young et al., 2010). On the opposite side, expression changes in several microRNAs that have been observed after SCI may attenuate the activation of NF-κB pathway, contributing to the attempts of the damaged spinal cord to recover homeostasis (Bareyre and Schwab, 2003). These changes include the increased expression of miR-146a at 7 days after injury (Liu et al., 2009; Yunta et al., 2012), which negatively regulates NF-κB expression (Taganov et al., 2006; Ma et al., 2010). Interestingly, miR-146a expression is induced by NF-κB and, thus, its overexpression at 7 days after injury may be consequence of the increased levels of NF-κB in the previous days (Bethea et al., 1998), forming a negative feedback that may cause the inactivation of NF-κB pathway.

A second group of factors with a prominent role in inflammation after SCI are the complement proteins (Brennan et al., 2012). Complement activation is involved in the removal of cellular debris, but it may also promote clearance of mildly damaged cells contributing to secondary cell death and demyelination. Complement protein C1qb increases its expression in the first day after injury and persist upregulated at least 5 weeks later (Aimone et al., 2004). C1q knockout mice show improved locomotor recovery and reduced secondary tissue damage after contusive SCI (Galvan et al., 2008). Interestingly, C1qb is a predicted target of miR-103 (Perri et al., 2012), which appears downregulated in the first week after injury (Liu et al., 2009; Yunta et al., 2012). Thus, miR-103 downregulation could be responsible for the overexpression of the complement protein C1qb and its associated deleterious effects.

Inflammation is also stimulated through the inhibition of anti-inflammatory pathways, such as the downregulation of pSMAD2, SMAD4, and TGFBR2 by observed upregulation of members of the miR-17-92 microRNA cluster (Mestdagh et al., 2010) or the silencing of the anti-inflammatory neuroprotective cytokine IL-10 by miR-98, miR-106a (Sharma et al., 2009; Liu et al., 2011). Many other microRNAs have been related to inflammation in SCI based on *in silico* predictions. Bioinformatics analyses predict that anti-inflammatory mRNAs annexin A1, annexin A2 and annexin A7 mRNAs are potential targets of the SCI, upregulated microRNAs miR-221, miR-1, and miR-323, respectively (Liu et al., 2009; Hu et al., 2013a). The list also includes miR-127, miR-411, and miR-34a, significantly downregulated after SCI in adult rats and which according to Liu et al. (2009) should lead to increased inflammation. Other pro-inflammatory microRNAs, such as miR-152, miR-214, miR-206, and miR-221, show significant changes in isolated studies or even show opposite expression trend (i.e., miR-1) in different studies (Liu et al., 2009; Strickland et al., 2011; Yunta et al., 2012). All these results will require further assays to elucidate the role in the inflammatory process of the SCI.

MicroRNA REGULATION OF CELL DEATH REGULATION IN SCI

Cell death is a hallmark of the pathophysiology of SCI (Crowe et al., 1997; Liu et al., 1997). The programed cell death (apoptosis) that characterizes the SCI secondary damage is a gene-controlled process that is stimulated or inhibited by a variety of regulatory factors including several microRNAs (Wang, 2010). Previous studies have shown that SCI alters the transcription levels of a substantial number of genes associated with the regulation of apoptosis (Aimone et al., 2004). The resulting scenario is complex, combining both temporal and spatial changes in the expression of both pro and anti-apoptotic signals. In agreement, many microRNAs have been proposed to promote or inhibit cell death during the course of SCI, with discrepancies among microRNA expression profiling studies. These discrepancies highlight the intricate roles that miRNAs play in the regulation of cellular processes and the difficulty to identify the precise activity of dysregulated microRNAs. However, two recent studies have provided direct evidence of microRNAs involvement in cell death modulation following SCI (**Figure 1**).

The first study deals with miR-20a, which shows an increased expression early after injury (24 h) that persists at least for 1 week (Liu et al., 2009; Jee et al., 2012b). miR-20a inhibits the expression of Ngn1, a protein with a key role in maintenance of cell survival, self-renewal, and neurogenesis in normal and injured spinal cords. Silencing Ngn1 by siNgn1 or infusion of miR-20a into uninjured mouse spinal cord reproduced SCI-like symptoms including apoptotic death of neural cells, whereas the administration of anti-miR-20a decreased apoptosis, reduced tissue damage and functional deficits were significantly ameliorated (Liu et al., 2009; Jee et al., 2012b). In a similar way, miR-486 is upregulated at 7 days after injury (Jee et al., 2012a). miR-486 represses neurogenic differentiation 6 (NeuroD6), a protein that promotes neuronal survival by increased expression of the ROS scavenger proteins (Jee et al., 2012a). Infusion of miR-486 into the normal spinal cord of mice reproduces SCI symptoms including increased neuronal death, whereas silencing miR-486 after SCI produced a decrease in the magnitude of neuronal death and led to a significant improvement in motor recovery. Therefore upregulation of miR-486 following SCI promotes neurodegeneration by suppressing NeuroD6, pointing to this microRNA as a potential target for therapeutic interventions (Jee et al., 2012a).

Further evidences of the roles of microRNAs on secondary cell death come from microRNA expression changes that are accompanied by changes in the expression of their apoptotic gene targets. Several pro and anti-apoptotic microRNAs act on key apoptosis molecules, such as caspases, Fas/CD95, c-Myc, TNF-α, or members of the BCL-2 family. For example, the decreased expression of the let-7/miR-98 family members miR-96 and miR-146a (Liu et al., 2009; Strickland et al., 2011; Yunta et al., 2012) would promote apoptosis by increasing the expression of their targets, the pro-apoptotic proteins caspase 3 (Citron et al., 2000; Aimone et al., 2004) and Fas/CD95 (Casha et al., 2001). On the contrary, overexpression of miR-21 would protect neural cells from death by repressing the expression of the pro-apoptotic molecules Fas ligand (Buller et al., 2010), TPM1 and PTEN (Hafez et al., 2012; Han et al., 2012), and PDCD4 (Frankel et al., 2008). BCL-2 modulation is highly representative of the complexity of microRNA regulation of cell death in SCI. Upregulation of miR-15b (Liu et al., 2009) would decrease BCL-2 (Cimmino et al., 2005; Saito et al., 2006) and induce apoptosis. However, upregulation of miR-15b is counteracted by the decreased expression during the first week of miR-138 and miR-148b, which also target BCL-2 (Liu et al., 2009; Yunta et al., 2012). Downregulation of these microRNAs is broadly consistent with the increase in the number of BCL-2-positive cells present 3 days after injury (Saito et al., 2000; however, see Qiu et al., 2001), although microRNA downregulation extends throughout the 7-day period after injury, which is the time-point when the number of BCL-2-positive cells is progressively reduced. Other microRNAs targeting BCL-2 appear dysregulated after SCI. Regulation of BCL-2 by miR-107 was discussed in the profiling study by Liu et al. (2009). These authors observed a miR-107 upregulation 4 h after injury, which they proposed should decrease BCL-2 levels and induce apoptosis, to be later downregulated at 7 dpi (also observed in Yunta et al., 2012) promoting cell survival. miR-1 represents a puzzling case that appears upregulated in Liu et al. (2009) and downregulated in the analyses by Strickland et al. (2011) and Yunta et al. (2012).

In addition to modulation of genes that regulate apoptosis, microRNAs also participate in the disruption of the calcium signaling or the oxidative stress events triggered after SCI that contribute to secondary cell death. Expression of the gene coding for the Ca^{2+}-related genes such as Ca^{2+} pump, voltage-gated (L-type) Ca^{2+} channels or Ca^{2+}-permeable ionotropic glutamate (AMPA) channels, is decreased with injury and post-transcriptionally regulated by microRNAs. Several studies have shown that upregulated miR-223 reduces the expression of the NR2B and GluR2 subunits of the NMDA and AMPA receptors, respectively (Kaur et al., 2012). Similarly, decreased expression of voltage-gated (L-type) Ca^{2+} channels may be result of upregulated miR-21 (Carrillo et al., 2011). These could cause an increment of intracellular Ca^{2+} concentration level that accompanies traumatic SCI, and could trigger mechanisms of secondary cell death, such as calpain activation. MicroRNAs also play an important role in the regulation of oxidative stress, a hallmark of the secondary damage of SCI that has received much attention in the attempts to develop effective therapies (Jia et al., 2012). Recent reports have demonstrated that miR-486 repress the expression of NeuroD6, a neuroprotective protein that promotes the expression of ROS scavenger proteins, such as GPX3, selenoprotein-N, and thioredoxin (Jee et al., 2012a). Upregulation of miR-486 – observed in motor neurons at 7 days after injury in murine models of SCI – leads to the repression of NeuroD6 expression, and consequently to a decrease in the expression of ROS scavenger proteins and increased neurodegeneration mediated by oxidative stress (Jee et al., 2012a).

Microarray analyses revealed increased expression of genes associated with anti-oxidant actions, such as SOD1, SOD2, catalase, and GPX (Di Giovanni et al., 2003; Aimone et al., 2004). This overexpression of the mitochondrial SOD2 gene (*sod2*) 7 days after injury (Santoscoy et al., 2002; Sugawara et al., 2002) is consistent with the downregulation of its modulator miR-145 (Dharap et al., 2009) described in Yunta et al. (2012). However, the bioinformatics analysis performed by Liu et al. (2009) revealed that some anti-oxidant genes such as SOD1 and catalase gene are potential targets of the upregulated miR-206, miR-152, and miR-214. Moreover, it has been proposed that downregulation of miR-1 and miR-129, which regulate transcription, differentiation or prevent post-mitotic cells from re-entering the cell cycle, could cause neural cells to become aberrantly mitotic, increasing the number of apoptotic cells observed at the injury site after SCI (Bhalala et al., 2013).

MicroRNA MODULATION OF ASTROCYTE REACTIVITY AND GLIAL SCAR

Astrogliosis is another hallmarks of the cellular response to SCI. It consists in an early hypertrophic neuroprotective phase followed by a hyperplasic phase characterized by the formation of a dense glial scar that inhibits CNS regeneration during the subacute and chronic phases of the SCI (Sofroniew, 2009). Recent genomic analyses have shown reactive astrogliosis is associated to a rapid, but quickly attenuated, induction of gene expression

(Zamanian et al., 2012). Increasing evidence supports the involvement of several microRNAs in the regulation of the astrocyte response to injury, including four microRNAs that appear dysregulated in studies of SCI. The best characterized is miR-21. Its expression increases in a time-dependent manner following SCI (Liu et al., 2009; Bhalala et al., 2012; Yunta et al., 2012; Hu et al., 2013b) and is highly expressed in astrocytes during the chronic stage (Bhalala et al., 2012). miR-21 expression after SCI shows a marked spatial pattern, with highest expression in the astrocytes adjacent to the lesion area (Bhalala et al., 2012). The role of miR-21 in astrogliosis has been studied in detail using transgenic mice that overexpress in astrocytes either miR-21 or a miRNA sponge designed to inhibit miR-21 function (Bhalala et al., 2012). The results from these studies demonstrate that miR-21 overexpression in astrocytes abrogates the hypertrophic astrocytic response after severe SCI, which is consistent with previous studies *in vitro* (Sahni et al., 2010; Sayed and Abdellatif, 2011). On the contrary, miR-21 inhibition enhances the hypertrophic response in early and chronic stages after SCI (Bhalala et al., 2012). BMP signaling following SCI mediates the miR-21 and astrocytic response through the opposing effects of the BMP receptors BMPR1a and BMPR1b (Sahni et al., 2010). BMPR1a signaling decreases levels of miR-21 and induces reactive astrocytic hypertrophy, whereas BMPR1b signaling increases miR-21 levels and negatively regulates astrogliosis. These findings point to the BMP–BMPR–miR-21 axis as a key regulator of astrocytic hypertrophy and glial scar progression after SCI, modulating the pro-reactive effects of the inflammatory signaling.

A second microRNA that has been related to astrogliosis is miR-125b. Overexpression of miR-125b correlates with the overexpression of the astrogliosis markers GFAP and vimentin in several neurological disorders (Pogue et al., 2010). *In vitro* studies show that miR-125b downregulation in IL-6 stimulated reactive astrocytes increases the expression of its target cyclin-dependent kinase inhibitor 2A (CDKN2A), a negative regulator cell growth, and attenuates cell proliferation. Thus, evidences indicate that miRNA-125b upregulation contributes to astrogliosis. However, contrary to expectations, miR-125b appears downregulated during the first week after injury (Yunta et al., 2012), which would contribute to inhibit astrocyte proliferation and astrogliosis.

The miR-181 family of miRNAs is another candidate for post-transcriptional regulation of neuroinflammation and reactive gliosis (Hutchison et al., 2013). miR-181s are constitutively expressed in astrocytes but inflammation causes its downregulation, in agreement with *in vivo* observations following SCI (Liu et al., 2009; Yunta et al., 2012). Genetic studies demonstrated that miR-181 inhibits the production of multiple pro-inflammatory cytokines (TNF-α, IL-6, IL-1β, IL-8, LIF, and HMGB1) and increases the levels of the anti-inflammatory cytokine IL-10 (Hutchison et al., 2013) in cultured astrocytes under LPS inflammatory exposure. Thus, miR-181s act as negative regulators of astrogliosis, reducing the expression of reactivity promoters such as pro-inflammatory cytokines (Balasingam et al., 1994; Sofroniew, 2009) and FGF2 (Goddard et al., 2002), and increasing the expression of reactivity inhibitors, such as IL-10 (Balasingam and Yong, 1996).

Similarly to miR-181s, miR-146a is a negative regulator of the astrocyte response to inflammation and, consequently, a negative regulator of astrogliosis (Iyer et al., 2012). miR-146a is expressed in reactive astrocytes in the areas of prominent gliosis (Iyer et al., 2012), and appears upregulated 7 dpi after SCI (Liu et al., 2009; Strickland et al., 2011; Yunta et al., 2012) as well as in several neurodegenerative pathologies (Junker et al., 2009; Cui et al., 2010; Iyer et al., 2012). Studies with astroglioma cell lines and primary astrocytes have shown that IL-1β stimulation induces a prominent upregulation of miR-146a expression. Overexpression of miR-146a has anti-inflammatory effects and significantly reduces the expression of signaling molecules downstream IL-1β, such as IRAK-1, IRAK-2, and TRAF-6 and inhibits the release of pro-reactive and pro-inflammatory factors, including IL-6 and COX-2 (Iyer et al., 2012). Thus, miR-146a forms a negative feedback of the IL-1β signaling, being induced by IL-1β but blocking the expression of its downstream response. Overexpression of miR-146a following SCI adds to the overexpression of miR-21 and miR-125b to limit astrocyte reactivity. On the contrary, downregulation of miR-181 family members would promote astrocyte reactivity, indicating a fairly complex regulation of the astrocyte response. It is interesting to note that according to recent studies, the disruption of microRNA biogenesis by deletion of Dicer leads to an altered mature astroglial transcriptome signature that resembles to a reactive state (Tao et al., 2011), which adds a further layer of complexity to the whole picture.

THE ROLES OF microRNAs IN AXONAL REGENERATION, MYELINATION, AND OTHER PROCESSES

Although less studied, microRNAs also seem to contribute to the regulation of other pivotal processes in the SCI pathophysiology, such as axonal regeneration, remyelination, or pain. As we mentioned before, failure to produce a sustained regenerative response is one of the critical features of the CNS. Local environmental clues are largely responsible for the lack of regeneration but intracellular specific features associated to neural cell maturation are also involved (see, for example, Goldberg, 2003). Different evidences indicate that microRNAs can contribute to these changes. In fact, microRNAs have a critical role in neurite outgrowth in post-mitotic neurons as demonstrated in Dicer conditional knockout mice. In this animals, silencing of Dicer and the subsequent inhibition of the microRNA biogenesis causes defects in neurite outgrowth and decreased soma size but has not influence in neurogenesis, cortical patterning or cell survival (Hong et al., 2013). Additional evidences have been obtained from the zebrafish, a model of spontaneous axonal regeneration in the damaged spinal cord (Becker et al., 1997). In this fish, miR-133b is overexpressed in regenerating neurons following SCI and its inhibition using antisense morpholinos result in reduced axonal regeneration (Yu et al., 2011). Functionally, miR-133b contributes to spinal cord regeneration through the downregulation of its target RhoA, a small GTPase that inhibits axonal growth. Contrary to zebrafish, miR-133b shows a significant downregulation at 1 and 7 days after contusive SCI in mammals (Liu et al., 2009; Yunta et al., 2012), which may contribute to their reduced neuroregenerative capacity. miRNA-124 presents a somehow similar behavior that may also contribute to reduce axonal regeneration after SCI. Previous studies have shown that miR-124 overexpression in differentiating mouse P19 cells promotes neurite outgrowth, while miR-124 inhibition reduces it (Yu et al., 2008). Thus the observed miR-124 downregulation after SCI may also contribute to hinder the axonal regenerative capacities of spinal cord neurons. However, microRNAs may also contribute to the activation of pro-regenerative gene programs after injury. Di Giovanni et al. (2005a) described the overexpression at 7 and 28 days after SCI of a gene cluster that comprise known promoters of the neural plasticity and the neurite outgrowth, including synaptotagmin-1. Interestingly, synaptotagmin-1 is a target of miR-34a (Agostini et al., 2011), and its upregulation after SCI is consistent with the observed downregulation of miR-34a at 3 and 7 after injury (Liu et al., 2009; Yunta et al., 2012).

The progressive loss of myelin in the areas surrounding the injury is another critical feature of the SCI that results from the combined effects of damage to oligodendrocytes and remyelination failure. Evidences have confirmed that microRNA loss of function due to Dicer1 ablation in mature oligodendrocytes causes demyelination, gliosis, and neuronal degeneration (Shin et al., 2009; Dugas et al., 2010). More precisely, Shin et al. (2009) identified miR-219 as a central actor in myelin maintenance and remyelination. miR-219 is highly expressed in mature oligodendrocytes and when is lost due to Dicer1 ablation, miR-219 target ELOVL7 increases its expression resulting in lipid accumulation in myelin-rich areas and disrupting the stability of the membranes (Shin et al., 2009). Strikingly, miR-219 abundance is markedly reduced after SCI (Liu et al., 2009; Yunta et al., 2012) although this decrease may also reflect the loss of spinal cord oligodendrocytes that takes place after injury. Further studies are needed to determine the contribution of microRNAs in demyelination and remyelination and to evaluate their use as therapeutic tools in the SCI and other CNS pathologies.

In addition to their direct roles in most processes implicated in the pathophysiology of the SCI, microRNAs are also involved in the functional consequences of SCI, including the neuropathic pain. Neuropathic pain is the manifestation of maladaptive plasticity in the nervous system characterized by pain in the absence of a stimulus and reduced nociceptive thresholds (Scholz and Woolf, 2007). It is a debilitating accompaniment of SCI that affects up to 50% SCI patients and limit their ability to achieve an optimal level of activity (Mann et al., 2013). Plastic changes in sensory neuron excitability are considered the cellular basis of neuropathic pain, although a growing body of evidence also implicates activated microglia and astrocytes as key players in the development of pain (Scholz and Woolf, 2007). Although information on the roles of miRNAs in neuropathic pain following SCI is very restricted, available evidences indicate that microRNAs expression at the spinal cord respond to pain induction (Kusuda et al., 2011; Genda et al., 2013; Li et al., 2013), although evidences are sometimes contradictory (Brandenburger et al., 2012). There are also evidences of the contribution of microRNAs in the development of central neuropathic pain. Recently, Im et al. (2012) demonstrated that SCI reduced the expression of miR-23b in GABAergic neurons from the spinal cord while increasing the levels of NADPH oxidase 4 (NOX4), a target of miR-23b and a key factor in the production of ROS and pain induction. Reduction of NOX4 expression and neuropathic pain was observed after infusion of miR-23b to the spinal cord confirming the involvement of this microRNA in pain regulation. Similarly, intrathecal administration of miR-124 inhibits the activation of spinal cord microglia, reducing inflammation and preventing neuropathic pain (Willemen et al., 2012). Many other microRNAs have been described to affect neuropathic pain at different levels, particularly at the dorsal root ganglia. However, a review of this complex system lies beyond the scope of the present article.

CLINICAL APPLICATIONS: microRNA-BASED THERAPEUTIC AND DIAGNOSTIC TOOLS

The capability of individual microRNAs to reduce the expression of numerous components of cellular networks supposes an opportunity to modulate the cell phenotypes by manipulating the expression or function of microRNAs. The possibility of a therapeutic use of the miRNAs is highly appealing due to their capability to modulate entire gene programs though tuning, not blunting, the expression of their targets (Hydbring and Badalian-Very, 2013). Moreover, microRNA deregulation has a critical role in a wide range of pathologies, and, indeed, several studies have identified specific deregulated microRNAs that can constitute potential targets of therapeutic approaches in a wide range of pathologies. As a consequence, in the short time from its discovery in humans, a microRNA-based therapeutic for suppression of hepatitis C virus has already entered phase II clinical trial and several others are on their way (see review in Hydbring and Badalian-Very, 2013).

Therapeutic approaches are based on local or systemic administration of either antagonists (anti-miRs) of endogenous microRNAs that show a gain-of-function in diseased tissues or mimics that replace downregulated microRNAs. Both modulators incorporate chemical modifications (phosphorothionate backbones, locked nucleic acids or LNAs, etc.) to confer resistance to nucleases, increase stability during delivery, and facilitate cellular uptake. Anti-miRs are siRNAs designed to inhibit miRNAs through complementary base pairing, in a similar way to siRNA. Since binding is irreversible, the resulting miRNA duplex cannot be processed by RISC and/or degraded. Anti-miRs are synthesized as short single-stranded oligonucleotides of small size that make delivery possible without vehicle-systems. On the contrary, administration of microRNA mimics, also known as "miRNA replacement therapy," aims to re-introduce miRNAs into diseased cells that are normally expressed in healthy cells. miRNA mimics is expected to re-activate pathways required for normal cellular welfare and block those driving disease. To be processed correctly by the cellular RNAi-machinery, miRNA mimics need to be double-stranded, which confer them greater chemical complexity and larger size. Thus, miRNA mimics require delivery techniques similar to those employed in siRNA therapeutics, including microvesicles, exosomes or adeno-associated viruses, which increase the complexity of replacement therapies.

The critical contribution of the phenotypic changes in the neural, immune, and vascular cells in the pathophysiology of the SCI and the capabilities of miRNAs to modulate these changes (see previous sections) make miRNA therapeutics a highly promising approach to be explored. Although no microRNA-based therapy has entered clinical trials for SCI up to now, preclinical assays provide the necessary proof of concept. Experimental treatments with anti-miRs have demonstrated that inhibition of specific dysregulated microRNAs back to pre-injury levels can effectively reduce cell death. For example, Jee et al. (2012b) showed that local infusion of miR-20a inhibitor in the injured spinal cord reduced the expression of pro-apoptotic genes, and promoted neuron survival and functional recovery. Similarly, Hu et al. (2013b) also employed microRNA inhibition to explore the neuroprotective role of miR-21. Intrathecal infusion of miR-21 antagomir resulted in over-expression of pro-apoptotic genes, increased cell death and reduced recovery of the hindlimb motor function. On the other hand, two articles have proven that miRNA replacement can be also a viable therapeutic approach. Willemen et al. (2012) showed that intrathecal administration of miR-124 prevents persistent pain in rats, probably due to its modulation of microglial activation (Ponomarev et al., 2011). Im et al. (2012) reported similar results infusing miR-23b intrathecally to a murine model of neuropathic pain. According to these authors, restoring the normal levels of miR-23b reduced the expression of inflammatory proteins, particularly NOX4 in GABAergic neurons, protecting them from cell death, and ameliorating the neuropathic pain derived from SCI. These preclinical data strongly supports the feasibility of microRNA-based therapeutics in SCI treatment, although key aspects –including timing and side effects – remain to be elucidated. Detailed analysis characterizing the beneficial effects and determining the underlying mechanisms are strongly needed before microRNAs can reach the clinic in the treatment of the SCI.

Another clinically relevant but yet unexplored topic concerns how SCI alters the profiles of circulating microRNAs, and how information on these alterations can be used for diagnostic and prognostic purposes. Circulating or cell-free microRNAs are released to the body fluids either actively by secretion in exosomes or microvesicles or in association with RNA-binding proteins such as AGO2 and HDL; or passively, within apoptotic bodies liberated from dying cells (Chen et al., 2012; Zampetaki and Mayr, 2012). Encapsulation within lipid vesicles or association to binding proteins confers high stability to circulating microRNAs, despite the presence of large amounts of RNase in the body fluids (Chen et al., 2012; Li et al., 2012). Stability of circulating microRNAs together with the changes in microRNA expression in pathological states make circulating microRNAs promising biomarkers. In fact, since their discovery in all body fluids in 2008, nearly 500 articles have proposed several circulating microRNAs as biomarkers for different pathologies, including cancer, cardiovascular pathologies, and CNS injuries, among others (Laterza et al., 2009; Kosaka et al., 2010; Zhang et al., 2011; Pritchard et al., 2012). For example, analysis of the expression of circulating microRNAs after a traumatic brain injury has identified several potential biomarkers in humans (Redell et al., 2010) and rats (Balakathiresan et al., 2012). Also, it has been shown that the plasma concentration of neuron marker miR-124 becomes significantly increased after acute stroke (Laterza et al., 2009). However, quantification of circulating microRNAs can be challenging due to (i) their low concentrations, (ii) the effects of cell contaminants, and iii) the absence of endogenous controls for normalization. Low concentrations of circulating microRNAs suppose a technical challenge for microRNA extraction and quantification, and also increase the risk that microRNAs from contaminant cells, which are at much higher concentrations, would mask or confound the circulating microRNA profile (Kirschner et al., 2011).

Circulating microRNAs are also highly interesting due to their possible role as paracrine regulators. Circulating microRNAs can be transferred to neighboring or distant cells, altering the expression of target genes and regulating various functions, including proliferation, death or even tumor cell invasion (see Zhu and Fan, 2011, and references therein). Interestingly, microRNA transfer occurs when microRNAs are wrapped in exosomes, microvesicles, or apoptotic bodies, as well as when packaged with proteins (Zhu and Fan, 2011). Although most available evidence deals with circulating microRNA transfer in immune and vascular cells, a recent article has also demonstrated that miRNA transfer occurs between neural cells. According to Morel et al. (2013), neurons are able to secrete exosomes containing miR-124a, which are internalized by astrocytes causing an increase in the glutamate transporter GLT1.

CONCLUDING REMARKS

Spinal cord injury is a complex pathology that induces strong cellular and molecular changes in the nervous, immune, and vascular systems. These changes alter the expression of the microRNAs - small non-coding RNAs that post-transcriptionally regulate the expression of thousands of genes- to different degrees up to a general downregulation of the microRNA expression. Bioinformatic analyses of the microRNA and mRNA expression profiles in the injured spinal cord have predicted that microRNA dysregulation strongly affects processes developing after the SCI. However, much more research analyzing the expression of specific cell populations and evaluating the effects of microRNA dysregulation is still needed if we want to validate the bioinformatic predictions, and to precisely characterize the changes in microRNA expression after SCI as well as their causes and their functional consequences. The pioneering studies developed up to now have been able to demonstrate the active role of individual microRNAs in the regulation of key processes of the SCI, such as cell death, inflammation, and astrogliosis. These results strongly suggest that microRNAs can be highly valuable therapeutic targets to modulate the deleterious events that follow SCI and to promote regenerative responses that will contribute to reduce the functional deficits associated to the SCI.

AUTHOR CONTRIBUTIONS

All authors contributed in the conception and design of the present review, as well as in drafting and revising the manuscript. All authors have given full approval to the present version for its publication.

ACKNOWLEDGMENTS

We would like to thank Dr. Tommaso Pizzorusso for the invitation to contribute to the present volume, and to two anonymous reviewers for their useful comments. Present contribution has been funded by Instituto de Salud Carlos III (MINECO), PI

12/28282. Rosa Navarro-Ruiz is funded by FISCAM (grant PI 2010/19) and Ángela del Águila by La Marato de TV3 foundation (grant exp.112131).

REFERENCES

Agostini, M., Tucci, P., Steinert, J. R., Shalom-Feuerstein, R., Rouleau, M., Aberdam, D., et al. (2011). microRNA-34a regulates neurite outgrowth, spinal morphology, and function. *Proc. Natl. Acad. Sci. U.S.A.* 108, 21099–21104. doi: 10.1073/pnas.1112063108

Aimone, J. B., Leasure, J. L., Perreau, V. M., and Thallmair, M. (2004). Spatial and temporal gene expression profiling of the contused rat spinal cord. *Exp. Neurol.* 189, 204–221. doi: 10.1016/j.expneurol.2004.05.042

Baek, D., Villen, J., Shin, C., Camargo, F. D., Gygi, S. P., and Bartel, D. P. (2008). The impact of microRNAs on protein output. *Nature* 455, 64–71. doi: 10.1038/nature07242

Bak, M., Silahtaroglu, A., Moller, M., Christensen, M., Rath, M. F., Skryabin, B., et al. (2008). MicroRNA expression in the adult mouse central nervous system. *RNA* 14, 432–444. doi: 10.1261/rna.783108

Balakathiresan, N., Bhomia, M., Chandran, R., Chavko, M., McCarron, R. M., and Maheshwari, R. K. (2012). MicroRNA let-7i is a promising serum biomarker for blast-induced traumatic brain injury. *J. Neurotrauma* 29, 1379–1387. doi: 10.1089/neu.2011.2146

Balasingam, V., Tejada-Berges, T., Wright, E., Bouckova, R., and Yong, V. W. (1994). Reactive astrogliosis in the neonatal mouse brain and its modulation by cytokines. *J. Neurosci.* 14, 846–856.

Balasingam, V., and Yong, V. W. (1996). Attenuation of astroglial reactivity by interleukin-10. *J. Neurosci.* 16, 2945–2955.

Bareyre, F. M., and Schwab, M. E. (2003). Inflammation, degeneration and regeneration in the injured spinal cord: insights from DNA microarrays. *Trends Neurosci.* 26, 555–563. doi: 10.1016/j.tins.2003.08.004

Bazzoni, F., Rossato, M., Fabbri, M., Gaudiosi, D., Mirolo, M., Mori, L., et al. (2009). Induction and regulatory function of miR-9 in human monocytes and neutrophils exposed to proinflammatory signals. *Proc. Natl. Acad. Sci. U.S.A.* 106, 5282–5287. doi: 10.1073/pnas.0810909106

Beck, K. D., Nguyen, H. X., Galvan, M. D., Salazar, D. L., Woodruff, T. M., and Anderson, A. J. (2010). Quantitative analysis of cellular inflammation after traumatic spinal cord injury: evidence for a multiphasic inflammatory response in the acute to chronic environment. *Brain* 133, 433–447. doi: 10.1093/brain/awp322

Becker, T., Wullimann, M. F., Becker, C. G., Bernhardt, R. R., and Schachner, M. (1997). Axonal regrowth after spinal cord transection in adult zebrafish. *J. Comp. Neurol.* 377, 577–595. doi: 10.1002/(SICI)1096-9861(19970127)377:4<577::AID-CNE8>3.0.CO;2-#

Bethea, J. R., Castro, M., Keane, R. W., Lee, T. T., Dietrich, W. D., and Yezierski, R. P. (1998). Traumatic spinal cord injury induces nuclear factor-κB activation. *J. Neurosci.* 18, 3251–3260.

Bhalala, O. G., Pan, L., Sahni, V., McGuire, T. L., Gruner, K., Tourtellotte, W. G., et al. (2012). microRNA-21 regulates astrocytic response following spinal cord injury. *J. Neurosci.* 32, 17935–17947. doi: 10.1523/JNEUROSCI.3860-12.2012

Bhalala, O. G., Srikanth, M., and Kessler, J. A. (2013). The emerging roles of microRNAs in CNS injuries. *Nat. Rev. Neurol.* 9, 328–339. doi: 10.1038/nrneurol.2013.67

Biering-Sorensen, E., Pedersen, V., and Clausen, S. (1990). Epidemiology of spinal cord lesions in Denmark. *Paraplegia* 28, 105–118. doi: 10.1038/sc.1990.13

Brandenburger, T., Castoldi, M., Brendel, M., Grievink, H., Schlosser, L., Werdehausen, R., et al. (2012). Expression of spinal cord microRNAs in a rat model of chronic neuropathic pain. *Neurosci. Lett.* 506, 281–286. doi: 10.1016/j.neulet.2011.11.023

Brennan, F. H., Anderson, A. J., Taylor, S. M., Woodruff, T. M., and Ruitenberg, M. J. (2012). Complement activation in the injured central nervous system: another dual-edged sword? *J. Neuroinflammation* 9, 137. doi: 10.1186/1742-2094-9-137

Buller, B., Liu, X., Wang, X., Zhang, R. L., Zhang, L., Hozeska-Solgot, A., et al. (2010). MicroRNA-21 protects neurons from ischemic death. *FEBS J.* 277, 4299–4307. doi: 10.1111/j.1742-4658.2010.07818.x

Byrnes, K. R., Garay, J., Di Giovanni, S., De Biase, A., Knoblach, S. M., Hoffman, E. P., et al. (2006). Expression of two temporally distinct microglia-related gene clusters after spinal cord injury. *Glia* 53, 420–433. doi: 10.1002/glia.20295

Callari, M., Dugo, M., Musella, V., Marchesi, E., Chiorino, G., Grand, M. M., et al. (2012). Comparison of microarray platforms for measuring differential microRNA expression in paired normal/cancer colon tissues. *PLoS ONE* 7:e45105. doi: 10.1371/journal.pone.0045105

Carmel, J. B., Galante, A., Soteropoulos, P., Tolias, P., Recce, M., Young, W., et al. (2001). Gene expression profiling of acute spinal cord injury reveals spreading inflammatory signals and neuron loss. *Physiol. Genomics* 7, 201–213.

Carrillo, E. D., Escobar, Y., Gonzalez, G., Hernandez, A., Galindo, J. M., Garcia, M. C., et al. (2011). Posttranscriptional regulation of the β2-subunit of cardiac L-type Ca^{2+} channels by MicroRNAs during long-term exposure to isoproterenol in rats. *J. Cardiovasc. Pharmacol.* 58, 470–478. doi: 10.1097/FJC.0b013e31822a789b

Casha, S., Yu, W. R., and Fehlings, M. G. (2001). Oligodendroglial apoptosis occurs along degenerating axons and is associated with FAS and p75 expression following spinal cord injury in the rat. *Neuroscience* 103, 203–218. doi: 10.1016/S0306-4522(00)00538-8

Chamankhah, M., Eftekharpour, E., Karimi-Abdolrezaee, S., Boutros, P. C., San-Marina, S., and Fehlings, M. G. (2013). Genome-wide gene expression profiling of stress response in a spinal cord clip compression injury model. *BMC Genomics* 14:583. doi: 10.1186/1471-2164-14-583

Chang, T. C., Yu, D., Lee, Y. S., Wentzel, E. A., Arking, D. E., West, K. M., et al. (2008). Widespread microRNA repression by Myc contributes to tumorigenesis. *Nat. Genet.* 40, 43–50. doi: 10.1038/ng.2007.30

Chen, C. Z., Schaffert, S., Fragoso, R., and Loh, C. (2013). Regulation of immune responses and tolerance: the microRNA perspective. *Immunol. Rev.* 253, 112–128. doi: 10.1111/imr.12060

Chen, R., Alvero, A. B., Silasi, D. A., Kelly, M. G., Fest, S., Visintin, I., et al. (2008). Regulation of IKKβ by miR-199a affects NF-κB activity in ovarian cancer cells. *Oncogene* 27, 4712–4723. doi: 10.1038/onc.2008.112

Chen, X., Liang, H., Zhang, J., Zen, K., and Zhang, C. Y. (2012). Secreted microRNAs: a new form of intercellular communication. *Trends Cell Biol.* 22, 125–132. doi: 10.1016/j.tcb.2011.12.001

Cimmino, A., Calin, G. A., Fabbri, M., Iorio, M. V., Ferracin, M., Shimizu, M., et al. (2005). miR-15 and miR-16 induce apoptosis by targeting BCL2. *Proc. Natl. Acad. Sci. U.S.A.* 102, 13944–1399. doi: 10.1073/pnas.0506654102

Citron, B. A., Arnold, P. M., Sebastian, C., Qin, F., Malladi, S., Ameenuddin, S., et al. (2000). Rapid upregulation of caspase-3 in rat spinal cord after injury: mRNA, protein, and cellular localization correlates with apoptotic cell death. *Exp. Neurol.* 166, 213–226. doi: 10.1006/exnr.2000.7523

Clarke, J., Seo, P., and Clarke, B. (2010). Statistical expression deconvolution from mixed tissue samples. *Bioinformatics* 26, 1043–1049. doi: 10.1093/bioinformatics/btq097

Cochella, L., and Hobert, O. (2012). Diverse functions of microRNAs in nervous system development. *Curr. Top. Dev. Biol.* 99, 115–143. doi: 10.1016/B978-0-12-387038-4.00005-7

Crowe, M. J., Bresnahan, J. C., Shuman, S. L., Masters, J. N., and Beattie, M. S. (1997). Apoptosis and delayed degeneration after spinal cord injury in rats and monkeys. *Nat. Med.* 3, 73–76. doi: 10.1038/nm0197-73

Cui, J. G., Li, Y. Y., Zhao, Y., Bhattacharjee, S., and Lukiw, W. J. (2010). Differential regulation of interleukin-1 receptor-associated kinase-1 (IRAK-1) and IRAK-2 by microRNA-146a and NF-kappaB in stressed human astroglial cells and in Alzheimer disease. *J. Biol. Chem.* 285, 38951–38960. doi: 10.1074/jbc.M110.178848

David, S., and Aguayo, A. J. (1981). Axonal elongation into peripheral nervous system "bridges" after central nervous system injury in adult rats. *Science* 214, 931–933. doi: 10.1126/science.6171034

Davis, B. N., Hilyard, A. C., Nguyen, P. H., Lagna, G., and Hata, A. (2010). Smad proteins bind a conserved RNA sequence to promote microRNA maturation by Drosha. *Mol. Cell* 39, 373–384. doi: 10.1016/j.molcel.2010.07.011

De Biase, A., Knoblach, S. M., Di Giovanni, S., Fan, C., Molon, A., Hoffman, E. P., et al. (2005). Gene expression profiling of experimental traumatic spinal cord injury as a function of distance from impact site and injury severity. *Physiol. Genomics* 22, 368–381. doi: 10.1152/physiolgenomics.00081.2005

Deo, M., Yu, J. Y., Chung, K. H., Tippens, M., and Turner, D. L. (2006). Detection of mammalian microRNA expression by in situ hybridization with RNA oligonucleotides. *Dev. Dyn.* 235, 2538–2548. doi: 10.1002/dvdy.20847

Dharap, A., Bowen, K., Place, R., Li, L. C., and Vemuganti, R. (2009). Transient focal ischemia induces extensive temporal changes in rat cerebral microRNAome. *J. Cereb. Blood Flow Metab.* 29, 675–687. doi: 10.1038/jcbfm.2008.157

Di Giovanni, S., De Biase, A., Yakovlev, A., Finn, T., Beers, J., Hoffman, E. P., et al. (2005a). *In vivo* and *in vitro* characterization of novel neuronal plasticity factors identified following spinal cord injury. *J. Biol. Chem.* 280, 2084–2091. doi: 10.1074/jbc.M411975200

Di Giovanni, S., Faden, A. I., Yakovlev, A., Duke-Cohan, J. S., Finn, T., Thouin, M., et al. (2005b). Neuronal plasticity after spinal cord injury: identification of a gene cluster driving neurite outgrowth. *FASEB J.* 19, 153–154.

Di Giovanni, S., Knoblach, S. M., Brandoli, C., Aden, S. A., Hoffman, E. P., and Faden, A. I. (2003). Gene profiling in spinal cord injury shows role of cell cycle in neuronal death. *Ann. Neurol.* 53, 454–468. doi: 10.1002/ana.10472

Donnelly, D. J., and Popovich, P. G. (2008). Inflammation and its role in neuroprotection, axonal regeneration and functional recovery after spinal cord injury. *Exp. Neurol.* 209, 378–388. doi: 10.1016/j.expneurol.2007.06.009

Dugas, J. C., Cuellar, T. L., Scholze, A., Ason, B., Ibrahim, A., Emery, B., et al. (2010). Dicer1 and miR-219 Are required for normal oligodendrocyte differentiation and myelination. *Neuron* 65, 597–611. doi: 10.1016/j.neuron.2010.01.027

Dumont, R. J., Okonkwo, D. O., Verma, S., Hurlbert, R. J., Boulos, P. T., Ellegala, D. B., et al. (2001). Acute spinal cord injury, part I: pathophysiologic mechanisms. *Clin. Neuropharmacol.* 24, 254–264. doi: 10.1097/00002826-200109000-00002

Ebert, M. S., and Sharp, P. A. (2012). Roles for microRNAs in conferring robustness to biological processes. *Cell* 149, 515–524. doi: 10.1016/j.cell.2012.04.005

Faulkner, J. R., Herrmann, J. E., Woo, M. J., Tansey, K. E., Doan, N. B., and Sofroniew, M. V. (2004). Reactive astrocytes protect tissue and preserve function after spinal cord injury. *J. Neurosci.* 24, 2143–2155. doi: 10.1523/JNEUROSCI.3547-03.2004

Fawcett, J. W., and Asher, R. A. (1999). The glial scar and central nervous system repair. *Brain Res. Bull.* 49, 377–391. doi: 10.1016/S0361-9230(99)00072-6

Fehlings, M. G., and Tator, C. H. (1995). The relationships among the severity of spinal cord injury, residual neurological function, axon counts, and counts of retrogradely labeled neurons after experimental spinal cord injury. *Exp. Neurol.* 132, 220–228. doi: 10.1016/0014-4886(95)90027-6

Fleming, J. C., Norenberg, M. D., Ramsay, D. A., Dekaban, G. A., Marcillo, A. E., Saenz, A. D., et al. (2006). The cellular inflammatory response in human spinal cords after injury. *Brain* 129, 3249–3269. doi: 10.1093/brain/awl296

Frankel, L. B., Christoffersen, N. R., Jacobsen, A., Lindow, M., Krogh, A., and Lund, A. H. (2008). Programmed cell death 4 (PDCD4) is an important functional target of the microRNA miR-21 in breast cancer cells. *J. Biol. Chem.* 283, 1026–1033. doi: 10.1074/jbc.M707224200

Friedman, R. C., Farh, K. K., Burge, C. B., and Bartel, D. P. (2009). Most mammalian mRNAs are conserved targets of microRNAs. *Genome Res.* 19, 92–105. doi: 10.1101/gr.082701.108

Galvan, M. D., Luchetti, S., Burgos, A. M., Nguyen, H. X., Hooshmand, M. J., Hamers, F. P., et al. (2008). Deficiency in complement C1q improves histological and functional locomotor outcome after spinal cord injury. *J. Neurosci.* 28, 13876–13888. doi: 10.1523/JNEUROSCI.2823-08.2008

Gangaraju, V. K., and Lin, H. (2009). MicroRNAs: key regulators of stem cells. *Nat. Rev. Mol. Cell Biol.* 10, 116–125. doi: 10.1038/nrm2621

Genda, Y., Arai, M., Ishikawa, M., Tanaka, S., Okabe, T., and Sakamoto, A. (2013). microRNA changes in the dorsal horn of the spinal cord of rats with chronic constriction injury: a TaqMan(R) Low Density Array study. *Int. J. Mol. Med.* 31, 129–137. doi: 10.3892/ijmm.2012.1163

Git, A., Dvinge, H., Salmon-Divon, M., Osborne, M., Kutter, C., Hadfield, J., et al. (2010). Systematic comparison of microarray profiling, real-time PCR, and next-generation sequencing technologies for measuring differential microRNA expression. *RNA* 16, 991–1006. doi: 10.1261/rna.1947110

Goddard, D. R., Berry, M., Kirvell, S. L., and Butt, A. M. (2002). Fibroblast growth factor-2 induces astroglial and microglial reactivity *in vivo*. *J. Anat.* 200, 57–67. doi: 10.1046/j.0021-8782.2001.00002.x

Goldberg, J. L. (2003). How does an axon grow? *Genes Dev.* 17, 941–958. doi: 10.1101/gad.1062303

Goldie, B. J., and Cairns, M. J. (2012). Post-transcriptional trafficking and regulation of neuronal gene expression. *Mol. Neurobiol.* 45, 99–108. doi: 10.1007/s12035-011-8222-0

Gosink, M. M., Petrie, H. T., and Tsinoremas, N. F. (2007). Electronically subtracting expression patterns from a mixed cell population. *Bioinformatics* 23, 3328–3334. doi: 10.1093/bioinformatics/btm508

Grossman, S. D., Rosenberg, L. J., and Wrathall, J. R. (2001). Temporal-spatial pattern of acute neuronal and glial loss after spinal cord contusion. *Exp. Neurol.* 168, 273–282. doi: 10.1006/exnr.2001.7628

Guedes, J., Cardoso, A. L., and Pedroso de Lima, M. C. (2013). Involvement of microRNA in microglia-mediated immune response. *Clin. Dev. Immunol.* 2013, 186872. doi: 10.1155/2013/186872

Guo, H., Ingolia, N. T., Weissman, J. S., and Bartel, D. P. (2010). Mammalian microRNAs predominantly act to decrease target mRNA levels. *Nature* 466, 835–840. doi: 10.1038/nature09267

Hafez, M. M., Hassan, Z. K., Zekri, A. R., Gaber, A. A., Al Rejaie, S. S., Sayed-Ahmed, M. M., et al. (2012). MicroRNAs and metastasis-related gene expression in Egyptian breast cancer patients. *Asian Pac. J. Cancer Prev.* 13, 591–598. doi: 10.7314/APJCP.2012.13.2.591

Han, M., Liu, M., Wang, Y., Chen, X., Xu, J., Sun, Y., et al. (2012). Antagonism of miR-21 reverses epithelial–mesenchymal transition and cancer stem cell phenotype through AKT/ERK1/2 inactivation by targeting PTEN. *PLoS ONE* 7:e39520. doi: 10.1371/journal.pone.0039520

Harris, T. A., Yamakuchi, M., Ferlito, M., Mendell, J. T., and Lowenstein, C. J. (2008). MicroRNA-126 regulates endothelial expression of vascular cell adhesion molecule 1. *Proc. Natl. Acad. Sci. U.S.A.* 105, 1516–1521. doi: 10.1073/pnas.0707493105

Hausmann, O. N. (2003). Post-traumatic inflammation following spinal cord injury. *Spinal Cord* 41, 369–378. doi: 10.1038/sj.sc.3101483

Hong, J., Zhang, H., Kawase-Koga, Y., and Sun, T. (2013). MicroRNA function is required for neurite outgrowth of mature neurons in the mouse postnatal cerebral cortex. *Front. Cell. Neurosci.* 7:151. doi: 10.3389/fncel.2013.00151

Hu, J. R., Lv, G. H., and Yin, B. L. (2013a). Altered microRNA expression in the ischemic-reperfusion spinal cord with atorvastatin therapy. *J. Pharmacol. Sci.* 121, 343–346. doi: 10.1254/jphs.12235SC

Hu, J. Z., Huang, J. H., Zeng, L., Wang, G., Cao, M., and Lu, H. B. (2013b). Anti-apoptotic effect of microRNA-21 after contusion spinal cord injury in rats. *J. Neurotrauma* 30, 1349–1360. doi: 10.1089/neu.2012.2748

Hutchison, E. R., Kawamoto, E. M., Taub, D. D., Lal, A., Abdelmohsen, K., Zhang, Y., et al. (2013). Evidence for miR-181 involvement in neuroinflammatory responses of astrocytes. *Glia* 61, 1018–1028. doi: 10.1002/glia.22483

Hydbring, P., and Badalian-Very, G. (2013). Clinical applications of microRNAs. *F1000Research* 2, 136. doi: 10.12688/f1000research.2-136.v3

Iliopoulos, D., Hirsch, H. A., and Struhl, K. (2009). An epigenetic switch involving NF-kappaB, lin28, Let-7 microRNA, and IL6 links inflammation to cell transformation. *Cell* 139, 693–706. doi: 10.1016/j.cell.2009.10.014

Iliopoulos, D., Jaeger, S. A., Hirsch, H. A., Bulyk, M. L., and Struhl, K. (2010). STAT3 activation of miR-21 and miR-181b-1 via PTEN and CYLD are part of the epigenetic switch linking inflammation to cancer. *Mol. Cell* 39, 493–506. doi: 10.1016/j.molcel.2010.07.023

Im, Y. B., Jee, M. K., Choi, J. I., Cho, H. T., Kwon, O. H., and Kang, S. K. (2012). Molecular targeting of NOX4 for neuropathic pain after traumatic injury of the spinal cord. *Cell Death Dis.* 3, e426. doi: 10.1038/cddis.2012.168

Iyer, A., Zurolo, E., Prabowo, A., Fluiter, K., Spliet, W. G., van Rijen, P. C., et al. (2012). MicroRNA-146a: a key regulator of astrocyte-mediated inflammatory response. *PLoS ONE* 7:e44789. doi: 10.1371/journal.pone.0044789

Izumi, B., Nakasa, T., Tanaka, N., Nakanishi, K., Kamei, N., Yamamoto, R., et al. (2011). MicroRNA-223 expression in neutrophils in the early phase of secondary damage after spinal cord injury. *Neurosci. Lett.* 492, 114–118. doi: 10.1016/j.neulet.2011.01.068

Jee, M. K., Jung, J. S., Choi, J. I., Jang, J. A., Kang, K. S., Im, Y. B., et al. (2012a). MicroRNA 486 is a potentially novel target for the treatment of spinal cord injury. *Brain* , 135, 1237–1252. doi: 10.1093/brain/aws047

Jee, M. K., Jung, J. S., Im, Y. B., Jung, S. J., and Kang, S. K. (2012b). Silencing of miR20a is crucial for Ngn1-mediated neuroprotection in injured spinal cord. *Hum. Gene Ther.* 23, 508–520. doi: 10.1089/hum.2011.121

Jeyaseelan, K., Lim, K. Y., and Armugam, A. (2008). MicroRNA expression in the blood and brain of rats subjected to transient focal ischemia by middle cerebral artery occlusion. *Stroke* 39, 959–966. doi: 10.1161/STROKEAHA.107.500736

Jia, Z., Zhu, H., Li, J., Wang, X., Misra, H., and Li, Y. (2012). Oxidative stress in spinal cord injury and antioxidant-based intervention. *Spinal Cord* 50, 264–274. doi: 10.1038/sc.2011.111

Jones, T. B., McDaniel, E. E., and Popovich, P. G. (2005). Inflammatory-mediated injury and repair in the traumatically injured spinal cord. *Curr. Pharm. Des.* 11, 1223–1236. doi: 10.2174/1381612053507468

Junker, A., Krumbholz, M., Eisele, S., Mohan, H., Augstein, F., Bittner, R., et al. (2009). MicroRNA profiling of multiple sclerosis lesions identifies modulators of the regulatory protein CD47. *Brain* 132, 3342–3352. doi: 10.1093/brain/awp300

Kaur, P., Armugam, A., and Jeyaseelan, K. (2012). MicroRNAs in neurotoxicity. *J. Toxicol.* 2012, 870150. doi: 10.1155/2012/870150

Kim, Y. K., Yu, J., Han, T. S., Park, S. Y., Namkoong, B., Kim, D. H., et al. (2009). Functional links between clustered microRNAs: suppression of cell-cycle inhibitors by microRNA clusters in gastric cancer. *Nucleic Acids Res.* 37, 1672–1681. doi: 10.1093/nar/gkp002

Kirschner, M. B., Kao, S. C., Edelman, J. J., Armstrong, N. J., Vallely, M. P., van Zandwijk, N., et al. (2011). Haemolysis during sample preparation alters microRNA content of plasma. *PLoS ONE* 6:e24145. doi: 10.1371/journal.pone.0024145

Kosaka, N., Iguchi, H., and Ochiya, T. (2010). Circulating microRNA in body fluid: a new potential biomarker for cancer diagnosis and prognosis. *Cancer Sci.* 101, 2087–2092. doi: 10.1111/j.1349-7006.2010.01650.x

Kosik, K. S. (2006). The neuronal microRNA system. *Nat. Rev. Neurosci.* 7, 911–920. doi: 10.1038/nrn2037

Kosik, K. S. (2010). MicroRNAs and cellular phenotypy. *Cell* 143, 21–26. doi: 10.1016/j.cell.2010.09.008

Kozomara, A., and Griffiths-Jones, S. (2011). miRBase: integrating microRNA annotation and deep-sequencing data. *Nucleic Acids Res.* 39, D152–D157. doi: 10.1093/nar/gkq1027

Krek, A., Grun, D., Poy, M. N., Wolf, R., Rosenberg, L., Epstein, E. J., et al. (2005). Combinatorial microRNA target predictions. *Nat. Genet.* 37, 495–500. doi: 10.1038/ng1536

Krichevsky, A. M. (2007). MicroRNA profiling: from dark matter to white matter, or identifying new players in neurobiology. *ScientificWorldJournal* 7, 155–166. doi: 10.1100/tsw.2007.201

Krichevsky, A. M., King, K. S., Donahue, C. P., Khrapko, K., and Kosik, K. S. (2003). A microRNA array reveals extensive regulation of microRNAs during brain development. *RNA* 9, 1274–1281. doi: 10.1261/rna.5980303

Krichevsky, A. M., Sonntag, K. C., Isacson, O., and Kosik, K. S. (2006). Specific microRNAs modulate embryonic stem cell-derived neurogenesis. *Stem Cells* 24, 857–864. doi: 10.1634/stemcells.2005-0441

Krol, J., Loedige, I., and Filipowicz, W. (2010). The widespread regulation of microRNA biogenesis, function and decay. *Nat. Rev. Genet.* 11, 597–610. doi: 10.1038/nrg2843

Kusuda, R., Cadetti, F., Ravanelli, M. I., Sousa, T. A., Zanon, S., De Lucca, F. L., et al. (2011). Differential expression of microRNAs in mouse pain models. *Mol. Pain* 7, 17. doi: 10.1186/1744-8069-7-17

Laterza, O. F., Lim, L., Garrett-Engele, P. W., Vlasakova, K., Muniappa, N., Tanaka, W. K., et al. (2009). Plasma MicroRNAs as sensitive and specific biomarkers of tissue injury. *Clin. Chem.* 55, 1977–1983. doi: 10.1373/clinchem.2009.131797

Lau, P., Verrier, J. D., Nielsen, J. A., Johnson, K. R., Notterpek, L., and Hudson, L. D. (2008). Identification of dynamically regulated microRNA and mRNA networks in developing oligodendrocytes. *J. Neurosci.* 28, 11720–11730. doi: 10.1523/JNEUROSCI.1932-08.2008

Lee, B. B., Cripps, R. A., Fitzharris, M., and Wing, P. C. (2013). The global map for traumatic spinal cord injury epidemiology: update 2011, global incidence rate. *Spinal Cord* 110–116. doi: 10.1038/sc.2012.158

Lee, E. J., Baek, M., Gusev, Y., Brackett, D. J., Nuovo, G. J., and Schmittgen, T. D. (2008). Systematic evaluation of microRNA processing patterns in tissues, cell lines, and tumors. *RNA* 14, 35–42. doi: 10.1261/rna.804508

Lee, R. C., Feinbaum, R. L., and Ambros, V. (1993). The *C. elegans* heterochronic gene lin-4 encodes small RNAs with antisense complementarity to lin-14. *Cell* 75, 843–854. doi: 10.1016/0092-8674(93)90529-Y

Li, H., Huang, S., Guo, C., Guan, H., and Xiong, C. (2012). Cell-free seminal mRNA and microRNA exist in different forms. *PLoS ONE* 7:e34566. doi: 10.1371/journal.pone.0034566

Li, H., Shen, L., Ma, C., and Huang, Y. (2013). Differential expression of miRNAs in the nervous system of a rat model of bilateral sciatic nerve chronic constriction injury. *Int. J. Mol. Med.* 32, 219–226. doi: 10.3892/ijmm.2013.1381

Li, X., and Jin, P. (2010). Roles of small regulatory RNAs in determining neuronal identity. *Nat. Rev. Neurosci.* 11, 329–338. doi: 10.1038/nrn2739

Lim, L. P., Lau, N. C., Garrett-Engele, P., Grimson, A., Schelter, J. M., Castle, J., et al. (2005). Microarray analysis shows that some microRNAs downregulate large numbers of target mRNAs. *Nature* 433, 769–773. doi: 10.1038/nature03315

Lindsay, M. A. (2008). microRNAs and the immune response. *Trends Immunol.* 29, 343–351. doi: 10.1016/j.it.2008.04.004

Liu, N. K., Wang, X. F., Lu, Q. B., and Xu, X. M. (2009). Altered microRNA expression following traumatic spinal cord injury. *Exp. Neurol.* 219, 424–429. doi: 10.1016/j.expneurol.2009.06.015

Liu, X. Z., Xu, X. M., Hu, R., Du, C., Zhang, S. X., McDonald, J. W., et al. (1997). Neuronal and glial apoptosis after traumatic spinal cord injury. *J. Neurosci.* 17, 5395–5406.

Liu, Y., Chen, Q., Song, Y., Lai, L., Wang, J., Yu, H., et al. (2011). MicroRNA-98 negatively regulates IL-10 production and endotoxin tolerance in macrophages after LPS stimulation. *FEBS Lett.* 585, 1963–1968. doi: 10.1016/j.febslet.2011.05.029

Liverman, C. T., Altevogt, B. M., Joy, J. E., and Johnson, R. T. (2005). *Spinal Cord Injury: Progress, Promise, and Priorities.* Washington, DC: National Academies Press.

Lu, J., Getz, G., Miska, E. A., Alvarez-Saavedra, E., Lamb, J., Peck, D., et al. (2005). MicroRNA expression profiles classify human cancers. *Nature* 435, 834–838. doi: 10.1038/nature03702

Lu, P., Nakorchevskiy, A., and Marcotte, E. M. (2003). Expression deconvolution: a reinterpretation of DNA microarray data reveals dynamic changes in cell populations. *Proc. Natl. Acad. Sci. U.S.A.* 100, 10370–10375. doi: 10.1073/pnas.1832361100

Ma, X., Becker Buscaglia, L. E., Barker, J. R., and Li, Y. (2010). MicroRNAs in NF-κB signaling. *J. Mol. Cell Biol.* 3, 159–166. doi: 10.1093/jmcb/mjr007

Makeyev, E. V., Zhang, J., Carrasco, M. A., and Maniatis, T. (2007). The MicroRNA miR-124 promotes neuronal differentiation by triggering brain-specific alternative pre-mRNA splicing. *Mol. Cell* 27, 435–448. doi: 10.1016/j.molcel.2007.07.015

Mann, R., Schaefer, C., Sadosky, A., Bergstrom, F., Baik, R., Parsons, B., et al. (2013). Burden of spinal cord injury-related neuropathic pain in the United States: retrospective chart review and cross-sectional survey. *Spinal Cord* 51, 564–570. doi: 10.1038/sc.2013.34

Mautes, A. E., Weinzierl, M. R., Donovan, F., and Noble, L. J. (2000). Vascular events after spinal cord injury: contribution to secondary pathogenesis. *Phys. Ther.* 80, 673–687.

McTigue, D. M., Popovich, P. G., Morgan, T. E., and Stokes, B. T. (2000). Localization of transforming growth factor-beta1 and receptor mRNA after experimental spinal cord injury. *Exp. Neurol.* 163, 220–230. doi: 10.1006/exnr.2000.7372

Merkerova, M., Belickova, M., and Bruchova, H. (2008). Differential expression of microRNAs in hematopoietic cell lineages. *Eur. J. Haematol.* 81, 304–310. doi: 10.1111/j.1600-0609.2008.01111.x

Mestdagh, P., Bostrom, A. K., Impens, F., Fredlund, E., Van Peer, G., De Antonellis, P., et al. (2010). The miR-17-92 microRNA cluster regulates multiple components of the TGF-β pathway in neuroblastoma. *Mol. Cell* 40, 762–773. doi: 10.1016/j.molcel.2010.11.038

Meza-Sosa, K. F., Valle-Garcia, D., Pedraza-Alva, G., and Perez-Martinez, L. (2012). Role of microRNAs in central nervous system development and pathology. *J. Neurosci. Res.* 90, 1–12. doi: 10.1002/jnr.22701

Miska, E. A., Alvarez-Saavedra, E., Townsend, M., Yoshii, A., Sestan, N., Rakic, P., et al. (2004). Microarray analysis of microRNA expression in the developing mammalian brain. *Genome Biol.* 5, R68. doi: 10.1186/gb-2004-5-9-r68

Morel, L., Regan, M., Higashimori, H., Ng, S. K., Esau, C., Vidensky, S., et al. (2013). Neuronal exosomal miRNA-dependent translational regulation of astroglial glutamate transporter GLT1. *J. Biol. Chem.* 288, 7105–7116. doi: 10.1074/jbc.M112.410944

Nakanishi, K., Nakasa, T., Tanaka, N., Ishikawa, M., Yamada, K., Yamasaki, K., et al. (2010). Responses of microRNAs 124a and 223 following spinal cord injury in mice. *Spinal Cord* 48, 192–196. doi: 10.1038/sc.2009.89

Oyinbo, C. A. (2011). Secondary injury mechanisms in traumatic spinal cord injury: a nugget of this multiply cascade. *Acta Neurobiol. Exp. (Wars)* 71, 281–299.

Pekny, M., and Pekna, M. (2004). Astrocyte intermediate filaments in CNS pathologies and regeneration. *J. Pathol.* 204, 428–437. doi: 10.1002/path.1645

Perri, R., Nares, S., Zhang, S., Barros, S. P., and Offenbacher, S. (2012). MicroRNA modulation in obesity and periodontitis. *J. Dent. Res.* 91, 33–38. doi: 10.1177/0022034511425045

Pogue, A. I., Cui, J. G., Li, Y. Y., Zhao, Y., Culicchia, F., and Lukiw, W. J. (2010). Micro RNA-125b (miRNA-125b) function in astrogliosis and glial cell proliferation. *Neurosci. Lett.* 476, 18–22. doi: 10.1016/j.neulet.2010.03.054

Ponomarev, E. D., Veremeyko, T., Barteneva, N., Krichevsky, A. M., and Weiner, H. L. (2011). MicroRNA-124 promotes microglia quiescence and suppresses EAE by deactivating macrophages via the C/EBP-alpha-PU.1 pathway. *Nat. Med.* 17, 64–70. doi: 10.1038/nm.2266

Pritchard, C. C., Cheng, H. H., and Tewari, M. (2012). MicroRNA profiling: approaches and considerations. *Nat. Rev. Genet.* 13, 358–369. doi: 10.1038/nrg3198

Profyris, C., Cheema, S. S., Zang, D., Azari, M. F., Boyle, K., and Petratos, S. (2004). Degenerative and regenerative mechanisms governing spinal cord injury. *Neurobiol. Dis.* 15, 415–436. doi: 10.1016/j.nbd.2003.11.015

Qiu, J., Nesic, O., Ye, Z., Rea, H., Westlund, K. N., Xu, G. Y., et al. (2001). Bcl-xL expression after contusion to the rat spinal cord. *J. Neurotrauma* 18, 1267–1278. doi: 10.1089/089771501317095304

Redell, J. B., Moore, A. N., Ward, N. H. III, Hergenroeder, G. W., and Dash, P. K. (2010). Human traumatic brain injury alters plasma microRNA levels. *J. Neurotrauma* 27, 2147–2156. doi: 10.1089/neu.2010.1481

Rowland, J. W., Hawryluk, G. W., Kwon, B., and Fehlings, M. G. (2008). Current status of acute spinal cord injury pathophysiology and emerging therapies: promise on the horizon. *Neurosurg. Focus* 25, E2. doi: 10.3171/FOC.2008.25.11.E2

Sahni, V., Mukhopadhyay, A., Tysseling, V., Hebert, A., Birch, D., McGuire, T. L., et al. (2010). BMPR1a and BMPR1b signaling exert opposing effects on gliosis after spinal cord injury. *J. Neurosci.* 30, 1839–1855. doi: 10.1523/JNEUROSCI.4459-09.2010

Saito, N., Yamamoto, T., Watanabe, T., Abe, Y., and Kumagai, T. (2000). Implications of p53 protein expression in experimental spinal cord injury. *J. Neurotrauma* 17, 173–182. doi: 10.1089/neu.2000.17.173

Saito, Y., Liang, G., Egger, G., Friedman, J. M., Chuang, J. C., Coetzee, G. A., et al. (2006). Specific activation of microRNA-127 with downregulation of the proto-oncogene BCL6 by chromatin-modifying drugs in human cancer cells. *Cancer Cell* 9, 435–443. doi: 10.1016/j.ccr.2006.04.020

Santoscoy, C., Rios, C., Franco-Bourland, R. E., Hong, E., Bravo, G., Rojas, G., et al. (2002). Lipid peroxidation by nitric oxide supplements after spinal cord injury: effect of antioxidants in rats. *Neurosci. Lett.* 330, 94–98. doi: 10.1016/S0304-3940(02)00716-4

Saugstad, J. A. (2010). MicroRNAs as effectors of brain function with roles in ischemia and injury, neuroprotection, and neurodegeneration. *J. Cereb. Blood Flow Metab.* 30, 1564–1576. doi: 10.1038/jcbfm.2010.101

Saugstad, J. A. (2013). MicroRNAs as effectors of brain function. *Stroke* 44(Suppl. 1), S17–S19. doi: 10.1161/STROKEAHA.113.000985

Sayed, D., and Abdellatif, M. (2011). MicroRNAs in development and disease. *Physiol. Rev.* 91, 827–887. doi: 10.1152/physrev.00006.2010

Scholz, J., and Woolf, C. J. (2007). The neuropathic pain triad: neurons, immune cells and glia. *Nat. Neurosci.* 10, 1361–1368. doi: 10.1038/nn1992

Selbach, M., Schwanhausser, B., Thierfelder, N., Fang, Z., Khanin, R., and Rajewsky, N. (2008). Widespread changes in protein synthesis induced by microRNAs. *Nature* 455, 58–63. doi: 10.1038/nature07228

Sempere, L. F., Freemantle, S., Pitha-Rowe, I., Moss, E., Dmitrovsky, E., and Ambros, V. (2004). Expression profiling of mammalian microRNAs uncovers a subset of brain-expressed microRNAs with possible roles in murine and human neuronal differentiation. *Genome Biol.* 5, R13. doi: 10.1186/gb-2004-5-3-r13

Sharma, A., Kumar, M., Aich, J., Hariharan, M., Brahmachari, S. K., Agrawal, A., et al. (2009). Posttranscriptional regulation of interleukin-10 expression by hsa-miR-106a. *Proc. Natl. Acad. Sci. U.S.A.* 106, 5761–5766. doi: 10.1073/pnas.0808743106

Sheedy, F. J., Palsson-McDermott, E., Hennessy, E. J., Martin, C., O'Leary, J. J., Ruan, Q., et al. (2010). Negative regulation of TLR4 via targeting of the proinflammatory tumor suppressor PDCD4 by the microRNA miR-21. *Nat. Immunol.* 11, 141–147. doi: 10.1038/ni.1828

Shin, D., Shin, J. Y., McManus, M. T., Ptacek, L. J., and Fu, Y. H. (2009). Dicer ablation in oligodendrocytes provokes neuronal impairment in mice. *Ann. Neurol.* 66, 843–857. doi: 10.1002/ana.21927

Shu, J., Kren, B. T., Xia, Z., Wong, P. Y., Li, L., Hanse, E. A., et al. (2011). Genomewide microRNA down-regulation as a negative feedback mechanism in the early phases of liver regeneration. *Hepatology* 54, 609–619. doi: 10.1002/hep.24421

Silver, J., and Miller, J. H. (2004). Regeneration beyond the glial scar. *Nat. Rev. Neurosci.* 5, 146–156. doi: 10.1038/nrn1326

Sluijter, J. P. G. (2013). MicroRNAs in cardiovascular regenerative medicine: directing tissue repair and cellular differentiation. *ISRN Vasc. Med.* 2013, 16.

Smirnova, L., Grafe, A., Seiler, A., Schumacher, S., Nitsch, R., and Wulczyn, F. G. (2005). Regulation of miRNA expression during neural cell specification. *Eur. J. Neurosci.* 21, 1469–1477. doi: 10.1111/j.1460-9568.2005.03978.x

Smith, B., Treadwell, J., Zhang, D., Ly, D., McKinnell, I., Walker, P. R., et al. (2010). Large-scale expression analysis reveals distinct microRNA profiles at different stages of human neurodevelopment. *PLoS ONE* 5:e11109. doi: 10.1371/journal.pone.0011109

Sofroniew, M. V. (2005). Reactive astrocytes in neural repair and protection. *Neuroscientist* 11, 400–407. doi: 10.1177/1073858405278321

Sofroniew, M. V. (2009). Molecular dissection of reactive astrogliosis and glial scar formation. *Trends Neurosci.* 32, 638–647. doi: 10.1016/j.tins.2009.08.002

Song, G., Cechvala, C., Resnick, D. K., Dempsey, R. J., and Rao, V. L. (2001). GeneChip analysis after acute spinal cord injury in rat. *J. Neurochem.* 79, 804–815. doi: 10.1046/j.1471-4159.2001.00626.x

Sonkoly, E., and Pivarcsi, A. (2009). microRNAs in inflammation. *Int. Rev. Immunol.* 28, 535–561. doi: 10.3109/08830180903208303

Stefani, G., and Slack, F. J. (2008). Small non-coding RNAs in animal development. *Nat. Rev. Mol. Cell Biol.* 9, 219–230. doi: 10.1038/nrm2347

Strickland, E. R., Hook, M. A., Balaraman, S., Huie, J. R., Grau, J. W., and Miranda, R. C. (2011). MicroRNA dysregulation following spinal cord contusion: implications for neural plasticity and repair. *Neuroscience* 186, 146–160. doi: 10.1016/j.neuroscience.2011.03.063

Sugawara, T., Lewen, A., Gasche, Y., Yu, F., and Chan, P. H. (2002). Overexpression of SOD1 protects vulnerable motor neurons after spinal cord injury by attenuating mitochondrial cytochrome c release. *FASEB J.* 16, 1997–1999.

Taganov, K. D., Boldin, M. P., Chang, K. J., and Baltimore, D. (2006). NF-κB-dependent induction of microRNA miR-146, an inhibitor targeted to signaling proteins of innate immune responses. *Proc. Natl. Acad. Sci. U.S.A.* 103, 12481–12486. doi: 10.1073/pnas.0605298103

Tao, J., Wu, H., Lin, Q., Wei, W., Lu, X. H., Cantle, J. P., et al. (2011). Deletion of astroglial dicer causes non-cell-autonomous neuronal dysfunction and degeneration. *J. Neurosci.* 31, 8306–8319. doi: 10.1523/JNEUROSCI.0567-11.2011

Taoka, Y., Okajima, K., Uchiba, M., Murakami, K., Kushimoto, S., Johno, M., et al. (1997). Role of neutrophils in spinal cord injury in the rat. *Neuroscience* 79, 1177–1182. doi: 10.1016/S0306-4522(97)00011-0

Tili, E., Michaille, J. J., Cimino, A., Costinean, S., Dumitru, C. D., Adair, B., et al. (2007). Modulation of miR-155 and miR-125b levels following lipopolysaccharide/TNF-alpha stimulation and their possible roles in regulating the response to endotoxin shock. *J. Immunol.* 179, 5082–5089.

Treiber, T., Treiber, N., and Meister, G. (2012). Regulation of microRNA biogenesis and function. *Thromb. Haemost.* 107, 605–610. doi: 10.1160/TH11-12-0836

Tsang, J. S., Ebert, M. S., and van Oudenaarden, A. (2010). Genome-wide dissection of microRNA functions and cotargeting networks using gene set signatures. *Mol. Cell* 38, 140–153. doi: 10.1016/j.molcel.2010.03.007

Tyor, W. R., Avgeropoulos, N., Ohlandt, G., and Hogan, E. L. (2002). Treatment of spinal cord impact injury in the rat with transforming growth factor-beta. *J. Neurol. Sci.* 200, 33–41. doi: 10.1016/S0022-510X(02)00113-2

Velardo, M. J., Burger, C., Williams, P. R., Baker, H. V., Lopez, M. C., Mareci, T. H., et al. (2004). Patterns of gene expression reveal a temporally orchestrated wound healing response in the injured spinal cord. *J. Neurosci.* 24, 8562–8576. doi: 10.1523/JNEUROSCI.3316-04.2004

Visvanathan, J., Lee, S., Lee, B., Lee, J. W., and Lee, S. K. (2007). The microRNA miR-124 antagonizes the anti-neural REST/SCP1 pathway during embryonic CNS development. *Genes Dev.* 21, 744–749. doi: 10.1101/gad.1519107

Wang, J., Gu, Z., Ni, P., Qiao, Y., Chen, C., Liu, X., et al. (2011). NF-κB P50/P65 hetero-dimer mediates differential regulation of CD166/ALCAM expression via interaction with micoRNA-9 after serum deprivation, providing evidence for a novel negative auto-regulatory loop. *Nucleic Acids Res.* 39, 6440–6455. doi: 10.1093/nar/gkr302

Wang, M., Master, S. R., and Chodosh, L. A. (2006). Computational expression deconvolution in a complex mammalian organ. *BMC Bioinformatics* 7:328. doi: 10.1186/1471-2105-7-328

Wang, Z. (2010). MicroRNA: a matter of life or death. *World J. Biol. Chem.* 1, 41–54. doi: 10.4331/wjbc.v1.i4.41

Willemen, H. L., Huo, X. J., Mao-Ying, Q. L., Zijlstra, J., Heijnen, C. J., and Kavelaars, A. (2012). MicroRNA-124 as a novel treatment for persistent hyperalgesia. *J. Neuroinflammation* 9, 143. doi: 10.1186/1742-2094-9-143

Wu, C. I., Shen, Y., and Tang, T. (2009). Evolution under canalization and the dual roles of microRNAs: a hypothesis. *Genome Res.* 19, 734–743. doi: 10.1101/gr.084640.108

Wu, H., Neilson, J. R., Kumar, P., Manocha, M., Shankar, P., Sharp, P. A., et al. (2007). miRNA profiling of naive, effector and memory CD8 T cells. *PLoS ONE* 2:e1020. doi: 10.1371/journal.pone.0001020

Wu, X., Yoo, S., and Wrathall, J. R. (2005). Real-time quantitative PCR analysis of temporal-spatial alterations in gene expression after spinal cord contusion. *J. Neurochem.* 93, 943–952. doi: 10.1111/j.1471-4159.2005.03078.x

Xiao, Q., Du, Y., Wu, W., and Yip, H. K. (2010). Bone morphogenetic proteins mediate cellular response and, together with Noggin, regulate astrocyte differentiation after spinal cord injury. *Exp. Neurol.* 221, 353–366. doi: 10.1016/j.expneurol.2009.12.003

Yang, L., Jones, N. R., Blumbergs, P. C., Van Den Heuvel, C., Moore, E. J., Manavis, J., et al. (2005). Severity-dependent expression of pro-inflammatory cytokines in traumatic spinal cord injury in the rat. *J. Clin. Neurosci.* 12, 276–284. doi: 10.1016/j.jocn.2004.06.011

Young, M. R., Santhanam, A. N., Yoshikawa, N., and Colburn, N. H. (2010). Have tumor suppressor PDCD4 and its counteragent oncogenic miR-21 gone rogue? *Mol. Interv.* 10, 76–79. doi: 10.1124/mi.10.2.5

Yu, J. Y., Chung, K. H., Deo, M., Thompson, R. C., and Turner, D. L. (2008). MicroRNA miR-124 regulates neurite outgrowth during neuronal differentiation. *Exp. Cell Res.* 314, 2618–2633. doi: 10.1016/j.yexcr.2008.06.002

Yu, Y. M., Gibbs, K. M., Davila, J., Campbell, N., Sung, S., Todorova, T. I., et al. (2011). MicroRNA miR-133b is essential for functional recovery after spinal cord injury in adult zebrafish. *Eur. J. Neurosci.* 33, 1587–1597. doi: 10.1111/j.1460-9568.2011.07643.x

Yunta, M., Nieto-Diaz, M., Esteban, F. J., Caballero-Lopez, M., Navarro-Ruiz, R., Reigada, D., et al. (2012). MicroRNA dysregulation in the spinal cord following traumatic injury. *PLoS ONE* 7:e34534. doi: 10.1371/journal.pone.0034534

Zamanian, J. L., Xu, L., Foo, L. C., Nouri, N., Zhou, L., Giffard, R. G., et al. (2012). Genomic analysis of reactive astrogliosis. *J. Neurosci.* 32, 6391–6410. doi: 10.1523/JNEUROSCI.6221-11.2012

Zampetaki, A., and Mayr, M. (2012). Analytical challenges and technical limitations in assessing circulating miRNAs. *Thromb. Haemost.* 108, 592–598. doi: 10.1160/TH12-02-0097

Zhang, K. H., Xiao, H. S., Lu, P. H., Shi, J., Li, G. D., Wang, Y. T., et al. (2004). Differential gene expression after complete spinal cord transection in adult rats: an analysis focused on a subchronic post-injury stage. *Neuroscience* 128, 375–388. doi: 10.1016/j.neuroscience.2004.07.008

Zhang, Y., Liao, Y., Wang, D., He, Y., Cao, D., Zhang, F., et al. (2011). Altered expression levels of miRNAs in serum as sensitive biomarkers for early diagnosis of traumatic injury. *J. Cell. Biochem.* 112, 2435–2442. doi: 10.1002/jcb.23168

Zhao, C., Sun, G., Li, S., Lang, M. F., Yang, S., Li, W., et al. (2010a). MicroRNA let-7b regulates neural stem cell proliferation and differentiation by targeting nuclear receptor TLX signaling. *Proc. Natl. Acad. Sci. U.S.A.* 107, 1876–1881. doi: 10.1073/pnas.0908750107

Zhao, X., He, X., Han, X., Yu, Y., Ye, F., Chen, Y., et al. (2010b). MicroRNA-mediated control of oligodendrocyte differentiation. *Neuron* 65, 612–626. doi: 10.1016/j.neuron.2010.02.018

Zhu, H., and Fan, G. C. (2011). Extracellular/circulating microRNAs and their potential role in cardiovascular disease. *Am. J. Cardiovasc. Dis.* 1, 138–149.

Ziu, M., Fletcher, L., Savage, J. G., Jimenez, D. F., Digicaylioglu, M., and Bartanusz, V. (2013). Spatial and temporal expression levels of specific microRNAs in a spinal cord injury mouse model and their relationship to the duration of compression. *Spine J.* 14, 353–360. doi: 10.1016/j.spinee.2013.08.015

11

Non-coding RNA interact to regulate neuronal development and function

Bharat R. Iyengar[1,2], Ashwani Choudhary[3], Mayuresh A. Sarangdhar[3], K. V. Venkatesh[2], Chetan J. Gadgil[1] and Beena Pillai[3]*

[1] *CSIR-National Chemical Laboratory, Chemical Engineering and Process Development Division, Pune, India*
[2] *Department of Chemical Engineering, Indian Institute of Technology Bombay, Mumbai, India*
[3] *Functional Genomics, CSIR-Institute of Genomics and Integrative Biology, Delhi, India*

Correspondence:
Beena Pillai, Functional Genomics, CSIR-Institute of Genomics and Integrative Biology, Mathura Road, Delhi 110020, India
e-mail: beena@igib.in

The human brain is one of the most complex biological systems, and the cognitive abilities have greatly expanded compared to invertebrates without much expansion in the number of protein coding genes. This suggests that gene regulation plays a very important role in the development and function of nervous system, by acting at multiple levels such as transcription and translation. In this article we discuss the regulatory roles of three classes of non-protein coding RNAs (ncRNAs)—microRNAs (miRNAs), piwi-interacting RNA (piRNAs) and long-non-coding RNA (lncRNA), in the process of neurogenesis and nervous function including control of synaptic plasticity and potential roles in neurodegenerative diseases. miRNAs are involved in diverse processes including neurogenesis where they channelize the cellular physiology toward neuronal differentiation. miRNAs can also indirectly influence neurogenesis by regulating the proliferation and self renewal of neural stem cells and are dysregulated in several neurodegenerative diseases. miRNAs are also known to regulate synaptic plasticity and are usually found to be co-expressed with their targets. The dynamics of gene regulation is thus dependent on the local architecture of the gene regulatory network (GRN) around the miRNA and its targets. piRNAs had been classically known to regulate transposons in the germ cells. However, piRNAs have been, recently, found to be expressed in the brain and possibly function by imparting epigenetic changes by DNA methylation. piRNAs are known to be maternally inherited and we assume that they may play a role in early development. We also explore the possible function of piRNAs in regulating the expansion of transposons in the brain. Brain is known to express several lncRNA but functional roles in brain development are attributed to a few lncRNA while functions of most of the them remain unknown. We review the roles of some known lncRNA and explore the other possible functions of lncRNAs including their interaction with miRNAs.

Keywords: miRNA, piRNA, lncRNA, network-motifs, gene expression regulation

BACKGROUND

The complexity of the nervous system is evident at the organ-system level, cellular level and at the molecular level. The systems-level complexity of the neuronal system is due to the highly connected neuronal network wherein each neuron connects to many other neurons by establishing synapses. At the cellular level, the complexity of the neuronal system arises from the cellular heterogeneity of the vertebrate brain, carrying at least four distinctly different cell types-neurons including several bio-chemically diverse sub-classes, astrocytes, oligodendrocytes and microglia; that have specialized but interdependent functions. At the molecular level, the complexity arises from the ability to create functional diversity from the genome through mechanisms like alternative splicing and RNA editing that are more prevalent in the nervous system as compared to other tissues; which makes the brain have the most complex transcriptome (Ramsköld et al., 2009), compared to other organs. The fact that brain capacity and cognitive abilities have greatly expanded from invertebrates to humans with a much lesser increase in the number of protein coding genes, indicates that gene regulation plays a major role in the development and function of the nervous system.

It was a long held idea that proteins are the versatile catalysts of life processes and RNAs serve the role of relaying the genetic message for the protein output. However, some of the key cellular processes including the very process of protein synthesis, is controlled by RNAs and studies, over the years, have shown that the functional ability of RNAs is much more than what was previously assumed. The diverse class of non-protein coding RNAs (ncRNAs), including microRNAs (miRNA), piwi-interacting RNA (piRNA), long-non-coding RNA (lncRNA) etc, are mainly involved in regulation of gene expression and are thus integral parts of the gene regulatory network (GRN). The recent evidences demonstrating wide-spread transcription throughout the genome suggest that the non-coding RNA form a sizeable component of the transcriptome of a eukaryotic cell (Jacquier, 2009; Clark et al., 2011). Several recent reviews have comprehensively cataloged these regulatory ncRNAs and provide a wealth of emerging evidence regarding their biogenesis, interacting partners and ability to regulate key target genes (Liu and Paroo, 2010).

Here, after a brief introduction to these classes of non-coding RNAs, we focus on two critical aspects of non-coding RNA function in the development of the vertebrate nervous system: their expression pattern and the network architecture of their interactions with other genes. The regulatory nature of these interactions is derived as much from the inherent features of the network as from the identity and functions of the genes that form the network. This review therefore draws on the principles of systems biology to explore the network of non-coding RNA and target interactions in the context of the nervous system.

CLASSES OF NON-CODING RNAs

Currently, these non-coding RNAs are classified into functional groups, on the basis of the rather arbitrary criteria of size and a limited knowledge of their functional roles in the cell. The major classes of ncRNAs are lncRNA (Mercer et al., 2009), piRNA, endogeneous small interfering RNA (endo-siRNA) and miRNAs.

miRNAs in their mature form are, on an average, 22 nt long and repress mRNAs which harbor miRNA "target sites" or miRNA recognition elements (MRE) in their 3′UTRs. These target sites are partially complementary to the miRNA and interact with the latter by Watson-Crick type base pairing. Functional miRNAs are bound to Argonaute (Ago) proteins and constitute a ribonucleoprotein complex called RNA Induced Silencing Complex (RISC), that is tethered to mRNAs by the miRNA-mRNA interaction. miRNAs arise from longer transcripts, called pri-miRNAs (primary miRNAs). Stem-loop like structures on pri-miRNA are identified by Drosha-DGCR8 (microprocessor) complex and are liberated from the long transcript by ribonucleolytic cleavage, to give rise to precursor miRNA (pre-miRNA). Pre-miRNA is exported to cytoplasm by Exportin-5 where it is again cleaved by Dicer to produce an imperfect RNA duplex. One or both the strands of the duplex is incorporated into Ago proteins to form a functional RISC (**Figure 1A**). Alternatively, miRNAs can also arise from introns of other transcripts as a result of splicing and subsequent cleavage by Dicer and these intronic regions are referred to as mirtrons (Filipowicz et al., 2008). The expression of miRNA can, therefore, be regulated at transcriptional or post-transcriptional levels (Winter et al., 2009). Even though the MREs are partially complementary to the miRNA, a 7-8mer region, called the seed, corresponding to 2nd–9th position of the miRNA, is essential for miRNA mediated regulation (Filipowicz et al., 2008). However, the partial complementarity allows the miRNA to target several mRNAs simultaneously (Chi et al., 2009; Helwak et al., 2013), forming a network motif called single input module (SIM) (**Figure 1D**). This may help in canalization of the gene regulation program (Hornstein and Shomron, 2006).

piRNAs are slightly longer than miRNA (24–32 nt long) and associate with Piwi family of proteins which include Piwi, Aubergine (Aub) and Ago3 in Drosophila and MIWI, MILI, and MIWI2 in mouse. Even though the binding partners of piRNAs are structurally similar to the miRNA-binding Ago proteins, the piRNA biosynthetic pathway is very different from that of miRNA. piRNAs arise from specific genomic loci known as piRNA clusters and check transposon expansion. Initially piRNAs were reported in the Drosophila and Mouse germline (Ishizu et al., 2012); subsequently they were also reported in somatic tissues like ovarian follicular cells of Drosophila and nervous system of mouse (Lee et al., 2011) and Aplysia (Rajasethupathy et al., 2012). Another class of piRNAs is predominantly expressed in mouse spermatids during pachytene stage of meiosis I. This class of piRNA is expressed in high abundance in these cells but its functions and putative targets, remain unknown. piRNA clusters store transposon derived sequences; transcripts arising from these clusters associate with Piwi-proteins (Piwi and Aub in Drosophila and MIWI and MILI in mouse) and are trimmed from the 3′ end to generate primary piRNAs. The 3′ end is 2′-O-methylated which makes the piRNA stable. Primary piRNA can undergo a cycle of amplification, called ping-pong cycle, to generate secondary piRNAs (Ishizu et al., 2012). Unlike Drosophila where cleavage is sufficient to repress transposons, piRNA-mediated transposon repression predominantly happens via DNA methylation in mouse (Aravin et al., 2008; Watanabe et al., 2011). The exact mechanism of this process is yet to be explored.

lncRNAs are a diverse set that are loosely defined as ncRNAs longer than 200 nt that lack apparent protein coding ability due to the absence of a relatively long uninterrupted open reading frame. Therefore, unlike miRNAs or piRNAs, the lncRNAs differ greatly from each other with respect to size, interacting partners and mode of action. Most lncRNA regulate gene expression by affecting chromatin dynamics or providing scaffold/tether to regulatory proteins (Mercer et al., 2009). lncRNAs typically have the same structural features as mRNAs such as the 5′ cap, polyadenylated 3′ tail and undergo splicing to give rise to the final product. They are localized both to the nucleus and cytoplasm, but the signals that drive their localization are not known. The genomic loci of lncRNA can provide clues to their regulatory targets as it is observed that genes that are regulated by an lncRNA are usually located very proximal to it on the genome. Unlike miRNAs, they are not highly conserved and their primary sequence has not provided much information about their function. Recently, it has been shown that several lncRNAs maybe spliced at their 5′ and 3′ ends to form circular RNAs (Memczak et al., 2013). However the functional importance of circularization, presumably for increased stability, has not been established.

miRNAs can interact with lncRNA (Jalali et al., 2013) and circular RNAs (Hansen et al., 2013; Memczak et al., 2013) besides their mRNA targets suggesting that in the cell, these ncRNAs may exist as a network of mutually regulating entities. They can possibly serve as sinks that sequester each other temporarily, or even target each other for degradation by the formation of dsRNA.

There are several lines of evidence which suggest that some of these ncRNAs have functional roles in the brain. Regulation by miRNAs is well known in the brain where they regulate neurogenesis and synaptic plasticity. Moreover, mRNAs in brain have extended 3′UTRs, which suggests that the component of regulation by miRNA or other forms of post-transcriptional mechanisms is higher in the brain compared to other tissues (Ramsköld et al., 2009; Miura et al., 2013). Brain also expresses several lncRNAs (Mercer et al., 2008) and is the only non-germline associated somatic tissue presently known to express piRNAs (Lee et al., 2011; Rajasethupathy et al., 2012). In this article we discuss how these three classes of ncRNAs regulate development of nervous system and maintenance of its activities. We primarily emphasize on the role of these ncRNAs as a part of the GRN and how their connectivity determines the functional output. We shed light on the effects of miRNA mediated regulation when they are present in certain types of network motifs.

NETWORK MOTIFS

In network terminology, each interacting entity is called a node and the interactions are called edges. A GRN is a directed network of gene products (including proteins and RNAs), in which certain genes control the expression of other genes. Since the interaction can either activate (positive) or repress (negative) the "target" gene, the edges of a GRN carry a sign along with direction. It is evident that for a given set of nodes several theoretically possible networks can be defined by taking all the combinations of edges from one gene to the other. However, real networks form a small subset of this large number of theoretically possible networks. Network motifs are the patterns of connections that are highly prevalent in real networks compared to what would be expected in a random network with the same set of nodes. This indicates that network motifs were selected over other patterns of connections because of the unique functions that the former can perform as a result of their structure. Network motifs form functional modules in a real network such as GRN: some common network motifs in the GRN include feedback loops (FBL) (autoregulation), feedforward loops (FFL), SIM, multiple input modules and dense overlapping regulons (Alon, 2007).

A gene "X" can regulate a target gene "Y" via multiple intermediates; the sign of the path from X to Y is the product of the signs of all the intermediate edges. If there is a path from a gene back to itself then the resultant network is called a FBL and based on the sign of this path there are two types of FBL: positive and negative, which perform distinct functions (**Figures 1B,C**).

In a FFL a node targets another node via two parallel branches. If the sign of both the branches are similar then the FFL is called coherent; otherwise incoherent. There are four types each of coherent and incoherent FFLs. Some types of FFL are more commonly observed than the others and are therefore well studied (**Figures 1E,F**). Like in the case of FBL, each type of FFL is associated with a unique function.

SIM is a network motif in which one node targets at least two nodes (**Figure 1D**). This is exemplified by one transcription factor or miRNA regulating many genes simultaneously. (Readers are encouraged to refer to Alon, 2007 for details on network motifs in GRN).

Since a gene is a part of a network, its regulation (or the regulation it exerts) cannot be studied in isolation. The study of the entire GRN would be cumbersome and intensive; however, because of the modular nature of the network motifs, they can be studied in isolation and their dynamic effect on the GRN can be predicted. Most of the network motifs discussed in this article are local; these in turn can be a part of a larger motif.

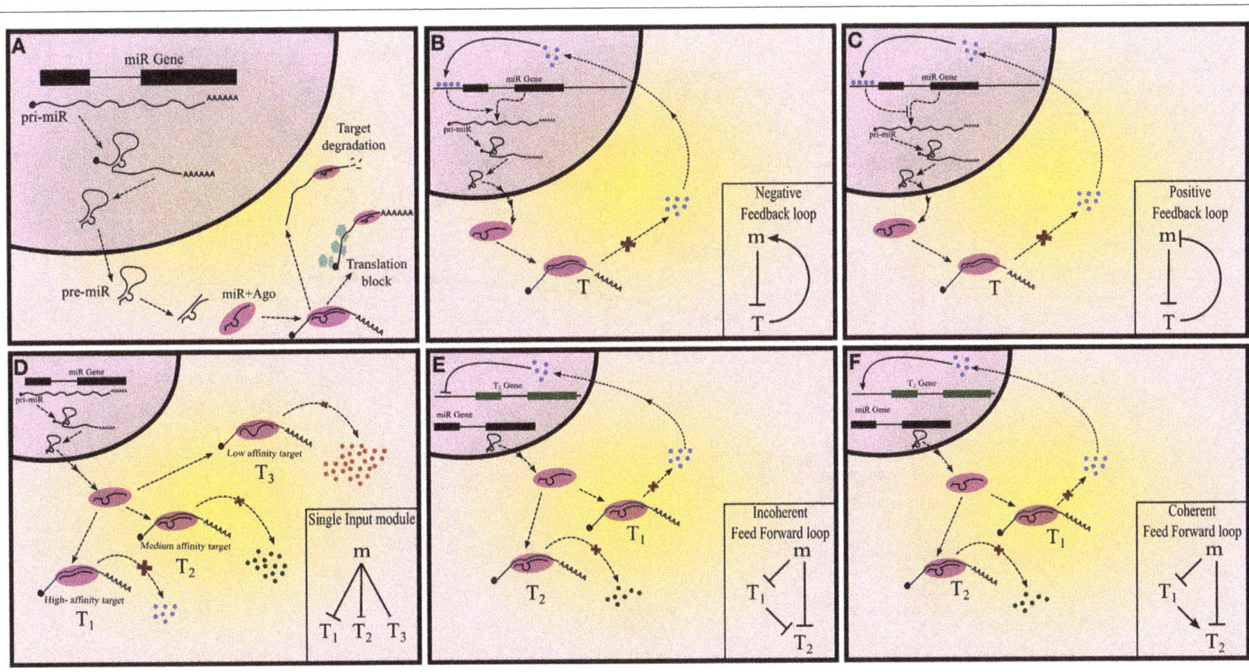

FIGURE 1 | Summary of different types of network motifs in miRNA mediated gene regulatory networks. (A) Summary of miRNA biogenesis and mechanism of action. **(B)** Positive and **(C)** negative feedback loops, with a miRNA and a transcription factor. **(D)** Single input module with miRNA regulating three target nodes. The extent of regulation can differ between different targets. Feed-forward loops **(E)** Incoherent and **(F)** coherent feedforward loops with a miRNA regulating the target-T_2.

miRNAs

miRNAs and transcription factors are the best studied components of the GRNs that underlie many developmental gene expression programs. Both of them can modulate the expression of multiple targets, alter cell fate and are often engaged in mutually reinforcing functions. However, miRNAs differ from transcription factors in many critical ways (Hobert, 2008). Firstly, almost all the known miRNAs are repressors while transcription factors are either repressors or activators and in some rare cases can act as both depending on the target and interacting partners. Secondly, miRNAs usually bring about downregulation of their targets by a post-transcriptional mechanism, by degrading the target RNA or blocking its translation. Transcription factor interaction with target DNA is largely mediated through structural elements while miRNA interaction with targets is largely governed by the rules of nucleic acid complementarity and are therefore more easily predicted. When a particular gene is targeted by a transcription factor there is usually a single or at most a few tandemly repeated sites present at that locus. However, a typical miRNA-target interaction is characterized by miRNA molecules that have to bind to several messenger RNA molecules. Lastly, transcription factors are usually not consumed in the transcription factor-DNA interactions and may indeed engage in multiple rounds of regulation. The fate of the miRNA engaged in miRNA-target complexes is not understood with similar clarity.

A general principle derived from empirical studies is that, usually, the lifetime of a response is inversely correlated with the response speed. Cell signaling responses, which usually rely on post-translational modifications or conformational changes of proteins, are fast but transient whereas transcriptional or epigenetic responses are long-lived but have a slow response. Post-transcriptional mechanisms, such as miRNA-mediated regulation, fall between these two extremes; faster than transcriptional regulation and relatively stable compared to cell signaling responses. The slow response time of transcriptional repression also results because of the continued presence of stable messenger RNAs since the already existing mRNAs continue to produce proteins. Indeed RNA degradation signals have evolved to ensure rapid turn-over of certain messenger RNAs but they do not allow regulation of the turn-over. miRNAs, can accelerate the response by rapidly clearing these mRNAs along with minimizing the effect of leaky transcription (Hornstein and Shomron, 2006). Therefore miRNA mediated regulation may be preferred over transcriptional regulation in certain situations while, in other situations it may by used along with the latter as a reinforcement.

The miRNAs that play an important role in regulation of the neuronal system act at three levels that in turn correspond to three different developmental time scales. During the earliest stages of development of the nervous system, the numbers of neural stem cells are determined through a wave of neural stem cell proliferation followed by a phase of massive apoptosis (Buss and Oppenheim, 2004). Several miRNAs regulate the development of nervous system by either promoting cell division by repressing pro-apoptotic genes or later promote apoptosis by shutting down pro-survival signals during this early phase of development. miR-29b targets multiple BH3 family of pro-apoptotic genes such as Bim, Bmf, Puma, Bak, and Hrk during early neural differentiation (**Figure 2**). miR-29b mediated repression of apoptosis in the surviving healthy neurons is essential for neural development (Kole et al., 2011).

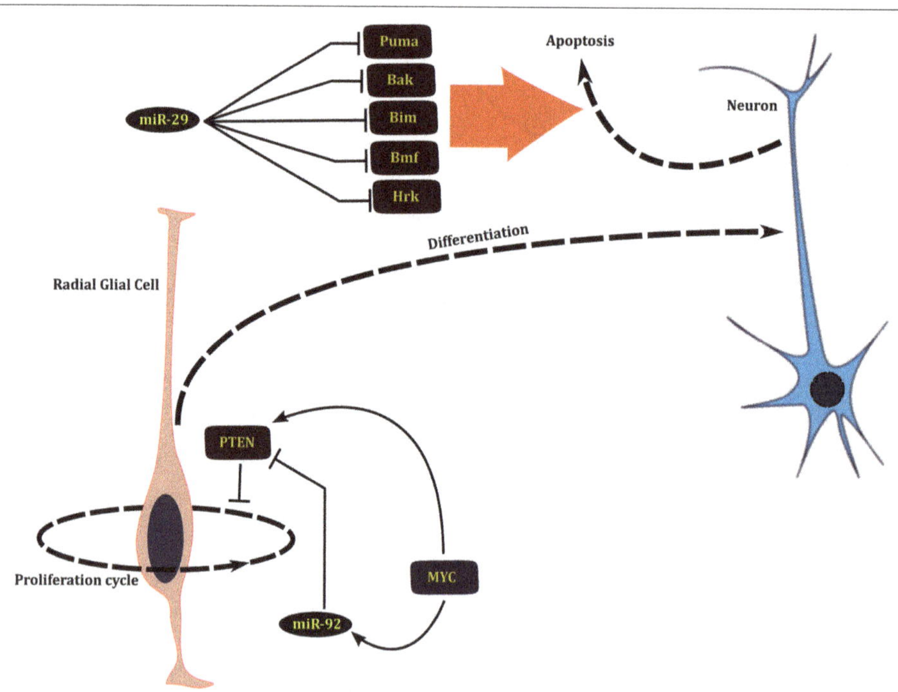

FIGURE 2 | miRNAs affect the development of nervous system by regulating proliferation of neural progenitors and apoptosis of young neurons.

A second set of miRNAs regulate the development of nervous system by either promoting differentiation (developmental function) or allowing the initial expansion of neural progenitors (maintenance function). miR-124 and miR-9 are classical examples of miRNAs associated with developmental functions. miR-124 targets several genes including Poly-Pyrimidine Tract Binding Protein-1 (PTBP1) (Makeyev et al., 2007), Small C-terminal domain Phosphatase 1 (SCP1/CTDSP1) (Visvanathan et al., 2007), Laminin-γ (LAMC1) and Integrin-β1 (ITGB1) (Cao et al., 2007), to promote neuronal differentiation (**Figure 3**). This type of interaction (also the previously discussed case of miR-29b) forms a network motif called SIM in which a single factor acts on multiple downstream genes. This network architecture allows coordinated regulation of a set of targets that are perhaps simultaneously required to be cleared. Each of these targets in turn may target several genes thus amplifying the scope of regulation. An interesting case is that of PTBP1, a splicing factor, whose downregulation by miR-124 causes a global change in alternative splicing patterns, leading to expression of several neuronal transcript variants. In transcription factor based networks, it has been shown that as the concentration of the transcription factor increases over time following an activating signal, the targets maybe switched on, one after the other in the order of their affinity for the factor (Kalir et al., 2001). Although such an evidence of temporal regulation does not exist for miRNA encoded SIMs, the understanding of the properties of a SIM allows a general extrapolation. When the expression of an miRNA is knocked down partially, the targets with the lowest affinity are likely to be relieved of repression while high affinity targets may continue to be repressed. Attempts to target miRNAs for therapeutic applications have to consider this aspect of miRNA mediated targeting.

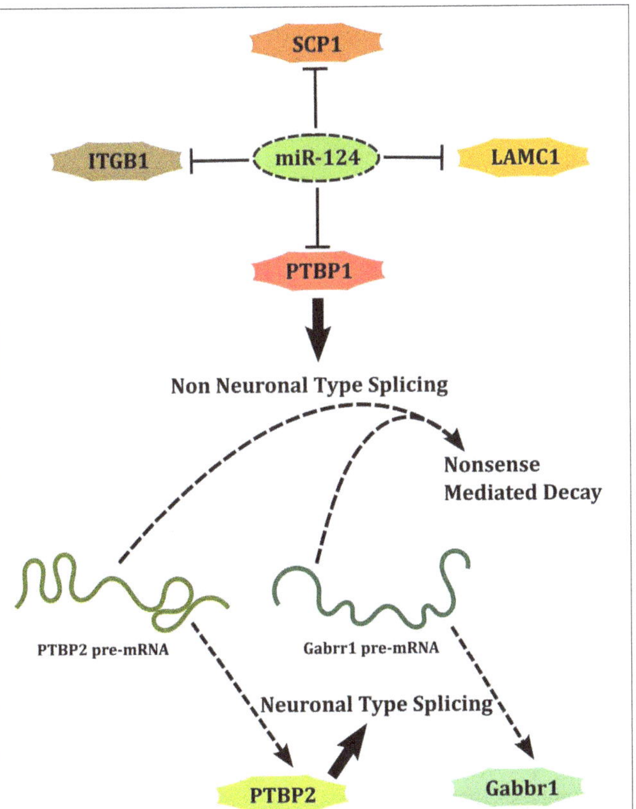

FIGURE 3 | miR-124 promotes neuronal differentiation by acting through a SIM. PTBP1 is downstream of miR-124 and is a part of another SIM.

The products of the miR-9 precursor—miR-9-3p and miR-9-5p—target the transcription factors REST and CoREST, respectively (Packer et al., 2008). In the proliferating progenitors, REST-CoREST, transcriptionally repress all the miR-9 genes, miR-9-1/2/3, and other neuronal genes. This mutual repression between miR-9 and REST-CoREST gives rise to a positive FBL (PFBL). miR-9 is also involved in a PFBL with TLX (**Figure 4**); a factor that regulates proliferation of neural progenitors (Zhao et al., 2009). It can be observed that developmental functions of miRNAs are associated with network motifs like SIM and PFBL. Multiple targets of a miRNA in a SIM allows simultaneous action on several genes thereby canalizing the cell toward differentiation. PFBLs give rise to bistability; existence of two stable steady states, i.e., differentiated and stem cell state. Examples of PFBL mediated switching behavior is also evident in case of transcriptional regulation; the most famous example would be the switching between lytic and lysogenic phenotypes in λ-phage.

Neural development is also indirectly affected by regulation of self-renewal and expansion of neural progenitors. Phosphatidylinsositide 3-kinase (PI3K)/Akt pathway is involved in growth and self renewal of stem cells whose dysregulation is implicated in several cancers. This pathway is also involved in regulation of neurogenesis; brains of *Akt3* knockout mice are greatly reduced in size (Easton et al., 2005). PTEN, which is a negative regulator of this pathway, is in turn regulated by the miR-17–92 cluster of miRNAs and loss of these miRNAs leads to suppression of neural stem cell expansion (Bian et al., 2013). Network analysis by El Baroudi et al. (2011) reveals that both the miR-17–2 cluster and PTEN are positively regulated by MYC, constituting a type 1 incoherent FFL (1I-FFL) (**Figure 2**). One of the functions that miRNAs perform as a part of 1I-FFL is to buffer transcriptional noise (Osella et al., 2011).

miRNA are also involved in maintenance of neuronal function by regulating synaptic plasticity. Since neurons are highly polarized cells with the nucleus quite distant from the dendritic spines, a local regulatory mechanism is required near the synapses to control protein synthesis at these regions. In other words, a transcriptional regulation in response to synaptic signals would be delayed and therefore miRNA mediated regulation is of great importance in neurons. miR-134 (Schratt et al., 2006) and miR-132 (Wayman et al., 2008; Mellios et al., 2011) are known to regulate synaptic plasticity and the morphology of dendritic spines. miR-134 is also shown to localize at the dendritic spines and repress LIMK1 (Schratt et al., 2006). It is to be noticed that under these conditions, the miRNA mediated regulation doesn't cause transcript degradation but rather, causes a translational repression. RNA binding proteins such as Dnd1 (Kedde et al., 2007) and HuR (Kundu et al., 2012) are reported to reverse miRNA mediated translational repression in germline and liver tissue. Banerjee et al. (2009) have reported that MOV10, a component of RISC,

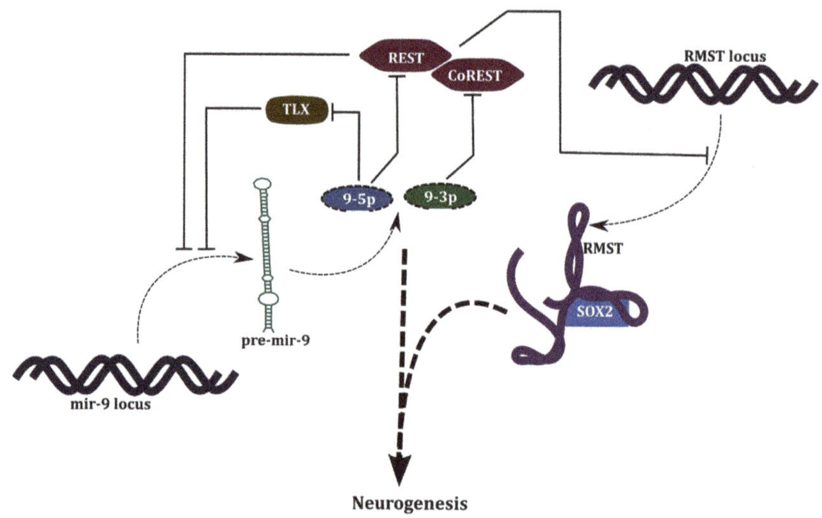

FIGURE 4 | Regulation of neurogenesis by miR-9 and lncRNA- RMST.

is rapidly degraded via NMDA-receptor mediated signaling, in dendritic spines. This relieves certain mRNAs, including LIMK1 and LYPA1, from miRNA mediated regulation. miRNAs have also been shown to specifically localize in the axons (Sasaki et al., 2013; Hancock et al., 2014); however, the list of axonally enriched miRNAs reported by these two studies are non-overlapping. Hancock et al. have found that miR-132 promotes axonal extension in mouse dorsal root ganglionic (DRG) neurons, by targeting Rasa1. In other studies it has been shown that certain miRNAs like miR-9 (Dajas-Bailador et al., 2012) and miR-138 (Liu et al., 2013) inhibit axonal extension by targeting Map1b and SIRT1, respectively. miRNAs are also implicated in regulation of axon regeneration, post-injury. Injury to sciatic nerve leads to upregulation of miR-21 and miR-431 in the DRG. Also, it was shown that miR-21 and miR-431 promote neurite outgrowth in cultured DRG neurons by targeting Spry2 and Kremen1, respectively (Strickland et al., 2011; Wu and Murashov, 2013a). Taken together, these facts indicate that miRNAs can perform contrasting roles in axonal regulation. Kaplan et al. (2013) and Wu and Murashov (2013b) have extensively reviewed this aspect of miRNA function in the nervous system. Many miRNA are known to co-express with their targets in the neurons suggesting that they might be controlled by a common regulator (Tsang et al., 2007). The fact that miRNAs and their targets are spatiotemporally co-expressed suggests that, in neurons, miRNAs are preferred over transcriptional mechanisms for dynamic gene regulation.

piRNA

piRNAs are a relatively new class of small non-coding RNAs originally discovered in mouse germline tissues. piRNAs are known to suppress transposable elements in the germline tissues, thereby protecting the germline DNA from deleterious mutations; dysregulation of piRNA pathway results in defects in germ cell proliferation and hence resulting in the loss of fertility. Although most studies on piRNA have been on its role in the germline, a few studies have reported their presence and function in somatic cells (Malone et al., 2009; Lee et al., 2011; Rajasethupathy et al., 2012).

The first evidence of piRNA in nervous system was reported by Lee et al. in which piRNAs in the mouse hippocampus were detected by deep sequencing of small RNA libraries and applying stringent criteria to filter other small RNA sequences including miRNAs (Lee et al., 2011). Some candidate sequences were also found to be associated with MIWI by real-time PCR. Further they showed the presence of the abundant piRNA complexes in the dendritic spines and the knockdown of piRNAs resulted in reduced spine density in the axons.

In another report it was shown that approximately 300 genomic regions encode for piRNAs in the neurons of the Aplysia (Rajasethupathy et al., 2012). It was shown that certain piRNAs are induced by serotonin (5-HT) signaling. Subsequently, using Piwi knockdown studies, it was found that piRNA pathway leads to methylation of CREB2, thereby reducing its expression and promoting memory formation. Even though Rajasethupathy et al. argue that the previous report of piRNA in the brain by Lee et al. is a misclassification and may have arisen because of RNA impurities, a careful analysis from multiple model systems is required to fully comprehend the role of piRNAs in the nervous system.

Despite these reports, the presence of piRNA in the brain is not fully justified. A possible clue about the functions of piRNA in the brain comes from the discovery of the L1 retrotransposons in the brain. These elements have been shown to be regulated during neuronal differentiation and hypothesized to give rise to neuronal heterogeneity and somatic mosacism in brain (Muotri et al., 2005; Coufal et al., 2009). It has been already shown that L1 retrotransposons are regulated by piRNAs in the germline tissues. The presence of both piRNAs and L1 retrotransposons in the brain suggests that the former may regulate the latter in the brain as well.

Recently, it has been shown that the there is extensive transposon expression in the αβ neurons of mushroom bodies in the Drosophila brain, compared to the adjacent neurons (Perrat et al.,

2013). In contrast Ago3 and Aub show a low expression in the αβ neurons compared to the rest of the brain. Moreover, mutants of different piRNA pathway components, i.e., Aub, Ago3, and Armi showed elevated levels of transposon expression in the brain. Considering all these observations it can be proposed, though not conclusively stated, that piRNAs are present in the brain for controlling transposons and repeat derived RNAs, and thereby regulating somatic heterogeneity.

lncRNA

lncRNAs have been reported in the brain and known to be associated with specific regions (Mercer et al., 2008). Many of these are found to be specifically expressed during the development of the brain and neural cell differentiation (Ng et al., 2012).

Although it is difficult to classify lncRNAs based on their structural or mechanistic features, lncRNAs are associated with specific roles that they play in the development and functioning of the nervous system therefore allowing a functional classification. There are two functional groups of lncRNAs associated with the development of nervous system—lncRNAs that promote either the self-renewal of neural stem cells or neural differentiation. Another group of lncRNAs are involved in the maintenance of the functioning of nervous system, such as regulation of synaptic activity.

In the previously mentioned study by Ng et al., it was found that three lncRNAs, designated as lncRNA_ES1, lncRNA_ES2, and lncRNA_ES3, are specifically associated with pluripotent stem cells (Ng et al., 2012) lncRNA_ES1 and lncRNA_ES3 had binding sites for the pluripotency associated transcription factors OCT4 and NANOG, and just NANOG respectively; it was further confirmed that knockdown of these proteins reduced the levels of these lncRNAs. The role of these lncRNAs in maintenance of pluripotency was confirmed when their knockdown resulted in reduced percentage of pluripotent cells. These lncRNA_ES1/2 were found to be associated with the PRC2 component SUZ12, suggesting that they indirectly regulate pro-differentiation genes by repressing their transcription.

In the same study four lncRNAs- RMST, lncRNA_N1, lncRNA_N2, and lncRNA_N3, were identified to be associated with neuronal differentiation and their knockdown resulted in reduction in number of neurons in culture along with a reduced expression of neuronal markers and increased expression of glial markers. Out of these, lncRNA_N2 was found to harbor neurogenesis associated miRNAs- miR-125b and let-7 in its intronic regions. In a subsequent study by the same group it was shown that RMST is transcriptionally repressed by REST (**Figure 4**). Also, it was shown that RMST associates with SOX2 and tethers it to promoters of neurogenetic genes like DLX1, NEUROG2 and ASCL1, thereby inducing their expression (Ng et al., 2013). DLX1 locus also encodes an antisense-lncRNA, DLX1AS which is expressed during neurogenesis in the subventricular zone of hippocampus, and positively regulates the expression of DLX1 and DLX2 (Ramos et al., 2013).

lncRNAs that are involved in maintenance activities regulate the general functioning of neurons and control processes such as synaptic signaling. BC1 which is a cytoplasmic lncRNA, localizes to dendrites and is involved in regulating the post-synaptic signaling, by repressing metabotropic glutamate receptor signaling (mGluR) induced local protein synthesis. BC1 represses translation initiation by interacting with eIF4A and poly-A binding protein (PABP), thereby disallowing the recruitment of the small ribosomal subunit to the mRNA (Wang et al., 2005). Loss of BC1 results in hyperexcitation of the neurons (Zhong et al., 2009) and is implicated in the mouse models of epilepsy (Gitaí et al., 2011). One of the genes induced by mGluR is Fragile-X mental retardation protein (FMRP), which is significantly upregulated in BC1 knockouts (Zhong et al., 2009). However, FMRP is also involved in controlling hyperexcitability of neurons by regulating protein synthesis and it has been shown that double knockout of FMRP and BC1 results in a more severe epileptic phenotype (Zhong et al., 2010) This suggests that FMRP supplements BC1 and may rescue any imbalance caused by fluctuations in BC1 activity.

BACE1 is a membrane protease which is implicated in Alzheimer's Disease by promoting cleavage of Amyloid Precursor Protein (APP) to form Amyloid-Beta 1-42 (Abeta 1-42) peptide. BACE1-Anti Sense (BACE1AS) RNA is partially complementary to BACE1 coding region (CDS) and renders stability to the mRNA, thereby leading to upregulation of Abeta 1-42. BACE1AS

Table 1 | Summary of lncRNAs involved in the development of the nervous system.

lncRNA	Biological function	Mechanism	References
Gomafu	Neurogenesis, oligodendrocyte lineage specification	Binds to QKI and SRSF1 and regulates splicing	Tsuiji et al., 2011; Qureshi et al., 2010
Anti-NOS2A	Neuronal differentiation	Represses NOS2A	Korneev et al., 2008
MALAT-1	Synaptogenesis	Splicing regulation	Bernard et al., 2010
EVF-2	Differentiation of GABAergic neurons	Activates Dlx-5/6	Bond et al., 2009
TUG1	Retinal differentiation	–	Young et al., 2005
NEAT1	Neuronal/oligodendrocyte differentiation	Paraspeckle integrity	Mercer et al., 2010
Sox8OT	Oligodendrocyte lineage commitment	–	Mercer et al., 2010
Nkx2.2AS	Oligodendrocyte differentiation	–	Tochitani and Hayashizaki, 2008
HAR1F	Neural development	Reelin upregulation	Pollard et al., 2006
HOTAIRM	Neuronal differentiation	–	Lin et al., 2011
SIX3OS	Retinal differentiation	Recruiting Ezh2	Rapicavoli et al., 2011
POU3F2	Neural stem cell proliferation	–	Ramos et al., 2013

is in turn upregulated because of the cellular stress due to Abeta 1-42, thereby further increasing Abeta 1-42 via BACE1. This results in a PFBL (Faghihi et al., 2008), however, in this study the authors have called it a feedforward regulation. It had been subsequently shown that BACE1AS stabilizes BACE1 mRNA by masking a non-canonical target site for miR-485-5p in the CDS of BACE1 mRNA (Faghihi et al., 2010).

In another contrasting case of antisense lncRNA mediated regulation, BDNF-AS represses Brain Derived Neurotrophic Factor (BDNF) and results in restriction of neurite growth. Also, this regulation occurs at the level of transcription where BDNF-AS helps in recruiting EZH2, which is a part of Polycomb Repressive Complex 2 (PRC2) and marks histones with repressive lysine methylation- H3k4me3 (Modarresi et al., 2012).

There are many other lncRNAs implicated in the development and function of nervous system but the targets and mechanisms are unknown for a majority of them; **Table 1** summarizes these different lncRNAs. In many cases lncRNAs emerge from the same genomic locus as their targets; this targeting is based on simple base pairing can happen at the level of either DNA or RNA. Some lncRNAs such as RMST act on several genes by tethering transcription factors to their promoters or serving as a scaffold for the assembly of RNA-binding proteins.

CONCLUDING REMARKS

Recent studies have revealed the importance of RNA mediated gene regulation in diverse biological processes. There are some advantages of having ncRNAs as gene expression regulators compared to an exclusively protein-regulated GRN. Since there is no step of translation, the cost as well the time required for making an ncRNA would be less compared to that of a protein. ncRNAs can target genes based on simple base pairing interactions; therefore evolution of such a regulator has a higher likelihood.

miRNA based regulation has a special importance in the highly polarized neurons as they control local translation at the dendrites thereby preventing the delay that can arise in transcriptional responses because of RNA synthesis and transport to distant cellular regions. Even though the exact importance of piRNAs in the brain is not understood it is highly likely that they regulate retrotransposons. Unlike miRNAs and piRNAs that are mostly repressors, lncRNAs can either activate or repress a gene. Since the dsDNA has limited ability to adopt distinctive structures, the DNA binding specificity of transcription factors and other DNA binding proteins relies on a limited repertoire of DNA binding domains. Long RNAs on the other hand are structured and proteins can bind to specific structures more effectively. The sequence information in the RNA can provide additional specificity to the binding. Thus lncRNAs may efficiently bridge the interactions between protein and DNA. lncRNAs can also mark large genomic regions for epigenetic regulation as in the case of XIST. It has also been argued that it is the act of transcription and not the product per-se, that causes the regulation (Berretta and Morillon, 2009).

Although these regulatory RNAs act via different mechanisms, usually their roles are convergent with that of the protein based transcriptional regulation to ensure an efficient and foolproof control of gene expression. As evident in many studies, blocking the activity of these regulatory RNAs affects the gene regulation to different extents. Therefore it is undeniable that ncRNAs supplement the gene regulation by proteins and are not merely redundant pathways. A systems-level analysis of ncRNAs is essential to understand their precise roles and the ability to confer robustness to the GRN.

ACKNOWLEDGMENTS

Bharat R. Iyengar and Ashwani Choudhary acknowledge the Council of Scientific and Industrial Research (CSIR), India and Mayuresh A. Sarangdhar acknowledges the University Grants Commission (UGC), India for research fellowships. The authors acknowledge CSIR-Institute of Genomics and Integrative Biology projects BSC0123 and BSC0124 for funding and for approving the manuscript for publication.

REFERENCES

Alon, U. (2007). Network motifs: theory and experimental approaches. *Nat. Rev. Genet.* 8, 450–461. doi: 10.1038/nrg2102

Aravin, A. A., Sachidanandam, R., Bourc'his, D., Schaefer, C., Pezic, D., Toth, K. F., et al. (2008). A piRNA pathway primed by individual transposons is linked to *de novo* DNA methylation in mice. *Mol. Cell* 31, 785–799. doi: 10.1016/j.molcel.2008.09.003

Banerjee, S., Neveu, P., and Kosik, K. S. (2009). A coordinated local translational control point at the synapse involving relief from silencing and MOV10 degradation. *Neuron* 64, 871–884. doi: 10.1016/j.neuron.2009.11.023

Bernard, D., Prasanth, K. V., Tripathi, V., Colasse, S., Nakamura, T., Xuan, Z., et al. (2010). A long nuclear-retained non-coding RNA regulates synaptogenesis by modulating gene expression. *EMBO J.* 29, 3082–3093. doi: 10.1038/emboj.2010.199

Berretta, J., and Morillon, A. (2009). Pervasive transcription constitutes a new level of eukaryotic genome regulation. *EMBO Rep.* 10, 973–982. doi: 10.1038/embor.2009.181

Bian, S., Hong, J., Li, Q., Schebelle, L., Pollock, A., Knauss, J. L., et al. (2013). MicroRNA cluster miR-17-92 regulates neural stem cell expansion and transition to intermediate progenitors in the developing mouse neocortex. *Cell Rep.* 3, 1398–1406. doi: 10.1016/j.celrep.2013.03.037

Bond, A. M., Vangompel, M. J., Sametsky, E. A., Clark, M. F., Savage, J. C., Disterhoft, J. F., et al. (2009). Balanced gene regulation by an embryonic brain ncRNA Is critical for adult hippocampal GABA circuitry. *Nat. Neurosci.* 12, 1020–1027. doi: 10.1038/nn.2371

Buss, R. R., and Oppenheim, R. W. (2004). Role of programmed cell death in normal neuronal development and function. *Anat. Sci. Int.* 79, 191–197. doi: 10.1111/j.1447-073x.2004.00088.x

Cao, X., Pfaff, S. L., and Gage, F. H. (2007). A functional study of miR-124 in the developing neural tube. *Genes Dev.* 21, 531–536. doi: 10.1101/gad.1519207

Chi, S. W., Zang, J. B., Mele, A., and Darnell, R. B. (2009). Argonaute HITS-CLIP decodes microRNA-mRNA interaction maps. *Nature* 460, 479–486. doi: 10.1038/nature08170

Clark, M. B., Amaral, P. P., Schlesinger, F. J., Dinger, M. E., Taft, R. J., Rinn, J. L., et al. (2011). The reality of pervasive transcription. *PLoS Biol.* 9:e1000625. doi: 10.1371/journal.pbio.1000625

Coufal, N. G., Garcia-Perez, J. L., Peng, G. E., Yeo, G. W., Mu, Y., Lovci, M. T., et al. (2009). L1 retrotransposition in human neural progenitor cells. *Nature* 460, 1127–1131. doi: 10.1038/nature08248

Dajas-Bailador, F., Bonev, B., Garcez, P., Stanley, P., Guillemot, F., and Papalopulu, N. (2012). microRNA-9 regulates axon extension and branching by targeting map1b in mouse cortical neurons. *Nat. Neurosci.* 15, 697–699. doi: 10.1038/nn.3082

Easton, R. M., Cho, H., Roovers, K., Shineman, D. W., Mizrahi, M., Forman, M. S., et al. (2005). Role for Akt3/protein kinase Bγ in attainment of normal brain size. *Mol. Cell. Biol.* 25, 1869–1878. doi: 10.1128/MCB.25.5.1869-1878.2005

El Baroudi, M., Corà, D., Bosia, C., Osella, M., and Caselle, M. (2011). A curated database of miRNA mediated feed-forward loops involving MYC as master regulator. *PLoS ONE* 6:e14742. doi: 10.1371/journal.pone.0014742

Faghihi, M. A., Modarresi, F., Khalil, A. M., Wood, D. E., Sahagan, B. G., Morgan, T. E., et al. (2008). Expression of a noncoding RNA is elevated in Alzheimer's disease and drives rapid feed-forward regulation of [beta]-secretase. *Nat. Med.* 14, 723–730. doi: 10.1038/nm1784

Faghihi, M. A., Zhang, M., Huang, J., Modarresi, F., Van der Brug, M. P., Nalls, M. A., et al. (2010). Evidence for natural antisense transcript-mediated inhibition of microRNA function. *Genome Biol.* 11, R56. doi: 10.1038/nm1784

Filipowicz, W., Bhattacharyya, S. N., and Sonenberg, N. (2008). Mechanisms of post-transcriptional regulation by microRNAs: are the answers in sight? *Nat. Rev. Genet.* 9, 102–114. doi: 10.1038/nrg2290

Gitaí, D. L., Fachin, A. L., Mello, S. S., Elias, C. F., Bittencourt, J. C., Leite, J. P., et al. (2011). The Non-coding RNA BC1 Is down-regulated in the hippocampus of Wistar Audiogenic Rat (WAR) strain after audiogenic kindling. *Brain Res.* 1367, 114–121. doi: 10.1016/j.brainres.2010.10.069

Hancock, M. L., Preitner, N., Quan, J., and Flanagan, J. G. (2014). MicroRNA-132 is enriched in developing axons, locally regulates Rasa1 mRNA, and promotes axon extension. *J. Neurosci.* 34, 66–78. doi: 10.1523/JNEUROSCI.3371-13.2014

Hansen, T. B., Jensen, T. I., Clausen, B. H., Bramsen, J. B., Finsen, B., Damgaard, C. K., et al. (2013). Natural RNA circles function as efficient microRNA sponges. *Nature* 495, 384–388. doi: 10.1038/nature11993

Helwak, A., Kudla, G., Dudnakova, T., and Tollervey, D. (2013). Mapping the human miRNA interactome by CLASH reveals frequent noncanonical binding. *Cell* 153, 654–665. doi: 10.1016/j.cell.2013.03.043

Hobert, O. (2008). Gene regulation by transcription factors and microRNAs. *Science* 319, 1785–1786. doi: 10.1126/science.1151651

Hornstein, E., and Shomron, N. (2006). Canalization of development by microRNAs. *Nat. Genet.* 38, S20–S24. doi: 10.1038/ng1803

Ishizu, H., Siomi, H., and Siomi, M. C. (2012). Biology of PIWI-interacting RNAs: new insights into biogenesis and function inside and outside of germlines. *Genes Dev.* 26, 2361–2373. doi: 10.1101/gad.203786.112

Jacquier, A. (2009). The complex eukaryotic transcriptome: unexpected pervasive transcription and novel small RNAs. *Nat. Rev. Genet.* 10, 833–844. doi: 10.1038/nrg2683

Jalali, S., Bhartiya, D., Lalwani, M. K., Sivasubbu, S., and Scaria, V. (2013). Systematic transcriptome wide analysis of lncRNA-miRNA interactions. *PLoS ONE* 8:e53823. doi: 10.1371/journal.pone.0053823

Kalir, S., McClure, J., Pabbaraju, K., Southward, C., Ronen, M., Leibler, S., et al. (2001). Ordering Genes in a flagella pathway by analysis of expression kinetics from living bacteria. *Science* 292, 2080–2083. doi: 10.1126/science.1058758

Kaplan, B. B., Kar, A. N., Gioio, A., and Aschrafi, A. (2013). MicroRNAs in the axon and presynaptic nerve terminal. *Front. Cell. Neurosci.* 7:126. doi: 10.3389/fncel.2013.00126

Kedde, M., Strasser, M. J., Boldajipour, B., Oude Vrielink, J. A. F., Slanchev, K., le Sage, C., et al. (2007). RNA-binding protein Dnd1 inhibits microRNA access to target mRNA. *Cell* 131, 1273–1286. doi: 10.1016/j.cell.2007.11.034

Kole, A. J., Swahari, V., Hammond, S. M., and Deshmukh, M. (2011). miR-29b is activated during neuronal maturation and targets BH3-only genes to restrict apoptosis. *Genes Dev.* 25, 125–130. doi: 10.1101/gad.1975411

Korneev, S. A., Korneeva, E. I., Lagarkova, M. A., Kiselev, S. L., Critchley, G., and O'Shea, M. (2008). Novel noncoding antisense RNA transcribed from human anti-NOS2A locus is differentially regulated during neuronal differentiation of embryonic stem cells. *RNA* 14, 2030–2037. doi: 10.1261/rna.1084308

Kundu, P., Fabian, M. R., Sonenberg, N., Bhattacharyya, S. N., and Filipowicz, W. (2012). HuR protein attenuates miRNA-mediated repression by promoting miRISC dissociation from the target RNA. *Nucleic Acids Res.* 40, 5088–5100. doi: 10.1093/nar/gks148

Lee, E. J., Banerjee, S., Zhou, H., Jammalamadaka, A., Arcila, M., Manjunath, B. S., et al. (2011). Identification of piRNAs in the central nervous system. *RNA* 17, 1090–1099. doi: 10.1261/rna.2565011

Lin, M., Pedrosa, E., Shah, A., Hrabovsky, A., Maqbool, S., Zheng, D., et al. (2011). RNA-Seq of human neurons derived from iPS cells reveals candidate long non-coding RNAs involved in neurogenesis and neuropsychiatric disorders. *PLoS ONE* 6:e23356. doi: 10.1371/journal.pone.0023356

Liu, C.-M., Wang, R.-Y., Saijilafu, Jiao, Z.-X., Zhang, B.-Y., and Zhou, F.-Q. (2013). MicroRNA-138 and SIRT1 form a mutual negative feedback loop to regulate mammalian axon regeneration. *Genes Dev.* 27, 1473–1483. doi: 10.1101/gad.209619.112

Liu, Q., and Paroo, Z. (2010). Biochemical principles of small RNA pathways. *Annu. Rev. Biochem.* 79, 295–319. doi: 10.1146/annurev.biochem.052208.151733

Makeyev, E. V., Zhang, J., Carrasco, M. A., and Maniatis, T. (2007). The MicroRNA miR-124 promotes neuronal differentiation by triggering brain-specific alternative pre-mRNA splicing. *Mol. Cell* 27, 435–448. doi: 10.1016/j.molcel.2007.07.015

Malone, C. D., Brennecke, J., Dus, M., Stark, A., McCombie, W. R., Sachidanandam, R., et al. (2009). Specialized piRNA pathways act in germline and somatic tissues of the Drosophila ovary. *Cell* 137, 522–535. doi: 10.1016/j.cell.2009.03.040

Mellios, N., Sugihara, H., Castro, J., Banerjee, A., Le, C., Kumar, A., et al. (2011). miR-132, an experience-dependent microRNA, is essential for visual cortex plasticity. *Nat. Neurosci.* 14, 1240–1242. doi: 10.1038/nn.2909

Memczak, S., Jens, M., Elefsinioti, A., Torti, F., Krueger, J., Rybak, A., et al. (2013). Circular RNAs are a large class of animal RNAs with regulatory potency. *Nature* 495, 333–338. doi: 10.1038/nature11928

Mercer, T., Qureshi, I., Gokhan, S., Dinger, M., Li, G., Mattick, J., et al. (2010). Long noncoding RNAs in neuronal-glial fate specification and oligodendrocyte lineage maturation. *BMC Neurosci.* 11:14. doi: 10.1186/1471-2202-11-14

Mercer, T. R., Dinger, M. E., and Mattick, J. S. (2009). Long non-coding RNAs: insights into functions. *Nat. Rev. Genet.* 10, 155–159. doi: 10.1038/nrg2521

Mercer, T. R., Dinger, M. E., Sunkin, S. M., Mehler, M. F., and Mattick, J. S. (2008). Specific expression of long noncoding RNAs in the mouse brain. *Proc. Natl. Acad. Sci. U.S.A.* 105, 716–721. doi: 10.1073/pnas.0706729105

Miura, P., Shenker, S., Andreu-Agullo, C., Westholm, J. O., and Lai, E. C. (2013). Widespread and extensive lengthening of 3' UTRs in the mammalian brain. *Genome Res.* 23, 812–825. doi: 10.1101/gr.146886.112

Modarresi, F., Faghihi, M. A., Lopez-Toledano, M. A., Fatemi, R. P., Magistri, M., Brothers, S. P., et al. (2012). Inhibition of natural antisense transcripts *in vivo* results in gene-specific transcriptional upregulation. *Nat. Biotechnol.* 30, 453–459. doi: 10.1038/nbt.2158

Muotri, A. R., Chu, V. T., Marchetto, M. C. N., Deng, W., Moran, J. V., and Gage F. H. (2005). Somatic mosaicism in neuronal precursor cells mediated by L1 retrotransposition. *Nature* 435, 903–910. doi:10.1038/nature03663

Ng, S.-Y., Bogu, G. K., Soh, B. S., and Stanton, L. W. (2013). The long noncoding RNA RMST interacts with SOX2 to regulate neurogenesis. *Mol. Cell* 51, 349–359. doi:10.1016/j.molcel.2013.07.017

Ng, S.-Y., Johnson, R., and Stanton, L. W. (2012). Human long non-coding RNAs promote pluripotency and neuronal differentiation by association with chromatin modifiers and transcription factors. *EMBO J.* 31, 522–533. doi: 10.1038/emboj.2011.459

Osella, M., Bosia, C., Corá, D., and Caselle, M. (2011). The role of incoherent microRNA-mediated feedforward loops in noise buffering. *PLoS Comput. Biol.* 7:e1001101. doi: 10.1371/journal.pcbi.1001101

Packer, A. N., Xing, Y., Harper, S. Q., Jones, L., and Davidson, B. L. (2008). The bifunctional microRNA miR-9/miR-9* regulates REST and CoREST and is downregulated in Huntington's disease. *J. Neurosci.* 28, 14341–14346. doi: 10.1523/JNEUROSCI.2390-08.2008

Perrat, P. N., DasGupta, S., Wang, J., Theurkauf, W., Weng, Z., Rosbash, M., et al. (2013). Transposition-driven genomic heterogeneity in the Drosophila brain. *Science* 340, 91–95. doi: 10.1126/science.1231965

Pollard, K. S., Salama, S. R., Lambert, N., Lambot, M.-A., Coppens, S., Pedersen, J. S., et al. (2006). An RNA gene expressed during cortical development evolved rapidly in humans. *Nature* 443, 167–172. doi: 10.1038/nature05113

Qureshi, I. A., Mattick, J. S., and Mehler, M. F. (2010). Long non-coding RNAs in nervous system function and disease. *Brain Res.* 1338, 20–35. doi:10.1016/j.brainres.2010.03.110

Rajasethupathy, P., Antonov, I., Sheridan, R., Frey, S., Sander, C., Tuschl, T., et al. (2012). A role for neuronal piRNAs in the epigenetic control of memory-related synaptic plasticity. *Cell* 149, 693–707. doi: 10.1016/j.cell.2012.02.057

Ramos, A. D., Diaz, A., Nellore, A., Delgado, R. N., Park, K.-Y., Gonzales-Roybal, G., et al. (2013). Integration of genome-wide approaches identifies lncRNAs of adult neural stem cells and their progeny *in vivo*. *Cell Stem Cell* 12, 616–628. doi: 10.1016/j.stem.2013.03.003

Ramsköld, D., Wang, E. T., Burge, C. B., and Sandberg, R. (2009). An abundance of ubiquitously expressed genes revealed by tissue transcriptome sequence data. *PLoS Comput. Biol.* 5:e1000598. doi: 10.1371/journal.pcbi.1000598

Rapicavoli, N., Poth, E., Zhu, H., and Blackshaw, S. (2011). The long noncoding RNA Six3OS acts in trans to regulate retinal development by modulating Six3 activity. *Neural Dev.* 6:32. doi: 10.1186/1749-8104-6-32

Sasaki, Y., Gross, C., Xing, L., Goshima, Y., and Bassell, G. J. (2013). Identification of axon-enriched microRNAs localized to growth cones of cortical neurons. *Dev. Neurobiol.* doi: 10.1002/dneu.22113. [Epub ahead of print].

Schratt, G. M., Tuebing, F., Nigh, E. A., Kane, C. G., Sabatini, M. E., Kiebler, M., et al. (2006). A brain-specific microRNA regulates dendritic spine development. *Nature* 439, 283–289. doi: 10.1038/nature04367

Strickland, I. T., Richards, L., Holmes, F. E., Wynick, D., Uney, J. B., and Wong, L.-F. (2011). Axotomy-induced miR-21 promotes axon growth in adult dorsal root ganglion neurons. *PLoS ONE* 6:e23423. doi: 10.1371/journal.pone.0023423

Tochitani, S., and Hayashizaki, Y. (2008). Nkx2.2 antisense RNA overexpression enhanced oligodendrocytic differentiation. *Biochem. Biophys. Res. Commun.* 372, 691–696. doi: 10.1016/j.bbrc.2008.05.127

Tsang, J., Zhu, J., and van Oudenaarden, A. (2007). MicroRNA-mediated feedback and feedforward loops are recurrent network motifs in mammals. *Mol. Cell* 26, 753–767. doi:10.1016/j.molcel.2007.05.018

Tsuiji, H., Yoshimoto, R., Hasegawa, Y., Furuno, M., Yoshida, M., and Nakagawa, S. (2011). Competition between a noncoding exon and introns: gomafu contains tandem UACUAAC repeats and associates with splicing factor-1. *Genes Cells* 16, 479–490. doi: 10.1111/j.1365-2443.2011.01502.x

Visvanathan, J., Lee, S., Lee, B., Lee, J. W., and Lee, S.-K. (2007). The microRNA miR-124 antagonizes the anti-neural REST/SCP1 pathway during embryonic CNS development. *Genes Dev.* 21, 744–749. doi: 10.1101/gad.1519107

Wang, H., Iacoangeli, A., Lin, D., Williams, K., Denman, R. B., Hellen, C. U. T., et al. (2005). Dendritic BC1 RNA in translational control mechanisms. *J. Cell Biol.* 171, 811–821. doi: 10.1083/jcb.200506006

Watanabe, T., Tomizawa, S.-I., Mitsuya, K., Totoki, Y., Yamamoto, Y., Kuramochi-Miyagawa, S., et al. (2011). Role for piRNAs and noncoding RNA in *de novo* DNA methylation of the imprinted mouse rasgrf1 locus. *Science* 332, 848–852. doi: 10.1126/science.1203919

Wayman, G. A., Davare, M., Ando, H., Fortin, D., Varlamova, O., Cheng, H.-Y. M., et al. (2008). An activity-regulated microRNA controls dendritic plasticity by down-regulating p250GAP. *Proc. Natl. Acad. Sci. U.S.A.* 105, 9093–9098. doi: 10.1073/pnas.0803072105

Winter, J., Jung, S., Keller, S., Gregory, R. I., and Diederichs, S. (2009). Many roads to maturity: microRNA biogenesis pathways and their regulation. *Nat. Cell Biol.* 11, 228–234. doi: 10.1038/ncb0309-228

Wu, D., and Murashov, A. K. (2013a). MicroRNA-431 regulates axon regeneration in mature sensory neurons by targeting the Wnt antagonist kremen1. *Front. Mol. Neurosci.* 6:35. doi:10.3389/fnmol.2013.00035

Wu, D., and Murashov, A. K. (2013b). Molecular mechanisms of peripheral nerve regeneration: emerging roles of microRNAs. *Front. Physiol.* 4:55. doi: 10.3389/fphys.2013.00055

Young, T. L., Matsuda, T., and Cepko, C. L. (2005). The noncoding RNA taurine upregulated gene 1 is required for differentiation of the murine retina. *Curr. Biol.* 15, 501–512. doi: 10.1016/j.cub.2005.02.027

Zhao, C., Sun, G., Li, S., and Shi, Y. (2009). A feedback regulatory loop involving microRNA-9 and nuclear receptor TLX in neural stem cell fate determination. *Nat. Struct. Mol. Biol.* 16, 365–371. doi: 10.1038/nsmb.1576

Zhong, J., Chuang, S.-C., Bianchi, R., Zhao, W., Lee, H., Fenton, A. A., et al. (2009). BC1 regulation of metabotropic glutamate receptor-mediated neuronal excitability. *J. Neurosci.* 29, 9977–9986. doi: 10.1523/JNEUROSCI.3893-08.2009

Zhong, J., Chuang, S.-C., Bianchi, R., Zhao, W., Paul, G., Thakkar, P., et al. (2010). Regulatory BC1 RNA and the fragile X mental retardation protein: convergent functionality in brain. *PLoS ONE* 5:e15509. doi: 10.1371/journal.pone.0015509

12

The role of microRNAs in regulating neuronal connectivity

Hui Chiu[†], Amel Alqadah and Chieh Chang*

Division of Developmental Biology, Cincinnati Children's Hospital Research Foundation, Cincinnati, OH, USA

Correspondence:
Chieh Chang, Division of Developmental Biology, Cincinnati Children's Hospital Research Foundation, 240 Albert Sabin Way, S3.419, Cincinnati, OH 45229-3039, USA
e-mail: chieh.chang1@gmail.com

[†]Present address:
Hui Chiu, Division of Biology and Biological Engineering and Howard Hughes Medical Institute, California Institute of Technology, Pasadena, CA 91125, USA

The assembly of functional neural circuits is critical for complex thoughts, behavior and general brain function. Precise construction of neural circuits requires orderly transition of sequential events from axon outgrowth, pathfinding, branching, to synaptogenesis. Each of these steps is required to be tightly regulated in order to achieve meticulous formation of neuronal connections. MicroRNAs (miRNAs), which silence gene expression post-transcriptionally via either inhibition of translation or destabilization of messenger RNAs, have emerged as key regulators of neuronal connectivity. The expression of miRNAs in neurons is often temporally and spatially regulated, providing critical timing and local mechanisms that prime neuronal growth cones for dynamic responses to extrinsic cues. Here we summarize recent findings of miRNA regulation of neuronal connectivity in a variety of experimental platforms.

Keywords: miRNAs, neuronal connectivity, axon pathfinding, axon branching, timing mechanisms, temporal regulation, heterochronic miRNAs, axon outgrowth

The diverse behaviors of organisms rely on fast information processing performed by the brain. Trillions of neurons comprising the brain form complex networks that enable animals to exhibit consciousness, accumulate memories, engage in learning, and adopt behaviors. The complexity of brain networks is greatly increased by the facts that one neuron can influence its target through multiple pathways (Gutierrez et al., 2013), and that common neurons shared by divergent circuits can modulate reciprocal inhibition between two mutually exclusive behaviors in response to environmental stimuli (Mann et al., 2013). The former case is achieved by the direct and indirect connections between two neurons via two or more synaptic routes and the latter depends on the appropriate information flow from sensory neurons to interneurons as well as from interneurons to motor neurons (Gutierrez et al., 2013; Mann et al., 2013). Both cases indicate the importance of precise connections between neurons to brain function. Precise neuronal connectivity is established through transition of sequential events from axon growth to synapse formation. Axons are attracted to targets, but upon arrival they must switch their responsiveness to guidance cues at the targets such that they are no longer sensitive to these cues, in order to stop outgrowth and form synaptic contacts (Tessier-Lavigne and Goodman, 1996; Stein and Tessier-Lavigne, 2001; Dickson, 2002; Chen et al., 2008). Miswiring of the nervous system can result in serious neurological deficits, such as autism, Parkinson's, and Alzheimer's diseases (Hoogland et al., 2003; Lesnick et al., 2007; Zikopoulos and Barbas, 2010). Thus, studying how neurons connect with each other to establish functional circuitry can help us better understand how animal behaviors go awry and may provide insights into potential therapeutic targets for neurological disorders.

NEURAL CIRCUIT ASSEMBLY

Neurons connect with targets through a series of events: axon initiation, axon pathfinding, axon branching, and synapse formation (Carmeliet and Tessier-Lavigne, 2005; Kolodkin and Tessier-Lavigne, 2011). A single axon grows out from the cell body, and forms a highly motile structure called the growth cone at its tip. The growth cone navigates along the stereotypical pathway via interactions with a variety of guidance cues present in the environment and travels a long distance to reach the target with remarkable precision. Upon reaching the target, the growth cone turns into a presynaptic terminal to form a connection with the target, and the axon starts branching extensively to establish an intricate pattern of connectivity. Each step of neuronal circuit assembly involves local protein synthesis (Campbell and Holt, 2001; Jung et al., 2012). Specific mRNAs are anterogradely transported from the cell body to the axon and to the growth cone to construct local transcriptomes (Zivraj et al., 2010; Gumy et al., 2011; Willis et al., 2011; Cajigas et al., 2012). The expression of mRNAs is tightly controlled by many post-transcriptional regulatory mechanisms, of which microRNA (miRNA)-mediated gene repression is one of them (Bushati and Cohen, 2007; Deglincerti and Jaffrey, 2012; Jung et al., 2012). The fast and dynamic changes in the local proteome enable growth cones to respond rapidly to diverse environmental cues, resulting in elongation, turning, or collapse of growth cones (Campbell and Holt, 2001; Hengst et al., 2009; Andreassi et al.,

2010; Zivraj et al., 2010). The post-transcriptional regulators, therefore, play a pivotal role in the establishment of neuronal connections.

miRNAs AS VERSATILE AND REVERSIBLE REGULATORS OF GENE EXPRESSION IN NEURONS

MiRNA-mediated gene regulation is involved in many aspects of neuronal development and function (Kosik, 2006; Schratt, 2009; McNeill and Van Vactor, 2012). Recent studies have worked out a few molecular mechanics of miRNA-mediated gene silencing (Fabian and Sonenberg, 2012). These small non-coding RNAs bind to the 3′UTR of target mRNAs and repress gene expression by interfering with stability or inhibiting translation of mRNAs (Bartel, 2009). The pleiotropy, speed, and reversibility are features that contribute to the unique regulatory niche of miRNA-based gene regulation in the nervous system (Hobert, 2008). First, individual miRNAs can target multiple genes at the same time to cause broad and significant changes in neuronal transcriptomes (Brennecke et al., 2005; Giraldez et al., 2006). On the other hand, each gene can be targeted by different miRNAs, and/or may contain more than one binding site of the same miRNA, allowing miRNAs to "fine-tune" the level of gene expression (Bartel and Chen, 2004; Hon and Zhang, 2007). Second, the effect of miRNA-mediated gene repression is instant because miRNAs can shut down protein synthesis of the target genes at ribosomes (Pillai et al., 2005). The small size and non-coding nature also allows fast production of miRNAs as compared to transcription factors (Hobert, 2008). Lastly, the miRNA-mediated gene repression can be easily relieved by translocating the targeted mRNA from a miRNA-hijacked ribosome to an active one (Bhattacharyya et al., 2006). In summary, miRNAs provide a local, versatile, fast and reversible mechanism that is sensitive to extracellular stimuli and provides exquisite control of local protein dynamics and axon development.

SPATIAL AND TEMPORAL ROLES OF miRNAs IN NEURONAL CONNECTIVITY

MiRNA expression is either spatially restricted or temporally regulated in neuronal development. The spatially restricted expression of miRNAs within neurons suggests roles for miRNAs in diverse differentiation events from axon pathfinding to synapse formation. Many miRNAs are expressed specifically in the nervous system, and even in distinct neuronal subsets, implying potentially unique roles in specific cell types. (Lagos-Quintana et al., 2002; He et al., 2012). Furthermore, miRNAs can be localized to subcellular compartments, such as axons, growth cones or synapses, to rapidly alter local gene expression profiles, but not much is known about the transport mechanisms that provide that specificity (Corbin et al., 2009; Natera-Naranjo et al., 2010; Kaplan et al., 2013; Sasaki et al., 2013). The temporally regulated expression of miRNAs within neurons suggests a role in the orderly transition of sequential differentiation events (Johnston and Hobert, 2003; Chang et al., 2004b; Hsieh et al., 2012; Zou et al., 2012, 2013; Chiu and Chang, 2013). Recent evidence indeed showed that miRNAs can provide timing mechanisms for orderly developmental events in neurons (Zou et al., 2012). Significant changes in the expression level of some brain-specific miRNAs during cortical neurogenesis have been reported previously (Krichevsky et al., 2003), suggesting that gene expression profiles may be controlled by the up- or down-regulation of certain miRNAs at each stage of brain development. Thus, the compartmentalized expression of miRNAs provides subcellular control of local gene expression for specific neuronal differentiation events while the temporal constraint of miRNA expression allows for the correct transition timing of sequential differentiation events.

CONTROL OF AXON OUTGROWTH BY miRNAs

The neural circuit assembly begins with axon outgrowth. In the early phase of neuronal development, a neuron first forms multiple naïve neurites around the soma. One of the neurites will be specified as an axon and extend further while the remaining become dendrites (Craig and Banker, 1994). Actin and microtubule dynamics are required for the neurite formation and elongation (Bradke and Dotti, 1999; Inagaki et al., 2001). Therefore, it is not surprising that miRNAs affect axon initiation or elongation by targeting regulators of the cytoskeleton (**Table 1**). miR-132, for example, induces neurite sprouting of cortical neurons. It does so by inhibiting the p250 GTPase-activating protein that acts upstream of small GTPases Cdc42 and RhoA, to regulate neuronal morphogenesis (Nakazawa et al., 2003; Vo et al., 2005). miRNAs can also regulate axon outgrowth by modulating local protein synthesis. miR-9 locally represses the translation of the microtubule-associated protein 1b (Map1b) in axons to control axon elongation of mouse cortical neurons (Dajas-Bailador et al., 2012). Overexpression of miR-9 decreases the Map1b regulatory effects on axonal microtubules, resulting in the reduction of axon length (Dajas-Bailador et al., 2012; Tymanskyj et al., 2012). miR-19a, a major member of the miR-17-92 cluster, acts in axons to down-regulate the protein level of phosphatase and tension homolog (PTEN) and activate phosphorylated mammalian target of rapamycin (mTOR) pathway (Zhang et al., 2013). mTOR activity is known to be required for local protein synthesis in axonal development and regeneration (Campbell and Holt, 2001; Park et al., 2008). Thus, miR-17-92 cluster promotes axon outgrowth by activating local protein synthesis (Zhang et al., 2013). Although several miRNAs have been shown to affect axon development, few have been shown to play a role specifically in the axon compartment (Aschrafi et al., 2008; Dajas-Bailador et al., 2012; Zhang et al., 2013). In addition, miRNAs also contribute to the temporal regulation of axon outgrowth. In *Caenorhabditis elegans*, the hermaphrodite specific neuron (HSN) projects a single axon to the ventral nerve cord in the fourth larva (L4) stage (Adler et al., 2006). The heterochronic miRNA *lin-4* acts cell-autonomously in HSN neurons to control the timing of axon formation (Olsson-Carter and Slack, 2010). No axon is extended at the L4 stage in *lin-4* mutants while precocious axon outgrowth at the third larval stage occurs in animals over-expressing *lin-4* in HSN neurons (Olsson-Carter and Slack, 2010). The targets of the *lin-4* miRNA, *lin-14* and *lin-28*, inhibit differentiation of HSN neurons. Thus, the *lin-4* miRNA signals axon outgrowth only after HSN neuronal fate is committed (Olsson-Carter and Slack, 2010).

miRNA REGULATION OF AXON PATHFINDING

Axons are directed to their synaptic targets via the guidance of attractive or repellent cues presented in the environment

Table 1 | Summary of miRNA functions in axon development.

MicroRNAs	Functions	Targets	Reference
Axon outgrowth			
miR-132	Promote axon outgrowth	p250 GTPase-activating protein	Vo et al. (2005)
miR-9	Inhibit axon outgrowth	Microtubule-associated protein 1b (Map1b)	Dajas-Bailador et al. (2012)
miR-17-92 cluster	Promote axon outgrowth	Phosphatase and tensin homolog (PTEN)	Zhang et al. (2013)
lin-4	Promote axon outgrowth	LIN-14 and LIN-28 transcription factors	Olsson-Carter and Slack (2010)
Axon guidance			
lin-4	Turn off the growth cone sensitivity to Netrin	LIN-14 transcription factor	Zou et al. (2012)
miR-124	Turn on the growth cone sensitivity to Sema3A	CoREST	Baudet et al. (2012, 2013)
Axon branching			
miR-9	Promote axon branching	Map1b	Dajas-Bailador et al. (2012)
miR-124	Promote axon branching	Small GTPase RhoG	Franke et al. (2012)

(Tessier-Lavigne and Goodman, 1996). The sensitivity of axons to guidance cues is determined by the expression of the corresponding receptors in growth cones (Dickson, 2002). To prevent the axon from stalling at intermediate targets or overshooting, the receptor expression needs to be tightly controlled in a timely manner (Zou et al., 2000; Stein and Tessier-Lavigne, 2001). Here we discuss the role of miRNAs in regulating the growth cone responsiveness to two prominent guidance molecules, netrins and semaphorins, during axon pathfinding.

Netrins are highly conserved guidance molecules that can function as both attractants and repellents in many stage-dependent biological events, such as axon guidance and motile cell migration (Hedgecock et al., 1990; Ishii et al., 1992; Chan et al., 1996; Kolodkin and Tessier-Lavigne, 2011), but the timing mechanism that controls the responsiveness of growth cones or migrating cells to Netrins at precise times is not fully understood. The axon of the *C. elegans* anterior ventral microtubule (AVM) sensory neurons is guided to the ventral midline through combined actions of Slit repulsion from the dorsal body wall muscles and netrin attraction to the ventral nerve cord (Chang et al., 2004a). Once reaching the ventral midline, the AVM axon projects anteriorly to the nerve ring where it stops outgrowth and forms synapses (**Figure 1A**). An unexpected role was recently reported for the conserved heterochronic miRNA *lin-4* and its target the LIN-14 transcription factor in AVM neuronal connectivity (Zou et al., 2012). Through genetic analysis of a well-characterized AVM axon ventral guidance event and a less characterized AVM synapse formation event, it was shown that *lin-4* functions as a potent and specific negative regulator of netrin signaling in AVM neuronal connectivity by targeting the LIN-14 transcription factor to control the availability of the netrin receptor UNC-40/DCC (Deleted in Colorectal Cancer; **Figure 1B**; Zou et al., 2012). It was well known that heterochronic genes are used in timing mitotic cell development required for molting in worms and embryonic stem cells self-renewal in mice. These results show that these heterochronic genes are re-used in postmitotic neurons to time their differentiation events.

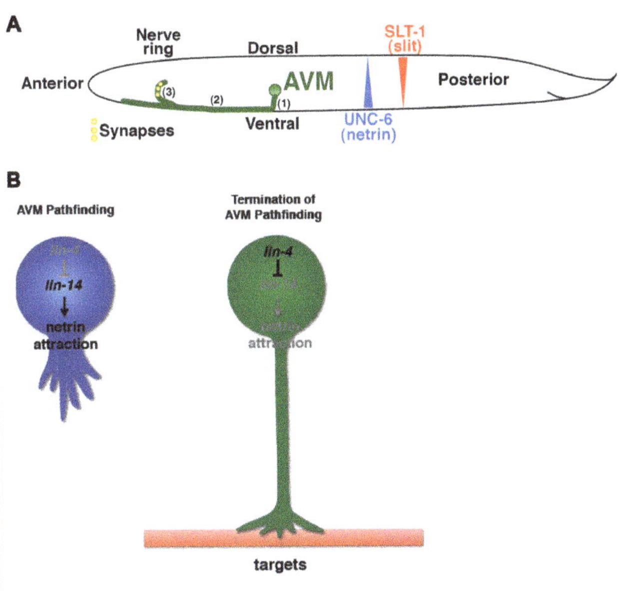

FIGURE 1 | Identification of the timing mechanism for orderly AVM axon connectivity. (A) Sequential events of AVM axon outgrowth and synapse formation in the first larval (L1) stage of *C. elegans*. (1) Axon grows ventrally. (2) Axon grows anteriorly. (3) End of axon pathfinding and initiation of synapse formation in the nerve ring. **(B)** The *lin-4–lin-14* regulatory circuit signals the end of axon pathfinding.

The Semaphorin family contains both secreted and transmembrane proteins that can function in long- or short-range guidance (Yazdani and Terman, 2006; Kolodkin and Tessier-Lavigne, 2011). Many Semaphorins bind the major receptor, Plexins, solely to mediate axonal repulsion. However, some of the secreted Semaphorins, such as Sema3A, bind to the co-receptor Neuropilins, instead (Kolodkin and Tessier-Lavigne, 2011). It has been shown that Sema3A is able to induce growth cone collapse at a specific stage of retinal ganglion cell (RGC) development in *Xenopus* (Campbell et al., 2001). The Sema3A responsiveness depends on the up-regulation of neuropilin-1 (NPR-1) receptor, which is indirectly controlled by the miRNA, miR-124, in a timely manner (Campbell et al., 2001; Baudet et al., 2012, 2013). The Repressor element-1 silencing transcription factor (REST) works with the REST corepressor 1 (CoREST) to inhibit the NPR-1 expression in young RGCs (Baudet et al., 2012, 2013). As the development progresses, the up-regulation of miR-124 accelerates the decay of CoREST mRNA, thereby attenuating the repression of NPR-1 expression (Baudet et al., 2012, 2013). The onset of Sema3A sensitivity of RGC growth cones is delayed in miR-124 knockdown, which is attributed to the retarded expression of NPR-1 (Baudet et al., 2012, 2013). Thus, miR-124 acts as an intrinsic timer to turn on the responsiveness of RGC growth cone to Sema3A by up-regulating NPR-1.

Slit is another key guidance molecule that is able to elicit axonal repulsion from a distance (Kolodkin and Tessier-Lavigne, 2011). The miRNA regulation of Slit signaling has been reported in the context of vascular patterning, but whether miRNAs control Slit signaling at specific times is unknown (Small et al., 2010). Even though no evidence has been shown that the Slit signaling is subject to the miRNA regulation in the context of axon guidance, it is likely that miRNAs may modulate Slit-mediated axon guidance since many molecular mechanisms are shared between vascular and axonal patterning (Carmeliet and Tessier-Lavigne, 2005).

UNIQUE ROLES OF miRNAs IN AXON BRANCHING

Once axons are in the vicinity of synaptic targets, they slow down outgrowth and branch out to form elaborate neural networks (Acebes and Ferrús, 2000). Similar to axon outgrowth, axon branching relies on cytoskeleton rearrangement, so cytoskeletal regulators likely coordinate both events in response to environmental cues. As mentioned above, miR-9 regulates microtubule dynamics by targeting the Map1b to control axon outgrowth (Dajas-Bailador et al., 2012). The miR-9 level in mouse cortical neurons is regulated by the brain-derived neurotrophic factor (BDNF) that functions as a chemoattractant and also a branching factor (Hoshino et al., 2010; Panagiotaki et al., 2010). In the initial phase of cortical neuron development *in vitro*, shorter exposure to BDNF results in reduced miR-9 expression, which leads to high level of Map1b expression and steady axon outgrowth. Prolonged exposure to BDNF, which could mimic the target recognition phase *in vivo*, results in elevated miR-9 expression, which leads to axon branching as a result of the repressed Map1b expression (Dajas-Bailador et al., 2012). In hippocampal neurons, it was shown that miR-124 regulates axon and dendrite branching by targeting the small GTPase RhoG (Franke et al., 2012). The RhoG activity inhibits axon branching via the ELMO/Dock180/Rac1 pathway, while reducing dendrite branching through the Cdc42 signaling. Therefore, expression of miR-124 in hippocampal neurons promotes axon and dendrite branching (Franke et al., 2012).

CONCLUDING REMARKS

The exquisite precision with which neural circuits are assembled is crucial for proper brain function, as inappropriate wiring in the nervous system results in various debilitating neurological diseases. Neurons are able to form appropriate connections using processes that involve spatial and temporal regulatory mechanisms, which ensure rapid responses to diverse environmental cues and faithful transition of sequential events in neuronal connectivity. miRNAs have proven to be essential and efficient regulators at several steps of this integral process due to their spatiotemporal specificity, versatile targeting, speed of gene repression, and ease of reversibility. Further study on how miRNAs contribute to the formation of neural circuits will ultimately provide insights into how mis-wiring by miRNA mis-regulation can lead to diseases.

ACKNOWLEDGMENTS

This work was funded by grants from the Whitehall Foundation, the March of Dimes Foundation, and by NSF grant IOS-1257023 to Chieh Chang.

REFERENCES

Acebes, A., and Ferrús, A. (2000). Cellular and molecular features of axon collaterals and dendrites. *Trends Neurosci.* 23, 557–565. doi: 10.1016/S0166-2236(00)01646-5

Adler, C. E., Fetter, R. D., and Bargmann, C. I. (2006). UNC-6/Netrin induces neuronal asymmetry and defines the site of axon formation. *Nat. Neurosci.* 9, 511–518. doi: 10.1038/nn1666

Andreassi, C., Zimmermann, C., Mitter, R., Fusco, S., De Vita, S., Saiardi, A., et al. (2010). An NGF-responsive element targets myo-inositol monophosphatase-1 mRNA to sympathetic neuron axons. *Nat. Neurosci.* 13, 291–301. doi: 10.1038/nn.2486

Aschrafi, A., Schwechter, A. D., Mameza, M. G., Natera-Naranjo, O., Gioio, A. E., and Kaplan, B. B. (2008). MicroRNA-338 regulates local cytochrome c oxidase IV mRNA levels and oxidative phosphorylation in the axons of sympathetic neurons. *J. Neurosci.* 28, 12581–12590. doi: 10.1523/JNEUROSCI.3338-08.2008

Bartel, D. P. (2009). MicroRNAs: target recognition and regulatory functions. *Cell* 136, 215–233. doi: 10.1016/j.cell.2009.01.002

Bartel, D. P., and Chen, C. Z. (2004). Micromanagers of gene expression: the potentially widespread influence of metazoan microRNAs. *Nat. Rev. Genet.* 5, 396–400. doi: 10.1038/nrg1328

Baudet, M. L., Bellon, A., and Holt, C. E. (2013). Role of microRNAs in Semaphorin function and neural circuit formation. *Semin. Cell Dev. Biol.* 24, 146–155. doi: 10.1016/j.semcdb.2012.11.004

Baudet, M. L., Zivraj, K. H., Abreu-Goodger, C., Muldal, A., Armisen, J., Blenkiron, C., et al. (2012). miR-124 acts through CoREST to control onset of Sema3A sensitivity in navigating retinal growth cones. *Nat. Neurosci.* 15, 29–38. doi: 10.1038/nn.2979

Bhattacharyya, S. N., Habermacher, R., Martine, U., Closs, E. I., and Filipowicz, W. (2006). Relief of microRNA-mediated translational repression in human cells subjected to stress. *Cell* 125, 1111–1124. doi: 10.1016/j.cell.2006.04.031

Bradke, F., and Dotti, C. G. (1999). The role of local actin instability in axon formation. *Science* 283, 1931–1934. doi: 10.1126/science.283.5409.1931

Brennecke, J., Stark, A., Russell, R. B., and Cohen, S. M. (2005). Principles of microRNA-target recognition. *PLoS Biol.* 3:e85. doi: 10.1371/journal.pbio.0030085

Bushati, N., and Cohen, S. M. (2007). MicroRNA functions. *Annu. Rev. Cell Dev. Biol.* 23, 175–205. doi: 10.1146/Annurev.Cellbio.23.090506.123406

Cajigas, I. J., Tushev, G., Will, T. J., Tom Dieck, S., Fuerst, N., and Schuman, E. M. (2012). The local transcriptome in the synaptic neuropil revealed by deep sequencing and high-resolution imaging. *Neuron* 74, 453–466. doi: 10.1016/j.neuron.2012.02.036

Campbell, D. S., and Holt, C. E. (2001). Chemotropic responses of retinal growth cones mediated by rapid local protein synthesis and degradation. *Neuron* 32, 1013–1026. doi: 10.1016/S0896-6273(01)00551-7

Campbell, D. S., Regan, A. G., Lopez, J. S., Tannahill, D., Harris, W. A., and Holt, C. E. (2001). Semaphorin 3A elicits stage-dependent collapse, turning, and branching in Xenopus retinal growth cones. *J. Neurosci.* 21, 8538–8547.

Carmeliet, P., and Tessier-Lavigne, M. (2005). Common mechanisms of nerve and blood vessel wiring. *Nature* 436, 193–200. doi: 10.1038/nature03875

Chan, S. S., Zheng, H., Su, M. W., Wilk, R., Killeen, M. T., Hedgecock, E. M., et al. (1996). UNC-40, a *C. elegans* homolog of DCC (Deleted in Colorectal Cancer), is required in motile cells responding to UNC-6 netrin cues. *Cell* 87, 187–195. doi: 10.1016/S0092-8674(00)81337-9

Chang, C., Yu, T. W., Bargmann, C. I., and Tessier-Lavigne, M. (2004a). Inhibition of Netrin-mediated axon attraction by a receptor protein tyrosine phosphatase. *Science* 305, 103–106. doi: 10.1126/science.1096983

Chang, S., Johnston, R. J., Frokjaer-Jensen, C., Lockery, S., and Hobert, O. (2004b). MicroRNAs act sequentially and asymmetrically to control chemosensory laterality in the nematode. *Nature* 430, 785–789. doi: 10.1038/Nature02752

Chen, Z., Gore, B. B., Long, H., Ma, L., and Tessier-Lavigne, M. (2008). Alternative splicing of the Robo3 axon guidance receptor governs the midline switch from attraction to repulsion. *Neuron* 58, 325–332. doi: 10.1016/j.neuron.2008.02.016

Chiu, H., and Chang, C. (2013). Rejuvenating nerve cells in adults. *Aging* 5, 485–486.

Corbin, R., Olsson-Carter, K., and Slack, F. (2009). The role of microRNAs in synaptic development and function. *BMB Rep.* 42, 131–135.

Craig, A. M., and Banker, G. (1994). Neuronal polarity. *Annu. Rev. Neurosci.* 17, 267–310. doi: 10.1146/annurev.ne.17.030194.001411

Dajas-Bailador, F., Bonev, B., Garcez, P., Stanley, P., Guillemot, F., and Papalopulu, N. (2012). microRNA-9 regulates axon extension and branching by targeting Map1b in mouse cortical neurons. *Nat. Neurosci.* 15, 697–699. doi: 10.1038/nn.3082

Deglincerti, A., and Jaffrey, S. R. (2012). Insights into the roles of local translation from the axonal transcriptome. *Open Biol.* 2, 120079. doi: 10.1098/rsob.120079

Dickson, B. J. (2002). Molecular mechanisms of axon guidance. *Science* 298, 1959–1964. doi: 10.1126/science.1072165

Fabian, M. R., and Sonenberg, N. (2012). The mechanics of miRNA-mediated gene silencing: a look under the hood of miRISC. *Nat. Struct. Mol. Biol.* 19, 586–593. doi: 10.1038/nsmb.2296

Franke, K., Otto, W., Johannes, S., Baumgart, J., Nitsch, R., and Schumacher, S. (2012). miR-124-regulated RhoG reduces neuronal process complexity via ELMO/Dock180/Rac1 and Cdc42 signalling. *EMBO J.* 31, 2908–2921. doi: 10.1038/emboj.2012.130

Giraldez, A. J., Mishima, Y., Rihel, J., Grocock, R. J., Van Dongen, S., Inoue, K., et al. (2006). Zebrafish MiR-430 promotes deadenylation and clearance of maternal mRNAs. *Science* 312, 75–79. doi: 10.1126/science.1122689

Gumy, L. F., Yeo, G. S. H., Tung, Y.-C. L., Zivraj, K. H., Willis, D., Coppola, G., et al. (2011). Transcriptome analysis of embryonic and adult sensory axons reveals changes in mRNA repertoire localization. *RNA* 17, 85–98. doi: 10.1261/rna.2386111

Gutierrez, G. J., O'Leary, T., and Marder, E. (2013). Multiple mechanisms switch an electrically coupled, synaptically inhibited neuron between competing rhythmic oscillators. *Neuron* 77, 845–858. doi: 10.1016/j.neuron.2013.01.016

He, M., Liu, Y., Wang, X., Zhang, M. Q., Hannon, G. J., and Huang, Z. J. (2012). Cell-type-based analysis of microRNA profiles in the mouse brain. *Neuron* 73, 35–48. doi: 10.1016/j.neuron.2011.11.010

Hedgecock, E. M., Culotti, J. G., and Hall, D. H. (1990). The unc-5, unc-6, and unc-40 genes guide circumferential migrations of pioneer axons and mesodermal cells on the epidermis in *C. elegans*. *Neuron* 4, 61–85. doi: 10.1016/0896-6273(90)90444-K

Hengst, U., Deglincerti, A., Kim, H. J., Jeon, N. L., and Jaffrey, S. R. (2009). Axonal elongation triggered by stimulus-induced local translation of a polarity complex protein. *Nat. Cell Biol.* 11, 1024–1030. doi: 10.1038/ncb1916

Hobert, O. (2008). Gene regulation by transcription factors and microRNAs. *Science* 319, 1785–1786. doi: 10.1126/science.1151651

Hon, L. S., and Zhang, Z. (2007). The roles of binding site arrangement and combinatorial targeting in microRNA repression of gene expression. *Genome Biol.* 8, R166. doi: 10.1186/gb-2007-8-8-r166

Hoogland, P. V., Van Den Berg, R., and Huisman, E. (2003). Misrouted olfactory fibres and ectopic olfactory glomeruli in normal humans and in Parkinson and Alzheimer patients. *Neuropathol. Appl. Neurobiol.* 29, 303–311. doi: 10.1046/j.1365-2990.2003.00459.x

Hoshino, N., Vatterott, P., Egwiekhor, A., and Rochlin, M. W. (2010). Brain-derived neurotrophic factor attracts geniculate ganglion neurites during embryonic targeting. *Dev. Neurosci.* 32, 184–196. doi: 10.1159/000313902

Hsieh, Y. W., Chang, C., and Chuang, C. F. (2012). The microRNA mir-71 inhibits calcium signaling by targeting the TIR-1/Sarm1 adaptor protein to control stochastic L/R neuronal asymmetry in *C. elegans*. *PLoS Genet.* 8:e1002864. doi: 10.1371/journal.pgen.1002864

Inagaki, N., Chihara, K., Arimura, N., Menager, C., Kawano, Y., Matsuo, N., et al. (2001). CRMP-2 induces axons in cultured hippocampal neurons. *Nat. Neurosci.* 4, 781–782. doi: 10.1038/90476

Ishii, N., Wadsworth, W. G., Stern, B. D., Culotti, J. G., and Hedgecock, E. M. (1992). UNC-6, a laminin-related protein, guides cell and pioneer axon migrations in *C. elegans*. *Neuron* 9, 873–881. doi: 10.1016/0896-6273(92)90240-E

Johnston, R. J., and Hobert, O. (2003). A microRNA controlling left/right neuronal asymmetry in *Caenorhabditis elegans*. *Nature* 426, 845–849. doi: 10.1038/nature02255

Jung, H., Yoon, B. C., and Holt, C. E. (2012). Axonal mRNA localization and local protein synthesis in nervous system assembly, maintenance and repair. *Nat. Rev. Neurosci.* 13, 308–324. doi: 10.1038/nrn3210

Kaplan, B. B., Kar, A. N., Gioio, A. E., and Aschrafi, A. (2013). MicroRNAs in the axon and presynaptic nerve terminal. *Front. Cell. Neurosci.* 7:126. doi: 10.3389/fncel.2013.00126

Kolodkin, A. L., and Tessier-Lavigne, M. (2011). Mechanisms and molecules of neuronal wiring: a primer. *Cold Spring Harb. Perspect. Biol.* 3, pii: a001727. doi: 10.1101/cshperspect.a001727

Kosik, K. S. (2006). The neuronal microRNA system. *Nat. Rev. Neurosci.* 7, 911–920. doi: 10.1038/nrn2037

Krichevsky, A. M., King, K. S., Donahue, C. P., Khrapko, K., and Kosik, K. S. (2003). A microRNA array reveals extensive regulation of microRNAs during brain development. *RNA* 9, 1274–1281. doi: 10.1261/rna.5980303

Lagos-Quintana, M., Rauhut, R., Yalcin, A., Meyer, J., Lendeckel, W., and Tuschl, T. (2002). Identification of tissue-specific microRNAs from mouse. *Curr. Biol.* 12, 735–739. doi: 10.1016/S0960-9822(02)00809-6

Lesnick, T. G., Papapetropoulos, S., Mash, D. C., Ffrench-Mullen, J., Shehadeh, L., De Andrade, M., et al. (2007). A genomic pathway approach to a complex disease: axon guidance and Parkinson disease. *PLoS Genet.* 3:e98. doi: 10.1371/journal.pgen.0030098

Mann, K., Gordon, M. D., and Scott, K. (2013). A pair of interneurons influences the choice between feeding and locomotion in *Drosophila*. *Neuron* 79, 754–765. doi: 10.1016/j.neuron.2013.06.018

McNeill, E., and Van Vactor, D. (2012). MicroRNAs shape the neuronal landscape. *Neuron* 75, 363–379. doi: 10.1016/j.neuron.2012.07.005

Nakazawa, T., Watabe, A. M., Tezuka, T., Yoshida, Y., Yokoyama, K., Umemori, H., et al. (2003). p250GAP, a novel brain-enriched GTPase-activating protein for Rho family GTPases, is involved in the N-methyl-d-aspartate receptor signaling. *Mol. Biol. Cell* 14, 2921–2934. doi: 10.1091/mbc.E02-09-0623

Natera-Naranjo, O., Aschrafi, A., Gioio, A. E., and Kaplan, B. B. (2010). Identification and quantitative analyses of microRNAs located in the distal axons of sympathetic neurons. *RNA* 16, 1516–1529. doi: 10.1261/rna.1833310

Olsson-Carter, K., and Slack, F. J. (2010). A developmental timing switch promotes axon outgrowth independent of known guidance receptors. *PLoS Genet.* 6:pii: e1001054. doi: 10.1371/journal.pgen.1001054

Panagiotaki, N., Dajas-Bailador, F., Amaya, E., Papalopulu, N., and Dorey, K. (2010). Characterisation of a new regulator of BDNF signalling, Sprouty3, involved in axonal morphogenesis in vivo. *Development* 137, 4005–4015. doi: 10.1242/dev.053173

Park, K. K., Liu, K., Hu, Y., Smith, P. D., Wang, C., Cai, B., et al. (2008). Promoting axon regeneration in the adult CNS by modulation of the PTEN/mTOR pathway. *Science* 322, 963–966. doi: 10.1126/science.1161566

Pillai, R. S., Bhattacharyya, S. N., Artus, C. G., Zoller, T., Cougot, N., Basyuk, E., et al. (2005). Inhibition of translational initiation by Let-7 MicroRNA in human cells. *Science* 309, 1573–1576. doi: 10.1126/science.1115079

Sasaki, Y., Gross, C., Xing, L., Goshima, Y., and Bassell, G. J. (2013). Identification of axon-enriched MicroRNAs localized to growth cones of cortical neurons. *Dev. Neurobiol.* doi: 10.1002/dneu.22113 [Epub ahead of print].

Schratt, G. (2009). microRNAs at the synapse. *Nat. Rev. Neurosci.* 10, 842–849. doi: 10.1038/nrn2763

Small, E. M., Sutherland, L. B., Rajagopalan, K. N., Wang, S., and Olson, E. N. (2010). MicroRNA-218 regulates vascular patterning by modulation of Slit-Robo signaling. *Circ. Res.* 107, 1336–1344. doi: 10.1161/CIRCRESAHA.110.227926

Stein, E., and Tessier-Lavigne, M. (2001). Hierarchical organization of guidance receptors: silencing of netrin attraction by slit through a Robo/DCC receptor complex. *Science* 291, 1928–1938. doi: 10.1126/science.1058445

Tessier-Lavigne, M., and Goodman, C. S. (1996). The molecular biology of axon guidance. *Science* 274, 1123–1133. doi: 10.1126/science.274.5290.1123

Tymanskyj, S. R., Scales, T. M., and Gordon-Weeks, P. R. (2012). MAP1B enhances microtubule assembly rates and axon extension rates in developing neurons. *Mol. Cell. Neurosci.* 49, 110–119. doi: 10.1016/j.mcn.2011.10.003

Vo, N., Klein, M. E., Varlamova, O., Keller, D. M., Yamamoto, T., Goodman, R. H., et al. (2005). A cAMP-response element binding protein-induced microRNA regulates neuronal morphogenesis. *Proc. Natl. Acad. Sci. U.S.A.* 102, 16426–16431. doi: 10.1073/pnas.0508448102

Willis, D. E., Xu, M., Donnelly, C. J., Tep, C., Kendall, M., Erenstheyn, M., et al. (2011). Axonal Localization of transgene mRNA in mature PNS and CNS neurons. *J. Neurosci.* 31, 14481–14487. doi: 10.1523/JNEUROSCI.2950-11.2011

Yazdani, U., and Terman, J. R. (2006). The semaphorins. *Genome Biol.* 7, 211. doi: 10.1186/gb-2006-7-3-211

Zhang, Y., Ueno, Y., Liu, X. S., Buller, B., Wang, X., Chopp, M., et al. (2013). The MicroRNA-17-92 cluster enhances axonal outgrowth in embryonic cortical neurons. *J. Neurosci.* 33, 6885–6894. doi: 10.1523/JNEUROSCI.5180-12.2013

Zikopoulos, B., and Barbas, H. (2010). Changes in prefrontal axons may disrupt the network in autism. *J. Neurosci.* 30, 14595–14609. doi: 10.1523/JNEUROSCI.2257-10.2010

Zivraj, K. H., Tung, Y. C. L., Piper, M., Gumy, L., Fawcett, J. W., Yeo, G. S. H., et al. (2010). Subcellular profiling reveals distinct and developmentally regulated repertoire of growth cone mRNAs. *J. Neurosci.* 30, 15464–15478. doi: 10.1523/jneurosci.1800-10.2010

Zou, Y., Chiu, H., Domenger, D., Chuang, C. F., and Chang, C. (2012). The lin-4 microRNA targets the LIN-14 transcription factor to inhibit netrin-mediated axon attraction. *Sci. Signal.* 5, ra43. doi: 10.1126/scisignal.2002437

Zou, Y., Chiu, H., Zinovyeva, A., Ambros, V., Chuang, C. F., and Chang, C. (2013). Developmental decline in neuronal regeneration by the progressive change of two intrinsic timers. *Science* 340, 372–376. doi: 10.1126/Science.1231321

Zou, Y., Stoeckli, E., Chen, H., and Tessier-Lavigne, M. (2000). Squeezing axons out of the gray matter: a role for slit and semaphorin proteins from midline and ventral spinal cord. *Cell* 102, 363–375. doi: 10.1016/S0092-8674(00)00041-6

13

The involvement of microRNAs in neurodegenerative diseases

Simona Maciotta[1,2], Mirella Meregalli[1] and Yvan Torrente[1]*

[1] *Stem Cell Laboratory, Department of Pathophysiology and Transplantation, Centro Dino Ferrari, Università degli Studi di Milano, Fondazione IRCCS Cà Granda Ospedale Maggiore Policlinico, Milan, Italy*
[2] *Diabetes Research Institute, University of Miami Miller School of Medicine, Miami, FL, USA*

Correspondence:
Yvan Torrente, Stem Cell Laboratory, Department of Pathophysiology and Transplantation, Centro Dino Ferrari, Università degli Studi di Milano, Fondazione IRCCS Cà Granda Ospedale Maggiore Policlinico, Via Francesco Sforza 35, 20122 Milan, Italy
e-mail: yvan.torrente@unimi.it

Neurodegenerative diseases (NDDs) originate from a loss of neurons in the central nervous system and are severely debilitating. The incidence of NDDs increases with age, and they are expected to become more common due to extended life expectancy. Because no cure is available, these diseases have become a major challenge in neurobiology. The increasing relevance of microRNAs (miRNAs) in biology has prompted investigation into their possible involvement in neurodegeneration in order to identify new therapeutic targets. The idea of using miRNAs as therapeutic targets is not far from realization, but important issues need to be addressed before moving into the clinics. Here, we review what is known about the involvement of miRNAs in the pathogenesis of NDDs. We also report the miRNA expression levels in peripheral tissues of patients affected by NDDs in order to evaluate their application as biomarkers of disease. Finally, discrepancies, innovations, and the effectiveness of collected data will be elucidated and discussed.

Keywords: microRNA, neurodegenerative diseases, biomarker, Parkinson's disease, Alzheimer's disease, amyotrophic lateral sclerosis, Huntington's disease

INTRODUCTION

Neurodegenerative diseases (NDDs) are a family of disorders characterized by progressive loss of neuronal function and structure, resulting in neuronal death in the nervous system. Different types of NDDs exist, depending on the neuron population affected; the most common are Alzheimer's disease (AD), Parkinson's disease (PD), Huntington's disease (HD), and amyotrophic lateral sclerosis (ALS). A commonality of NDDs is that they are not monogenic or polygenic diseases, and they are even more complicated because several events take part in the pathogenesis independent of genetic mutations. The molecular events responsible for neurodegeneration include oxidative stress, axonal transport deficits, protein oligomerization and aggregation, calcium deregulation, mitochondrial dysfunction, neuron–glial interactions, neuroinflammation, DNA damage, and aberrant RNA processing. The greatest risk factor for neurodegeneration is advancing age in combination with mitochondrial DNA mutation and oxidative stress damage. Other possible causes include gender, poor education, endocrine conditions, oxidative stress, inflammation, stroke, hypertension, diabetes, smoking, head trauma, depression, infection, tumors, vitamin deficiencies, immune and metabolic conditions, and chemical exposure. Because the pathogenesis of many of these diseases remains unknown, the role of environmental factors needs to be considered.

In the last few decades, NDDs have become a major challenge in neurobiology due to their enormous and growing social and economic implications in society. For the same reason, increasing research efforts have investigated the underlying molecular mechanisms in order to find a cure. Based on the latest evidence reviewed here, miRNA deregulation is emerging as a contributor to neurodegeneration by influencing most of the mechanisms responsible for NDDs. Neurodegeneration can also be considered to be an RNA disorder (Johnson et al., 2012) in which microRNAs play a major role. Studying miRNA involvement in NDDs might also provide targets for innovative therapies. Until now, patients affected by NDDs have been surgically and pharmacologically treated without obtaining a resolute therapy, which is due primarily to the fact that therapeutic approaches for NDDs require the modulation of multiple targets and molecular pathways because they are multigenic diseases. Based on the evidence that a single miRNA can influence several target genes, a whole disease phenotype could potentially be modified by modulating a single miRNA molecule, which makes these RNA molecules very intriguing from a therapeutic point of view. Furthermore, the identification of deregulated miRNAs in patients affected by NDDs or any other disease might allow earlier diagnosis and the monitoring of disease progress. The main challenge of using proteins as targets for routine diagnostics is low sensitivity, reproducibility, and specificity (Johnson et al., 2012). In conclusion, the aim of this review is to elucidate the broad implications of miRNAs in NDDs, but also to point out the need to overcome technical difficulties related to the study of miRNAs in NDDs. Finally, we also report in detail what has been discovered thus far regarding the involvement of miRNAs in different NDDs in order to evaluate their potential as therapeutic targets.

NON-CODING RNAs

The sequencing of the human genome has demonstrated that the transcriptional output of the human genome is extremely rich in non-coding RNAs (ncRNAs) (Lipovich et al., 2010). Since this discovery, expectations regarding ncRNAs have increased exponentially. More importantly, the expectations have been supported by the development of next-generation sequencing technologies, which have revealed thousands of unknown ncRNAs. The vocabulary for ncRNAs is still far from saturated. The fascination of functional non-protein coding RNAs is that they represent a means for an organism's cells (cells that are genetically identical) to develop unique identities and functions. RNA is part of a mechanism that exerts control over DNA to guarantee the expression of a specific repertoire of genes at the appropriate level and with the appropriate timing. Two important classes of functional RNAs can be distinguished: long non-coding RNAs (lncRNAs) and small RNAs. LncRNAs account for the majority of transcription, they have no unifying structure or function, and they are solely defined as RNA transcripts greater than 200 nucleotides in length with no coding potential (Ponting et al., 2009). Relatively few lncRNAs have been characterized functionally, but increasing evidence suggests important roles for the thousands of uncharacterized transcripts. LncRNAs have been shown to target proteins to specific genomic loci, affecting transcription patterns (Plath et al., 2003; Silva et al., 2003; Kohlmaier et al., 2004; Zhao et al., 2008); to modulate the activity of protein-binding partners (Dreyfuss et al., 2002; Allen et al., 2004; Espinoza et al., 2004; Feng et al., 2006; Shamovsky et al., 2006; Mariner et al., 2008); to function as precursors for small RNAs (Kapranov et al., 2007; Fejes-Toth et al., 2009) to affect the processing of other RNAs (Hellwig and Bass, 2008); and to modulate translation, DNA methylation, and chromatin.

In contrast to lncRNAs, the biogenesis and function of small RNAs is well known and can be divided into five classes: (i) short interfering (si) RNAs (Elbashir et al., 2001a), (ii) small temporal (st) RNAs (Pasquinelli et al., 2000), (iii) heterochromatic siRNAs (Reinhart and Bartel, 2002), (iv) tiny non-coding RNAs (Ambros et al., 2003), and (v) micro (mi) RNAs (Lagos-Quintana et al., 2001; Lau et al., 2001; Lee et al., 2001).These small RNAs are processed from longer precursors and loaded into an Argonaute (Ago) family member within a large effector protein complex. The typical function of small RNAs is to mediate the post-transcriptional gene silencing (PTGS) of target RNA transcripts. The best understood class of small RNAs is miRNAs, which were first discovered by Lee et al. (1993). miRNAs are 21–22nt single-stranded RNA molecules that inhibit gene expression by binding to a complementary sequence in the 3'UTR of target genes (Bartel, 2004). These molecules originate from longer transcripts (pri-miRNA) that are processed by Drosha nuclease to yield a short hairpin "pre-miRNA," which is then processed by Dicer to generate a double-stranded RNA of 21–22nt. Only one of the two strands is loaded into the RNA-induced silencing complex (RISC) that identifies target mRNA based on sequence complementarity with the miRNA. One of the core components of RISC is member of the Argonaute (Ago) protein family, in particular Ago1 and Ago2. After association with RISC, the choice of post-transcriptional repression is determined by sequence complementarity of the miRNA with its binding sequence on the 3′UTR of target mRNA: mRNA cleavage will happen when there is sufficient complementarity, otherwise inhibition of protein translation will occur. (Hammond et al., 2000; Elbashir et al., 2001a,b; Nykanen et al., 2001; Martinez et al., 2002; Schwarz et al., 2002). The relevance of miRNAs has increased with time; they are currently known to be involved in almost all biological processes and developmental programs (Bartel and Bartel, 2003; Carrington and Ambros, 2003; Hunter and Poethig, 2003). The first evidence that ncRNAs play a key role in neurodevelopment is the widespread transcription of ncRNAs in the developing mammalian brain (Lagos-Quintana et al., 2002; Krichevsky et al., 2003; Sempere et al., 2004; Smirnova et al., 2005; Bak et al., 2008). Next generation sequencing allowed the identification of a group of miRNAs that are enriched in the brain and whose expression varies according to area of the brain (Landgraf et al., 2007). In particular, neuronal-specific miRNAs have been demonstrated to control neuronal differentiation, excitability, and function. These brain-enriched miRNAs play a role in a wide range of neurodegenerative pathologies as disease-causing genes, biomarkers, or actors in pathogenesis. The idea of using miRNAs as therapeutic targets is not far from being realized. Two miRNA-based therapeutic approaches can be applied: miRNA mimics and anti-miRNAs. miRNA mimics are small RNA molecules with the same sequence as the mature miRNA of interest that are used to down-regulate the expression of target proteins mimicking the miRNA of interest. The desired effect is over-expression of miRNAs and down-regulation of their target mRNA, which can be used as a protective therapeutic strategy. This strategy has some important challenges that need to be overcome before moving into the clinic. First, the possibility exists that many out off object proteins might also be down-regulated because they are targets of the miRNA of interest. Second, the half-lives of mimics *in vivo* are not well known. Third, treating the brain with miRNA mimics is difficult because they need to pass through the blood-brain barrier (BBB). The second approach is to deliver RNA molecules with a sequence complementary to the miRNA of interest. Stoffel's group designed "antagomirs," RNA snippets conjugated to cholesterol molecules that help the RNA enter a cell (Krutzfeldt et al., 2005). The limit of antagomirs as a possible tool for treating NDDs is that they are not able to cross the BBB and require a local injection. Another strategy to inhibit endogenous miRNAs is to deliver synthetic sponge mRNA, which contains several complementary binding sites for the miRNA of interest (Kluiver et al., 2012a,b). Certain long ncRNAs are able to base-pair with small RNAs, inhibiting the ability of miRNAs to bind to their targets. Therefore, lncRNAs are analogous to how artificial miRNA sponges function (Ebert et al., 2007). This hypothesis was demonstrated by Franco-Zorrilla et al. (2007) with the long ncRNA induced by phosphate starvation 1 (IPS1) in *Arabidopsis thaliana* (Catarecha et al., 2007). Future prospects regarding the administration of miRNAs as therapeutics for NDDs will be discussed later.

NEURODEGENERATIVE DISEASES AND miRNAs

miRNAs IN PARKINSON'S DISEASE (PD)

PD is the second most common NDD, estimated to occur in approximately 1% of individuals >60 years of age, with 4.1–4.6 million people affected worldwide. PD is a progressive neurodegenerative disorder characterized clinically by bradykinesia, tremor, rigidity, and eventually postural instability (Shtilbans and Henchcliffe, 2012). These symptoms are attributed to a loss of dopaminergic neurons of the substantia nigra. The pathology spreads to involve other brain regions, including the amygdala, cingulate gyrus, and higher cortical regions, resulting in the development of dementia and psychosis. The disease itself is quite heterogeneous, and symptom progression is variable (Mouradian, 2012).

Despite rigorous research efforts, patient management and clinical research are still hampered by suboptimal methods for diagnosis, refining the prognosis, predicting individual responses to therapeutic interventions, and tracking disease progression. The critical reliance of dopaminergic neurons on a functioning miRNA network has been demonstrated in both cultured cells and *in vivo* (Kim et al., 2007). The miRNA machinery is important in NDDs in general and in PD in particular because the recognition of the amount of certain pathogenic proteins in specific neuronal populations is critical for the survival of neurons involved in the pathogenesis of disease. No cure is currently available for PD, and ongoing therapies are only directed at treating the most bothersome symptoms. Treatment approaches include medication (dopaminergic administration) and surgical therapy. Other strategies include general lifestyle modifications (rest and exercise), physical therapy, support groups, occupational therapy, and speech therapy. Nevertheless, new experimental therapies are under investigation and ongoing clinical trials are testing the efficacy of anti-inflammatory (pioglitazone) and parasympathomimetic (rivastigmine) drugs, ganglioside administration, and stemcell-based therapies. Even though PD is a multigenic disease, one of the most promising therapeutic approaches is to compensate biologically for the genetic defects responsible for PD pathogenesis. Some efforts have been made in this direction in the field of miRNAs, and the results are encouraging, even if far from clinical implementation.

miR-7/miR-153 regulation of α-synuclein

A negative correlation has been reported with specific miRNAs for two of the genes involved in PD: α-synuclein (SNCA) and leucine-rich repeat kinase2 (LRRK2). SNCA localizes in presynaptic terminals, where it associates with the plasma membrane. The protein is widely expressed in the adult brain, particularly the neocortex, hippocampus, and substantia nigra (Jakes et al., 1994; Mori et al., 2002; Wislet-Gendebien et al., 2008). The 3′UTR of the human protein is more than twice as long as the coding sequence and highly conserved (Sotiriou et al., 2009). This reports simply a relevant role for the 3′in stabilizing SNCA mRNAs and regulating its translation into protein. Point mutations and gene duplication and triplication events in the SNCA locus have been identified in a number of families with autosomal dominant early onset PD (Singleton et al., 2003; Wood-Kaczmar et al., 2006). Higher expression of wild-type SNCA and expression of the three mutant forms of SNCA give rise to insoluble aggregates that constitute the main structure of the Lewy Bodies (Masliah et al., 2000; Tan and Skipper, 2007; Saiki et al., 2011). Thus, downregulation of SNCA represents a possible mechanism for resolving PD. Two miRNAs have been demonstrated to inhibit the expression of SNCA: miR-7 and miR-153 (Junn et al., 2009; Doxakis, 2010) (**Table 1**). Both miRNAs are highly enriched in the brain (Bak et al., 2008), and their sequences are conserved among different organisms. miR-153, in particular, is conserved across vertebrate species. Both miRNAs inhibit SNCA mRNA and protein (Junn et al., 2009; Doxakis, 2010), with an additive effect (Doxakis, 2010). Interestingly, the expression profile of these two miRNAs in the brain of post-natal day 1 mice is similar to α-synuclein protein and mRNA, and has been localized primarily to the neurons of the midbrain, hippocampus, and cortex (Junn et al., 2009; Doxakis, 2010). Co-localization of a miRNA with its target gene suggests tight control of the amount of the target gene produced.

miR-205/let-7/miR-184 regulation of LRRK2*

LRRK2 is a member of the leucine-rich repeat kinase family and is present largely in the cytoplasm, but also associates with

Table 1 | Specific target genes of miRNAs involved in neurodegeneration are listed.

NDDs	miRNAs	Target genes	References
PD	miR-7	DP	Junn et al., 2009; Doxakis, 2010
	miR-153	E2F1	Doxakis, 2010
	let-7	LRRK2	Junn et al., 2009; Gehrke et al., 2010
	miR-184*	LRRK2	Gehrke et al., 2010
	miR-433	FGF20	Davis et al., 2005; Wang et al., 2008a,b
	miR-205	LRRK2	Cho et al., 2013
AD	miR-106a, -520c	APP	Patel et al., 2008
	miR-20a, -106a/b, -17	APP	Hebert and De Strooper, 2009
	miR-16, -101	APP	Long and Lahiri, 2011
	miR-147, -655, -323-3p, -644, -153	APP	Delay et al., 2011
	miR-124	APP splicing	Smith et al., 2011
	miR-29a, -29b-1, -9	BACE1	Hebert and De Strooper, 2009
	miR-298, -328, -195	BACE1	Boissonneault et al., 2009; Zhang, 2012
	miR-124	BACE1	Fang et al., 2012
	miR-98	IGF1	Hu et al., 2013
	miR-181c, -137	SPTLC1	Geekiyanage and Chan, 2011
	miR-29a, -29b-1, -9	SPTLC2	Geekiyanage and Chan, 2011
	miR-34a	TAU	Dickson et al., 2013
ALS	miR-206	HDAC4	Williams et al., 2009
	miR-9	NEFH	Haramati et al., 2010
HD	miR-9	REST	Juliano et al., 2008
	miR-9*	CoREST	Juliano et al., 2008
	miR-196a	mut-Htt	Cheng et al., 2013

NDDs, neurodegenerative diseases; PD, Parkinson's Disease; AD, Alzheimer Disease; ALS, Amiotrophic Lateral Sclerosis; HD, Huntington's disease.

the mitochondrial outer membrane. It is highly expressed in the brain, with the highest levels of expression in the hippocampus and striatum (Galter et al., 2006; Melrose et al., 2006). LRRK2 is involved in the early development of neuronal processes (Parisiadou et al., 2009) and gain-of-function mutations cause familial as well as sporadic PD (Zimprich et al., 2004). Recent investigations in flies have demonstrated that the mutated form of LRRK2 (mut-LRRK2) is responsible for a reduced miRNA-mediated gene repression. This is due to the fact that mut-LRKK2 physically interacts with Ago1 and Ago2—two components of the RISC—inducing their down-regulation in aged Drosophila Melanogaster (Gehrke et al., 2010). Gehrke et al. also investigated the possible target mRNAs whose translation is induced by mut-LRRK2 and identified E2F1 and DP. Flies expressing mut-LRRK2 were in fact characterized by higher expression levels of E2F1 and DP, and down-regulation of E2F1 and DP suppressed the death of dopaminergic neurons. Finally Gehrke S et al. demonstrated that miR-184* and let-7, respectively, repressed E2F1 and DP (**Table 1**) and that inhibition of these miRNAs in wild-type animals was sufficient to phenocopy pathogenic LRRK2. In line with this, both let-7 and miR-184* have been demonstrated to regulate dopaminergic survival and activity (Junn et al., 2009; Gehrke et al., 2010). Regardless the role of mut-LRRK2 in PD, latest studies investigated the consequences of wild-type LRRK2 deregulation in PD pathogenesis. In particular LRRK2 gene locus was identified as a genetic risk factor for the more common sporadic PD (Satake et al., 2009; Simon-Sanchez et al., 2009), indicating that alteration of its expression might be part of PD etiology. Moreover, up-regulation of LRKK2 in an animal model of PD quickened neurodegeneration (Lin et al., 2009). Basing on these evidences, Cho et al. analyzed the expression levels of LRKK2 (protein and mRNA) in the frontal cortex tissue of 8 sporadic PD patients and relative control subjects. No differences in the mRNA levels were found but affected brains were characterized by higher expression levels of LRRK2 protein, suggesting a miRNA-mediated regulation of this protein. *In silico* analysis has demonstrated a predicted binding site for miR-205 in the 3′UTR of LRKK2 and *in vitro* experiments confirmed a direct inhibition of LRKK2 via miR-205. Finally they demonstrated that transfection of miR-205 in the neurons expressing a PD-related LRKK2 R1441G mutant prevented the neurite outgrowth defects (Cho et al., 2013).

miR-433 regulation of FGF20

Fibroblast growth factor 20 (FGF20) is a neurotrophic factor preferentially expressed in the substantia nigra that sustains the survival of dopaminergic neurons (Ohmachi et al., 2000, 2003). In contrast to this pro-survival activity, FGF20 treatment of human neuroblastoma cell line SH-SY5Y increases the amount of endogenous SNCA, demonstrating an anti-survival role of FGF20 in dopaminergic neurons. Single nucleotide polymorphisms (SNPs) in the 3′UTR of this gene (i.e., rs1721100, ss20399075, and rs12720208) have been found to be associated with PD (Wang et al., 2008a). Importantly, the latest polymorphism is within the miR-433 binding site (Davis et al., 2005),which is highly enriched in the brain. Wang et al. demonstrated that SNP rs12720208 avoids inhibition by FGF20 through miR-433 (Wang et al., 2008a). Finally, subsequent investigations failed to confirm a relationship between the rs12720208 genotype, FGF20, and SNCA. These discrepancies are often related to the ethnic origins or genetic backgrounds of PD patients.

miRNAs in the peripheral tissues of PD patients

The use of biomarkers in PD is a moot point, and no reliable biomarker exists for this NDD, with the exception of the monogenetic form of PD. With the increasing relevance of miRNAs in NDDs, some efforts have been made to investigate the possibility of miRNAs as biomarkers. In particular, qRT-PCR analyses of peripheral blood isolated from eight untreated PD patients (NT) and eight control subjects (CTR) showed that the expression levels of three miRNAs (miR-1, miR-22*, and miR-29a) distinguish NT from CTR (Margis et al., 2011) (**Table 2**). A second study was based on qRT-PCR analyses of plasma obtained from 31 NT and 25 CTR (Cardo et al., 2013) and identified seven over-expressed miRNAs (miR-181c, miR-331-5p, miR-193a-3p, miR-196b, miR-454, miR-125a-3p, and miR-137) in NT (**Table 2**). Discrepancies may be attributed to intrinsic differences between the sample types (**Table 2**).

miRNAs IN ALZHEIMER'S DISEASE (AD)

AD is the most common form of dementia in people over 65 years of age. The disease is characterized by progressive neuronal loss and inflammation affecting memory, language, behavior, and cognition. The disease is characterized by amyloid-β (Aβ) deposition, neurofibrillary tangle (NFT) formation, and extensive neuronal degeneration in the brain. Aβ is derived from the sequential cleavage of amyloid precursor protein (APP) by beta-site APP-cleaving enzyme 1 (BACE1) and the γ-secretase complex. The precise pathological mechanisms underlying AD are currently unknown. Clinical and research evidence indicates that aberrant regulation of miRNA-dependent gene expression is closely associated with molecular events responsible for Aβ production, NFT formation, and neurodegeneration (Hebert and De Strooper, 2007, 2009; Hebert et al., 2008; Wang et al., 2008b). The regulation of APP is complex but represents a great challenge in the treatment of AD patients. Current drug discovery approaches in AD have focused on (i) preventing Aβ formation or increasing "normal" APP processing through the inhibition of γ- and β-secretase or the activation of α-secretase activity (Palop and Mucke, 2010; Saido and Leissring, 2012; Schenk et al., 2012); removing existing amyloid deposits via immunotherapeutic approaches,e.g., antibodies or vaccines against amyloid (Schenk et al., 2012). The miRNA field has moved in the same direction, and miRNAs have been discovered to regulate APP expression in three different ways: directly, indirectly, and by regulating the alternative splicing of its mRNA.

Direct inhibition of APP via miRNAs

Direct regulation of APP is mediated by miRNA binding to a specific sequence in the 3'UTR. Several miRNAs that inhibit APP expression *in vitro* have been identified, including miR-106a and miR-520c; members of the miR-20a family (e.g., miR-20a, miR-106a/b, miR-17) (Hebert and De Strooper, 2009); miR-16 and miR-101 (Vilardo et al., 2010; Long and Lahiri, 2011); and miR-147, miR-655, miR-323-3p, miR-644, and miR-153 (Delay et al.,

Table 2 | miRNAs deregulation in NDDs patients.

NDD	miRNAs	Source	Changes	Patients (P) and controls (C)	References
PD	miR-133b	SNC	Down-regulation	3P, 5C	Kim et al., 2007
	miR-34b/c	SNC	Down-regulation	11P, 6C	Minones-Moyano et al., 2011
	miR-1, -22*, -29a	Peripheral blood	Down-regulation	8P, 8C	Margis et al., 2011
	miR-181c, -331-5p, -193a-p, -196b, -454, -125a-3p, -137	Plasma	Over-expression	31P,25 C	Cardo et al., 2013
AD	miR-34a, -181b	PBMC	Over-expression	16P, 16C	Schipper et al., 2007
	miR -26a, -27b, -30e-5p, -34a, -92, -125, -145, -200c, -381, -422a, -423	Hippocampus, cerebellum, medial frontal gyrus	Over-expression	15P, 12C	Cogswell et al., 2008
	miR-9, -132, -146b, -212		Down-regulation		
	let-7f, miR-105, -125a, -135a, -138, -141, -151, -186, -191, -197, -204, -205,- 216, -302b, -30a-5p, -30a-3p, -30b, -30c, -30d, -32, -345, -362, -371, -374, -375, -380-3p, -429, -448, -449, -494, -501, -517, -517b, -518b, 518f, 520a*, 526a	Cerebrospinal fluid	Over-expression	10P, 10C	
	miR-10a, -10b, -125, -126*, -127, 142-5p, -143, -146b, -154, -15b, -181a, -181c, -194, -195, -199a*, -214, -221, -328, -422b, -451, -455, -497, -99a		Down-regulation		
	miR-9, -125b, -146a, 155	Cerebrospinal fluid and brain tissue derived extracellular fluid	Over-expression	3P, 3C	Lukiw, 2007
	miR-26b	Substanzia nigra	Over-expression	10P, 8C	Absalon et al., 2013
ALS	miR-338-3p	Whole blood	Over-expression	12P, 8C	De Felice et al., 2012
	miR-451, -1275, -328, -638, -149, -665, -583		Down-regulation		
	miR-27a, -155, -146a, -32-3p	$CD14^{+}CD16^{-}$ monocytes	Over-expression	8P, 8C	Butovsky et al., 2012
	miR-146*, -524-5p, 582-3p	Spinal cord	Over-expression	5P, 3C	Campos-Melo et al., 2013
	miR-24-2*, -142-3p, -142-5p, -1461, -146b, -155	Spinal cord	Over-expression	16P, 12C	Koval et al., 2013
HD	miR-29a, -330	Brodmann's area 4	Over-expression		Johnson et al., 2008
	miR-132		Down-regulation		
	miR-132, -196, -486	Brodmann's area 4	Over-expression	19P, 7C	Packer et al., 2008
	miR-9, -9*, -124, - 29b, 17-3p, -22, -485-5p, 500, -222		Down-regulation	19P, 7C	
	miR-100, -151-3p,-16, -219-2-3p, -27b, -451, -92a	Frontal cortex and striatum	Over-expression	11P, 11C	Marti et al., 2010
	miR-128, -139-3p,-222,-382,-433,-483-3p	Frontal cortex and striatum	Down-regulation	11P, 11C	Marti et al., 2010
	miR-34b	Plasma	Over-regulation	27P, 12C	Gaughwin et al., 2011

NDDs, neurodegenerative diseases; PD, Parkinson's Disease; AD, Alzheimer Disease; ALS, Amiotrophic Lateral Sclerosis; HD, Huntington's disease.

2011) (**Table 1**). Only a few of these miRNAs are deregulated in the brains of AD patients (Hebert et al., 2008; Nunez-Iglesias et al., 2010), and it is difficult to determine which of these miRNAs regulate APP *in vivo*.

Indirect inhibition of APP via miRNAs

Indirect inhibition of APP via miRNAs is through the direct down-regulation of genes in pathways regulating the expression, function, or processing of this protein. β-secretase BACE1, insulin-like growth factor 1 (IGF-1), and serine palmitoyltransferase (SPT) influence APP expression and are modulated by miRNAs.

BACE1 plays a pivotal role in regulating Aβ production by cleaving APP and releasing APPβ. Hebert et al. demonstrated the *in vitro* inhibition of BACE1 by miR-29a, miR-29b-1, and miR-9 and confirmed an association between the down-regulation of these miRNAs and AD (Hebert et al., 2008). Mice over-expressing miR-29c are characterized by the down-regulation of BACE1 levels, demonstrating an *in vivo* effect on BACE1 modulation (Zong et al., 2011). Other studies demonstrated a negative correlation between BACE1 and miR-298/miR-328/miR-195 in several animal models of AD and confirmed direct inhibition in different mouse cell lines (Boissonneault et al., 2009; Zhu et al., 2012). Finally, the most conserved and abundantly expressed nervous system-specific miR-124 has been shown to inhibit BACE1 expression in cultured rat PC12 cell lines and primary cultured hippocampal neurons, a cellular model of AD (Fang et al., 2012).

De-regulation of IGF-1-mediated signaling has been correlated with AD (Rosario, 2010). IGF-1 function in the brain includes Aβ clearance from the brain and phosphorylation of tau (Hong and Lee, 1997; Vargas et al., 2011). Hu et al. showed that the expression of miR-98 negatively correlates with the IGF-1 expression level in a mouse model of AD. Furthermore, over-expression of miR-98 in cellular models of AD is responsible for the down-regulation of IGF-1, enhanced Aβ production, and tau phosphorylation (Hu et al., 2013).

SPT, a heterodimer composed of serine palmitoyltransferase long chain 1 (SPTLC1) and serine palmitoyltransferase long chain 2 (SPTLC2), is the first rate-limiting enzyme in the de novo ceramide synthesis pathway (Hannun and Obeid, 2008). Membrane ceramides are known to contribute to AD pathology by facilitating the mislocation of BACE1 and γ-secretase to lipid rafts, thereby promoting Aβ formation (Lee et al., 1998; Vetrivel et al., 2005). Interestingly, SPT is increased in the brain of sporadic AD patients (Geekiyanage and Chan, 2011) with up-regulation of several miRNAs, including miR-137, miR-181c, miR-9, miR-29a, miR-29b-1, and miR-15. *In vitro* luciferase assay confirmed direct inhibition of SPTLC1 by miR-181c and miR-137 and of SPTLC2 by miR-29a, miR-29b1, and miR-9. Moreover, a negative correlation has been demonstrated between the expression levels of these miRNAs and their relative target genes, SPTLC1 and SPTLC2, in the frontal cortices of sporadic AD patients (Geekiyanage and Chan, 2011).

miRNAs regulating the alternative splicing of APP

Human APP exists as three major isoforms (APP751, APP770, and APP695) originating from alternative splicing. Isoforms APP751 and APP770 are widely expressed and contain the Kunitz protease inhibitor (KPI) domain encoded by exon7, but only APP770 contains the putative glycosylation domain OX2 encoded by exon8. The APP695 isoform is majorly expressed in neurons (Zhang et al., 2011) and contains neither the KPI nor OX2 domains. Changes in the expression profile of neuronal APP are associated with an increase in Aβ production (Donev et al., 2007). Higher expression of APP isoforms containing exons 7 and 8 is found in various areas of the brains of AD patients (Golde et al., 1990; Neve et al., 1990; Jacobsen et al., 1991; Tanzi et al., 1993; Rockenstein et al., 1995). To investigate the involvement of miRNAs in the regulation of APP splicing, Smith et al. created a forebrain-specific Dicer conditional knock-out mouse in which post-mitotic neurons were characterized as having increased levels of APP751 and APP770 isoforms. Because miR-124 plays a pivotal role in neuronal maintenance and splicing (Makeyev et al., 2007; Papagiannakopoulos and Kosik, 2009), Smith et al. induced the ectopic expression of miR-124 in Neuro2a cells, which was enough to induce the skipping of exons 7 and 8 by inhibiting polypyrimidine tract binding protein 1 (PTB1). In addition, and supporting this observation, lower expression of miR-124 was measured in the brains of AD patients (Smith et al., 2011).

miR-34a/miR-26b regulation of tau protein

The microtubule-associated protein tau promotes the assembly and stability of microtubules (Weingarten et al., 1975; Drubin and Kirschner, 1986). It is involved in many NDDs, collectively known as tauopathies (Lee et al., 2001). In the case of AD, tau is hyperphosphorylatated and accumulates in the cytoplasm where it gives origin to intraneuronal protein aggregates known as NFTs (Kosik et al., 1986; Nukina and Ihara, 1986; Wood et al., 1986). Although alterations in tau protein are not considered the earliest event in AD pathogenesis, reduction in its expression levels may be safe and beneficial to prevent or treat AD (Rapoport et al., 2002; Roberson et al., 2007; Ittner et al., 2010; Vossel et al., 2010). In this optics, Dickson et al. investigated the role of the 3′UTR of human tau mRNA in regulating tau expression. Using different prediction algorithms, they found several miRNA-binding sites and they were able to validate direct inhibition of human tau by miR-34a (Dickson et al., 2013). Another approach to inhibit NFT formation is represented by regulating the phosphorilation status of tau protein. Tau is in fact a phosphoprotein that contains more than 80 potential phosphorylation sites (Hanger and Noble, 2011). As mentioned above, hyperphosphorilation of tau causes insoluble aggregates into the cytoplasm of neurons. In regard, Absalon et al. identified a specific miRNA (miR-26b) that rises in the substantia nigra at early stages of AD (Braak III) and remains elevated in the pathological area of human AD brain during disease progression. A target mRNA of miR-26b was confirmed to be Retinoblastoma (Rb). Both over-expression of miR-26b and down-regulation of Rb in primary cortical neurons showed activation of cyclin-dependent kinase 5 (Cdk5) and enhanced tau phosphorylation, followed by apoptosis and neurodegeneration *in vitro* (Absalon et al., 2013). AntagomiR-26b based therapy might not only decrease tau phosphorylation and NTF formation, but also enhances neuronal survival.

miR-146 regulation of presenilin

As described by Haas et al. the APP undergoes successive proteolysis by β- and γ-secretases to produce the Aβ that characteristically deposits in AD brain (Hass et al., 2009). γ-Secretases is a large complex of four integral membrane proteins, with presenilin (PSEN) as the catalytic subunit. Dominant mutations in the genes encoding for presenilins (PSEN1 and PSEN2) are the most common cause of familial early-onset Alzheimer's disease (Brouwers et al., 2008). These mutations alter the biochemical character of the γ-secretase complex and its interaction with the APP substrate, so that a longer and aggregation-prone form of Aβ is produced (Mucke and Selkoe, 2011). It is also to note that presenilins function is likely to be relevant to the development of sporadic AD. For all above reasons, presenilins together with β- and γ-secretases are top targets for AD drug discovery. In addition to its role in Aβ generation, PSEN2 was demonstrated to modulate the microglia activity (Jayadev et al., 2013). More in detail, Jayadev et al. demonstrated that *in vivo* deficiency of PSEN2 associated with exaggerated pro-inflammatory state in microglia. Basing on this evidence, they hypothesized that presenilin disfunctions could contribute to AD neurotoxic inflammation (Jayadev et al., 2010). In order to elucidate the underlining molecular mechanisms, PSEN2 knockout (KO) and wt microglia were analyzed for differential miRNA expression. The expression profiles of several miRNAs involved in the regulation of innate immune signaling were perturbed in PSENKO microglia, including miR-146 that is a potent negative regulator of innate immunity. This observation suggested that PS2 modulates cytokine responses via inhibition of miR-146. In line with this evidence, the target mRNA of miR-146a IRAK-1 (interleukin-1 receptor-associated kinase-1) was increased in PS2KO microglia. One of the function of IRAK-1 is to be a mediator of IL-1 (interleukin-1) signaling (Cao et al., 1996) and a critical regulator of Toll-like receptor (TLR) signal transduction (Swantek et al., 2000). When activated, IRAK-1 binds to NFkB thereby promoting nuclear localization and transcriptional activity (Flannery and Bowie, 2010). Indeed PS2KO vs. wt. microglia showed increased NFkB activity upon stimulation with lipopolysaccharide (LPS). Jayadev et al. strongly demonstrated that PSEN2 influences microglia activity but the exact mechanism by which PSEN2 carries out this task via miR-146 modulation still need to be elucidated (Jayadev et al., 2013).

miRNA profile of the brain and peripheral tissues in AD

In most cases, AD can only be diagnosed by neuropsychological studies, neuroimaging, and clinical data from patients that allow characterization as probable or possible AD patients (Mckhann et al., 1984) with a sensitivity of 93% and specificity of 55%. Furthermore, diagnosis is far more difficult in early and unusual presentations of the disease. Several research efforts have examined miRNAs in order to identify potential biomarkers. In 2007, the first small-scale profiling of miRNAs was performed on the hippocampal region of fetal, adult, and AD brains (Lukiw, 2007). Since then, several large-scale analyses have been performed on different AD tissues, including brain, peripheral blood, and cerebrospinal fluid (CSF) (Schipper et al., 2007; Cogswell et al., 2008; Hebert et al., 2008; Wang et al., 2008a; Nunez-Iglesias et al., 2010; Shioya et al., 2010). Nevertheless, miRNA expression studies on AD patients have had either no or very little overlap in miRNA changes (**Table 2**). Schipper et al. analyzed blood mononuclear cells (BMC) from patients with sporadic AD using miRNA microarray analyses and found two miRNAs that are significantly up-regulated in AD subjects: miR-34a and miR-181b (Schipper et al., 2007) (**Table 2**). Cogswell et al. performed qRT-PCR analysis on brain tissue and CSF from AD patients, identifying a set of miRNAs, so-called AD-specific miRNAs, that are differentially expressed in the brain and altered in the CSF of AD patients (Cogswell et al., 2008) (**Table 2**). Finally, Lukiw et al. group recently characterized the miRNome of AD CSF and short post-mortem interval brain tissue-derived extracellular fluid (ECF) using fluorescent miRNA array, finding significant increases in miR-9, miR-125b, miR-146a, and miR-155 in AD CSF and ECF (Lukiw, 2007) (**Table 2**).

miRNAs IN AMYOTROPHIC LATERAL SCLEROSIS (ALS)

ALS is often referred to as "Lou Gehrig's Disease." It is a progressive, idiopathic, fatal NDD that affects nerve cells in the brain and spinal cord. Motor neuron loss gives rise to malfunctions in the muscle tissue, causing weakness, atrophy, and ultimately paralysis and death within 3 or 5 years of symptom onset. The disease occurs worldwide with an incidence of approximately 2×10^5 and a prevalence of approximately 6–8 $\times 10^5$. Currently, there is only one FDA-approved compound; riluzole does not resolve the disease, but slows progression and extends survival with modest effects. The discovery of small molecules that change the course of disease in ALS is desirable. With the increasing relevance of miRNAs, many recent research efforts have investigated the role of these small RNA molecules in the pathogenesis of ALS. The data that have been obtained are encouraging but still in their infancy, as they demonstrated an involvement but are far from proposing a solution. Nevertheless, if we are able to improve our understanding of the pathogenesis of ALS, it could lead to the development of early and specific diagnostic methods and extend the life expectancy of ALS patients. No definitive diagnostic tests or biomarkers exist for ALS, and neurologists rely on clinical criteria for diagnosis. The development of novel biomarkers to evaluate disease progression could give us the ability to refine the design of therapeutic trials and reduce the costs of clinical trials (Kiernan et al., 2011).

miR-206 and re-innervation

One of the most promising studies toward an innovative approach to cure ALS was conducted by Williams et al. (2009). miRNAs are involved in the stress response in skeletal muscle (Van Rooij and Olson, 2007). Because ALS is characterized by paralysis of the lower limbs, Williams et al. investigated the miRNome of muscles isolated from the lower limbs of an animal model of ALS, SOD1 transgenic mice. MyomiR-206 (Chen et al., 2006; Rao et al., 2006) was strongly induced, and its up-regulation coincided with the onset of symptoms. After severing the sciatic nerve of wild-type mice to induce denervation of the lower leg muscles, higher expression levels of miR-206 were observed 10 days after surgery in fast-twitch muscles, suggesting the involvement of this miRNA in re-innervation. This hypothesis was confirmed when miR-206 was knocked out in SOD1 transgenic mice, demonstrating accelerated progression of ALS and shortened survival (Williams et al., 2009). The underlying molecular mechanism was investigated and miR-206 was found to induce the secretion of fibroblast growth factor binding protein 1 (FGFBP1) from muscle by inhibiting Histone deacetylase 4 (HDAC4) translation. FGFBP1 potentiates the effect of FGFs in the promotion of presynaptic differentiation at the neuromuscular junction (Fox et al., 2007).

miRNA biogenesis and ALS

Multiple studies have identified several dominant mutations in the 43-kDa trans-activating response region (TAR) DNA-binding protein (TDP-43) in both sporadic and familial ALS patients that are associated with other NDDs (Kabashi et al., 2008; Sreedharan et al., 2008; Pesiridis et al., 2009; Lagier-Tourenne et al., 2010). A functionally related gene, fused in sarcoma/translocation in liposarcoma (FUS/TLS), is also mutated in ALS (Kwiatkowski et al., 2009; Vance et al., 2009). These two DNA/RNA-binding proteins physically interact with one another and are physiologically involved in the regulation of RNA transcription and splicing (Giordana et al., 2010; Lagier-Tourenne et al., 2010). The exact mechanism by which these proteins become pathogenic in ALS remains uncertain, but the most assessed hypothesis is related to their nuclear/cytoplasmic imbalance (Kwiatkowski et al., 2009; Vance et al., 2009; Giordana et al., 2010). Moreover, Ling et al. discovered that ALS-associated forms of TDP-43 have longer half-lives, contributing to TDP-43 aggregation in ALS patients, and they have an increased affinity for FUS/TLS (Ling et al., 2010).

By combining tandem-affinity purification and quantitative mass-spectrometry analysis, Ling et al. discovered that TDP-43 is associated with multiple hnRNP proteins and the Drosha microprocessing complex (Ling et al., 2010). Similarly, data indicated that Drosha protein is a putative FUS interactor (Gregory et al., 2004). Association with Drosha and mislocation of TDP-43 and FUS/TLS suggests de-regulation of miRNA biogenesis in ALS. Independent from this study, knocking down TDP-43 in the human Hep-3B cell line was later shown to replicate the changes occurring in the total miRNA population (Buratti et al., 2010). A relationship was also demonstrated between TDP-43 and brain-enriched miR-9; loss of Drosophila TDP-43 was characterized by down-regulation of miR-9a and TDP-43 influenced sensory organ precursor (SOP) cells in Drosophila through miR-9a (Li et al., 2013). Regarding FUS/TLS, its down-regulation in neuroblastoma cell line SK-N-BE affected the biogenesis of a large class of miRNAs, including neuronal isoforms. FUS/TLS is recruited at the chromatin, where it directly binds pri-miRNAs, facilitating Drosha loading (Morlando et al., 2012).

miR-9 regulation of neurofilaments

Neurofilaments are components of the neuronal cytoskeleton and provide structural support to the axons. They are assembled from light, medium, and heavy subunits, creating three different types of neurofilaments: light (NEFL), medium (NEFM), and heavy (NEFH). If the expression of neurofilaments is not well orchestrated, axonal cytoskeletal defects occur (Julien, 1999; Liem and Messing, 2009). Perturbation of the fine neurofilaments is associated with the development of human ALS (Figlewicz et al., 1994; Tomkins et al., 1998; Al-Chalabi et al., 1999). The 3′UTRs of neurofilament-encoding genes appear to interact with an uncharacterized trans-acting factor that is attenuated in ALS (Haramati et al., 2010), which might be miRNAs. In support of this hypothesis, ablation of Dicer1 in post-mitotic post-natal motor neurons fails to coordinate neurofilament subunit stoichiometry, but only the expression levels of NEFH were perturbed. Prediction analyses found one and nine binding sites for miR-9 in the 3′UTR of NEFL and NEFH, respectively. Direct inhibition of NEFH by miR-9 was confirmed by *in vitro* experiments (**Table 1**), but no luciferase assays were performed to validate the NEFL/miR-9 interaction. Thus, dysregulation of neurofilament stoichiometry in several motoneuron diseases is due to miR-9 loss (Haramati et al., 2010). No further efforts have been made to understand the involvement of miR-9 in ALS.

miRNA profile of the spinal cord in ALS

The first study aiming to characterize the miRNA profile in the spinal cord of sporadic ALS patients was conducted by Campos-Melo et al. (2013). They used a quantitative qRT-PCR-based array method to screen 664 human miRNAs from the spinal cords of three healthy controls and five ALS patients; they identified 246 down-regulated and 10 up-regulated miRNAs (**Table 2**). This was the only study reporting such a mass decrease in the miRNA profile for NDDs. Interestingly, many of the de-regulated miRNAs were predicted to have a binding site in the 3′UTR of NEFL, and consistent inhibition was demonstrated for miR-146*, miR-524-5p, and miR-582-3p (Campos-Melo et al., 2013). Around the same time, Koval et al. characterized the expression of 613 miRNAs using miRNA microarray experiments and the spinal cords of diseased rats and mice. Using individual assays, 11 miRNAs were confirmed in the diseased mice, 10 in $SOD1^{G93A}$ rats, and 6 in ALS patients (miR-24-2*, miR-142-3p, miR-142-5p, miR-1461, miR-146b, and miR-155) (**Table 2**). More importantly, miR-155 was increased in both sporadic and familial ALS patients, and when its expression was inhibited in the brain of $SOD1^{G93A}$ rats *in vivo*, both survival and disease duration were increased (Koval et al., 2013).

miRNAs in the peripheral tissues of ALS patients

De Felice et al. performed the first and only miRNA profiling of leukocytes isolated from blood to identify characteristic patterns in sporadic ALS patients (De Felice et al., 2012). Briefly, leukocytes were isolated from the blood of 8 patients and 12 healthy controls and screened for the expression of 911 human miRNAs using microarray technology. Eight miRNAs (miR-338-3p, miR-451, miR-1275, miR-328, miR-638, miR-149, miR-665, and miR-583) were de-regulated in ALS patients (**Table 2**). Among these miRNAs, miR-338-3p was previously found in brain tissue from ALS patients (Shioya et al., 2010).This study detected, for the first time, specific disease-related changes in miRNAs at an earlier stage of sporadic ALS.

Another study was performed on peripheral tissues from ALS patients; in particular, the analyses were restricted to a subgroup of monocytes ($CD14^{+}CD16^{-}$) isolated from ALS patients. This population was chosen because its murine analog ($Ly6^{Chi}$monocytes) isolated from SOD1 mice has a pronounced pro-inflammatory profile (gene and miRNA expression) prior to disease onset and is recruited to the spinal cord, where the cells proliferate during disease progression. The human $CD14^{+}CD16^{-}$monocytes isolated from ALS patients and $Ly6^{Chi}$ monocytes isolated from SOD1 mice had a unique inflammatory miRNA profile. $Ly6^{Chi}$ diseased monocytes were characterized by the up-regulation of let- 7, miR-15b, miR-16, miR-27a, miR-34a, miR-132, miR-146a, miR-155, miR-223, and miR-451 (**Table 2**). Human $CD14^{+}CD16^{-}$ALS monocytes had higher expression levels of miR-27a, miR-155, miR-146a, and miR-32-3p (Butovsky et al., 2012) (**Table 2**). Finally, the authors underlined the potential role of these miRNAs as biomarkers of ALS.

miRNAs AND HUNTINGTON'S DISEASE (HD)

HD is an incurable neurodegenerative condition caused by CAG repeat expansion in the huntingtin gene (Htt). HD patients manifest cognitive defects and motor control impairment due to neuronal dysfunction characterized by progressive loss of cortical and striatal neurons. Neuronal death happens due to the toxicity associated with the mutant Htt protein and loss of the neuroprotective effects of the wild-type protein (Cattaneo et al., 2005). Little is known about the function of Htt, but its mutant form affects cellular phenotype and viability (Zuccato et al., 2010). Several genes have been found to be altered in the brain of HD patients (Cha, 2007), and many transcription factors (TFs) interact with Htt and are recruited to the mutant Htt aggregates (Sugars and Rubinsztein, 2003) in the brain. Recruitment to Htt aggregates prevents TFs from binding to DNA and eliciting their functions. More importantly, mutant Htt inhibits the formation of processing bodies (P bodies) by interacting with Ago1 and Ago2, which are involved in miRNA biogenesis (Savas et al., 2008). Thus, miRNA dysregulation is expected in the brain of HD patients. Currently, no cure exists for HD; all of the treatments are palliative. RNA therapy has emerged as a powerful tool for modifying the disease course by targeting mutant HTT mRNA for degradation.

miRNA profile in the brain of HD patients

Htt was demonstrated to interact with repressor element 1 silencing transcription factor (REST), the essential transcriptional repressor also known as neuron-restrictive silencing factor (NRSF), in neurons (Zuccato et al., 2003; Ooi and Wood, 2007). In control individuals, Htt sequesters REST in the cytoplasm of neurons and prevents the repressor from binding to DNA; in HD patients the mutant Htt does not associate with REST, which relocates to the nucleus of HD neurons and represses many of its target genes. One of the target genes of REST is BDNF, which is essential for neuron survival (Zuccato et al., 2003).

Based on the presence of REST binding sites in the genome, Johnson et al. were able to identify a set of REST-target miRNAs in the human genome (miR-9-1, 9-3, 29a, 29b-1, 124a-1, 124a-2, 124a-3, 132, 135b, 139, 203, 204, 212, 330, and 346) that are also brain or neuron-specific (Johnson et al., 2008). Among these miRNAs, four (miR-29a, miR-124a, miR-132, and miR-330) were found to be decreased in the cortex of R6/2 mice, an animal model of HD. Furthermore, their known target mRNAs were increased in R6/2 mice (Johnson et al., 2008) Johnson et al. then analyzed the expression profile of miR-29a, miR-124a, miR-132, and miR-135b in parietal cortical tissues from control and HD individuals; only down-regulation of miR-132 was confirmed in the human samples (**Table 2**). Otherwise, the expression levels of miR-29a and miR-330 were increased and miR-124a did not differ between HD and control subjects (Johnson et al., 2008) (**Table 2**).

Packer et al. investigated whether miRNAs correlate with disease progression in HD patients by analyzing the expression profile of predicted REST-regulated miRNAs in Brodmann's area 4 (BA4) isolated from control and HD grade 1–4 brain samples (Packer et al., 2008). Five miRNAs (miR-9, miR-9*, miR-29b, miR-124a, and miR-132) were significantly different with increasing HD grade (Packer et al., 2008). Otherwise, no correlation with disease progression was observed for miR-139, miR-135b, and miR-212. Next, a qRT-PCR-based miRNA array platform was used to evaluate the expression profiles of 365 mature miRNAs in the BA4 cortex from control and early stage HD (grades 1 and 2) patients. The de-regulation of additional miRNAs, including miR-486, miR-196a, miR-17-3p, miR-22, miR-485-5p, miR-500, and miR-222, was found (Packer et al., 2008).

Finally, Marti et al. analyzed the expression profile of miRNAs in the frontal cortex and striatum of HD patients using three different techniques: RNA sequencing, microarray, and qRT-PCR. miR-100, miR-151-3p, miR-16, miR-219-2-3p, miR-27b, miR-451, and miR-92a were found to be over-expressed in diseased tissues in all three experiments (Marti et al., 2010). Similarly, miR-128, miR-139-3p, miR-222, miR-382, miR-433, and miR-483-3p were decreased in the HD brain tissue in all three experiments (Marti et al., 2010).

Based on the data above, 30 miRNAs are increased and 24 miRNAs are decreased in the brains of HD patients. De-regulation of 33 of the 54 miRNAs associated with HD can be attributed to four TFs that are altered in the HD brain; TP53, REST, E2F1, and GATA4 (Sinha et al., 2012). In particular, TP53 is involved in processing the primary miRNA transcript to the mature miRNA (Suzuki et al., 2009). Because intronic miRNAs are transcribed at the same levels as the host genes if oriented in the same direction (Baskerville and Bartel, 2005; Wang et al., 2009), Sinha et al. investigated a possible relationship between the host genes and intronic miRNAs in HD. Thirty-one of the 54 miRNAs deregulated in the brains of HD patients are encoded within the introns, and the expression of some of these miRNAs correlates with the expression levels of their host genes (Sinha et al., 2012).

miR-9/9 -REST/CoREST feedback in HD*

As mentioned above, the expression levels of miR-9 and miR9* are decreased in the cerebral cortex of HD-affected subjects. Interestingly these two miRNAs target REST and CoREST, respectively (Johnson and Bucley, 2009a). REST has been demonstrated to inhibit the expression of neuronal genes in non-neuronal cells, and under normal conditions it is retained in the cytoplasm by interacting with Htt. When Htt is mutated, REST no longer associates with Htt, which then relocates and accumulates in the nucleus, where it inhibits the expression of several genes (Zuccato et al., 2003). Decreased levels of miR-9/9* in HD would increase the transcription of REST, amplifying the accumulation of this protein in the presence of mutated Htt. This phenomenon is further magnified because miR-9/9* transcription depends on REST. Thus, the translocation of REST to the nucleus in HD brain tissues explains the reduced expression of miR-9/miR9* (Johnson et al., 2009b).

miR-196a and HTT expression

Based on the results published by Packer et al. (2008) and on unpublished microarray data from transgenic monkeys with HD, Cheng et al. identified miR-196a as a possible miRNA involved in the pathogenesis of HD. To further investigate the role of this miRNA in HD, they co-transfected human embryonic kidney and murine neuroblastoma cell lines with two constructs: miR-196a mimic and the mutant form of Htt. These *in vitro* experiments showed for the first time that miR-196a suppresses the expression of mutant Htt at the mRNA and protein levels. Furthermore, this inhibition was not due to the direct binding of miR-196a to the3′UTR of mutated Htt. Otherwise, miR-196a predominantly suppressed Htt expression through the inhibition of protein synthesis and partly through enhanced protein degradation. To confirm these results *in vivo*, Cheng et al. generated a miR-196a transgenic mouse and bred it with transgenic mice expressing mutant Htt fused to green fluorescent protein (GFP). The expression of miR-196a and mutant Htt were up- and down-regulated, respectively, in the brain of double transgenic mice, confirming the *in vitro* results. Moreover, inhibition by miR-196a also occurred at later stages of the disease in double transgenic mice when more Htt aggregates accumulated. Because the double transgenic mouse model represents a model of over-expression, Chen et al. evaluated the inhibition of mutated Htt via miR-196a by transfecting induced pluripotent stem cells derived from individuals with HD (HD-iPSCs) with lentiviral vector encoding for miR-196a. As expected, untreated cells accumulated more mutated Htt aggregates, whereas cells transfected with miR-196a were characterized by lower expression of mutated Htt, suggesting that miR-196a can alleviate the pathological phenotypes in human samples. The downstream effect of miR-196a over-expression on Htt metabolism was investigated; the ubiquitin-proteosome system, gliosis, cAMP response element-binding protein pathway, and several neuronal regulatory pathways were implicated (Cheng et al., 2013). All of these evidences suggest a potential therapeutic role of miR-196a in HD.

miRNAs in the peripheral tissues of HD patients

Even though the ultimate trait biomarker is represented by mutated Htt, many efforts have focused on identifying mRNAs or proteins with expression profiles that could correlate with disease progression. Gaughwin et al. developed a cell model of HD (HTT-Exon-1 over-expressing human cell line) in order to identify miRNA biomarkers. Briefly, they transfected an embryonal carcinoma-derived pluripotent cell line (NT2) capable of differentiating into neurons with Htt-Exon-1 construct carrying 23, 73, and 145 polyglutamine repeats. Microarray analysis revealed two known miRNAs (miR-34b and miR-1285) that are increased in the presence of 73Q-Htt and 145Q-Htt compared to23Q-Htt. Based on these data, they investigated the expression levels of miR-34b and miR-1285 in human plasma, demonstrating that they are detectable in human samples and bio-stable relative to proteins. When the investigation was expanded to plasma from HD patients, miR-34b was increased in pre-manifest HD plasma relative to age-matched controls (Gaughwin et al., 2011). In contrast, no correlation was found for miR-1285. These results suggest that miR-34b behaves as a potential biomarker of HD prior to symptom onset. Despite the novelty of the results obtained, a limitation of this study was the small patient cohort, which needs to be enlarged.

THERAPEUTIC miRNAs FOR NDDs

The essential properties of a drug are favorable bioavailability, a reasonable half-life, and few side effects. These requirements are dependent on the type of drug, the target organ, and on the delivery system used. An ideal vector for *in vivo* delivery of RNA molecules should be equipped with a cationic group for effective transfection, an endosomolytic group for endosomal escape, a surface modifier to decrease steric hindrance, which enhances circulation in the blood, and a targeting moiety to direct the delivery system at target cells or tissue (Whitehead et al., 2009). From the injection of miRNA agonists/antagonists and knockdown of target genes/endogenous miRNAs, physiological barriers represent the first obstacle to the efficacy of drug treatment. Many checkpoints are represented by glomerular filtration, hepatic metabolism, reticular endothelial system (RES) uptake, and endothelial barriers. If injected as naked molecules, RNA is subjected to nuclease degradation, which is responsible for 70% knockdown of drug efficacy within 1 min of administration (Mahato et al., 1995). To avoid the action of nucleases, chemical modification or non-viral carriers can be used (Borchard, 2001; Wang et al., 2002; Crooke, 2004; Juliano, 2005; Juliano et al., 2008). RNA particles >200 nm delivered to liposomes, lipoplexes, polyplexes, or nanoparticles are subjected to phagocytosis by RES (Alexis et al., 2008), and those smaller than 100 nm are the target of hepatic Kupffer cells. Conjugation with non-viral carriers might induce marked toxicity because RNA molecules will also enter the non-targeted cells due to an interaction between the negatively charged cellular membrane and cationic carriers (Uyechi et al., 2001). This effect might be reduced by coating carriers with hydrophilic molecules (polyethylene glycol) or by conjugation with a ligand (e.g., surface receptor-specific antibodies) (Balyasnikova et al., 2002). Furthermore, RNA molecules can be associated with aptamers, monoclonal antibodies, or peptides to target specific cell surface receptors and the desired target in the body (Juliano, 2005; Chu et al., 2006; Kumar et al., 2008). After RNA molecules have passed these physiological barriers, they have to enter the target cells to elicit their actions. This means that they have to cross the cell membrane, escape endosomes, and localize in the nucleus. Therefore, nuclear-localization signals and cell-penetrating and endosomal-release signal peptides can influence the duration of action of injected RNA molecules (Jere et al., 2009).

In vivo delivery of RNA can be achieved two ways: systematically and locally (**Figure 1**). A great amount of drug is required when it is injected systemically. In contrast, local delivery allows a small amount of drug to be administered with reduced side effects (Pardridge, 2007; Pushparaj et al., 2008; Shen, 2008). Notably, systemic delivery is preferred when the target organ is the liver as the majority of systemically administered drug molecules localize to the liver. Efforts have been made to deliver RNA molecules across

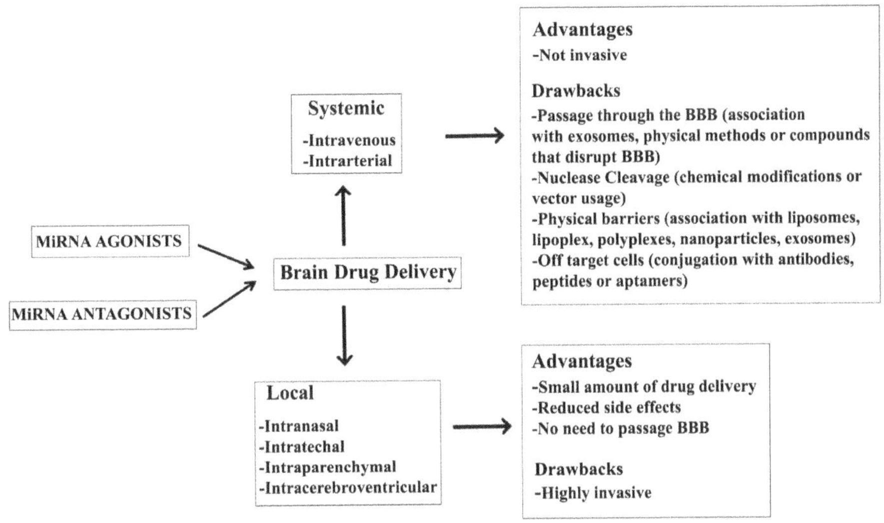

FIGURE 1 | Advantages and drawbacks of a miRNA-based therapy for the treatment of NDDs.

the BBB by *in vivo* systemic delivery, but it remains a major challenge in the treatment of NDDs. In particular, physical methods, such as ultrasound (Chen et al., 2010; Liu et al., 2010), and the intra-arterial infusion of compounds that disrupt the BBB (e.g., potassium channel agonists and minoxidil sulphate) increase the chances of overcoming the BBB (Ningaraj et al., 2007; Bidros et al., 2010). Recently, Alvarez-Erviti et al. experimented the delivery of RNA molecules associated with exosomes across the BBB. Exosomes are cell-derived vesicles that enable cell-to-cell communication by transferring RNA molecules and proteins. They have been shown to preserve mRNAs and miRNAs in the presence of RNase and subsequently deliver them to recipient cells (Valadi et al., 2007; Skog et al., 2008; Zomer et al., 2010). In particular, Alvarez-Erviti et al. isolated brain-targeting exosomes from dendritic cells bioengineered to express an exosomal membrane protein (Lamp 2b) fused to a ligand of the acetylcholine receptor. Exosomes were then loaded with siRNAs targeting BACE1 mRNA by electroporation and injected intravenously, resulting in a significant knock-down of BACE1 expression (Alvarez-Erviti et al., 2011).

Efficient local delivery strategies for the CNS are intranasal, intracerebroventricular, intrathechal, or intraparenchymal injection of naked RNAi formulated in isotonic saline buffer (Makimura et al., 2002). Adenoviral, lentiviral, and adeno-associated virus-based local delivery has also been performed in animal models of AD, HD (Harper et al., 2005), and ALS (Ralph et al., 2005), demonstrating significant improvement. Nevertheless, the strategy to locally deliver a drug to the brain is still far from normal practice because of the complexities associated with direct injection into the brain.

CONCLUSION

Following the discovery of miRNAs, their actions were investigated in almost all biological processes and, even more importantly, their central role in gene-expression regulation implicated in many human diseases (Subramanian et al., 2008; Thum et al., 2008; Eisenberg et al., 2009; Malumbres et al., 2009; Matkovich et al., 2009; Crist and Buckingham, 2010; Maciotta et al., 2012). miRNAs are of particular interest in understanding complex disorders, such as NDDs, because they can potentially regulate several pathways involved in the insurgence and progression of the disease. In the last few years, miRNAs have also been considered as biomarkers; they offer several advantages over mRNA or protein, including increased stability and biological relevance in many different diseases. In fact, miRNAs offer the possibility to link a biomarker with an altered biological process and therapy capable of targeting the pathological mechanism. miRNA-based therapeutic treatments for NDDs may follow two different strategies: miRNA over-expression (gain-of-function) or miRNA repression (loss-of-function) (**Figure 1**). The first approach might use miRNA-associated target gene specificity in order to down-regulate the expression of the aberrant gene within the cell of interest; the second should use miRNAs to directly influence the differentiation of neural stem cells (NSCs) (Palm et al., 2012).

In the last few years, the hypothesis that miRNAs could be involved in NDDs has gained support (Hebert and De Strooper, 2007) due to many experiments with different animal models, such as the fly and mouse. Much experimental data demonstrate that the miRNA network is necessary for neuron survival (Hebert and De Strooper, 2009). Experiments conducted in humans support the idea that changes in miRNA expression profiles or miRNA targets could increase the risk of major NDDs, such as AD and PD (**Tables 1, 2**).

miRNA research seems particularly promising for understanding not only the very prevalent and poorly understood sporadic forms of AD, but also forms of PD. The challenge now is to understand the role of specific miRNAs in biological models and translate this knowledge to clinical studies (Hebert and De Strooper, 2009).

The use of miRNAs as potential therapeutic targets remains controversial with regard to methods of delivery and target specificity. When considering a treatment for NDDs mediated by miRNA delivery, we have to evaluate its ability to pass through the BBB. In order to overcome the problem of the BBB, several siRNA delivery systems are being developed for *in vivo* purposes, including vector-based, chemically modified, and "packaged" RNA oligonucleotides (Kim and Rossi, 2007). Progress in the latter area will immediately translate into progress in the miRNA area because both are based on the same principles. Both small RNAs regulate at the post-transcriptional level; therefore, miRNAs and siRNAs are chemically identical. However, the big question is whether these different approaches will result in clinically feasible therapies because of bioavailability and toxicity issues inherent to all of these approaches, and the BBB constitutes an enormous hurdle for the effective delivery of these experimental drugs in the brain.

Oligonucleotides can be effectively deployed in animal models, and RNA complexity provides the opportunity to uncover novel regulatory mechanisms and biomarkers. A limit to clinical miRNA use is that much remains to be improved in the prediction of target genes for both miRNAs and lncRNAs (Johnson et al., 2012).The most effective way of interfering with ncRNA action is likely not by targeting the RNA/target gene interaction itself, but to target the recruited epigenetic apparatus; this offers the advantage of exploiting a growing array of chemical compounds aimed at the active sites of chromatin modifiers (Kelly et al., 2010). At the very least, this expanded view of the importance of RNA, both protein-coding and non-coding, both small and large, offers an abundance of novel interactions to target that are distinct from the current focus on protein regulation in neurodegeneration.

Small ncRNAs add a novel and exciting layer of complexity to molecular neuronal biology. In addition, publications will exponentially increase in the years to come, which will provide novel insights into this recently discovered field of research (Hebert and De Strooper, 2009). A "many to many" relationship exists between miRNAs and their target mRNAs. The ability of a single miRNA to potentially target as many as 200 different miRNAs is well documented, but there is also evidence of single mRNA being targets of multiple miRNAs. To put this complex "many to many" relationship in a biological context, a comprehensive analysis of all miRNA targets suggested to be regulated by a single miRNA generally constitutes a biological network of functionally associated molecules in human cells. This evidence may represent a limitation for the use of regulatory small RNAs as a biomarker in NDDs or for future clinical trials to treat NDDs. However, miRNAs might help extract some biologically relevant targets among the high number of "predicted targets" of individual miRNAs, and potentially serves as a filter when using pathway analysis tools to understand the functional pathways affected by miRNA profile changes in NDDs.

In conclusion, many scientific questions remain to be addressed before efficient delivery and/or modulation of miRNAs in the brain will be possible (Krutzfeldt et al., 2005, 2007).

ACKNOWLEDGMENTS

This work was supported in part by grants from EU's Framework Programme 7 Optistem 223098, the Associazione ProductIDLa Nostra FamigliaLa Nostra Famiglia Fondo DMD Gli Amici di Emanuele, and by the Associazione Amici del Centro Dino Ferrari.

REFERENCES

Absalon, S., Kochanek, D. M., Raghavan, V., and Krichevsky, A. M. (2013). MiR-26b, upregulated in Alzheimer's disease, activates cell cycle entry, tau-phosphorylation, and apoptosis in postmitotic neurons. *J. Neurosci.* 33, 14645–14659. doi: 10.1523/JNEUROSCI.1327-13.2013

Al-Chalabi, A., Andersen, P. M., Nilsson, P., Chioza, B., Andersson, J. L., Russ, C., et al. (1999). Deletions of the heavy neurofilament subunit tail in amyotrophic lateral sclerosis. *Hum. Mol. Genet.* 8, 157–164. doi: 10.1093/hmg/8.2.157

Alexis, F., Pridgen, E., Molnar, L. K., and Farokhzad, O. C. (2008). Factors affecting the clearance and biodistribution of polymeric nanoparticles. *Mol. Pharm.* 5, 505–515. doi: 10.1021/mp800051m

Allen, T. A., Von Kaenel, S., Goodrich, J. A., and Kugel, J. F. (2004). The SINE-encoded mouse B2 RNA represses mRNA transcription in response to heat shock. *Nat. Struct. Mol. Biol.* 11, 816–821. doi: 10.1038/nsmb813

Alvarez-Erviti, L., Seow, Y., Yin, H., Betts, C., Lakhal, S., and Wood, M. J. (2011). Delivery of siRNA to the mouse brain by systemic injection of targeted exosomes. *Nat. Biotechnol.* 29, 341–345. doi: 10.1038/nbt.1807

Ambros, V., Lee, R. C., Lavanway, A., Williams, P. T., and Jewell, D. (2003). MicroRNAs and other tiny endogenous RNAs in *C. elegans*. *Curr. Biol.* 13, 807–818. doi: 10.1016/S0960-9822(03)00287-2

Bak, M., Silahtaroglu, A., Moller, M., Christensen, M., Rath, M. F., Skryabin, B., et al. (2008). MicroRNA expression in the adult mouse central nervous system. *RNA* 14, 432–444. doi: 10.1261/rna.783108

Balyasnikova, I. V., Yeomans, D. C., Mcdonald, T. B., and Danilov, S. M. (2002). Antibody-mediated lung endothelium targeting: *in vivo* model on primates. *Gene Ther.* 9, 282–290. doi: 10.1038/sj.gt.3301657

Bartel, B., and Bartel, D. P. (2003). MicroRNAs: at the root of plant development? *Plant Physiol.* 132, 709–717. doi: 10.1104/pp.103.023630

Bartel, D. P. (2004). MicroRNAs: genomics, biogenesis, mechanism, and function. *Cell* 116, 281–297. doi: 10.1016/S0092-8674(04)00045-5

Baskerville, S., and Bartel, D. P. (2005). Microarray profiling of microRNAs reveals frequent coexpression with neighboring miRNAs and host genes. *RNA* 11, 241–247. doi: 10.1261/rna.7240905

Bidros, D. S., Liu, J. K., and Vogelbaum, M. A. (2010). Future of convection-enhanced delivery in the treatment of brain tumors. *Future Oncol.* 6, 117–125. doi: 10.2217/fon.09.135

Boissonneault, V., Plante, I., Rivest, S., and Provost, P. (2009). MicroRNA-298 and microRNA-328 regulate expression of mouse beta-amyloid precursor protein-converting enzyme 1. *J. Biol. Chem.* 284, 1971–1981. doi: 10.1074/jbc.M807530200

Borchard, G. (2001). Chitosans for gene delivery. *Adv. Drug Deliv. Rev.* 52, 145–150. doi: 10.1016/S0169-409X(01)00198-3

Brouwers, N., Sleegers, K., and Van Broeckhoven, C. (2008). Molecular genetics of Alzheimer's disease: an update. *Ann. Med.* 40, 562–583. doi: 10.1080/07853890802186905

Buratti, E., De Conti, L., Stuani, C., Romano, M., Baralle, M., and Baralle, F. (2010). Nuclear factor TDP-43 can affect selected microRNA levels. *FEBS J.* 277, 2268–2281. doi: 10.1111/j.1742-4658.2010.07643.x

Butovsky, O., Siddiqui, S., Gabriely, G., Lanser, A. J., Dake, B., Murugaiyan, G., et al. (2012). Modulating inflammatory monocytes with a unique microRNA gene signature ameliorates murine ALS. *J. Clin. Invest.* 122, 3063–3087. doi: 10.1172/JCI62636

Campos-Melo, D., Droppelmann, C. A., He, Z., Volkening, K., and Strong, M. J. (2013). Altered microRNA expression profile in amyotrophic lateral sclerosis: a role in the regulation of NFL mRNA levels. *Mol. Brain* 6, 26. doi: 10.1186/1756-6606-6-26

Cao, Z., Henzel, W. J., and Gao, X. (1996). IRAK: a kinase associated with the interleukin-1 receptor. *Science* 271, 1128–1131. doi: 10.1126/science.271.5252.1128

Cardo, L. F., Coto, E., De Mena, L., Ribacoba, R., Moris, G., Menendez, M., et al. (2013). Profile of microRNAs in the plasma of Parkinson's disease patients and healthy controls. *J. Neurol.* 260, 1420–1422. doi: 10.1007/s00415-013-6900-8

Carrington, J. C., and Ambros, V. (2003). Role of microRNAs in plant and animal development. *Science* 301, 336–338. doi: 10.1126/science.1085242

Catarecha, P., Segura, M. D., Franco-Zorrilla, J. M., Garcia-Ponce, B., Lanza, M., Solano, R., et al. (2007). A mutant of the Arabidopsis phosphate transporter PHT1;1 displays enhanced arsenic accumulation. *Plant Cell* 19, 1123–1133. doi: 10.1105/tpc.106.041871

Cattaneo, E., Zuccato, C., and Tartari, M. (2005). Normal huntingtin function: an alternative approach to Huntington's disease. *Nat. Rev. Neurosci.* 6, 919–930. doi: 10.1038/nrn1806

Cha, J. H. (2007). Transcriptional signatures in Huntington's disease. *Prog. Neurobiol.* 83, 228–248. doi: 10.1016/j.pneurobio.2007.03.004

Chen, J. F., Mandel, E. M., Thomson, J. M., Wu, Q., Callis, T. E., Hammond, S. M., et al. (2006). The role of microRNA-1 and microRNA-133 in skeletal muscle proliferation and differentiation. *Nat. Genet.* 38, 228–233. doi: 10.1038/ng1725

Chen, P. Y., Liu, H. L., Hua, M. Y., Yang, H. W., Huang, C. Y., Chu, P. C., et al. (2010). Novel magnetic/ultrasound focusing system enhances nanoparticle drug delivery for glioma treatment. *Neuro Oncol.* 12, 1050–1060. doi: 10.1093/neuonc/noq054

Cheng, P. H., Li, C. L., Chang, Y. F., Tsai, S. J., Lai, Y. Y., Chan, A. W., et al. (2013). miR-196a Ameliorates Phenotypes of Huntington Disease in Cell, Transgenic Mouse, and Induced Pluripotent Stem Cell Models. *Am. J. Hum. Genet.* 93, 306–312. doi: 10.1016/j.ajhg.2013.05.025

Cho, H. J., Liu, G., Jin, S. M., Parisiadou, L., Xie, C., Yu, J., et al. (2013). MicroRNA-205 regulates the expression of Parkinson's disease-related leucine-rich repeat kinase 2 protein. *Hum. Mol. Genet.* 22, 608–620. doi: 10.1093/hmg/dds470

Chu, T. C., Twu, K. Y., Ellington, A. D., and Levy, M. (2006). Aptamer mediated siRNA delivery. *Nucleic Acids Res.* 34:e73. doi: 10.1093/nar/gkl388

Cogswell, J. P., Ward, J., Taylor, I. A., Waters, M., Shi, Y., Cannon, B., et al. (2008). Identification of miRNA changes in Alzheimer's disease brain and CSF yields putative biomarkers and insights into disease pathways. *J. Alzheimers Dis.* 14, 27–41.

Crist, C. G., and Buckingham, M. (2010). Megarole for microRNA in muscle disease. *Cell Metab.* 12, 425–426. doi: 10.1016/j.cmet.2010.10.007

Crooke, S. T. (2004). Progress in antisense technology. *Annu. Rev. Med.* 55, 61–95. doi: 10.1146/annurev.med.55.091902.104408

Davis, E., Caiment, F., Tordoir, X., Cavaille, J., Ferguson-Smith, A., Cockett, N., et al. (2005). RNAi-mediated allelic trans-interaction at the imprinted Rtl1/Peg11 locus. *Curr. Biol.* 15, 743–749. doi: 10.1016/j.cub.2005.02.060

De Felice, B., Guida, M., Guida, M., Coppola, C., De Mieri, G., and Cotrufo, R. (2012). A miRNA signature in leukocytes from sporadic amyotrophic lateral sclerosis. *Gene* 508, 35–40. doi: 10.1016/j.gene.2012.07.058

Delay, C., Calon, F., Mathews, P., and Hebert, S. S. (2011). Alzheimer-specific variants in the 3'UTR of Amyloid precursor protein affect microRNA function. *Mol. Neurodegener.* 6, 70. doi: 10.1186/1750-1326-6-70

Dickson, J. R., Kruse, C., Montagna, D. R., Finsen, B., and Wolfe, M. S. (2013). Alternative polyadenylation and miR-34 family members regulate tau expression. *J. Neurochem.* 127, 739–749. doi: 10.1111/jnc.12437

Donev, R., Newall, A., Thome, J., and Sheer, D. (2007). A role for SC35 and hnRNPA1 in the determination of amyloid precursor protein isoforms. *Mol. Psychiatry* 12, 681–690. doi: 10.1038/sj.mp.4001971

Doxakis, E. (2010). Post-transcriptional regulation of alpha-synuclein expression by mir-7 and mir-153. *J. Biol. Chem.* 285, 12726–12734. doi: 10.1074/jbc.M109.086827

Dreyfuss, G., Kim, V. N., and Kataoka, N. (2002). Messenger-RNA-binding proteins and the messages they carry. *Nat. Rev. Mol. Cell Biol.* 3, 195–205. doi: 10.1038/nrm760

Drubin, D. G., and Kirschner, M. W. (1986). Tau protein function in living cells. *J. Cell Biol.* 103, 2739–2746. doi: 10.1083/jcb.103.6.2739

Ebert, M. S., Neilson, J. R., and Sharp, P. A. (2007). MicroRNA sponges: competitive inhibitors of small RNAs in mammalian cells. *Nat. Methods* 4, 721–726. doi: 10.1038/nmeth1079

Eisenberg, I., Alexander, M. S., and Kunkel, L. M. (2009). miRNAS in normal and diseased skeletal muscle. *J. Cell. Mol. Med.* 13, 2–11. doi: 10.1111/j.1582-4934.2008.00524.x

Elbashir, S. M., Lendeckel, W., and Tuschl, T. (2001a). RNA interference is mediated by 21- and 22-nucleotide RNAs. *Genes Dev.* 15, 188–200. doi: 10.1101/gad.862301

Elbashir, S. M., Martinez, J., Patkaniowska, A., Lendeckel, W., and Tuschl, T. (2001b). Functional anatomy of siRNAs for mediating efficient RNAi in *Drosophila melanogaster* embryo lysate. *EMBO J.* 20, 6877–6888. doi: 10.1093/emboj/20.23.6877

Espinoza, C. A., Allen, T. A., Hieb, A. R., Kugel, J. F., and Goodrich, J. A. (2004). B2 RNA binds directly to RNA polymerase II to repress transcript synthesis. *Nat. Struct. Mol. Biol.* 11, 822–829. doi: 10.1038/nsmb812

Fang, M., Wang, J., Zhang, X., Geng, Y., Hu, Z., Rudd, J. A., et al. (2012). The miR-124 regulates the expression of BACE1/beta-secretase correlated with cell death in Alzheimer's disease. *Toxicol. Lett.* 209, 94–105. doi: 10.1016/j.toxlet.2011.11.032

Fejes-Toth, K., Sotirova, V., Sachidanandam R., Assaf, G., Hannon, G., and Kapranov, P. (2009). Post-transcriptional processing generates a diversity of 5'-modified long and short RNAs. *Nature* 457, 1028–1032. doi: 10.1038/nature07759

Feng, J., Bi, C., Clark, B. S., Mady, R., Shah, P., and Kohtz, J. D. (2006). The Evf-2 noncoding RNA is transcribed from the Dlx-5/6 ultraconserved region and functions as a Dlx-2 transcriptional coactivator. *Genes Dev.* 20, 1470–1484. doi: 10.1101/gad.1416106

Figlewicz, D. A., Krizus, A., Martinoli, M. G., Meininger, V., Dib, M., Rouleau, G. A., et al. (1994). Variants of the heavy neurofilament subunit are associated with the development of amyotrophic lateral sclerosis. *Hum. Mol. Genet.* 3, 1757–1761. doi: 10.1093/hmg/3.10.1757

Flannery, S., and Bowie, A. G. (2010). The interleukin-1 receptor-associated kinases: critical regulators of innate immune signalling. *Biochem. Pharmacol.* 80, 1981–1991. doi: 10.1016/j.bcp.2010.06.020

Fox, M. A., Sanes, J. R., Borza, D. B., Eswarakumar, V. P., Fassler, R., Hudson, B. G., et al. (2007). Distinct target-derived signals organize formation, maturation, and maintenance of motor nerve terminals. *Cell* 129, 179–193. doi: 10.1016/j.cell.2007.02.035

Franco-Zorrilla, J. M., Valli, A., Todesco, M., Mateos, I., Puga, M. I., Rubio-Somoza, I., et al. (2007). Target mimicry provides a new mechanism for regulation of microRNA activity. *Nat Genet.* 39, 1033–1037. doi: 10.1038/ng2079

Galter, D., Westerlund, M., Carmine, A., Lindqvist, E., Sydow, O., and Olson, L. (2006). LRRK2 expression linked to dopamine-innervated areas. *Ann. Neurol.* 59, 714–719. doi: 10.1002/ana.20808

Gaughwin, P. M., Ciesla, M., Lahiri, N., Tabrizi, S. J., Brundin, P., and Bjorkqvist, M. (2011). Hsa-miR-34b is a plasma-stable microRNA that is elevated in pre-manifest Huntington's disease. *Hum. Mol. Genet.* 20, 2225–2237. doi: 10.1093/hmg/ddr111

Geekiyanage, H., and Chan, C. (2011). MicroRNA-137/181c regulates serine palmitoyltransferase and in turn amyloid beta, novel targets in sporadic Alzheimer's disease. *J. Neurosci.* 31, 14820–14830. doi: 10.1523/JNEUROSCI.3883-11.2011

Gehrke, S., Imai, Y., Sokol, N., and Lu, B. (2010). Pathogenic LRRK2 negatively regulates microRNA-mediated translational repression. *Nature* 466, 637–641. doi: 10.1038/nature09191

Giordana, M. T., Piccinini, M., Grifoni, S., De Marco, G., Vercellino, M., Magistrello, M., et al. (2010). TDP-43 redistribution is an early event in sporadic amyotrophic lateral sclerosis. *Brain Pathol.* 20, 351–360. doi: 10.1111/j.1750-3639.2009.00284.x

Golde, T. E., Estus, S., Usiak, M., Younkin, L. H., and Younkin, S. G. (1990). Expression of beta amyloid protein precursor mRNAs: recognition of a novel alternatively spliced form and quantitation in Alzheimer's disease using PCR. *Neuron* 4, 253–267. doi: 10.1016/0896-6273(90)90100-T

Gregory, R. I., Yan, K. P., Amuthan, G., Chendrimada, T., Doratotaj, B., Cooch, N., et al. (2004). The Microprocessor complex mediates the genesis of microRNAs. *Nature* 432, 235–240. doi: 10.1038/nature03120

Hammond, S. M., Bernstein, E., Beach, D., and Hannon, G. J. (2000). An RNA-directed nuclease mediates post-transcriptional gene silencing in Drosophila cells. *Nature* 404, 293–296. doi: 10.1038/35005107

Hanger, D. P., and Noble, W. (2011). Functional implications of glycogen synthase kinase-3-mediated tau phosphorylation. *Int. J. Alzheimers Dis.* 2011, 352805. doi: 10.4061/2011/352805

Hannun, Y. A., and Obeid, L. M. (2008). Principles of bioactive lipid signalling: lessons from sphingolipids. *Nat. Rev. Mol. Cell Biol.* 9, 139–150. doi: 10.1038/nrm2329

Haramati, S., Chapnik, E., Sztainberg, Y., Eilam, R., Zwang, R., Gershoni, N., et al. (2010). miRNA malfunction causes spinal motor neuron disease. *Proc. Natl. Acad. Sci. U.S.A.* 107, 13111–13116. doi: 10.1073/pnas.1006151107

Harper, S. Q., Staber, P. D., He, X., Eliason, S. L., Martins, I. H., Mao, Q., et al. (2005). RNA interference improves motor and neuropathological abnormalities in a Huntington's disease mouse model. *Proc. Natl. Acad. Sci. U.S.A.* 102, 5820–5825. doi: 10.1073/pnas.0501507102

Hass, M. R., Sato, C., Kopan, R., and Zhao, G. (2009). Presenilin: RIP and beyond. *Semin. Cell Dev. Biol.* 20, 201–210. doi: 10.1016/j.semcdb.2008.11.014

Hebert, S. S., and De Strooper, B. (2007). Molecular biology. miRNAs in neurodegeneration. *Science* 317, 1179–1180. doi: 10.1126/science.1148530

Hebert, S. S., and De Strooper, B. (2009). Alterations of the microRNA network cause neurodegenerative disease. *Trends Neurosci.* 32, 199–206. doi: 10.1016/j.tins.2008.12.003

Hebert, S. S., Horre, K., Nicolai, L., Papadopoulou, A. S., Mandemakers, W., Silahtaroglu, A. N., et al. (2008). Loss of microRNA cluster miR-29a/b-1 in sporadic Alzheimer's disease correlates with increased BACE1/beta-secretase expression. *Proc. Natl. Acad. Sci. U.S.A.* 105, 6415–6420. doi: 10.1073/pnas.0710263105

Hellwig, S., and Bass, B. L. (2008) A starvation-induced noncoding RNA modulates expression of Dicer-regulated genes. *Proc. Natl. Acad. Sci. U.S.A.* 105, 12897–12902 doi: 10.1073/pnas.0805118105

Hong, M., and Lee, V. M. (1997). Insulin and insulin-like growth factor-1 regulate tau phosphorylation in cultured human neurons. *J. Biol. Chem.* 272, 19547–19553. doi: 10.1074/jbc.272.31.19547

Hu, Y. K., Wang, X., Li, L., Du, Y. H., Ye, H. T., and Li, C. Y. (2013). MicroRNA-98 induces an Alzheimer's disease-like disturbance by targeting insulin-like growth factor 1. *Neurosci. Bull.* 29, 745–751. doi: 10.1007/s12264-013-1348-5

Hunter, C., and Poethig, R. S. (2003). miSSING LINKS: miRNAs and plant development. *Curr. Opin. Genet. Dev.* 13, 372–378. doi: 10.1016/S0959-437X(03)00081-9

Ittner, L. M., Ke, Y. D., Delerue, F., Bi, M., Gladbach, A., Van Eersel, J., et al. (2010). Dendritic function of tau mediates amyloid-beta toxicity in Alzheimer's disease mouse models. *Cell* 142, 387–397. doi: 10.1016/j.cell.2010.06.036

Jacobsen, J. S., Blume, A. J., and Vitek, M. P. (1991). Quantitative measurement of alternatively spliced amyloid precursor protein mRNA expression in Alzheimer's disease and normal brain by S1 nuclease protection analysis. *Neurobiol. Aging* 12, 585–592. doi: 10.1016/0197-4580(91)90090-7

Jakes, R., Spillantini, M. G., and Goedert, M. (1994). Identification of two distinct synucleins from human brain. *FEBS Lett.* 345, 27–32. doi: 10.1016/0014-5793(94)00395-5

Jayadev, S., Case, A., Alajajian, B., Eastman, A. J., Moller, T., and Garden, G. A. (2013). Presenilin 2 influences miR146 level and activity in microglia. *J. Neurochem.* 127, 592–599. doi: 10.1111/jnc.12400

Jayadev, S., Case, A., Eastman, A. J., Nguyen, H., Pollak, J., Wiley, J. C., et al. (2010). Presenilin 2 is the predominant gamma-secretase in microglia and modulates cytokine release. *PLoS ONE* 5:e15743. doi: 10.1371/journal.pone.0015743

Jere, D., Arote, R., Jiang, H. L., Kim, Y. K., Cho, M. H., and Cho, C. S. (2009). Bioreducible polymers for efficient gene and siRNA delivery. *Biomed. Mater.* 4:025020. doi: 10.1088/1748-6041/4/2/025020

Johnson, R. and Bucley, N. J. (2009a). Gene dysregulation in Huntington's disease: REST, microRNAs and beyond. *Neuromolecular Med.* 11, 183–99. doi: 10.1007/s12017-009-8063-4

Johnson, R., Teh CH., Jia H., Vanisri RR., Pandey T., Lu ZH., et al. (2009b) Regulation of neural macroRNAs by the transcriptional repressor REST. *RNA* 15, 85–96. doi: 10.1261/rna.1127009

Johnson, R., Noble, W., Tartaglia, G. G., and Buckley, N. J. (2012). Neurodegeneration as an RNA disorder. *Prog. Neurobiol.* 99, 293–315. doi: 10.1016/j.pneurobio.2012.09.006

Johnson, R., Zuccato, C., Belyaev, N. D., Guest, D. J., Cattaneo, E., and Buckley, N. J. (2008). A microRNA-based gene dysregulation pathway in Huntington's disease. *Neurobiol. Dis.* 29, 438–445. doi: 10.1016/j.nbd.2007.11.001

Juliano, R., Alam, M. R., Dixit, V., and Kang, H. (2008). Mechanisms and strategies for effective delivery of antisense and siRNA oligonucleotides. *Nucleic Acids Res.* 36, 4158–4171. doi: 10.1093/nar/gkn342

Juliano, R. L. (2005). Peptide-oligonucleotide conjugates for the delivery of antisense and siRNA. *Curr. Opin. Mol. Ther.* 7, 132–136.

Julien, J. P. (1999). Neurofilament functions in health and disease. *Curr. Opin. Neurobiol.* 9, 554–560. doi: 10.1016/S0959-4388(99)00004-5

Junn, E., Lee, K. W., Jeong, B. S., Chan, T. W., Im, J. Y., and Mouradian, M. M. (2009). Repression of alpha-synuclein expression and toxicity by microRNA-7. *Proc. Natl. Acad. Sci. U.S.A.* 106, 13052–13057. doi: 10.1073/pnas.0906277106

Kabashi, E., Valdmanis, P. N., Dion, P., Spiegelman, D., Mcconkey, B. J., Vande Velde, C., et al. (2008). TARDBP mutations in individuals with sporadic and familial amyotrophic lateral sclerosis. *Nat. Genet.* 40, 572–574. doi: 10.1038/ng.132

Kapranov, P., Cheng, J., Dike, S., Nix, D. A., Duttagupta, R., Willingham, A. T., et al. (2007). RNA maps reveal new RNA classes and a possible function for pervasive transcription. *Science* 316, 1484–1488. doi: 10.1126/science.1138341

Kelly, T. K., De Carvalho, D. D., and Jones, P. A. (2010). Epigenetic modifications as therapeutic targets. *Nat. Biotechnol.* 28, 1069–1078. doi: 10.1038/nbt.1678

Kiernan, M. C., Vucic, S., Cheah, B. C., Turner, M. R., Eisen, A., Hardiman, O., et al. (2011). Amyotrophic lateral sclerosis. *Lancet* 377, 942–955. doi: 10.1016/S0140-6736(10)61156-7

Kim, D. H., and Rossi, J. J. (2007). Strategies for silencing human disease using RNA interference. *Nat. Rev. Genet.* 8, 173–184. doi: 10.1038/nrg2006

Kim, J., Inoue, K., Ishii, J., Vanti, W. B., Voronov, S. V., Murchison, E., et al. (2007). A MicroRNA feedback circuit in midbrain dopamine neurons. *Science* 317, 1220–1224. doi: 10.1126/science.1140481

Kluiver, J., Gibcus, J. H., Hettinga, C., Adema, A., Richter, M. K., Halsema, N., et al. (2012a). Rapid generation of microRNA sponges for microRNA inhibition. *PLoS ONE* 7:e29275. doi: 10.1371/journal.pone.0029275

Kluiver, J., Slezak-Prochazka, I., Smigielska-Czepiel, K., Halsema, N., Kroesen, B. J., and Van Den Berg, A. (2012b). Generation of miRNA sponge constructs. *Methods* 58, 113–117. doi: 10.1016/j.ymeth.2012.07.019

Kohlmaier, A., Savarese, F., Lachner, M., Martens, J., Jenuwein, T., and Wutz, A. (2004). A chromosomal memory triggered by Xist regulates histone methylation in X inactivation. *PLoS Biol.* 2:E171. doi: 10.1371/journal.pbio.0020171

Kosik, K. S., Joachim, C. L., and Selkoe, D. J. (1986). Microtubule-associated protein tau (tau) is a major antigenic component of paired helical filaments in Alzheimer disease. *Proc. Natl. Acad. Sci. U.S.A.* 83, 4044–4048. doi: 10.1073/pnas.83.11.4044

Koval, E. D., Shaner, C., Zhang, P., Du Maine, X., Fischer, K., Tay, J., et al. (2013). Method for widespread microRNA-155 inhibition prolongs survival in ALS-model mice. *Hum. Mol. Genet.* 22, 4127–4135. doi: 10.1093/hmg/ddt261

Krichevsky, A. M., King, K. S., Donahue, C. P., Khrapko, K., and Kosik, K. S. (2003). A microRNA array reveals extensive regulation of microRNAs during brain development. *RNA* 9, 1274–1281. doi: 10.1261/rna.5980303

Krutzfeldt, J., Kuwajima, S., Braich, R., Rajeev, K. G., Pena, J., Tuschl, T., et al. (2007). Specificity, duplex degradation and subcellular localization of antagomirs. *Nucleic Acids Res.* 35, 2885–2892. doi: 10.1093/nar/gkm024

Krutzfeldt, J., Rajewsky, N., Braich, R., Rajeev, K. G., Tuschl, T., Manoharan, M., et al. (2005). Silencing of microRNAs *in vivo* with 'antagomirs'. *Nature* 438, 685–689. doi: 10.1038/nature04303

Kumar, P., Ban, H. S., Kim, S. S., Wu, H., Pearson, T., Greiner, D. L., et al. (2008). T cell-specific siRNA delivery suppresses HIV-1 infection in humanized mice. *Cell* 134, 577–586. doi: 10.1016/j.cell.2008.06.034

Kwiatkowski, T. J., Jr., Bosco, D. A., Leclerc, A. L., Tamrazian, E., Vanderburg, C. R., Russ, C., et al. (2009). Mutations in the FUS/TLS gene on chromosome 16 cause familial amyotrophic lateral sclerosis. *Science* 323, 1205–1208. doi: 10.1126/science.1166066

Lagier-Tourenne, C., Polymenidou, M., and Cleveland, D. W. (2010). TDP-43 and FUS/TLS: emerging roles in RNA processing and neurodegeneration. *Hum. Mol. Genet.* 19, R46–R64. doi: 10.1093/hmg/ddq137

Lagos-Quintana, M., Rauhut, R., Lendeckel, W., and Tuschl, T. (2001). Identification of novel genes coding for small expressed RNAs. *Science* 294, 853–858. doi: 10.1126/science.1064921

Lagos-Quintana, M., Rauhut, R., Yalcin, A., Meyer, J., Lendeckel, W., and Tuschl, T. (2002). Identification of tissue-specific microRNAs from mouse. *Curr. Biol.* 12, 735–739. doi: 10.1016/S0960-9822(02)00809-6

Landgraf, P., Rusu, M., Sheridan, R., Sewer, A., Iovino, N., Aravin, A., et al. (2007). A mammalian microRNA expression atlas based on small RNA library sequencing. *Cell* 129, 1401–1414. doi: 10.1016/j.cell.2007.04.040

Lau, N. C., Lim, L. P., Weinstein, E. G., and Bartel, D. P. (2001). An abundant class of tiny RNAs with probable regulatory roles in Caenorhabditis elegans. *Science* 294, 858–862. doi: 10.1126/science.1065062

Lee, R. C., Feinbaum, R. L., and Ambros, V. (1993). The C. *elegans* heterochronic gene lin-4 encodes small RNAs with antisense complementarity to lin-14. *Cell* 75, 843-854. doi: 10.1016/0092-8674(93)90529-Y

Lee, S. J., Liyanage, U., Bickel, P. E., Xia, W., Lansbury, P. T. Jr., and Kosik, K. S. (1998). A detergent-insoluble membrane compartment contains A beta *in vivo*. *Nat. Med.* 4, 730–734. doi: 10.1038/nm0698-730

Lee, V. M., Goedert, M., and Trojanowski, J. Q. (2001). Neurodegenerative tauopathies. *Annu. Rev. Neurosci.* 24, 1121–1159. doi: 10.1146/annurev.neuro.24.1.1121

Li, Z., Lu, Y., Xu, X. L., and Gao, F. B. (2013). The FTD/ALS-associated RNA-binding protein TDP-43 regulates the robustness of neuronal specification through microRNA-9a in Drosophila. *Hum. Mol. Genet.* 22, 218–225. doi: 10.1093/hmg/dds420

Liem, R. K., and Messing, A. (2009). Dysfunctions of neuronal and glial intermediate filaments in disease. *J. Clin. Invest.* 119, 1814–1824. doi: 10.1172/JCI38003

Lin, X., Parisiadou, L., Gu, X. L., Wang, L., Shim, H., Sun, L., et al. (2009). Leucine-rich repeat kinase 2 regulates the progression of neuropathology induced by Parkinson's-disease-related mutant alpha-synuclein. *Neuron* 64, 807–827. doi: 10.1016/j.neuron.2009.11.006

Ling, S. C., Albuquerque, C. P., Han, J. S., Lagier-Tourenne, C., Tokunaga, S., Zhou, H., et al. (2010). ALS-associated mutations in TDP-43 increase its stability and promote TDP-43 complexes with FUS/TLS. *Proc. Natl. Acad. Sci. U.S.A.* 107, 13318–13323. doi: 10.1073/pnas.1008227107

Lipovich, L., Johnson, R., and Lin, C. Y. (2010). MacroRNA underdogs in a microRNA world: evolutionary, regulatory, and biomedical significance of mammalian long non-protein-coding RNA. *Biochim. Biophys. Acta* 1799, 597–615. doi: 10.1016/j.bbagrm.2010.10.001

Liu, H. L., Hua, M. Y., Chen, P. Y., Chu, P. C., Pan, C. H., Yang, H. W., et al. (2010). Blood-brain barrier disruption with focused ultrasound enhances delivery of chemotherapeutic drugs for glioblastoma treatment. *Radiology* 255, 415–425. doi: 10.1148/radiol.10090699

Long, J. M., and Lahiri, D. K. (2011). MicroRNA-101 downregulates Alzheimer's amyloid-beta precursor protein levels in human cell cultures and is differentially expressed. *Biochem. Biophys. Res. Commun.* 404, 889–895. doi: 10.1016/j.bbrc.2010.12.053

Lukiw, W. J. (2007). Micro-RNA speciation in fetal, adult and Alzheimer's disease hippocampus. *Neuroreport* 18, 297–300. doi: 10.1097/WNR.0b013e3280148e8b

Maciotta, S., Meregalli, M., Cassinelli, L., Parolini, D., Farini, A., Fraro, G. D., et al. (2012). Hmgb3 is regulated by microRNA-206 during muscle regeneration. *PLoS ONE* 7:e43464. doi: 10.1371/journal.pone.0043464

Mahato, R. I., Kawabata, K., Takakura, Y., and Hashida, M. (1995). *In vivo* disposition characteristics of plasmid DNA complexed with cationic liposomes. *J. Drug Target.* 3, 149–157. doi: 10.3109/10611869509059214

Makeyev, E. V., Zhang, J., Carrasco, M. A., and Maniatis, T. (2007). The MicroRNA miR-124 promotes neuronal differentiation by triggering brain-specific alternative pre-mRNA splicing. *Mol. Cell* 27, 435–448. doi: 10.1016/j.molcel.2007.07.015

Makimura, H., Mizuno, T. M., Mastaitis, J. W., Agami, R., and Mobbs, C. V. (2002). Reducing hypothalamic AGRP by RNA interference increases metabolic rate and decreases body weight without influencing food intake. *BMC Neurosci.* 3:18. doi: 10.1186/1471-2202-3-18

Malumbres, R., Sarosiek, K. A., Cubedo, E., Ruiz, J. W., Jiang, X., Gascoyne, R. D., et al. (2009). Differentiation stage-specific expression of microRNAs in B lymphocytes and diffuse large B-cell lymphomas. *Blood* 113, 3754–3764. doi: 10.1182/blood-2008-10-184077

Margis, R., Margis, R., and Rieder, C. R. (2011). Identification of blood microRNAs associated to Parkinsonis disease. *J. Biotechnol.* 152, 96–101. doi: 10.1016/j.jbiotec.2011.01.023

Mariner, P. D., Walters, R. D., Espinoza, C. A., Drullinger, L. F., Wagner, S. D., Kugel, J. F., et al. (2008). Human Alu RNA is a modular transacting repressor of mRNA transcription during heat shock. *Mol. Cell* 29, 499–509. doi: 10.1016/j.molcel.2007.12.013

Marti, E., Pantano, L., Banez-Coronel, M., Llorens, F., Minones-Moyano, E., Porta, S., et al. (2010). A myriad of miRNA variants in control and Huntington's disease brain regions detected by massively parallel sequencing. *Nucleic Acids Res.* 38, 7219–7235. doi: 10.1093/nar/gkq575

Martinez, J., Patkaniowska, A., Urlaub, H., Luhrmann, R., and Tuschl, T. (2002). Single-stranded antisense siRNAs guide target RNA cleavage in RNAi. *Cell* 110, 563–574. doi: 10.1016/S0092-8674(02)00908-X

Masliah, E., Rockenstein, E., Veinbergs, I., Mallory, M., Hashimoto, M., Takeda, A., et al. (2000). Dopaminergic loss and inclusion body formation in alpha-synuclein mice: implications for neurodegenerative disorders. *Science* 287, 1265–1269. doi: 10.1126/science.287.5456.1265

Matkovich, S. J., Van Booven, D. J., Youker, K. A., Torre-Amione, G., Diwan, A., Eschenbacher, W. H., et al. (2009). Reciprocal regulation of myocardial microRNAs and messenger RNA in human cardiomyopathy and reversal of the microRNA signature by biomechanical support. *Circulation* 119, 1263–1271. doi: 10.1161/CIRCULATIONAHA.108.813576

Mckhann, G., Drachman, D., Folstein, M., Katzman, R., Price, D., and Stadlan, E. M. (1984). Clinical diagnosis of Alzheimer's disease: report of the NINCDS-ADRDA Work Group under the auspices of Department of Health and Human Services Task Force on Alzheimer's Disease. *Neurology* 34, 939–944. doi: 10.1212/WNL.34.7.939

Melrose, H., Lincoln, S., Tyndall, G., Dickson, D., and Farrer, M. (2006). Anatomical localization of leucine-rich repeat kinase 2 in mouse brain. *Neuroscience* 139, 791–794. doi: 10.1016/j.neuroscience.2006.01.017

Minones-Moyano, E., Porta, S., Escaramis, G., Rabionet, R., Iraola, S., Kagerbauer, B., et al. (2011). MicroRNA profiling of Parkinson's disease brains identifies early downregulation of miR-34b/c which modulate mitochondrial function. *Hum. Mol. Genet.* 20, 3067–3078. doi: 10.1093/hmg/ddr210

Mori, F., Anji, K., Oshimoto, M., Akahashi, H., and Wakabayashi, K. (2002). Demonstration of alpha-synuclein immunoreactivity in neuronal and glial cytoplasm in normal human brain tissue using proteinase K and formic acid pretreatment. *Exp. Neurol.* 176, 98–104. doi: 10.1006/exnr.2002.7929

Morlando, M., Dini Modigliani, S., Torrelli, G., Rosa, A., Di Carlo, V., Caffarelli, E., et al. (2012). FUS stimulates microRNA biogenesis by facilitating co-transcriptional Drosha recruitment. *EMBO J.* 31, 4502–4510. doi: 10.1038/emboj.2012.319

Mouradian, M. M. (2012). MicroRNAs in Parkinson's disease. *Neurobiol. Dis.* 46, 279–284. doi: 10.1016/j.nbd.2011.12.046

Mucke, L., and Selkoe, D. J. (2011). Neurotoxicity of amyloid beta-protein: synaptic and network dysfunction. *Cold Spring Harb. Perspect. Med.* 2:a006338. doi: 10.1101/cshperspect.a006338

Neve, R. L., Rogers, J., and Higgins, G. A. (1990). The Alzheimer amyloid precursor-related transcript lacking the beta/A4 sequence is specifically increased in Alzheimer's disease brain. *Neuron* 5, 329–338. doi: 10.1016/0896-6273(90)90169-G

Ningaraj, N. S., Salimath, B. P., Sankpal, U. T., Perera, R., and Vats, T. (2007). Targeted brain tumor treatment-current perspectives. *Drug Target Insights* 2, 197–207.

Nukina, N., and Ihara, Y. (1986). One of the antigenic determinants of paired helical filaments is related to tau protein. *J. Biochem.* 99, 1541–1544.

Nunez-Iglesias, J., Liu, C. C., Morgan, T. E., Finch, C. E., and Zhou, X. J. (2010). Joint genome-wide profiling of miRNA and mRNA expression in Alzheimer's disease cortex reveals altered miRNA regulation. *PLoS ONE* 5:e8898. doi: 10.1371/journal.pone.0008898

Nykanen, A., Haley, B., and Zamore, P. D. (2001). ATP requirements and small interfering RNA structure in the RNA interference pathway. *Cell* 107, 309–321. doi: 10.1016/S0092-8674(01)00547-5

Ohmachi, S., Mikami, T., Konishi, M., Miyake, A., and Itoh, N. (2003). Preferential neurotrophic activity of fibroblast growth factor-20 for dopaminergic neurons through fibroblast growth factor receptor-1c. *J. Neurosci. Res.* 72, 436–443. doi: 10.1002/jnr.10592

Ohmachi, S., Watanabe, Y., Mikami, T., Kusu, N., Ibi, T., Akaike, A., et al. (2000). FGF-20, a novel neurotrophic factor, preferentially expressed in the substantia nigra pars compacta of rat brain. *Biochem. Biophys. Res. Commun.* 277, 355–360. doi: 10.1006/bbrc.2000.3675

Ooi, L., and Wood, I. C. (2007). Chromatin crosstalk in development and disease: lessons from REST. *Nat. Rev. Genet.* 8, 544–554. doi: 10.1038/nrg2100

Packer, A. N., Xing, Y., Harper, S. Q., Jones, L., and Davidson, B. L. (2008). The bifunctional microRNA miR-9/miR-9* regulates REST and CoREST and is downregulated in Huntington's disease. *J. Neurosci.* 28, 14341–14346. doi: 10.1523/JNEUROSCI.2390-08.2008

Palm, T., Bahnassawy, L., and Schwamborn, J. (2012). MiRNAs and neural stem cells: a team to treat Parkinson's disease? *RNA Biol.* 9, 720–730. doi: 10.4161/rna.19984

Palop, J. J., and Mucke, L. (2010). Amyloid-beta-induced neuronal dysfunction in Alzheimer's disease: from synapses toward neural networks. *Nat. Neurosci.* 13, 812–818. doi: 10.1038/nn.2583

Papagiannakopoulos, T., and Kosik, K. S. (2009). MicroRNA-124: micromanager of neurogenesis. *Cell Stem Cell* 4, 375–376. doi: 10.1016/j.stem.2009.04.007

Pardridge, W. M. (2007). shRNA and siRNA delivery to the brain. *Adv. Drug Deliv. Rev.* 59, 141–152. doi: 10.1016/j.addr.2007.03.008

Parisiadou, L., Xie, C., Cho, H. J., Lin, X., Gu, X. L., Long, C. X., et al. (2009). Phosphorylation of ezrin/radixin/moesin proteins by LRRK2 promotes the rearrangement of actin cytoskeleton in neuronal morphogenesis. *J. Neurosci.* 29, 13971–13980. doi: 10.1523/JNEUROSCI.3799-09.2009

Pasquinelli, A. E., Reinhart, B. J., Slack, F., Martindale, M. Q., Kuroda, M. I., Maller, B., et al. (2000). Conservation of the sequence and temporal expression of let-7 heterochronic regulatory RNA. *Nature* 408, 86–89. doi: 10.1038/35040556

Patel, N., Hoang, D., Miller, N., Ansaloni, S., Huang, Q., Rogers, J. T., et al. (2008). MicroRNAs can regulate human APP levels. *Mol. Neurodegener.* 3:10. doi: 10.1186/1750-1326-3-10

Pesiridis, G. S., Lee, V. M., and Trojanowski, J. Q. (2009). Mutations in TDP-43 link glycine-rich domain functions to amyotrophic lateral sclerosis. *Hum. Mol. Genet.* 18, R156–R162. doi: 10.1093/hmg/ddp303

Plath, K., Fang, J., Mlynarczyk-Evans, S. K., Cao, R., Worringer, K. A., Wang, H., et al. (2003). Role of histone H3 lysine 27 methylation in X inactivation. *Science* 300, 131–135. doi: 10.1126/science.1084274

Ponting, C. P., Oliver, P. L., and Reik, W. (2009). Evolution and functions of long noncoding RNAs. *Cell* 136, 629–641. doi: 10.1016/j.cell.2009.02.006

Pushparaj, P. N., Aarthi, J. J., Manikandan, J., and Kumar, S. D. (2008). siRNA, miRNA, and shRNA: *in vivo* applications. *J. Dent. Res.* 87, 992–1003. doi: 10.1177/154405910808701109

Ralph, G. S., Radcliffe, P. A., Day, D. M., Carthy, J. M., Leroux, M. A., Lee, D. C., et al. (2005). Silencing mutant SOD1 using RNAi protects against neurodegeneration and extends survival in an ALS model. *Nat. Med.* 11, 429–433. doi: 10.1038/nm1205

Rao, P. K., Kumar, R. M., Farkhondeh, M., Baskerville, S., and Lodish, H. F. (2006). Myogenic factors that regulate expression of muscle-specific microRNAs. *Proc. Natl. Acad. Sci. U.S.A.* 103, 8721–8726. doi: 10.1073/pnas.0602831103

Rapoport, M., Dawson, H. N., Binder, L. I., Vitek, M. P., and Ferreira, A. (2002). Tau is essential to beta -amyloid-induced neurotoxicity. *Proc. Natl. Acad. Sci. U.S.A.* 99, 6364–6369. doi: 10.1073/pnas.092136199

Reinhart, B. J., and Bartel, D. P. (2002). Small RNAs correspond to centromere heterochromatic repeats. *Science* 297, 1831. doi: 10.1126/science.1077183

Roberson, E. D., Scearce-Levie, K., Palop, J. J., Yan, F., Cheng, I. H., Wu, T., et al. (2007). Reducing endogenous tau ameliorates amyloid beta-induced deficits in an Alzheimer's disease mouse model. *Science* 316, 750–754. doi: 10.1126/science.1141736

Rockenstein, E. M., Mcconlogue, L., Tan, H., Power, M., Masliah, E., and Mucke, L. (1995). Levels and alternative splicing of amyloid beta protein precursor (APP) transcripts in brains of APP transgenic mice and humans with Alzheimer's disease. *J. Biol. Chem.* 270, 28257–28267. doi: 10.1074/jbc.270.47.28257

Rosario, P. W. (2010). Normal values of serum IGF-1 in adults: results from a Brazilian population. *Arq. Bras. Endocrinol. Metabol.* 54, 477–481. doi: 10.1590/S0004-27302010000500008

Saido, T., and Leissring, M. A. (2012). Proteolytic degradation of amyloid beta-protein. *Cold Spring Harb. Perspect. Med.* 2:a006379. doi: 10.1101/cshperspect.a006379

Saiki, S., Sato, S., and Hattori, N. (2011). Molecular pathogenesis of Parkinson's disease: update. *J. Neurol. Neurosurg. Psychiatry* 83, 430–436. doi: 10.1136/jnnp-2011-301205

Satake, W., Nakabayashi, Y., Mizuta, I., Hirota, Y., Ito, C., Kubo, M., et al. (2009). Genome-wide association study identifies common variants at four loci as genetic risk factors for Parkinson's disease. *Nat. Genet.* 41, 1303–1307. doi: 10.1038/ng.485

Savas, J. N., Makusky, A., Ottosen, S., Baillat, D., Then, F., Krainc, D., et al. (2008). Huntington's disease protein contributes to RNA-mediated gene silencing through association with Argonaute and P bodies. *Proc. Natl. Acad. Sci. U.S.A.* 105, 10820–10825. doi: 10.1073/pnas.0800658105

Schenk, D., Basi, G. S., and Pangalos, M. N. (2012). Treatment strategies targeting amyloid beta-protein. *Cold Spring Harb. Perspect. Med.* 2:a006387. doi: 10.1101/cshperspect.a006387

Schipper, H. M., Maes, O. C., Chertkow, H. M., and Wang, E. (2007). MicroRNA expression in Alzheimer blood mononuclear cells. *Gene Regul. Syst. Biol.* 1, 263–274.

Schwarz, D. S., Hutvagner, G., Haley, B., and Zamore, P. D. (2002). Evidence that siRNAs function as guides, not primers, in the Drosophila and human RNAi pathways. *Mol. Cell* 10, 537–548. doi: 10.1016/S1097-2765(02)00651-2

Sempere, L. F., Freemantle, S., Pitha-Rowe, I., Moss, E., Dmitrovsky, E., and Ambros, V. (2004). Expression profiling of mammalian microRNAs uncovers a subset of brain-expressed microRNAs with possible roles in murine and human neuronal differentiation. *Genome Biol.* 5:R13. doi: 10.1186/gb-2004-5-3-r13

Shamovsky, I., Ivannikov, M., Kandel, E. S., Gershon, D., and Nudler, E. (2006). RNA-mediated response to heat shock in mammalian cells. *Nature* 440, 556–560. doi: 10.1038/nature04518

Shen, Y. (2008). Advances in the development of siRNA-based therapeutics for cancer. *IDrugs* 11, 572–578.

Shioya, M., Obayashi, S., Tabunoki, H., Arima, K., Saito, Y., Ishida, T., et al. (2010). Aberrant microRNA expression in the brains of neurodegenerative diseases: miR-29a decreased in Alzheimer disease brains targets neurone navigator 3. *Neuropathol. Appl. Neurobiol.* 36, 320–330. doi: 10.1111/j.1365-2990.2010.01076.x

Shtilbans, A., and Henchcliffe, C. (2012). Biomarkers in Parkinson's disease: an update. *Curr. Opin. Neurol.* 25, 460–465. doi: 10.1097/WCO.0b013e3283550c0d

Silva, J., Mak, W., Zvetkova, I., Appanah, R., Nesterova, T. B., Webster, Z., et al. (2003). Establishment of histone h3 methylation on the inactive X chromosome requires transient recruitment of Eed-Enx1 polycomb group complexes. *Dev. Cell* 4, 481–495. doi: 10.1016/S1534-5807(03)00068-6

Simon-Sanchez, J., Schulte, C., Bras, J. M., Sharma, M., Gibbs, J. R., Berg, D., et al. (2009). Genome-wide association study reveals genetic risk underlying Parkinson's disease. *Nat. Genet.* 41, 1308–1312. doi: 10.1038/ng.487

Singleton, A. B., Farrer, M., Johnson, J., Singleton, A., Hague, S., Kachergus, J., et al. (2003). alpha-Synuclein locus triplication causes Parkinson's disease. *Science* 302, 841. doi: 10.1126/science.1090278

Sinha, M., Mukhopadhyay, S., and Bhattacharyya, N. P. (2012). Mechanism(s) of alteration of micro RNA expressions in Huntington's disease and their possible contributions to the observed cellular and molecular dysfunctions in the disease. *Neuromolecular Med.* 14, 221–243. doi: 10.1007/s12017-012-8183-0

Skog, J., Wurdinger, T., Van Rijn, S., Meijer, D. H., Gainche, L., Sena-Esteves, M., et al. (2008). Glioblastoma microvesicles transport RNA and proteins that promote tumour growth and provide diagnostic biomarkers. *Nat. Cell Biol.* 10, 1470–1476. doi: 10.1038/ncb1800

Smirnova, L., Grafe, A., Seiler, A., Schumacher, S., Nitsch, R., and Wulczyn, F. G. (2005). Regulation of miRNA expression during neural cell specification. *Eur. J. Neurosci.* 21, 1469–1477. doi: 10.1111/j.1460-9568.2005.03978.x

Smith, P., Al Hashimi, A., Girard, J., Delay, C., and Hebert, S. S. (2011). *In vivo* regulation of amyloid precursor protein neuronal splicing by microRNAs. *J. Neurochem.* 116, 240–247. doi: 10.1111/j.1471-4159.2010.07097.x

Sotiriou, S. Gibney G., Baxevanis AD., and Nussbaum RL. (2009) A single nucleotide polymorphism in the 3'UTR of SNCA gene encoding alpha-synuclein is a new potential susceptibility locus for Parkinson's Disease. *Neurosci. Lett.* 461, 196–201 doi: 10.1016/j.neulet.2009.06.034

Sreedharan, J., Blair, I. P., Tripathi, V. B., Hu, X., Vance, C., Rogelj, B., et al. (2008). TDP-43 mutations in familial and sporadic amyotrophic lateral sclerosis. *Science* 319, 1668–1672. doi: 10.1126/science.1154584

Subramanian, S., Lui, W. O., Lee, C. H., Espinosa, I., Nielsen, T. O., Heinrich, M. C., et al. (2008). MicroRNA expression signature of human sarcomas. *Oncogene* 27, 2015–2026. doi: 10.1038/sj.onc.1210836

Sugars, K. L., and Rubinsztein, D. C. (2003). Transcriptional abnormalities in Huntington disease. *Trends Genet.* 19, 233–238. doi: 10.1016/S0168-9525(03)00074-X

Suzuki, H. I., Yamagata, K., Sugimoto, K., Iwamoto, T., Kato, S., and Miyazono, K. (2009). Modulation of microRNA processing by p53. *Nature* 460, 529–533. doi: 10.1038/nature08199

Swantek, J. L., Tsen, M. F., Cobb, M. H., and Thomas, J. A. (2000). IL-1 receptor-associated kinase modulates host responsiveness to endotoxin. *J. Immunol.* 164, 430–436.

Tan, E. K., and Skipper, L. M. (2007). Pathogenic mutations in Parkinson disease. *Hum. Mutat.* 28, 641–653. doi: 10.1002/humu.20507

Tanzi, R., Gaston, S., Bush, A., Romano, D., Pettingell, W., Peppercorn, J., et al. (1993). Genetic heterogeneity of gene defects responsible for familial Alzheimer disease. *Genetica* 91, 255–263. doi: 10.1007/BF01436002

Thum, T., Gross, C., Fiedler, J., Fischer, T., Kissler, S., Bussen, M., et al. (2008). MicroRNA-21 contributes to myocardial disease by stimulating MAP kinase signalling in fibroblasts. *Nature* 456, 980–984. doi: 10.1038/nature07511

Tomkins, J., Usher, P., Slade, J. Y., Ince, P. G., Curtis, A., Bushby, K., et al. (1998). Novel insertion in the KSP region of the neurofilament heavy gene in amyotrophic lateral sclerosis (ALS). *Neuroreport* 9, 3967–3970. doi: 10.1097/00001756-199812010-00036

Uyechi, L. S., Gagne, L., Thurston, G., and Szoka, F. C. Jr. (2001). Mechanism of lipoplex gene delivery in mouse lung: binding and internalization of fluorescent lipid and DNA components. *Gene Ther.* 8, 828–836. doi: 10.1038/sj.gt.3301461

Valadi, H., Ekstrom, K., Bossios, A., Sjostrand, M., Lee, J. J., and Lotvall, J. O. (2007). Exosome-mediated transfer of mRNAs and microRNAs is a novel mechanism of genetic exchange between cells. *Nat. Cell Biol.* 9, 654–659. doi: 10.1038/ncb1596

Vance, C., Rogelj, B., Hortobagyi, T., De Vos, K. J., Nishimura, A. L., Sreedharan, J., et al. (2009). Mutations in FUS, an RNA processing protein, cause familial amyotrophic lateral sclerosis type 6. *Science* 323, 1208–1211. doi: 10.1126/science.1165942

Van Rooij, E., and Olson, E. N. (2007). MicroRNAs: powerful new regulators of heart disease and provocative therapeutic targets. *J. Clin. Invest.* 117, 2369–2376. doi: 10.1172/JCI33099

Vargas, T., Martinez-Garcia, A., Antequera, D., Vilella, E., Clarimon, J., Mateo, I., et al. (2011). IGF-I gene variability is associated with an increased risk for AD. *Neurobiol. Aging* 32, 556 e553–e511. doi: 10.1016/j.neurobiolaging.2010.10.017

Vetrivel, K. S., Cheng, H., Kim, S. H., Chen, Y., Barnes, N. Y., Parent, A. T., et al. (2005). Spatial segregation of gamma-secretase and substrates in distinct membrane domains. *J. Biol. Chem.* 280, 25892–25900. doi: 10.1074/jbc.M503570200

Vilardo, E., Barbato, C., Ciotti, M., Cogoni, C., and Ruberti, F. (2010). MicroRNA-101 regulates amyloid precursor protein expression in hippocampal neurons. *J. Biol. Chem.* 285, 18344–18351. doi: 10.1074/jbc.M110.112664

Vossel, K. A., Zhang, K., Brodbeck, J., Daub, A. C., Sharma, P., Finkbeiner, S., et al. (2010). Tau reduction prevents Abeta-induced defects in axonal transport. *Science* 330, 198. doi: 10.1126/science.1194653

Wang, D., Lu, M., Miao, J., Li, T., Wang, E., and Cui, Q. (2009). Cepred: predicting the co-expression patterns of the human intronic microRNAs with their host genes. *PLoS ONE* 4:e4421. doi: 10.1371/journal.pone.0004421

Wang, G., Van Der Walt, J. M., Mayhew, G., Li, Y. J., Zuchner, S., Scott, W. K., et al. (2008a). Variation in the miRNA-433 binding site of FGF20 confers risk for Parkinson disease by overexpression of alpha-synuclein. *Am. J. Hum. Genet.* 82, 283–289. doi: 10.1016/j.ajhg.2007.09.021

Wang, W. X., Rajeev, B. W., Stromberg, A. J., Ren, N., Tang, G., Huang, Q., et al. (2008b). The expression of microRNA miR-107 decreases early in Alzheimer's disease and may accelerate disease progression through regulation of beta-site amyloid precursor protein-cleaving enzyme 1. *J. Neurosci.* 28, 1213–1223. doi: 10.1523/JNEUROSCI.5065-07.2008

Wang, J., Zhang, P. C., Lu, H. F., Ma, N., Wang, S., Mao, H. Q., et al. (2002). New polyphosphoramidate with a spermidine side chain as a gene carrier. *J. Control. Release* 83, 157–168. doi: 10.1016/S0168-3659(02)00180-3

Weingarten, M. D., Lockwood, A. H., Hwo, S. Y., and Kirschner, M. W. (1975). A protein factor essential for microtubule assembly. *Proc. Natl. Acad. Sci. U.S.A.* 72, 1858–1862. doi: 10.1073/pnas.72.5.1858

Whitehead, K. A., Langer, R., and Anderson, D. G. (2009). Knocking down barriers: advances in siRNA delivery. *Nat. Rev. Drug Discov.* 8, 129–138. doi: 10.1038/nrd2742

Williams, A. H., Valdez, G., Moresi, V., Qi, X., Mcanally, J., Elliott, J. L., et al. (2009). MicroRNA-206 delays ALS progression and promotes regeneration of neuromuscular synapses in mice. *Science* 326, 1549–1554. doi: 10.1126/science.1181046

Wislet-Gendebien, S., Visanji, N. P., Whitehead, S. N., Marsilio, D., Hou, W., Figeys, D., et al. (2008). Differential regulation of wild-type and mutant alpha-synuclein binding to synaptic membranes by cytosolic factors. *BMC Neurosci.* 9:92. doi: 10.1186/1471-2202-9-92

Wood, J. G., Mirra, S. S., Pollock, N. J., and Binder, L. I. (1986). Neurofibrillary tangles of Alzheimer disease share antigenic determinants with the axonal microtubule-associated protein tau (tau). *Proc. Natl. Acad. Sci. U.S.A.* 83, 4040–4043. doi: 10.1073/pnas.83.11.4040

Wood-Kaczmar, A., Gandhi, S., and Wood, N. W. (2006). Understanding the molecular causes of Parkinson's disease. *Trends Mol. Med.* 12, 521–528. doi: 10.1016/j.molmed.2006.09.007

Zhang, C. (2012). Natural compounds that modulate BACE1-processing of amyloid-beta precursor protein in Alzheimer's disease. *Discov. Med.* 14, 189–197.

Zhang, Y. W., Thompson, R., Zhang, H., and Xu, H. (2011). APP processing in Alzheimer's disease. *Mol. Brain* 4, 3. doi: 10.1186/1756-6606-4-3

Zhao, J., Sun, B. K., Erwin, J. A., Song, J. J., and Lee, J. T. (2008). Polycomb proteins targeted by a short repeat RNA to the mouse X chromosome. *Science* 322, 750–756. doi: 10.1126/science.1163045

Zhu, H. C., Wang, L. M., Wang, M., Song, B., Tan, S., Teng, J. F., et al. (2012). MicroRNA-195 downregulates Alzheimer's disease amyloid-beta production by targeting BACE1. *Brain Res. Bull.* 88, 596–601. doi: 10.1016/j.brainresbull.2012.05.018

Zimprich, A., Biskup, S., Leitner, P., Lichtner, P., Farrer, M., Lincoln, S., et al. (2004). Mutations in LRRK2 cause autosomal-dominant parkinsonism with pleomorphic pathology. *Neuron* 44, 601–607. doi: 10.1016/j.neuron.2004.11.005

Zomer, A., Vendrig, T., Hopmans, E. S., Van Eijndhoven, M., Middeldorp, J. M., and Pegtel, D. M. (2010). Exosomes: fit to deliver small RNA. *Commun. Integr. Biol.* 3, 447–450. doi: 10.4161/cib.3.5.12339

Zong, Y., Wang, H., Dong, W., Quan, X., Zhu, H., Xu, Y., et al. (2011). miR-29c regulates BACE1 protein expression. *Brain Res.* 1395, 108–115. doi: 10.1016/j.brainres.2011.04.035

Zuccato, C., Tartari, M., Crotti, A., Goffredo, D., Valenza, M., Conti, L., et al. (2003). Huntingtin interacts with REST/NRSF to modulate the transcription of NRSE-controlled neuronal genes. *Nat. Genet.* 35, 76–83. doi: 10.1038/ng1219

Zuccato, C., Valenza, M., and Cattaneo, E. (2010). Molecular mechanisms and potential therapeutical targets in Huntington's disease. *Physiol. Rev.* 90, 905–981. doi: 10.1152/physrev.00041.2009

14

A lentiviral sponge for miR-101 regulates RanBP9 expression and amyloid precursor protein metabolism in hippocampal neurons

Christian Barbato, Silvia Pezzola, Cinzia Caggiano, Martina Antonelli, Paola Frisone, Maria Teresa Ciotti and Francesca Ruberti*

Institute of Cell Biology and Neurobiology (IBCN), National Research Council (CNR), Rome, Italy

***Correspondence:**
Francesca Ruberti, Institute of Cell Biology and Neurobiology (IBCN), National Research Council (CNR), Via del Fosso di Fiorano 64/65, 00143 Rome, Italy
e-mail: francesca.ruberti@inmm.cnr.it; francesca.ruberti@cnr.it

Neurodegeneration associated with amyloid β (Aβ) peptide accumulation, synaptic loss, and memory impairment are pathophysiological features of Alzheimer's disease (AD). Numerous microRNAs regulate amyloid precursor protein (APP) expression and metabolism. We previously reported that miR-101 is a negative regulator of APP expression in cultured hippocampal neurons. In this study, a search for predicted APP metabolism-associated miR-101 targets led to the identification of a conserved miR-101 binding site within the 3′ untranslated region (UTR) of the mRNA encoding Ran-binding protein 9 (RanBP9). RanBP9 increases APP processing by β-amyloid converting enzyme 1 (BACE1), secretion of soluble APPβ (sAPPβ), and generation of Aβ. MiR-101 significantly reduced reporter gene expression when co-transfected with a RanBP9 3′-UTR reporter construct, while site-directed mutagenesis of the predicted miR-101 target site eliminated the reporter response. To investigate the effect of stable inhibition of miR-101 both *in vitro* and *in vivo*, a microRNA sponge was developed to bind miR-101 and derepress its targets. Four tandem bulged miR-101 responsive elements (REs), located downstream of the enhanced green fluorescence protein (EGFP) open reading frame and driven by the synapsin promoter, were placed in a lentiviral vector to create the pLSyn-miR-101 sponge. Delivery of the sponge to primary hippocampal neurons significantly increased both APP and RanBP9 expression, as well as sAPPβ levels in the conditioned medium. Importantly, silencing of endogenous RanBP9 reduced sAPPβ levels in miR-101 sponge-containing hippocampal cultures, indicating that miR-101 inhibition may increase amyloidogenic processing of APP by RanBP9. Lastly, the impact of miR-101 on its targets was demonstrated *in vivo* by intrahippocampal injection of the pLSyn-miR-101 sponge into C57BL6 mice. This study thus provides the basis for studying the consequences of long-term miR-101 inhibition on the pathology of AD.

Keywords: Alzheimer's disease, amyloid precursor protein, microRNA, miR-101, Ran-binding protein 9

INTRODUCTION

Alzheimer's disease (AD) is a progressive neurodegenerative disorder characterized by extracellular senile plaques, intracellular neurofibrillary tangles (Krstic and Knuesel, 2013), and memory loss. Increased amyloidogenic processing of amyloid precursor protein (APP), a type I transmembrane protein, and accumulation of its amyloid β (Aβ) peptide product have important implications for AD pathogenesis. The Aβ peptide is derived from the processing of APP through sequential cleavages by β and γ secretases (Nalivaeva and Turner, 2013). Cleavage by β secretase generates a large soluble fragment sAPPβ and a membrane anchored C-terminal fragment, CTFβ; the latter may be further cleaved by the γ-secretase complex and release Aβ as well as the APP intracellular domain AICD. The Aβ load during disease progression is thought to lead to neurological dysfunction (reviewed in Mucke and Selkoe, 2012).

The APP gene is linked to AD, and familial AD can be caused by increased expression of APP (and consequently Aβ) due to either genomic duplication or regulatory sequence alterations (Podlisny et al., 1987; Rovelet-Lecrux et al., 2006; Theuns et al., 2006).

RanBP9 interacts with APP and influences its trafficking and processing (Lakshmana et al., 2009). RanBP9 is a scaffolding protein involved in the modulation of neuronal functions for the maintenance of cell homeostasis (Suresh et al., 2012). RanBP9 interacts with low-density lipoprotein-related protein (LRP), APP, and BACE1, promoting BACE1-dependent cleavage of APP and Aβ generation both *in vitro* and *in vivo* (Lakshmana et al., 2009, 2012). Furthermore, RanBP9 is increased in mutant APP transgenic mice and in the degenerating brains of patients with AD (Lakshmana et al., 2010, 2012). In addition, RanBP9 overexpression promotes neuronal apoptosis and potentiates Aβ-induced neurotoxicity independently of its capacity to stimulate Aβ generation (Woo et al., 2012), whereas RanBP9 transgenic mice show a significantly increased incidence of synapse loss, neurodegeneration, and spatial memory deficits (Lakshmana et al., 2012; Woo et al., 2012). These various actions of RanBP9 may contribute to the pathogenesis of AD.

The microRNAs represent an emerging class of small non-coding RNA molecules which, in mammals, regulate gene expression primarily by imperfect base pairing with the 3′-untranslated region (UTR) of specific target mRNAs. Hence, microRNAs mediate post-transcriptional repression of target mRNAs (Sun and Lai, 2013). Changes of microRNA expression have been shown to be associated to AD (Tan et al., 2013) and to be deregulated in transgenic animal models of AD (Lee et al., 2012; Barak et al., 2013). MicroRNAs are among the molecules identified as physiological and pathological regulators of key genes involved in AD, including APP (Patel et al., 2008; Hebert et al., 2009; Liu et al., 2010; Vilardo et al., 2010; Long and Lahiri, 2011; Smith et al., 2011; Long et al., 2012; Liang et al., 2012), BACE1 (Hébert et al., 2008; Wang et al., 2008; Boissonneault et al., 2009; Fang et al., 2012; Zhu et al., 2012) and microtubule associated protein tau, MAPT (Hébert et al., 2010). Each microRNA has the potential to target a large number of mRNAs (Friedman et al., 2009) and miRNAs may reinforce their effect through the simultaneous and coherent regulation of multiple targets (reviewed in Inui et al., 2010). Indeed miRNAs that simultaneously regulate APP/BACE1 expression have recently been described (Fang et al., 2012; Ai et al., 2013).

Previously, we demonstrated that the 3′UTR of APP mRNA can functionally interact with miR-101, a brain-enriched microRNA, and that inhibition of endogenous miR-101 increases APP levels. On the other hand, lentivirus-mediated overexpression of miR-101 significantly reduced APP expression and the Aβ load in hippocampal neurons (Vilardo et al., 2010). Furthermore, miR-101 is downregulated in the human AD brain, suggesting that miR-101 expression levels may critically participate in the pathogenesis of AD (Hébert et al., 2008; Nunez-Iglesias et al., 2010).

Here searching for predicted APP metabolism-associated miR-101 targets we further investigated the action of endogenous miR-101 in hippocampal neurons. The hippocampus is affected during the early stages of AD, and changes in the hippocampus coincide with the memory deficits observed in AD patients. Therefore, study of hippocampal cells may improve our understanding of the role of miR-101 and other microRNAs in the gene regulation as well as the involvement of microRNAs in neurodegenerative processes associated with the progression of AD.

Our study provides evidence that miR-101 may regulate not only APP but also RanBP9 in hippocampal neurons both *in vitro* and *in vivo* and that miR-101-mediated post-transcriptional regulation of RanBP9 may modulate the amyloidogenic processing of APP.

MATERIALS AND METHODS

CELL CULTURE

Primary hippocampal neurons were prepared from day 17–18 embryos obtained from timed-pregnant Wistar rats (Charles River). Neurons were plated at a density of 1×10^6 cells/dish on 3.5-cm tissue culture dishes pre-coated with poly(D/L-lysine) and cultured in neurobasal medium supplemented with B-27 and GlutaMAX™ (Gibco). Half of the medium was changed every 3–4 days. The neurons were transduced at 7 days *in vitro* with 2×10^6 transducing units (TU)/mL of the pLSyn-miR-101 sponge vector (constructed as described below), or with a control pLSyn vector expressing only EGFP. Protein lysates were collected at 7 days post-transduction and used in Western blotting experiments, as described below.

SH-SY5Y neuroblastoma cells were cultured in Dulbecco's modified Eagle's medium (DMEM) containing 10% fetal bovine serum in a 5% CO_2-humidified incubator at 37°C. The cells were used in luciferase assays, as described below.

LUCIFERASE REPORTER GENE CONSTRUCTS AND LUCIFERASE ASSAY

The SC-RANBP9 3′UTR was purchased from Origene (SC210772). The SC control firefly vector was derived from the SC-RANBP9 3′UTR. The RANBP9 luciferase mutant constructs were generated by using the QuikChange® II Site-Directed Mutagenesis Kit (Stratagene) and the following synthetic oligonucleotides: RanBP9 3′UTR mut up, 5′-ATGGAAGAAATCATTTTT AATGTGTAGAGTAAAACTTGAAATACTCAGGAGCTG-3′; and RanBP9 3′UTR mut down, 5′-CAGCTCCTGAGTATTTCAAGTT TTACTCTACACATTAAAAATGATTTCTTCCAT-3′.

SH-SY5Y cells were plated at a density of 0.6×10^5 per well in 24-well plates and transfected after 24 h with 20 pmole of the indicated microRNA duplexes (Dharmacon) and 50 ng of the firefly luciferase expression vector conjugated to 0.5 µL Lipofectamine 2000 (Invitrogen) in Opti-MEM® reduced-serum medium (Gibco). Cells were lysed at 24 h after transfection, and luciferase assays were performed by using the Dual Luciferase Reporter Assay System (Promega) according to the manufacturer's protocol. The experiments were carried out in triplicate.

PREPARATION OF THE miR-101 SPONGE, miRNA AND SILENCING RNA LENTIVIRAL VECTORS, AND VIRAL PARTICLES

The pLSyn vector was described previously (Barbato et al., 2010). The miR-101 sponge was constructed by using the following synthetic oligonucleotides: S1 CATAATTCAGTTATCCAGTACT GTACGATTTCAGTTATCCAGTACTGTAACCGGT; AS1 TACA GTACTGGATAACTGAAATCGTACAGTACTGGATAACTGAAT TATGGTAC; S2 TT CAGTTATCCAGTACTGTATCACTTCAG TTATCCAGTACTGTACCCGGGGGTACCGAGCT; and AS2 CG GTACCCCCGGGTACAGTACTGGATAACTGAAGTGATACAG TACTGGATAACTGAAACCGG. Oligonucleotides S1 and S2, containing four tandem bulged miR-101 binding sites (at position 11), were annealed with AS1 and AS2, respectively, ligated, and digested with the KpnI restriction enzyme. The product was purified and cloned into the KpnI site of the pLSyn backbone, downstream of the woodchuck hepatitis virus post-transcriptional regulatory element. PLB-scr and pLB-101 lentiviral vector have been previously described (Vilardo et al., 2010).

RanBP9 downregulation was induced by using a lentiviral vector expressing a silencing (si) RNA that targets rat RanBP9 mRNA (sh-RanBP9, TRCN0000102112, Sigma-Aldrich), and a control vector expressing a siRNA that does not target rat mRNAs (SHC002, Sigma-Aldrich).

The preparation of the G glycoprotein vesicular stomatitis virus-pseudotyped lentiviral particles has been described previously (Barbato et al., 2010). Briefly, HEK293T cells were transduced with viral vectors, and the virus-containing medium was harvested 60 h later, filtered through a 0.45-mm Durapore Stericup unit, and concentrated by a two-step ultracentrifugation procedure. The titers of the viral vectors used in this study were in the range of $1–3 \times 10^9$ TU/ml.

ANIMALS

A total of 12 males C57BL/6Ncrl mice (Charles River, Italy) were used at the age of 6–7 weeks. All experiments were performed in accordance with European Community Directive 86/609/EC. Mice were unilaterally microinfused into the CA1 field of the hippocampus with lentiviral particles derived from the control pLSyn vector ($n = 6$) or the pLSyn-miR-101 sponge vector ($n = 6$), as described below.

INTRAHIPPOCAMPAL INJECTION OF LENTIVIRAL VECTORS

Mice were anesthetized with chloral hydrate (400 mg/kg, i.p.). Holes were drilled above the CA1 field of the hippocampus (anterior/posterior = -2.2, medial/lateral = ±1.8, ventral = -1.8) by using standard stereotaxic procedures. Control pLSyn vector or pLSyn-miR-101 sponge vector (1 μL) was unilaterally microinfused into the hippocampus via a stainless steel cannula (0.1 mm in diameter) connected to a Hamilton microsyringe. An infusion pump was maintained at an infusion rate of 0.2 μL/min, and the cannula was left in place for 5 min following completion of the infusion. Two weeks later, the hippocampi were removed and processed for subsequent analyses, as described below.

RNA EXTRACTION AND ANALYSIS

Total RNA was extracted from primary hippocampal neurons with TRIzol (Invitrogen) according to the manufacturer's instructions. RNA quantitation was performed via quantitative real-time PCR (RT-PCR). The total RNA was treated using the TURBO DNA-free™ Kit (Ambion), reverse-transcribed with SuperScript III reverse transcriptase (Invitrogen), and amplified by using the SensiMixPlus SYBR Kit (BioLine) and the 7900HT Fast Real-Time PCR System (Applied Biosystems). Oligonucleotides amplifying the TATA binding protein (TBP), APP, and RanBP9 were chosen from the Roche Universal Probe Library and were as follows:

rno-TBP-1029-1048FW CCCACCAGCAGTTCAGTAGC
rno-TBP-1081-1103RW CAATTCTGGGTTTGATCATTCTG
rno-APP-FW GCCTGAACTCGAATTAATATACA
rno-APP-RW GCTTCTTCTTCCTCAACATCG
rno-Ranbp9-675-693 FW TGCTTTCACCGACTTACCG
rno-Ranbp9-737-755 RW CCAAAGTTGGCATCAACCA

Relative changes in gene expression were quantified by applying the comparative threshold method (Ct) after determining the Ct values for the reference gene (TBP, the endogenous control) and the target genes in each sample set according to the $2^{-\Delta\Delta Ct}$ method. All reactions were performed in triplicate.

PROTEIN EXTRACTION AND WESTERN BLOT ANALYSIS

Hippocampal tissues or cultured cells were homogenized in buffer (1% Triton, 0.25% sodium dodecyl sulphate (SDS), 1% sodium deoxycholate, 2 mM EDTA, and 1 mM dithiothreitol) supplemented with a protease inhibitor mixture (Sigma-Aldrich) to yield total protein extracts. The standard 2X Laemmli loading buffer contained 4% SDS, 10% β-mercaptoethanol, 20% glycerol, and 0.04% bromophenol blue in 125 mM Tris-HCl, pH 6.8. Equal amounts of total protein extract were fractionated by electrophoresis in an 8% SDS-polyacrylamide gel and then transferred to a nitrocellulose membrane (Hybond-ECL, GE Healthcare). Membranes were incubated with the indicated primary antibody overnight at 4°C. Incubation with a secondary peroxidase-coupled anti-mouse or anti-rabbit antibody (GE Healthcare) was performed at room temperature for 1 h. Immunoreactivity was determined by using an enhanced chemiluminescence detection kit (Millipore). The following primary antibodies and dilutions were used: mouse monoclonal anti-APP (4G8, 1:500, Signet), rabbit polyclonal anti-sAPPβ (SIG-39138, 1:1000, Covance), rabbit polyclonal anti-RanBP9 (ab78127, 1:2000, Abcam), mouse monoclonal anti-GFP (1:2000, JL-8 632380 Clontech) and anti-glyceraldehyde 3-phosphate dehydrogenase (GAPDH) (1:6000, Covance).

RESULTS

RanBP9 IS A TARGET OF miR-101

To identify putative miR-101 target mRNAs associated with APP metabolism, we used several microRNA target prediction computational programs, such as TargetScan, Pictar, and miRanda (Gomes et al., 2013). Some features of these target prediction programs are: the ability to predict base-pairing patterns and the thermodynamic stability of microRNA-mRNA hybrids, as well as the capacity to perform comparative sequence analysis to evaluate sequence conservation and the individuation of multiple target sites.

Our analysis revealed a putative miR-101 RE within the 3′UTR of the mRNA encoding RanBP9 (seed location 507–513 bp), which is conserved among vertebrates (**Figure 1A**). The RanBP9 protein interacts with the cytoplasmic tails of LRP, APP and BACE1 proteins promoting BACE1-dependent cleavage of APP and Aβ generation both *in vitro* and *in vivo* (Lakshmana et al., 2009, 2012). To determine whether the RanBP9 gene is a target of miR-101, we introduced a firefly reporter vector containing the full-length RanBP9 3′UTR (883 bp) downstream of the luciferase open reading frame into SH-SY5Y neuroblastoma cells. SH-SY5Y cells were co-transfected with either a reporter construct containing the RanBP9 3′UTR or with a control firefly plasmid, in addition to a synthetic miR-101 precursor or a control microRNA (**Figures 1B,C**). The synthetic miR-101 precursor significantly reduced luciferase expression by more than 40% relative to the control microRNA. The repressive effect of miR-101 on the RanBP9 3′UTR was abrogated by site-directed mutagenesis of the nucleotides at positions 4 and 5 of the miR-101 RE at 507–513 bp. These data indicate that miR-101 negatively regulates RanBP9 expression.

A LENTIVIRAL SPONGE INDUCES THE EXPRESSION OF miR-101 TARGETS IN HIPPOCAMPAL NEURONS

To assay the effects of miR-101 on its target genes and their protein products in hippocampal neurons, we used a lentiviral

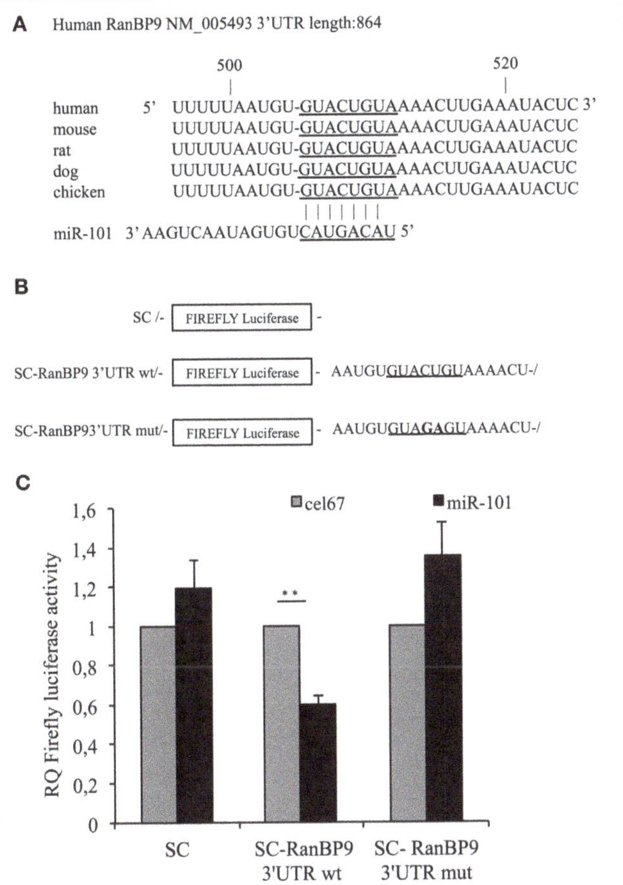

FIGURE 1 | The conserved miR-101 target site at the 507–513 bp region of the RanBP9 3′UTR is necessary for RanBP9 post-transcriptional regulation. (A) Ribonucleotide sequences of the conserved putative miR-101 RE within the RanBP9 3′UTR paired with the mature miR-101 sequence. **(B)** Schematic representation of the luciferase constructs used in this study. The miR-101 RE within the RanBP9 3′-UTR is underlined. In the mutant construct, the nucleotides at positions 4 and 5 of the miR-101 RE were mutated, as indicated in bold font. **(C)** SH-SY5Y neuroblastoma cells were transfected independently with the SC control plasmid or with each of two SC-RanBP9 luciferase reporter genes together with either miR-101 or a control microRNA (cel-miR-67) (100 nM). At 24 h post-transfection, luciferase activity was determined. Results are presented as the normalized activity of miR-101-transfected cells relative to that of cells transfected with cel-miR-67. Data are presented as the means ± the SE from three or four independent experiments (**$p < 0.01$, Student's *t*-test).

pLSyn-miR-101 sponge vector in which the synapsin promoter controlled the expression of four tandem bulged miR-101 REs located downstream of the EGFP open reading frame (**Figure 2**). Rat hippocampal cultures were transduced at 7 days *in vitro* with either the control pLSyn vector or the pLSyn-miR-101 sponge vector. Seven days later, the lentiviral vector-transduced hippocampal neurons expressed EGFP mRNA at a sub-saturating level, resulting in a notable reduction in EGFP fluorescence in the pLSyn-miR-101 sponge-containing neurons vs. the pLSyn vector-containing neurons (**Figure 2**).

We next evaluated the capacity of the miR-101 sponge to affect miR-101-mediated post-transcriptional regulation by measuring the protein expression levels of APP and RanBP9 in primary hippocampal neurons transduced with either the pLSyn-miR-101 sponge vector or the control pLSyn vector. Western blotting analysis showed that APP and RanBP9 proteins levels were significantly increased in neurons transduced with the pLSyn-miR-101 sponge vector compared with the control pLSyn vector (**Figures 3A,B**). However, no significant alterations in APP or RANBP9 mRNA levels were observed (**Figure 3C**). These results suggest that the increase in APP and RanBP9 expression is likely due to a relief of microRNA-mediated translational suppression. Consistently with these data we found that the over-expression of miR-101 in hippocampal neurons induced a significant downregulation of RanBP9 protein (**Figure S2**).

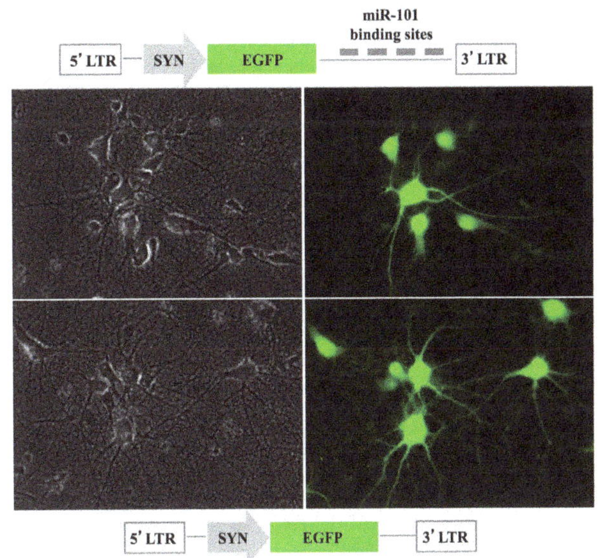

FIGURE 2 | Expression of the pLSyn-miR-101 sponge in primary hippocampal neurons. A schematic representation of the pLSyn-miR-101 sponge and the control pLSyn lentiviral vector is shown. The EGFP signal was slightly lower in the pLSyn-miR-101 sponge-containing neurons (top image) at 14 days post-transduction with respect to the pLSyn-containing neurons (bottom image). Left: phase contrast images, right: EGFP signal.

Because RanBP9 increases the amyloidogenic processing of APP to yield sAPPβ by modulation of BACE1 activity (Lakshmana et al., 2009), sAPPβ levels in the extracellular medium of lentiviral vector-transduced hippocampal neurons were next examined. The secretion of sAPPβ into the conditioned culture medium was significantly increased for neurons transduced with the pLSyn-miR-101 sponge vector relative to the control pLSyn vector (**Figure 3D**). This result demonstrates that the inhibition of miR-101 action on its target genes increases the amyloidogenic processing of APP.

SILENCING OF RanBP9 AFTER miR-101 INHIBITION MITIGATES sAPPβ OVERPRODUCTION

To evaluate the role of RanBP9 in sAPPβ overproduction, we analyzed the levels of sAPPβ in pLSyn-miR-101 sponge-containing hippocampal cultures in which RanBP9 was downregulated. Cultured hippocampal neurons expressing the miR-101 sponge

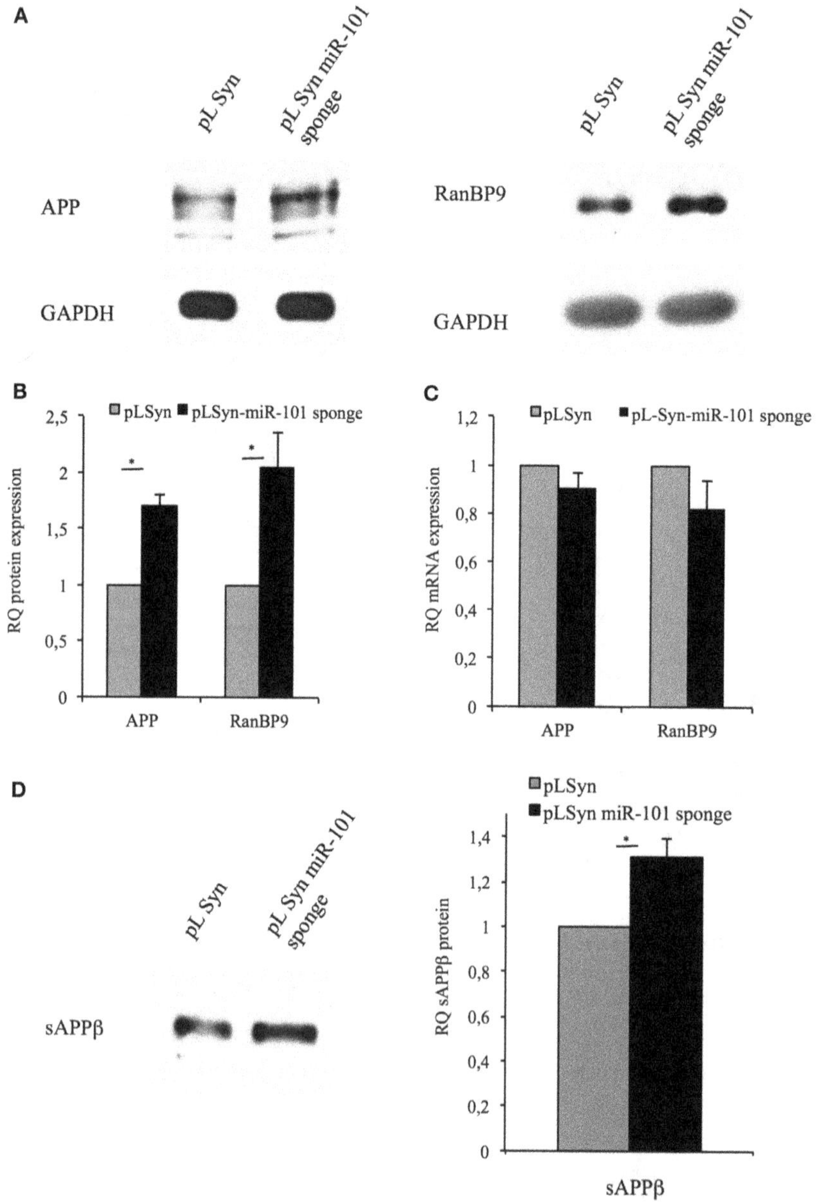

FIGURE 3 | Inhibition of miR-101 in neurons increases levels of endogenous RanBP9, full-length APP, and its secreted product, sAPPβ. (A) Representative Western blot analysis of protein extracts from lentiviral vector-transduced hippocampal neurons at 7 days post-infection with an antibody recognizing RanBP9, an antibody recognizing full-length APP (4G8), or an antibody recognizing GAPDH. Full blot for RanBP9 with multiple samples is shown in **Figure S1**. **(B)** The intensities of the bands were quantified by densitometry. The results obtained with the 4G8 antibody or the RanBP9 antibody were normalized to those obtained with the GAPDH antibody and expressed as arbitrary optical density (OD) units. The band intensities for miR-101 sponge-containing neurons were quantified relative to those for control pLSyn vector-containing neurons. **(C)** Quantitative RT-PCR for APP and RanBP9 mRNA, using hippocampal cell total RNA as the template. Expression levels in miR-101 sponge-transduced neurons relative to control pLSyn vector-transduced cells are shown. **(D)** Conditioned culture medium samples from lentivirus-transduced hippocampal neurons were collected from cells cultured in 35-mm dishes, normalized according to the protein content of the corresponding cell extracts, and analyzed by Western blotting with the sAPPβ antibody, which recognizes the secreted form of APP. Cultures expressing the pLSyn-miR-101 sponge exhibited sAPPβ levels that were 1.3-fold higher than the control levels found in pLSyn-transduced cells. Results in **(B–D)** are presented as the means ± the SE of three independent experiments (*$p < 0.05$, Student's *t*-test).

were transduced with a lentiviral vector containing RanBP9 siRNA under the control of the U6 promoter, or with a control lentiviral vector expressing a scrambled siRNA. The pLSyn vector-containing hippocampal neurons transduced with the scrambled lentiviral vector were used as the experimental control. Neurons were collected at 96 h after RanBP9 silencing and subjected to Western blot analysis for APP, RanBP9, and sAPPβ (**Figure 4**). The pLSyn-miR-101 sponge-containing neurons

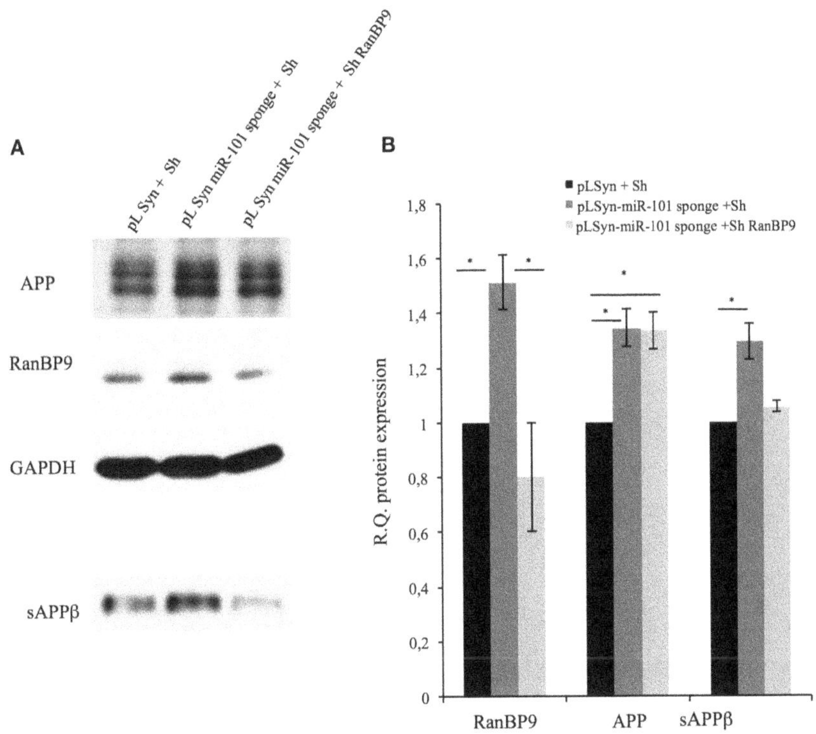

FIGURE 4 | Silencing of RanBP9 reverses oversecretion of sAPPβ into the conditioned medium of pLSyn-miR-101-containing hippocampal neurons. Hippocampal neurons at 7 days *in vitro* were infected with the control pLSyn vector or the pLSyn-miR-101 sponge vector. Seventy-two hours later, the cells were transduced with a lentiviral vector containing RanBP9 siRNA under the control of the U6 promoter, or with a control lentivirus expressing a scrambled siRNA. After 14 days, the neurons were collected for Western blot analysis. **(A)** Representative immunoblots of protein extracts from lentiviral vector-transduced neurons reacted with an antibody recognizing RanBP9, an antibody recognizing full-length APP (4G8), or an antibody recognizing GAPDH are shown. Alternatively, conditioned culture medium samples were collected from lentiviral vector-transduced hippocampal neurons cultured in 35-mm dishes, normalized according to the protein content of the corresponding cell extracts, and analyzed by Western blotting with the sAPPβ antibody. **(B)** Quantitative data are provided in the histogram. The data are expressed as means ± the SE of three independent experiments (*$p < 0.05$, Student's *t*-test).

transduced with the scrambled siRNA showed an increase in all three proteins compared with the control neurons. On the other hand, the pLSyn-miR-101 sponge-containing neurons with silenced RanBP9 showed a positive correlation between decreased RanBP9 expression and attenuated sAPPβ secretion into the conditioned medium (**Figure 4**). This observation suggests that RanBP9 upregulation may increase sAPPβ production when miR-101 is inhibited.

THE miR-101 SPONGE INDUCES APP AND RanBP9 EXPRESSION *IN VIVO*

The significance of miR-101-mediated post-transcriptional regulation on the expression of its targets was evaluated *in vivo* by unilaterally injecting lentiviral particles into the hippocampus of adult mice. Infection was monitored by western blot analysis of EGFP expression. Two weeks after injection, the right and left sides of the hippocampus were processed for biochemical analysis. Western blotting showed that the expression of the miR-101 sponge induced the upregulation of the APP and RanBP9 proteins in the injected side of the hippocampus relative to the non-injected side (**Figure 5**). The injection of the control lentivirus did not appreciably alter the expression of either miR-101 target (**Figure 5**). These findings indicate that miR-101-mediated post-transcriptional regulation is involved in the APP metabolism of adult neurons both *in vivo* and *in vitro*.

DISCUSSION

MicroRNAs are abundantly expressed in the brain, where they play important roles in neural development and function. MicroRNAs also feature predominantly in gene regulation under both normal and pathological conditions (Eacker et al., 2013). Changes in microRNA expression are found in the brains of patients affected by various neurological diseases, including AD. Several *in vitro* and *in vivo* studies explored the functional role of microRNAs in AD pathogenesis, and showed that these molecules are potentially involved in the regulation of APP metabolism (reviewed in Delay et al., 2012). Notably, aberrant processing of APP is implicated as a causative factor in AD (Nalivaeva and Turner, 2013).

Recently, we reported that miR-101 is among the microRNA species that target the APP gene (Vilardo et al., 2010). In addition, miR-101 is also downregulated in the human AD cerebral cortex (Hébert et al., 2008; Nunez-Iglesias et al., 2010). Here, we demonstrate that the RanBP9 gene is a novel target of miR-101, and that miR-101 is involved in the amyloidogenic processing

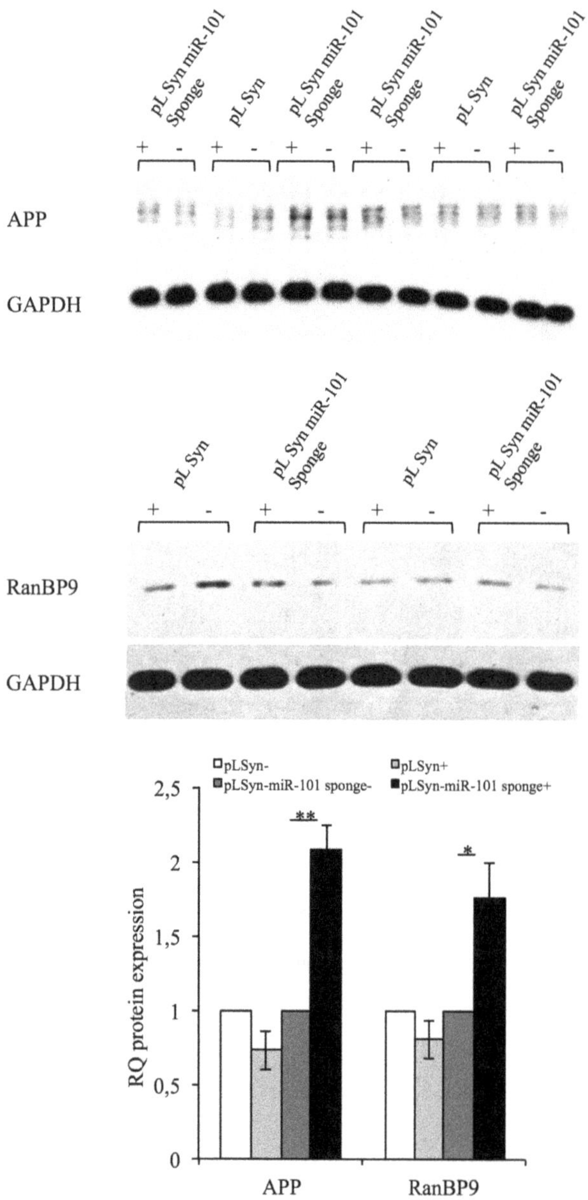

FIGURE 5 | Full-length APP and RanBP9 are targets of miR-101 in mouse hippocampal neurons *in vivo*. Western blotting was performed of hippocampal tissues injected and non-injected with lentiviral vectors. Effective expression of the lentiviral vector was revealed by the presence of EGFP (data not shown). Expression of the miR-101 lentiviral sponge resulted in an increase in the protein expression levels of the miR-101 targets, APP and RanBP9, with respect to non-injected tissue. APP and RanBP9 band intensities were quantified by densitometry, normalized to the GAPDH signal, and expressed as arbitrary OD units. The relative ratio of APP (pLSyn $n = 3$; pLSyn-miR-101 sponge $n = 4$) and RanBP9 (pLSyn $n = 3$; pLSyn-miR-101 sponge $n = 4$) expression in injected vs. non-injected tissue is shown. Results are presented as the means ± the SE ($^{*}p < 0.05$; $^{**}p < 0.01$, Student's *t*-test).

of APP by downregulating the expression of the RanBP9 protein. RanBP9 regulates Aβ peptide production in several cell lines and primary neuronal cultures and exerts its actions by forming protein complexes with APP, LRP, and BACE1, leading to the increased proteolytic processing of APP, secretion of sAPPβ, and generation of Aβ, which is present in excessive amounts in the brains of AD patients. Through the use of computational prediction programs, we found a putative conserved miR-101 RE within the RanBP9 mRNA 3′UTR. Furthermore, luciferase assays and site-directed mutagenesis experiments demonstrated a functional interaction between the RanBP9 3′UTR and miR-101.

It is worth mentioning that beyond miR-101, among several microRNAs reported to regulate APP expression, miR-153 (Long et al., 2012) is also predicted to target human and mouse, but not rat, RanBP9 3′UTR. However, the miR-153 binding site is very close to the RanBP9 open reading frame suggesting that the efficiency of targeting should be low (Grimson et al., 2007).

Next, we demonstrated the specific relevance of miR-101-mediated post-transcriptional regulation of the RanBP9 gene to APP metabolism in hippocampal neurons. We first took advantage of the neuron-selective synapsin promoter (Kügler et al., 2003) to express a lentiviral miR-101 sponge in cultured neurons. This sponge interferes with the actions of miR-101 on its targets, including the RanBP9 gene. Inhibition of miR-101 via delivery of the sponge increased protein expression levels of APP and RanBP9, as well as the secretion of sAPPβ. Moreover, the overproduction of sAPPβ in the extracellular medium of pLSyn-miR-101 sponge-containing neurons was reversed by RanBP9 silencing. Intrahippocampal injection of lentiviral sponge particles in adult mice also demonstrated that the APP and RanBP9 genes are regulated by miR-101 in adult hippocampal neurons *in vivo*.

Our data indicate that RanBP9 translation may be modulated by microRNA post-transcriptional regulation. On the other hand a recent study suggests that additional pathways may regulate RanBP9 protein expression (Wang et al., 2013). Indeed RanBP9 protein half-life is increased by COPS5, a novel RanBP9-interacting protein that increases the stability of its interacting proteins most likely through an action on the ubiquitin-proteosome system (Wang et al., 2013).

APP expression is extensively regulated at post-transcriptional level by several microRNAs and different RNA binding proteins (reviewed by Ruberti et al., 2010). To date, however, interactions between these regulatory mechanisms on APP expression have not been evidenced. The Fragile X Mental Retardation Protein (FMRP) binds APP mRNA and represses its translation (Westmark and Malter, 2007). Interestingly RanBP9 may interact with FMRP and inhibit its RNA binding activity (Menon et al., 2004). It would therefore be tempting to speculate that APP protein levels may be influenced by miR-101 post-transcriptional regulation of FMRP/RanBP9 complex. Since RANBP9 silencing in pLSyn-miR-101 sponge neurons did not reverse APP protein overexpression we can exclude that RANBP9 protein levels were indirectly modulating APP translation.

Our data showed that miR-101 regulates two target genes that are closely associated with AD, Further investigations are required to determine whether alteration of this regulatory mechanism may affect AD pathogenesis. Importantly, experimental evidence suggests that if the amyloidogenic processing of APP could be halted or decelerated, the devastating effects of AD might be mitigated. Thus, the elucidation of which microRNAs act on APP metabolism provides researchers with a specific focus for the development of new drugs for the management of AD. Furthermore, the demonstration that RanBP9 is post-transcriptionally regulated by miR-101 might have interesting disease implications independently of its effects on amyloidogenic processing, because the overexpression of RanBP9 can induce neuronal apoptosis without generating Aβ peptides (Woo et al., 2012), and RanBP9 transgenic mice show synapse loss, neurodegeneration, and spatial memory deficits (Lakshmana et al., 2012; Woo et al., 2012).

Finally, miR-101 is downregulated in the hippocampus of very old vs. young wild-type mice, and in both very old and young mouse models of AD compared with their age-matched normal controls (Barak et al., 2013). Further studies in mouse models may therefore elucidate the consequences of long-term inhibition of miR-101 on AD pathology.

ACKNOWLEDGMENTS

The authors thank G Vetere and M Ammassari-Teule's group for advices and assistance with stereotaxic injection. This research was supported by "PNR-CNR Aging Program 2012–2014," and in collaboration with Distretto Tecnologico delle Bioscienze Regione Lazio. Silvia Pezzola and Paola Frisone were supported from FILAS Regione Lazio Funds for "Sviluppo della Ricerca su Cervello."

SUPPLEMENTARY MATERIAL

Figure S1 | The gel blot of RanBP9 protein level in three independent hippocampal cultured neurons expressing the miR-101 sponge construct (pLSyn-miR-101 sponge) and the parental control vector (pLSyn). Two exposure time of RanBP9 are shown.

Figure S2 | Reduction of RanBP9 protein levels by miR-101 overexpression. **(A)** Western immunoblots show the expression of RanBP9 and APP in hippocampal neurons that were transduced with either a control lentiviral vector (pLB-scr) expressing a control microRNA or a lentiviral vector expressing a mature miR-101 (pLB-101) **(B)** GAPDH-relative expressions are shown in the histogram. Data are presented as the means ± the *SD* ($^*p < 0.05$; $^{**}p < 0.01$, Student's *t*-test; $n = 3$).

REFERENCES

Ai, J., Sun, L. H., Che, H., Zhang, R., Zhang, T. Z., Wu, W. C., et al. (2013). MicroRNA-195 protects against dementia induced by chronic brain hypoperfusion via its anti-amyloidogenic effect in rats. *J. Neurosci.* 33, 3989–4001. doi: 10.1523/JNEUROSCI.1997-12.2013

Barak, B., Shvarts-Serebro, I., Modai, S., Gilam, A., Okun, E., Michaelson, D. M., et al. (2013). Opposing actions of environmental enrichment and Alzheimer's disease on the expression of hippocampal microRNAs in mouse models. *Transl. Psychiatry* 3, e304. doi: 10.1038/tp.2013.77

Barbato, C., Ruberti, F., Pieri, M., Vilardo, E., Costanzo, M., Ciotti, M. T., et al. (2010). MicroRNA-92 modulates K(+) Cl(-) co-transporter KCC2 expression in cerebellar granule neurons. *J. Neurochem.* 113, 591–600. doi: 10.1111/j.1471-4159.2009.06560.x

Boissonneault, V., Plante, I., Rivest, S., and Provost, P. (2009). MicroRNA-298 and microRNA-328 regulate expression of mouse beta-amyloid precursor protein-converting enzyme 1. *J. Biol. Chem.* 284, 1971–1981. doi: 10.1074/jbc.M807530200

Delay, C., Mandemakers, W., and Hébert, S. S. (2012). MicroRNAs in Alzheimer's disease. *Neurobiol. Dis.* 46, 285–290. doi: 10.1016/j.nbd.2012.01.003

Eacker, S. M., Dawson, T. M., and Dawson, V. L. (2013). The interplay of microRNA and neuronal activity in health and disease. *Front. Cell. Neurosci.* 7:136. doi: 10.3389/fncel.2013.00136

Fang, M., Wang, J., Zhang, X., Geng, Y., Hu, Z., Rudd, J. A., et al. (2012). The miR-124 regulates the expression of BACE1/beta-secretase correlated with cell death in Alzheimer's disease. *Toxicol. Lett.* 209, 94–105. doi: 10.1016/j.toxlet.2011.11.032

Friedman, R. C., Farh, K. K., Burge, C. B., and Bartel, D. P. (2009). Most mammalian mRNAs are conserved targets of microRNAs. *Genome Res.* 19, 92–105. doi: 10.1101/gr.082701.108

Gomes, C. P., Cho, J. H., Hood, L., Franco, O. L., Pereira, R. W., and Wang, K. (2013). A review of computational tools in microRNA discovery. *Front. Genet.* 4:81. doi: 10.3389/fgene.2013.00081

Grimson, A., Farh, K. K., Johnston, W. K., Garrett-Engele, P., Lim, L. P., and Bartel, D. P. (2007). MicroRNA targeting specificity in mammals: determinants beyond seed pairing. *Mol. Cell.* 27, 91–105. doi: 10.1016/j.molcel.2007.06.017

Hebert, S. S., Horre, K., Nicolai, L., Bergmans, B., Papadopoulou, A. S., Delacourte, A., et al. (2009). MicroRNA regulation of Alzheimer's Amyloid precursor protein expression. *Neurobiol. Dis.* 33, 422–428. doi: 10.1016/j.nbd.2008.11.009

Hébert, S. S., Horré, K., Nicolaï, L., Papadopoulou, A. S., Mandemakers, W., Silahtaroglu, A. N., et al. (2008). Loss of microRNA cluster miR-29a/b-1 in sporadic Alzheimer's disease correlates with increased BACE1/beta-secretase expression. *Proc. Natl. Acad. Sci. U.S.A.* 105, 6415–6420. doi: 10.1073/pnas.0710263105

Hébert, S. S., Papadopoulou, A. S., Smith, P., Galas, M. C., Planel, E., Silahtaroglu, A. N., et al. (2010). Genetic ablation of Dicer in adult forebrain neurons results in abnormal tau hyperphosphorylation and neurodegeneration. *Hum. Mol. Genet.* 19, 3959–3969. doi: 10.1093/hmg/ddq311

Inui, M., Martello, G., and Piccolo, S. (2010). MicroRNA control of signal transduction. *Nat. Rev. Mol. Cell Biol.* 11, 252–263. doi: 10.1038/nrm2868

Krstic, D., and Knuesel, I. (2013). Deciphering the mechanism underlying late-onset Alzheimer disease. *Nat. Rev. Neurol.* 9, 25–34. doi: 10.1038/nrneurol.2012.236

Kügler, S., Kilic, E., and Bähr, M. (2003). Human synapsin 1 gene promoter confers highly neuron-specific long-term transgene expression from an adenoviral vector in the adult rat brain depending on the transduced area. *Gene Ther.* 10, 337–347. doi: 10.1038/sj.gt.3301905

Lakshmana, M. K., Chung, J. Y., Wickramarachchi, S., Tak, E., Bianchi, E., Koo, E. H., et al. (2010). A fragment of the scaffolding protein RanBP9 is increased in Alzheimer's disease brains and strongly potentiates amyloid-beta peptide generation. *FASEB J.* 24, 119–127. doi: 10.1096/fj.09-136457

Lakshmana, M. K., Hayes, C. D., Bennett, S. P., Bianchi, E., Reddy, K. M., Koo, E. H., et al. (2012). Role of RanBP9 on amyloidogenic processing of APP and synaptic protein levels in the mouse brain. *FASEB J.* 26, 2072–2083. doi: 10.1096/fj.11-196709

Lakshmana, M. K., Yoon, I. S., Chen, E., Bianchi, E., Koo, E. H., and Kang, D. E. (2009). Novel role of RanBP9 in BACE1 processing of amyloid precursor protein and amyloid beta peptide generation. *J. Biol. Chem.* 284, 11863–11872. doi: 10.1074/jbc.M807345200

Lee, S. T., Chu,K., Jung,K. H., Kim, J. H., Huh, J. Y., Yoon,H., et al. (2012). miR-206 regulates brain-derived neurotrophic factor in Alzheimer disease model. *Ann. Neurol.* 72, 269–277. doi: 10.1002/ana.23588

Liang, C., Zhu, H., Xu, Y., Huang, L., Ma, C., Deng, W., et al. (2012). MicroRNA-153 negatively regulates the expression of amyloid precursor protein and amyloid precursor-like protein 2. *Brain Res.* 1455, 103–113. doi: 10.1016/j.brainres.2011.10.051

Liu, W., Liu, C., Zhu, J., Shu, P., Yin, B., Gong, Y., et al. (2010). MicroRNA-16 targets amyloid precursor protein to potentially modulate Alzheimer's-associated pathogenesis in SAMP8 mice. *Neurobiol. Aging* 33, 522–534. doi: 10.1016/j.neurobiolaging.2010.04.034

Long, J. M., and Lahiri, D. K. (2011). MicroRNA-101 downregulates Alzheimer's amyloid-beta precursor protein levels in human cell cultures and is differentially expressed. *Biochem. Biophys. Res. Commun.* 404, 889–895. doi: 10.1016/j.bbrc.2010.12.053

Long, J. M., Ray, B., and Lahiri, D. K. (2012). MicroRNA-153 physiologically inhibits expression of amyloid-beta precursor protein in cultured human fetal brain cells and is dysregulated in a subset of Alzheimer disease patients. *J. Biol. Chem.* 287, 31298–31310. doi: 10.1074/jbc.M112.366336.

Menon, R. P., Gibson, T. J., and Pastore, A. (2004). The C terminus of fragile X mental retardation protein interacts with the multi-domain Ran-binding protein in the microtubule-organising centre. *J. Mol. Biol.* 343, 43–53. doi: 10.1016/j.jmb.2004.08.024

Mucke, L., and Selkoe, D. J. (2012). Neurotoxicity of amyloid β-protein: synaptic and network dysfunction. *Cold Spring Harb. Perspect. Med.* 2, a006338. doi: 10.1101/cshperspect.a006338

Nalivaeva, N. N., and Turner, A. J. (2013). The amyloid precursor protein: a biochemical enigma in brain development, function and disease. *FEBS Lett.* 587, 2046–2054. doi: 10.1016/j.febslet.2013.05.010

Nunez-Iglesias, J., Liu, C. C., Morgan, T. E., Finch, C. E., and Zhou, X. J. (2010). Joint genome-wide profiling of miRNA and mRNA expression in Alzheimer's disease cortex reveals altered miRNA regulation. *PLoS ONE* 5:e8898. doi: 10.1371/journal.pone.0008898

Patel, N., Hoang, D., Miller, N., Ansaloni, S., Huang, Q., Rogers, J. T., et al. (2008). MicroRNAs can regulate human APP levels. *Mol. Neurodegener.* 3, 10. doi: 10.1186/1750-1326-3-10

Podlisny, M. B., Lee, G., and Selkoe, D. J. (1987). Gene dosage of the amyloid beta precursor protein in Alzheimer's disease. *Science* 238, 669–671. doi: 10.1126/science.2960019

Rovelet-Lecrux, A., Hannequin, D., Raux, G., Le Meur, N., Laquerrière, A., Vital, A., et al. (2006). APP locus duplication causes autosomal dominant early-onset Alzheimer disease with cerebral amyloid angiopathy. *Nat. Genet.* 38, 24–26. doi: 10.1038/ng1718

Ruberti, F., Barbato, C., and Cogoni, C. (2010). Post-transcriptional regulation of amyloid precursor protein by microRNAs and RNA binding proteins. *Commun. Integr. Biol.* 3, 499–503. doi: 10.4161/cib.3.6.13172

Smith, P., Al Hashimi, A., Girare, J., Delay, C., and Hébert, S. S. (2011). *In vivo* regulation of amyloid precursor protein neuronal splicing by microRNAs. *J. Neurochem.* 116, 240–247. doi: 10.1111/j.1471-4159.2010.07097.x

Sun, K., and Lai, E. C. (2013). Adult-specific functions of animal microRNAs. *Nat. Rev. Genet.* 14, 535–548. doi: 10.1038/nrg3471

Suresh, B., Ramakrishna, S., and Baek, K. H. (2012). Diverse roles of the scaffolding protein RanBPM. *Drug Discov. Today* 17, 379–387. doi: 10.1016/j.drudis.2011.10.030

Tan, L., Yu, J. T., Hu, N., and Tan, L. (2013). Non-coding RNAs in Alzheimer's disease. *Mol. Neurobiol.* 47, 382–393. doi: 10.1007/s12035-012-8359-5

Theuns, J., Brouwers, N., Engelborghs, S., Sleegers, K., Bogaerts, V., Corsmit, E., et al. (2006). Promoter mutations that increase amyloid precursor-protein expression are associated with Alzheimer disease. *Am. J. Hum. Genet.* 78, 936–946. doi: 10.1086/504044

Vilardo, E., Barbato, C., Ciotti, M. T., Cogoni, C., and Ruberti, F. (2010). MicroRNA-101 regulates amyloid precursor protein expression in hippocampal neurons. *J. Biol. Chem.* 285, 18344–18351. doi: 10.1074/jbc.M110.112664

Wang, H., Dey, D., Carrera, I., Minond, D., Bianchi, E., Xu, S., et al. (2013). COPS5 (Jab1) protein increases β site processing of amyloid precursor protein and amyloid β peptide generation by stabilizing RanBP9 protein levels. *J. Biol. Chem.* 288, 26668–26677. doi: 10.1074/jbc.M113.476689

Wang, H., Song, L., Laird, F., Wong, P. C., and Lee, H. K. (2008). BACE1 knock-outs display deficits in activity-dependent potentiation of synaptic transmission at mossy fiber to CA3 synapses in the hippocampus. *J. Neurosci.* 28, 8677–8681. doi: 10.1523/JNEUROSCI.2440-08.2008

Westmark, C. J., and Malter, J. S. (2007). FMRP mediates mGluR5-dependent translation of amyloid precursor protein. *PLoS Biol.* 5:e52. doi: 10.1371/journal.pbio.0050052

Woo, J. A., Jung, A. R., Lakshmana, M. K., Bedrossian, A., Lim, Y., Bu, J. H., et al. (2012). Pivotal role of the RanBP9-cofilin pathway in Aβ-induced apoptosis and neurodegeneration. *Cell Death Differ.* 19, 1413–1423. doi: 10.1038/cdd.2012.14

Zhu, H.C., Wang, L. M., Wang, M., Song, B., Tan, S., Teng, J. F., et al. (2012). MicroRNA-195 downregulates Alzheimer's disease amyloid-β production by targeting BACE1. *Brain Res. Bull.* 88, 596–601. doi: 10.1016/j.brainresbull.2012.05.018

15

miR-9: a versatile regulator of neurogenesis

Marion Coolen*, Shauna Katz and Laure Bally-Cuif*

Zebrafish Neurogenetics Team, Laboratory of Neurobiology and Development, Institute of Neurobiology Alfred Fessard, CNRS, Gif-sur-Yvette, France

Correspondence:
Marion Coolen and Laure Bally-Cuif, Zebrafish Neurogenetics Team, Laboratory of Neurobiology and Development, Institute of Neurobiology Alfred Fessard, CNRS, 1 Avenue de la Terrasse, 91198 Gif-sur-Yvette, France
e-mail: coolen@inaf.cnrs-gif.fr; bally-cuif@inaf.cnrs-gif.fr

Soon after its discovery, microRNA-9 (miR-9) attracted the attention of neurobiologists, since it is one of the most highly expressed microRNAs in the developing and adult vertebrate brain. Functional analyses in different vertebrate species have revealed a prominent role of this microRNA in balancing proliferation in embryonic neural progenitor populations. Key transcriptional regulators such as FoxG1, Hes1 or Tlx, were identified as direct targets of miR-9, placing it at the core of the gene network controlling the progenitor state. Recent data also suggest that this function could extend to adult neural stem cells. Other studies point to a role of miR-9 in differentiated neurons. Moreover miR-9 has been implicated in human brain pathologies, either displaying a protective role, such as in Progeria, or participating in disease progression in brain cancers. Altogether functional studies highlight a prominent feature of this highly conserved microRNA, its functional versatility, both along its evolutionary history and across cellular contexts.

Keywords: microRNA-9, neurogenesis, embryonic progenitors, neural stem cells, proliferation

microRNAs are small regulatory RNAs that modulate, generally negatively, the translation and/or stability of mRNA targets through complementary binding to their 3′ untranslated region (3′UTR; Bartel, 2009). microRNA genes are transcribed as primary transcripts (pri-miR), which are cleaved in the nucleus to generate precursor transcripts (pre-miR) (Yang and Lai, 2011). One characteristic of pre-miR is that they form a secondary hairpin structure. Pre-miR are exported to the cytoplasm where they are further cleaved by the enzyme Dicer. This cleavage gives rise to a duplex of short RNA strands (the 5′ and 3′ strands), one of which is then loaded into the RNA-induced silencing complex (RISC). The discovery of microRNAs unraveled a new layer of complexity of gene regulatory networks. Computational and experimental approaches have demonstrated that a single microRNA can regulate the expression of hundreds of mRNA targets. However, despite their large spectrum of action, loss of microRNA function often results in paradoxically subtle phenotypes, some of which are only apparent in a sensitized genomic or environmental context (Li et al., 2009). In the light of these findings, microRNAs are hypothesized to confer robustness to developmental programs, and to facilitate transitions between different cellular states (Takacs and Giraldez, 2010; Ebert and Sharp, 2012). Therefore, studying their implication during neurogenesis, which implies the transition of a neural progenitor to a differentiated neuronal cell, might shed new light on regulation of this process. microRNA-9 (miR-9) captured the attention of neurobiologists because of its high sequence conservation in bilaterian animals, and its high and specific expression in the central nervous system (CNS) of vertebrates. As its function and spectrum of action begins to be unraveled, this microRNA proves to be highly versatile, exerting various and sometimes opposite activities depending on the species and cellular context.

EVOLUTIONARY HISTORY OF *miR-9* GENES

STRUCTURAL EVOLUTION OF THE *miR-9* GENE FAMILY

The *miR-9* gene is ancient in animal evolution, as it appeared at the transition towards triploblasty (Wheeler et al., 2009). The genome of some extant animal species contains several copies of this gene (**Figure 1A**). In Vertebrates, the amplification of *miR-9* genes parallels the whole genome duplication events that occurred in the phylum and thus likely results from them. Independent duplications events also occurred in other phyla such as arthropods. This led in particular to the presence of five *miR-9* genes in *Drosophila*, three of which are clustered in the same gene complex (Lai et al., 2004). The level of sequence conservation of pre-miR-9 among animals is strikingly high, in particular at the level of both 5′ and 3′ mature microRNA strands. For instance the 5′ strand of drosophila *miR-9a* gene is identical to the one in human genes (**Figure 1B**). The retention in vertebrate genomes of multiple independent copies of a gene generating identical microRNA forms is quite surprising. It could be linked to differential expression of paralogous *miR-9* genes, leading to subfunctionalization between copies (Berezikov, 2011).

There is in contrast a high variability in strand preference among *miR-9* copies (see **Figure 1A**). Upon association of microRNA duplexes with the RISC complex, only one strand is retained while the other is discarded. For most microRNAs, one of the two arms, either the 5′ or 3′, is preferentially selected at this step (sometimes called guide strand), while the other tends to be used more infrequently (passenger strand or star strand). In the case of *miR-9* genes, the guide strand can be generated either from the 5′ (miR-9-5p) or the 3′ arm (miR-9-3p) depending on the gene considered. In deuterostomes, *miR-9* genes always show a preferential usage of the 5′ strand (miR-9-5p), although the 3′ strand (miR-9-3p) is still present at detectable levels. This explains

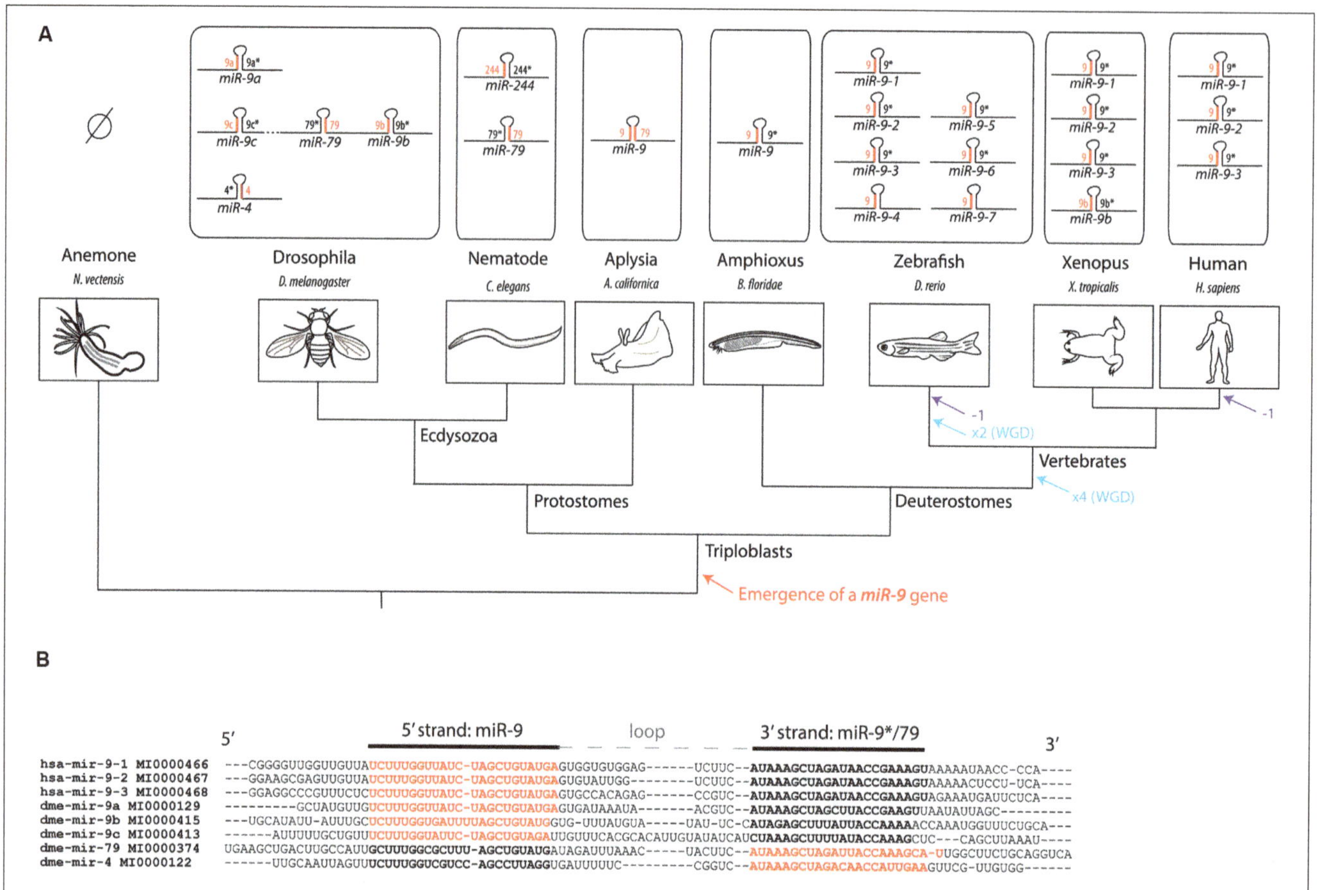

FIGURE 1 | History of the miR-9 gene family. **(A)** Phylogenetic tree showing the evolutionary relationships between different model species and the composition of the *miR-9* gene family in their respective genomes. The preferred microRNA strand is represented in red, while the non-preferred (or "star") is represented in black. No *miR-9* gene has been recovered so far from genomes of cnidarian species, such as the sea anemone or hydra, suggesting that the emergence of a *miR-9* gene occurred at the transition towards triploblasty. At the origin of jawed vertebrates, two rounds of whole genome duplications (WGD) have occurred. An additional WGD occurred in the teleost lineage. These duplication events likely account for the presence of multiple miR-9 genes in vertebrates. Eutherian mammals lost one class of *miR-9* genes (corresponding to *miR-9-4*, also called *miR-9b*). **(B)** Alignment of pre-miR-9 sequences from *Drosophila* and human. Sequences, names and reference numbers were retrieved from miRBase.[1] Nucleotides highlighted in bold correspond to the two microRNA strands, with the preferred strand in red, and the non-preferred one in black.

why miR-9-5p is often referred to as miR-9, while miR-9-3p is referred to as miR-9*. In *Drosophila* and nematode the strand bias is different for the different copies (Lim et al., 2003; Lai et al., 2004). For instance, for 3 of the 5 fly genes (*miR-9a*, *miR-9b* and *miR-9c*) the preferred strand is the 5′ strand, while it is the 3′ strand in the other two genes (*miR-4* and *miR-79*) (Lai et al., 2004). The bias in strand usage in this species is incidentally reflected in the gene nomenclature. Yet a different situation is observed in the marine snail *Aplysia californica*. In this species of mollusk there is only one *miR-9* gene with no preferential strand usage, mature microRNAs being equally recovered from both 5′ and 3′ strands of the duplex (Rajasethupathy et al., 2009). Altogether these data show that strand preference in *miR-9* genes has been quite labile during the course of evolution which certainly influenced the regulation and functional evolution of the gene family.

FUNCTIONAL EVOLUTION OF miR-9: IMPLICATION OF miR-9a IN FLY NEUROGENESIS

Large scale analysis of microRNAs expression revealed that miR-9 is highly enriched in both the developing and mature nervous system of vertebrates (Miska et al., 2004; Sempere et al., 2004; Wienholds et al., 2005; Heimberg et al., 2010). Functional analyses in vertebrate model species have highlighted a prominent role of miR-9 in regulating the behavior of neural progenitors, as well as the differentiation of some neuronal populations (see further sections). The expression of miR-9/9* in human fibroblasts, in synergy with miR-124, is sufficient to convert them into neurons, placing miR-9/9* at the core of the gene network controlling the neural fate (Yoo et al., 2011). The presence of miR-9 in nervous cells might be an ancestral characteristic of bilaterian animals, as it has been observed in cephalochordate and annelid species (Christodoulou et al., 2010; Candiani et al., 2011).

However, in *Drosophila*, although miR-9a does influence the development of peripheral nervous system sensory organs, its function is encoded negatively, through miR-9 restricted

[1]http://www.mirbase.org

expression in non-neural epidermal cells (Li et al., 2006). In wild-type flies sensory precursor (SOP) cells are specified in invariable numbers among ectodermal epithelial cells in a two-step process (Skeath and Carroll, 1994; **Figure 2A**). First, small groups of cells, the proneural clusters, acquire neural competence via the induction of proneural genes encoding basic helix-loop-helix (bHLH) proteins such as Achaete and Scute (Ac/Sc). Among cells of the proneural cluster, as a consequence of a lateral inhibition mechanism via the Notch signaling pathway, one cell will express higher levels of proneural genes and become a SOP (**Figure 2B**). Mutant *miR-9a* flies display a few ectopic sensory neurons in the embryo and in the adult, a phenotype resulting from the specification of an excessive number of SOP cells (Li et al., 2006). *miR-9a* mutant phenotype is however quite mild, and its penetrance is influenced

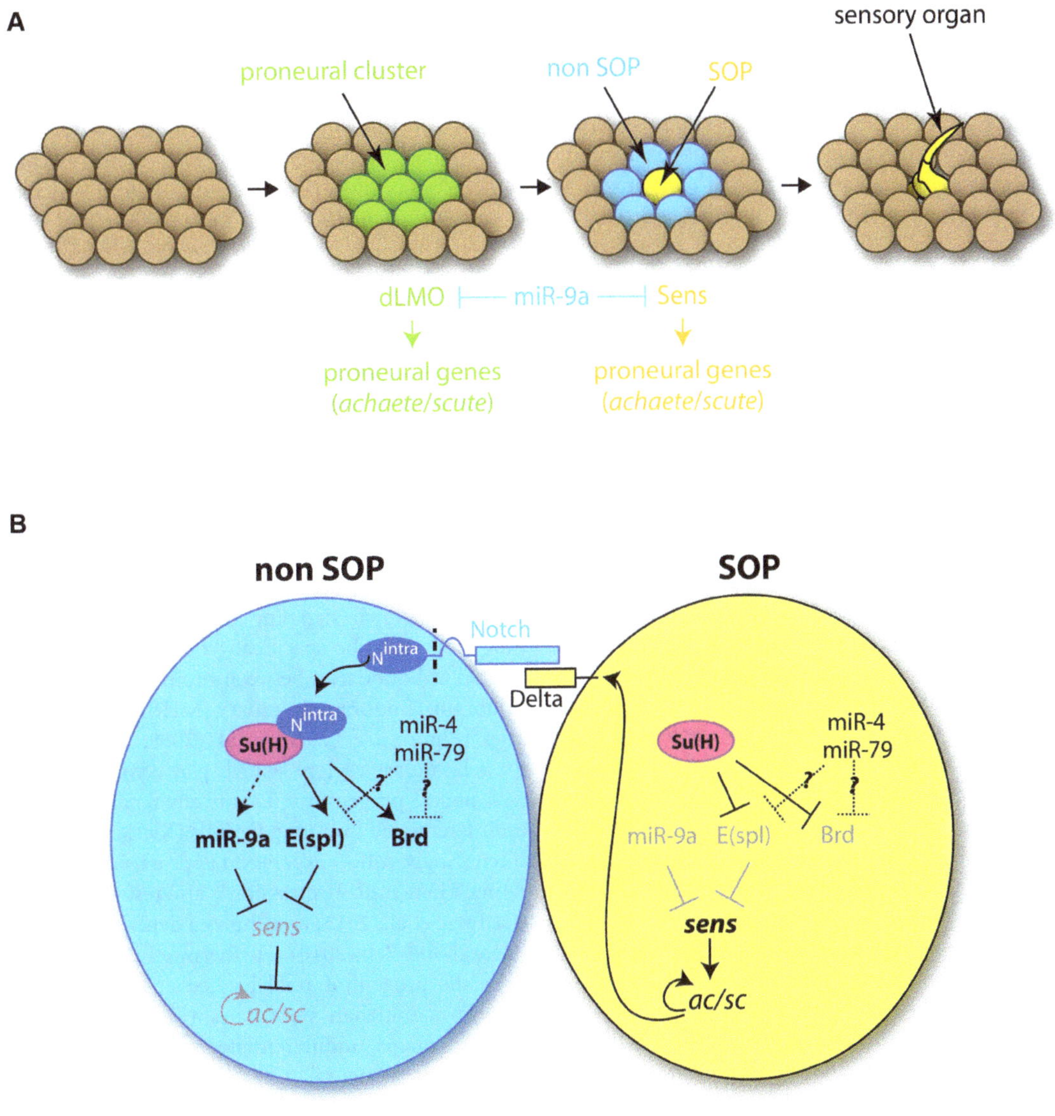

FIGURE 2 | Role of miR-9 in the development of drosophila sensory organs. (A) Different steps of the formation of sensory organs. Among the ectodermal tissue, groups of cells, called proneural clusters (green), acquire neural competence via the induction of proneural genes. The dLMO protein participates in the acquisition of this competence. Among competent cells, one will maintain high levels of proneural genes expression, notably of the *sense* gene, and become a SOP cell (SOP, yellow). Concomitantly the neural fate is inhibited in the neighboring cells (non-SOP, blue). The SOP cell later divides to give rise to a sensory organ. miR-9a is present in all ectodermal cells except the SOP cell, and inhibits dLMO and Sens protein expression. **(B)** Role of miR-9a in SOP cell specification. The SOP cell expresses high levels of the ligand Delta, which interacts with Notch receptors located at the surface of neighboring cells. This interaction leads to Notch cleavage, which releases Notch intracellular domain (N^{intra}) in non-SOP cells. N^{intra} interacts with the transcription factor Suppressor of Hairless Su(H), which induces *E(spl)* gene expression. *E(spl)* genes encode transcriptional repressors inhibiting the expression of proneural genes and in particular *sens*. In the SOP cell, in the absence of N^{intra}, Su(H) has an inhibitory effect on the transcription of *E(spl)* genes which allows for the expression of *sens*. Sens activates the expression of proneural genes of the *ac/scute* complex (*ac/sc*) which specify the SOP cell fate. miR-9a, expressed in non-SOP cells, prevents ectopic expression of *sens*, thereby conferring robustness to the developmental program. Other genes of the *miR-9* family might also play a role here, as miR-4 and miR-79 have been shown to regulate the expression Notch target genes, such as *E(spl)* or *Brd*.

by the genetic background (Li et al., 2006; Bejarano et al., 2010). miR-9a is therefore not a strong deterministic factor, but rather confers robustness to this developmental program, a role frequently undertaken by microRNAs (Ebert and Sharp, 2012). Remarkably miR-9a influences both steps of SOP specification, through the inhibition of two major targets, *drosophila LIM-only* (*dLMO*) and *senseless* (*sens*) (**Figure 2A**; Li et al., 2006; Biryukova et al., 2009; Bejarano et al., 2010). *dLMO* encodes a component of a multimeric transcriptional complex shown to participate in the initial induction of *ac/sc* expression in proneural clusters (Ramain et al., 2000; Asmar et al., 2008). Like *miR-9a* mutants, *dLMO* gain of function mutants display extra sensory bristles (Asmar et al., 2008). These *dLMO* mutants lack large portions of *dLMO* 3′UTR, which contains a miR-9a binding site, conserved among Drosophila species, and through which miR-9a was shown to directly repress the production of the dLMO protein (Biryukova et al., 2009; Bejarano et al., 2010). *sens* is first expressed in proneural cluster cells and later accumulates at high levels in the prospective SOP (Nolo et al., 2000). Sens acts as a binary switch factor: present at low levels in proneural cluster cells, it limits the expression of *ac*; in contrast, high levels of Sens activates proneural genes expression in the SOP cell, contributing to its specification (Jafar-Nejad et al., 2003). Similar to *dLMO*, *sens* 3′UTR harbors miR-9a putative binding sites and mediates an interaction with miR-9a, which impacts on Sens protein levels (Li et al., 2006). Heterozygosity of either *dLMO* or *sens* can partially rescue the excessive number of bristles in *miR-9a* mutants, demonstrating that de-repression of these targets contributes to this phenotype (Bejarano et al., 2010). Little is known however about the upstream regulators of *miR-9a* in flies and how its expression becomes restricted to non-neural cells. The only known miR-9a regulator is the RNA-binding protein transactive response DNA-binding protein 43 (TDP-43), which seems to stabilize miR-9a pri-miR (Li et al., 2013). However, the function of other *miR-9* genes, and in particular of *miR-4* and *miR-79*, which use the opposite strand, has yet to be directly addressed in drosophila. Both miR-4 and miR-79 have been shown to interact with Bearded (Brd) box, a sequence motif previously identified as enriched on the 3′UTR of Notch target genes such as *Enhancer-of-split* (*E(spl)*) or *Brd* (Lai and Posakony, 1997; Lai et al., 2005; **Figure 2B**). One could thus hypothesize a role of these microRNAs in neurogenesis through the deregulation of Notch target genes.

In sharp contrast with the situation in vertebrates, studies in drosophila thus point to an anti-neural role of miR-9a: expressed in non-neural epithelial cells, miR-9a restricts the number of specified SOP by dampening the expression of the proneural genes *dLMO* and *sens*. This suggests that, despite the fact that miR-9a sequence is strictly identical to its vertebrate counterparts, its function and its set of targets have been profoundly remodeled during evolution.

miR-9 REGULATION OF NEURAL DEVELOPMENT

In deuterostomes, *miR-9* genes demonstrate a strong evolutionary plasticity, in terms of strand usage and developmental function. In contrast, studies in vertebrate model species point to highly conserved functions of miR-9, especially in the regulation of neural progenitor proliferation.

miR-9 REGULATION OF NEURAL PROGENITORS

miR-9 expression is preferentially associated with neurogenic progenitors

The first large scale microRNA expression profiles performed in vertebrates soon identified miR-9 as a brain enriched microRNA (Lagos-Quintana et al., 2002; Krichevsky et al., 2003; Miska et al., 2004; Sempere et al., 2004). In particular, its expression levels were shown to be dynamically regulated during brain development, and during *in vitro* induced neurogenesis (Miska et al., 2004; Sempere et al., 2004; Krichevsky et al., 2006). miR-9*, derived from the 3′ strand of *miR-9* genes, is also present at detectable levels in vertebrate neural tissues. *In situ* hybridization analyses in different vertebrate model organisms have revealed very similar spatiotemporal patterns of miR-9 expression during (CNS) development (Darnell et al., 2006; Deo et al., 2006; Leucht et al., 2008; Shibata et al., 2008; Walker and Harland, 2008). miR-9 expression starts at mid-embryogenesis stages, after the specification of the major brain subdivisions and the development of the primary neuronal scaffold. Its expression is first induced in the telencephalon, and later spreads to more posterior brain regions and spinal cord. All along the CNS, miR-9 expression is predominantly associated with ventricular neural progenitors areas (Darnell et al., 2006; Leucht et al., 2008; Shibata et al., 2008, 2011; Bonev et al., 2011; Coolen et al., 2012), although some differentiated neurons also express miR-9, notably in the dorsal telencephalon and spinal cord (Leucht et al., 2008; Otaegi et al., 2011; Shibata et al., 2011). Its expression characterizes active neurogenic areas and its expression is dependent on the activity of Notch signaling (Coolen et al., 2012). In contrast, miR-9 seems to be specifically excluded from progenitor pools located at boundaries between brain compartments, such as the Midbrain-Hindbrain Boundary (MHB) or rhombomeres boundaries (**Figure 3A**; Leucht et al., 2008; Coolen et al., 2012). In these boundary regions, which play a role as late signaling centers, neural progenitors do not enter neurogenesis and remain undifferentiated over long periods (Kiecker and Lumsden, 2005). Interestingly, miR-9 expression appears similarly regulated in the retina. There miR-9 expression is also restricted to late progenitors (La Torre et al., 2013) and shows a dependence on Notch activity (Georgi and Reh, 2010). Furthermore it appears to be excluded from the progenitor pool located at the ciliary marginal zone in non-mammalian vertebrates (Kapsimali et al., 2007). This pool maintains undifferentiated progenitors over a long time, reminiscent of neural tube boundary regions. miR-9 was also detected in adult brain neurogenic areas, in both fish and mouse (Deo et al., 2006; Kapsimali et al., 2007; Tozzini et al., 2012), and in primary cultures of mouse adult stem cells (Zhao et al., 2009). However a precise characterization of miR-9-positive cells in adult brains remains to be performed.

Regulation of neural progenitors proliferation by miR-9

As the expression of miR-9 suggests, functional analyses uncovered a prominent role of miR-9 in the regulation of embryonic neural progenitors states. In zebrafish embryos, miR-9 was shown to participate in the late patterning of the midbrain/hindbrain region. The activity of miR-9 on both sides of the MHB restricts the extent of the pool of non-neurogenic progenitors located

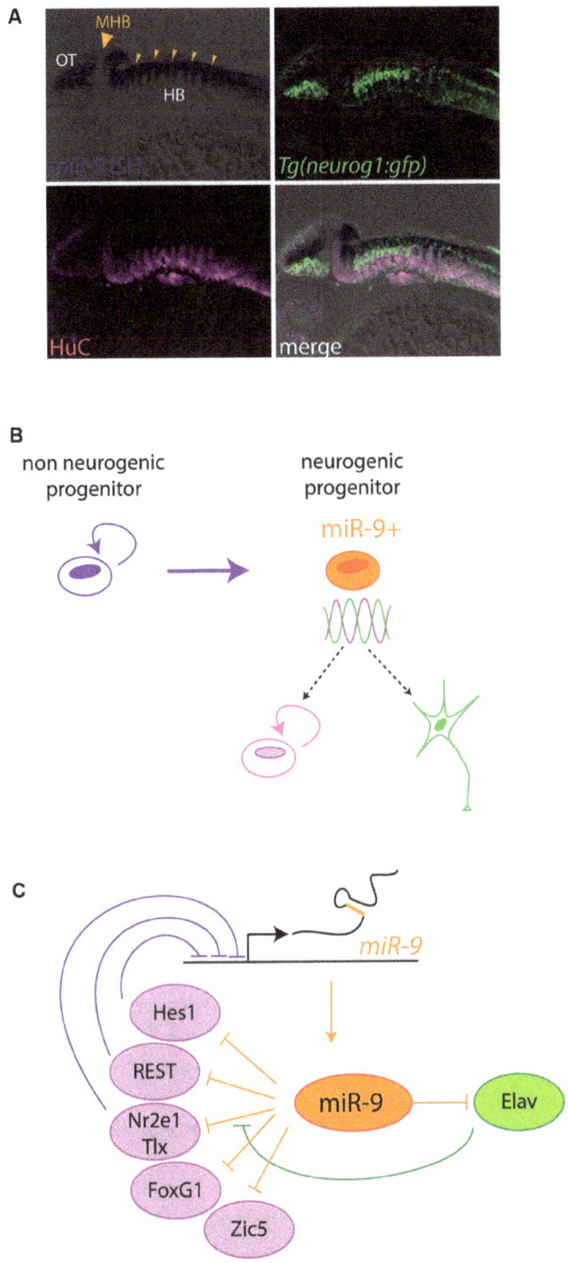

FIGURE 3 | miR-9 regulates progenitor states in Vertebrates. (A) miR-9 is expressed in active neurogenic zones. Sagittal section through a zebrafish embryo at 48 h post fertilization, showing the expression of miR-9 as revealed by *in situ* hybridization (blue). miR-9 is expressed at the ventricular zone, and excluded from differentiated neurons expressing the protein HuC (magenta). Its expression is induced in neurogenic areas, where the expression of proneural genes such as *neurogenin1* (*neurog1*) is detected (green). In contrast, miR-9 is excluded specifically from boundary regions, containing long-lasting neural progenitors, such as the MHB (big arrowhead) or rhombomere boundaries (small arrowheads). **(B)** Functional data suggest that miR-9 promotes the transition from a non-neurogenic progenitor, expressing high levels of Hes1, to a neurogenic progenitor, in which Hes1 levels oscillate. The miR-9 expressing neurogenic progenitor is in an ambivalent state, poised to respond to proliferation or differentiation cues. **(C)** Scheme representing negative feedback loops between miR-9 and its targets, some of which promoting proliferation (purple) and others promoting differentiation (green).

at this boundary (Leucht et al., 2008). However, miR-9 has a more general influence on the behavior of neurogenic progenitors along the neural tube. Overexpression of miR-9/9* duplexes in the zebrafish embryo (Leucht et al., 2008), mouse embryonic cortex (Zhao et al., 2009), and chick spinal cord (Yoo et al., 2011) leads to a reduction in the number of proliferating progenitors. This effect is accompanied by precocious neuronal differentiation (Leucht et al., 2008; Zhao et al., 2009). miR-9/9* was also shown to promote differentiation of adult neural stem cells *in vitro*, albeit only if they were primed for differentiation beforehand using forskolin or retinoic acid (Zhao et al., 2009). Additionally, infecting human neonatal fibroblasts with lentiviral vectors containing miR-9/9* and miR-124 induces their conversion into postmitotic neurons. However, this conversion is dependent on the expression on all three microRNAs (Yoo et al., 2011). Thus, these *in vitro* data show that miR-9 alone is not sufficient to induce neuronal differentiation. Conversely, miR-9 loss-of-function consistently induces an increased proliferation of embryonic neural progenitors (Bonev et al., 2011; Shibata et al., 2011; Coolen et al., 2012) or mouse adult neural stem cells (Zhao et al., 2009). However neural progenitors resume differentiation even under miR-9 depletion conditions, their cell cycle exit being only delayed (Shibata et al., 2011; Coolen et al., 2012). Altogether this data suggests that miR-9 does not act as a necessary and sufficient differentiation switch, but rather could favor the transition of progenitors from a proliferative mode to a neurogenic mode. Of note, in over-expression experiments or in mouse mutants, the effects observed result from the combined gain or loss of both miR-9 strands. In contrast, in depletion experiments using antisense oligonucleotides, like the one performed in zebrafish or Xenopus embros, only miR-9 (miR-9-5p) is down-regulated. The individual role of the other miR-9* (miR-9-3p) has yet to be assessed. Moreover, in human embryonic stem cell-derived neural progenitors, and rat embryonic cortical progenitors, miR-9 was shown to have a completely opposite role (Delaloy et al., 2010). In this study, inhibition of miR-9 led to a decrease in neural progenitor proliferation, concomitant with increased migratory capacities. The different effects observed on neural progenitors in culture might be linked to a different timing of miR-9 depletion during *in vitro* differentiation (Zhao et al., 2009; Delaloy et al., 2010). These results indicate that miR-9 can inversely impact the proliferation of neural progenitors depending on the cellular context. Differential expression of mRNA targets or the synergy between miR-9 and other mRNA regulating factors could account for this phenomenon. For instance the RNA binding proteins Elavl1 and Musashi1 can synergize with miR-9 to increase the expression of some of its targets (Shibata et al., 2011). A better appreciation of the spatial and temporal variations of miR-9 function *in vivo* awaits the development of more refined conditional knock-down tools.

miR-9 targets in neural progenitors reveal a complex interacting network

A better understanding of miR-9 function will certainly arise from the characterization of its set of targets and the analysis of the impact of these interactions *in vivo*. *In silico* algorithms predict several hundred targets for miR-9, a high figure typical of ancient microRNAs (Bartel, 2009). So far, only a few of these interactions have been confirmed *in vitro* or *in vivo*, but these studies have shed light on the complex mode of action of miR-9 in neural progenitors.

A first set of miR-9 targets are members of the *Hes* gene family (Leucht et al., 2008; Bonev et al., 2011, 2012; Coolen et al., 2012). *Hes* genes are the main Notch signaling effectors and encode transcriptional repressors (Kageyama et al., 2008). Expressed in neural progenitors, they inhibit differentiation by repressing proneural genes such as *ascl1*, a vertebrate homolog of *Drosophila ac/sc* complex genes. Some of them are also highly expressed at boundaries and help in maintaining slow cycling non-neurogenic progenitors at these locations (Kageyama et al., 2008; Stigloher et al., 2008). Among miR-9 targets is *her5*, which in zebrafish embryos is specifically expressed at the MHB. In this area miR-9 restricts the size of the MHB progenitor pool through repressing *her5* while simultaneously limiting the signaling activity of the MHB progenitors by repressing Fibroblast growth factor (FGF) pathway genes (Leucht et al., 2008). *Hes1/her6* genes also harbor a miR-9 binding site in their 3′UTR, which is conserved across vertebrates. In zebrafish and frog embryos, target protector morpholinos (Choi et al., 2007) that block the miR-9 binding site on the *hes1/her6* 3′UTR, induce an increased proliferation, mimicking the effect of miR-9 blockade (Bonev et al., 2011; Coolen et al., 2012) and thus demonstrate that miR-9 targeting of this gene is crucial to properly balance progenitor proliferation. Interestingly, *Hes1* was previously shown to be expressed in neural progenitors both at boundary regions and inside brain compartments. However, live imaging using a *Hes1* luciferase reporter demonstrated that at boundaries, *Hes1* expression is high and stable, whereas it displays ultradian oscillations inside brain compartments (Shimojo et al., 2008). This difference in *Hes1* expression mode is thought to parallel the non-neurogenic versus neurogenic properties of these two kinds of progenitors (Kageyama et al., 2008). In an *in vitro* model, the dampening of *Hes1* expression by miR-9 was shown to be necessary for oscillations of *Hes1* to occur (Bonev et al., 2012; Tan et al., 2012). miR-9 could therefore promote a transition towards neurogenesis via influencing the mode of *Hes1* expression.

Several other validated targets of miR-9 are also transcription factors that were previously shown to promote progenitor proliferation. They include notably the forkhead transcription factor FoxG1 (Shibata et al., 2008, 2011), the homeobox factor Gsx2 (Shibata et al., 2011), the orphan nuclear receptor Tlx/Nr2e1 (Biryukova et al., 2009; Bonev et al., 2011) and the zinc finger transcription factor Zic5 (Coolen et al., 2012). The repression of these transcription factors by miR-9 could explain the anti-proliferative effect it exerts in neural progenitors, while their up-regulation could participate in miR-9 the depletion phenotype. Thus in *miR-9-2/3* double mutant mice, the clear increase in FoxG1 and Gsx2 protein levels could contribute to increasing proliferation of embryonic pallial and subpallial progenitor cells (Shibata et al., 2011). Moreover, the reduction of proliferation induced by miR-9 can be rescued by overexpressing TLX, suggesting that the inhibition of this target could participate in this phenotype (Zhao et al., 2009). Surprisingly however, the levels of TLX proteins are not up-regulated but down-regulated in *miR-9-2/3* double mutant mice (Shibata et al., 2011). This discrepancy could be linked to the presence of the RNA binding proteins Elavl1 or Msi1, which were shown *in vitro* to be able to convert miR-9 to an activator (Shibata et al., 2011). Alternatively, indirect effects of miR-9 depletion could also explain the reduction of TLX protein. Zic5 belongs to a family of Zinc finger transcription factors that act as inhibitors of neuronal differentiation during development (Aruga, 2004). In vertebrates, *Zic5* mRNA possesses a very conserved binding site for miR-9, and moreover, in the zebrafish embryonic hindbrain, injection of a target protector morpholino restricting binding to this site leads to an increase in progenitor proliferation (Coolen et al., 2012).

Other targets of miR-9 are linked with the epigenetic machinery, which is subjected to drastic remodeling during the course of neuronal differentiation. The 3′UTR of repressor-element-1 silencing transcription factor (REST) and the corepressor CoREST, were shown to harbor functional binding sites for miR-9 and miR-9* respectively (Packer et al., 2008). REST and CoREST act in a chromatin-bound protein complex, which recruits histone modifiers to repress the expression of neuronal genes in neural stem cells and progenitors (Ballas and Mandel, 2005). During neuronal differentiation, the complex is dismantled, which allows for the expression of neuronal genes. During the transition from progenitors to neurons, there is also an exchange of subunits within the Switch/Sucrose non fermentable (Swi/Snf) chromatin remodeling complex: the subunit BRG1- and BRM-associated factor 53a (BAF53a) present in neural progenitors is notably replaced by its homologous BAF53b. Interestingly, miR-9* seems to be able to facilitate this exchange, via repressing the expression of BAF53a (Yoo et al., 2009). miR-9 can also inhibit the expression of Sirt1, a member of the class III nicotinamide adenine dinucleotide (NAD+)-dependent histone deacetylases (Delaloy et al., 2010). Sirt1 associates with different repressor complexes and opposite influences of this factor have been observed during *in vitro* neurogenesis: Sirt1 can associate with Hes1 to repress proneural gene expression (Prozorovski et al., 2008), however, on the other hand, Sirt1 translocation to the nucleus was also shown to accompany neuronal differentiation of neural stem cells *in vitro* and accelerate this process via repressing Notch targets such as Hes1 (Hisahara et al., 2008). It is therefore hard to draw a conclusion on the potential functional consequences of miR-9 repression of Sirt1 at this stage. Importantly the significance of these microRNA-targets interactions remains to be directly assessed *in vivo*. Nevertheless they suggest exciting links between miR-9 and the epigenetic landscape of neural progenitor cells. Interestingly miR-9 could also participate in remodeling the microRNAs landscape in neural cells. Indeed miR-9 can inhibit the pluripotent factors Lin28A and Lin28B, RNA binding proteins that block the processing of some microRNAs, including let-7 (Eda et al., 2009; La Torre et al., 2013).

miR-9 can promote neural differentiation via the inhibition of proliferation factors and progenitor specific epigenetic factors. Surprisingly however, miR-9 was shown to also downregulate the expression of genes with differentiation promoting activities. For instance, using target protector morpholinos, a cryptic role of miR-9 in inhibiting *elavl3*, a proneural differentiation factor, was revealed in zebrafish embryos (Coolen et al., 2012). In doing this, miR-9 dampens the expression of factors favoring antagonist fates. Thereby it seems to favor an ambivalent progenitor state, poised to respond to both progenitor maintenance and commitment cues (**Figure 3B**). This ambivalent state could possibly correspond to the previously described "oscillating" neurogenic progenitors in which the levels of opposite fate determinants like Hes1 and Ngn2 oscillate prior to commitment (Kageyama et al., 2008). Another striking feature emerging from the analyses of miR-9 targets is that they often exert feedback regulation on miR-9 (**Figure 3C**). Transcription of *miR-9* genes is repressed by Nr2e2/Tlx, Hes1 and REST, and its effect on mRNA targets can be modulated by Elavl proteins, also targeted by this microRNA (Zhao et al., 2009; Laneve et al., 2010; Shibata et al., 2011; Bonev et al., 2012). Feedback loops are recurring motifs in gene regulatory networks involving microRNAs, and they can stabilize cellular states and provide robustness to developmental programs (Peláez and Carthew, 2012). Altogether the study of miR-9 targets point to a role of this microRNA to facilitate, pace and stabilize the transition of progenitors towards neural differentiation. To obtain a full picture of its gene network a thorough characterization of miR-9 targets and validation of the impact of individual interactions should be conducted. This would help understanding the phenotype resulting from its absence, which combines the sometimes opposite effects of the deregulation of many mRNAs.

ADDITIONAL ROLES OF miR-9 IN NEURAL DEVELOPMENT: miR-9 IN POST-MITOTIC NEURONS

A few studies have unraveled additional functions of miR-9 at later steps of neural development, linked to its expression in some populations of post-mitotic neurons.

miR-9 is transiently expressed during the differentiation of spinal cord motoneurons (MN), located in the lateral motor column and innervating limb muscles, but not in neighboring MN (Otaegi et al., 2011). These MN are characterized by the expression of FoxP1 and Isl1/2, both of which are putative targets of miR-9. In this context, manipulating miR-9 levels impairs the differentiation and axonal projections of spinal motoneuron lineages, possibly through a de-regulation of FoxP1 protein levels.

The paralog gene *Foxp2* also possesses functional miR-9 binding sites on its 3′UTR. Foxp2 protein is expressed in the embryonic cortex, but its expression starts much later than miR-9. Furthermore, while miR-9 expression spans most layers of the cortex, being however enriched in ventricular progenitors, Foxp2 expression is restricted to post-migratory neurons (Shibata et al., 2011; Clovis et al., 2012). Both miR-9 putative binding sites can mediate the repression of a reporter transgene by endogenous miR-9 present in the cortex (Clovis et al., 2012). This suggests that miR-9 could prevent excessive expression of the protein FoxP2 in the cortex, which was shown to severely impair neuronal migration. Moreover excessive expression of FoxP2 also compromises maturation of cortical neurons.

A role of miR-9 in the maturation of cortical neurons was more directly demonstrated by another study in which miR-9 expression could be detected in axons and dendrites of differentiated neurons (Dajas-Bailador et al., 2012). Moreover, inhibition of miR-9 in cultured neurons increased axonal length and reduced axonal branching. Specific inhibition of miR-9 binding on the *Map1b* 3′UTR both *in vitro* and *in vivo* using target protectors could mimic this effect of miR-9. Thus miR-9 regulates neuronal maturation through modulating the expression level of this gene, which is an important regulator of microtubules dynamics.

IMPLICATION OF miR-9 IN HUMAN PATHOLOGIES

miR-9 IN CANCER

Studies in the developing brain demonstrated that miR-9 is deeply rooted in gene networks controlling the regulation of neural progenitors proliferation. It is therefore not surprising to see this microRNA implicated in the progression of brain cancers such as medulloblastoma and glioblastoma. As in the normal contexts, this microRNA demonstrates its versatility in the context of tumors.

Medulloblastomas (MB) are the most frequent form of pediatric brain cancers. They originate from cerebellar progenitors. miR-9 expression is reduced in MB samples compared to neighboring brain tissues (Ferretti et al., 2009). This could contribute to disease progression as inhibition of miR-9 in MB cell lines increases their proliferation. One target of miR-9, the truncated form of the neurotrophin receptor TrkC (t-TrkC), is up-regulated in MB and was shown to promote proliferation of MB cells. The deregulation of t-TrkC following down-regulation of miR-9 could therefore play a role in sustaining proliferation of MB cells. Conversely a high expression of miR-9 was detected in a subclass of glioblastoma, the most common but also the most aggressive type of adult brain tumors (Kim et al., 2011). Interestingly, miR-9 expression was particularly associated with tumor cells possessing stem-like features (Schraivogel et al., 2011). These cells, referred to as glioblastoma stem cells (GSC), are defined by long term self-renewal capacities thus endowing them with greater potential for cancer initiation and propagation (Huang et al., 2010). Several studies demonstrate that these cells are particularly resistant to radiotherapy and chemotherapy, and are therefore likely responsible for tumor resistance and recurrence. Reducing miR-9 expression in glioblastoma primary culture leads to a reduction of the number of cells with *in vitro* self-renewing potential (Schraivogel et al., 2011). This effect is mediated by an up-regulation of calmodulin-binding transcription activator 1 (CAMTA1), a tumor suppressor whose 3′UTR is targeted by miR-9. However another study suggests that miR-9* inhibits the expression of Sox2, a factor which, in contrast to CAMTA1, confers self-renewal properties and drug resistance to GSC (Jeon et al., 2011). miR-9 impact on GSCs and tumor growth seems therefore to be variable among glioblastoma samples, an observation likely to reflect the high heterogeneity of these tumors. It would however be particularly interesting to investigate further the link between miR-9 and GSCs properties and compare miR-9 action in normal versus tumoral stem cells.

Surprisingly, miR-9 was also linked with cancers originating outside the nervous system. In some cases, miR-9 behaves like an oncogene, in some others like a tumor suppressor. miR-9 is highly expressed and appears to favor progression of Hodgkin lymphomas (Leucci et al., 2012), breast cancers (Ma et al., 2010), cervical cancers (Wilting et al., 2013), colon cancers (Lu et al.,

2012) and stomach cancers (Rotkrua et al., 2011). The proximal causes of miR-9 up-regulation have been identified only in a few cases. Chromosomal amplifications can account for increased miR-9 expression in some cervical cancers (Wilting et al., 2013), while the up-regulation of *miR-9-3* transcription is caused by the MYC oncogene in some breast cancers (Ma et al., 2010). miR-9 has been shown to influence various tumorigenic processes, including cellular proliferation (Rotkrua et al., 2011; Wilting et al., 2013), migration (Ma et al., 2010; Lu et al., 2012) and inflammation (Leucci et al., 2012). A reduction of miR-9 expression compared to normal tissue was also observed in other types of cancer, including leukemia (Senyuk et al., 2013), lung cancers (Heller et al., 2012) and colon cancers (Bandres et al., 2009). The implication of miR-9 in tumorigenesis in such a variety of tissues suggests that miR-9 may regulate general processes and define a specific cellular state that could exist outside the nervous system.

miR-9 IN NEURODEGENERATIVE DISORDERS

Links between neurodegenerative disorders and microRNAs, especially brain enriched microRNAs such as miR-9, have started to emerge in the literature (Lau and de Strooper, 2010). Huntington's disease (HD) is an autosomal dominant neurodegenerative disease caused by trinucleotide repeat expansions in the *Huntingtin* gene (*Htt*). One hallmark of HD is an alteration of the transcriptome of some brain regions, linked to abnormal activity of the transcriptional repressor REST (Buckley et al., 2010). In contrast to the wild-type HTT, mutant HTT no longer traps REST in the cytoplasm, thus allowing it to translocate to the nucleus and excessively represses its targets. As previously mentioned, REST was shown to repress *miR-9* transcription and REST and its co-repressor coREST are targets of miR-9/9* (Packer et al., 2008; Laneve et al., 2010). In the brain of HD patients, miR-9/9* expression decreases with increasing disease grades (Packer et al., 2008). The down-regulation of miR-9/9* could be linked to the excessive activity of REST and may also amplify REST activity by increasing REST and coREST protein levels. Considering the number of targets of miR-9/9*, their down-regulation could also impact more widely the transcriptional landscape in HD patients brains. miR-9 was also found to be deregulated in other neurodegenerative disorders. It is down-regulated in the brain of Alzheimer's disease patients (Cogswell et al., 2008; Hébert et al., 2008) and up-regulated in the cortex of Parkinson's disease patients (Kim et al., 2007). Finally, miR-9 was suggested to participate in amyotrophic lateral sclerosis (ALS), a neurodegenerative disease affecting MN (Haramati et al., 2010). miR-9 was shown to be down-regulated in a mouse model of motoneuron disease and its over-expression can repress the expression of a neurofilament heavy subunit previously linked to motoneuron degeneration. Probing more directly the impact of miR-9 deregulation on neurodegenerative disease progression is a challenging task, which will need to be addressed in the future.

miR-9 PROTECTS NEURAL TISSUE FROM DELETERIOUS PROGERIN

Hutchinson-Gilford progeria syndrome (HGPS) is a rare disease whose symptoms resemble physiological ageing. It is caused by a de novo specific mutation in *LMNA* gene. This gene encodes two components of the nuclear lamina, lamin A and lamin C, as a result of alternative splicing (**Figure 4**). HGPS causing mutations affect only lamin A-encoding transcripts and generate a truncated form of this protein which is toxic to cells, referred to as Progerin. While most tissues and organs are affected by the presence of Progerin, the CNS of HGPS-affected patients is remarkably spared. This is most likely due to a lower expression of lamin A in neural cells, but the underlying mechanism

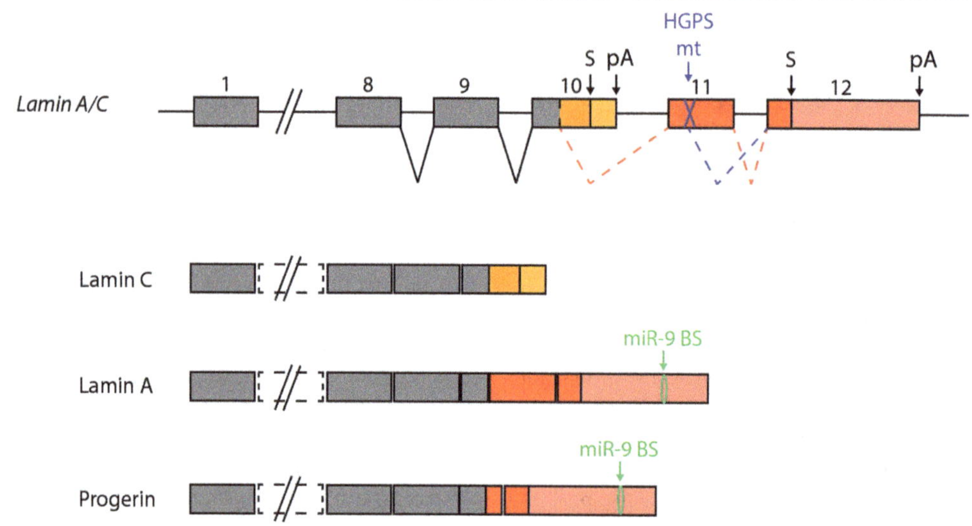

FIGURE 4 | miR-9 protects the brain from Progerin. Two alternative transcripts are generated from the the Lamin A/C gene, encoding Lamin C and Lamin A proteins. HGPS is caused by a mutation in exon 11, which is specific to Lamin A encoding transcripts. The mutation generates an additional splice site, which leads to the generation of a new transcript encoding a truncated form of Lamin A. The truncated protein is referred to as Progerin, and is toxic to cells. The presence of miR-9 in the central nervous system can explain, at least in part, the low levels of Lamin A detected in this tissue compared to Lamin C. In HGPS patients, miR-9 repression of Progerin expression protects the CNS from this harmful protein.

remained unknown. Two recent studies demonstrated a role of miR-9 in this process (Jung et al., 2012; Nissan et al., 2012). The first study confirmed that lamin A transcripts and proteins are less abundant than lamin C in mouse brains, whereas they are expressed at similar levels in other tissues (Jung et al., 2012). Low levels of Progerin were also found in the brain of knock-in mice harboring the HGPS mutant allele. The authors could show that the differential levels of lamin A versus lamin C in brain tissues was not linked to differences in alternative splicing, but rather that it is likely linked to the presence of miR-9 in neural tissues. Lamin A and C encoding transcripts possess different 3′UTR sequences, but only lamin A transcripts can be down-regulated by miR-9 through a functional binding site. Inhibition of miR-9 in neural cells *in vitro* lead to increased levels of lamin A transcripts. These results were confirmed to be relevant in human patients by the second study, in which neural cells differentiated from HGPS patient-induced pluripotent stem cells (iPSC) were analyzed (Nissan et al., 2012). Neural stem cells and neurons derived from patient iPSCs express lower levels of lamin A and Progerin transcripts compared to other iPSC derived cell types. These cells are also characterized by high levels of miR-9. Over-expression of miR-9 in mesenchymal cells of HGPS patients could reduce the levels of lamin A and progerin, an effect mediated by the 3′UTR of the lamin A transcripts. Altogether this suggests that miR-9 expression may account for the low expression of lamin A in the neural tissue, thus protecting it from the deleterious effects of Progerin in HGPS patients. This regulation could stimulate the development of new therapies for HGPS patients. The reason why lamin A expression would need to be restricted by miR-9 in a healthy brain remains to be discovered.

CONCLUSION

miR-9 is a very ancient microRNA and its function and set of targets seem to have undergone dramatic changes during the evolution of Bilateria. In drosophila, through its expression in non-neural cells miR-9a confers robustness to the developmental program of peripheral organs. In contrast, in vertebrates, miR-9 displays a conserved expression pattern in the CNS. During vertebrate evolution, miR-9 seemingly had the time to accumulate a large set of mRNA targets, and is deeply embedded in the gene network controlling the behavior of neural progenitors. Strikingly, functional studies of miR-9 point to a highly versatile action. Conditional depletion of miR-9 *in vivo*, using refined genetic tools, will help better characterizing this phenomenon *in vivo*. In addition, to better understand the full repertoire of miR-9 actions, it will be necessary to identify the set of miR-9 targets in different cellular contexts and evaluate the functional impact of these interactions individually. This will constitute a major challenge, especially since miR-9 targets are functionally interconnected. For most targets studied so far in vertebrates, miR-9 binding sites are highly conserved and are thus part of an ancestral set of miR-9 targets. It would be interesting now to start to explore species-specific targets of miR-9 and see how they could participate in the diversification of the nervous system. Finally, to investigate the variability of miR-9 actions, it will be of interest to identify its regulators. In vertebrates, the transcription factors that were shown to bind *miR-9* promoters are all repressors (Tlx, REST, Hes1); the factors that can induce miR-9 expression are still unknown. Further studying the link between miR-9 activity and RNA binding proteins, which can either regulate miR-9 expression and processing or alter its effect of mRNA targets, will refine our understanding of miR-9 action (Shibata et al., 2011; Xu et al., 2011; Li et al., 2013). Altogether, a comprehensive knowledge of how miR-9 function can be modulated across different species and cellular contexts will be necessary to unravel its contribution in human pathologies.

ACKNOWLEDGMENTS

The authors are grateful to past and present members of the Zebrafish Neurogenetics group for stimulating scientific discussions and valuable inputs. We thank William Norton for his critical reading of the manuscript. Shauna Katz is recipient of a PhD fellowship of the DIM Cerveau et Pensée and the Ecole des Neurosciences de Paris. Marion Coolen received support from the FP7 Marie Curie intraeuropean post-doctoral fellowship program and the EMBO long-term post-doctoral fellowship program. Work in the LBC laboratory at the CNRS is funded by the EU project ZF-Health (FP7/2010–2015 grant agreement no 242048), the ANR (grants ANR-08-CEX-08-000-01 and ANR-2012-BSV4-0004-01), the Ecole des Neurosciences de Paris, the FRM (FRP « Equipe » DEQ20120323692), and the ERC (AdG 322936 "SyStematics").

REFERENCES

Aruga, J. (2004). The role of Zic genes in neural development. *Mol. Cell. Neurosci.* 26, 205–221. doi: 10.1016/j.mcn.2004.01.004

Asmar, J., Biryukova, I., and Heitzler, P. (2008). Drosophila dLMO-PA isoform acts as an early activator of achaete/scute proneural expression. *Dev. Biol.* 316, 487–497. doi: 10.1016/j.ydbio.2008.01.040

Ballas, N., and Mandel, G. (2005). The many faces of REST oversee epigenetic programming of neuronal genes. *Curr. Opin. Neurobiol.* 15, 500–506. doi: 10.1016/j.conb.2005.08.015

Bandres, E., Agirre, X., Bitarte, N., Ramirez, N., Zarate, R., Roman-Gomez, J., et al. (2009). Epigenetic regulation of microRNA expression in colorectal cancer. *Int. J. Cancer.* 125, 2737–2743. doi: 10.1002/ijc.24638

Bartel, D. P. (2009). MicroRNAs: target recognition and regulatory functions. *Cell* 136, 215–233. doi: 10.1016/j.cell.2009.01.002

Bejarano, F., Smibert, P., and Lai, E. C. (2010). miR-9a prevents apoptosis during wing development by repressing Drosophila LIM-only. *Dev. Biol.* 338, 63–73. doi: 10.1016/j.ydbio.2009.11.025

Berezikov, E. (2011). Evolution of microRNA diversity and regulation in animals. *Nat. Rev. Genet.* 12, 846–860. doi: 10.1038/nrg3079

Biryukova, I., Asmar, J., Abdesselem, H., and Heitzler, P. (2009). Drosophila mir-9a regulates wing development via fine-tuning expression of the LIM only factor, dLMO. *Dev. Biol.* 327, 487–496. doi: 10.1016/j.ydbio.2008.12.036

Bonev, B., Pisco, A., and Papalopulu, N. (2011). MicroRNA-9 reveals regional diversity of neural progenitors along the anterior-posterior axis. *Dev. Cell* 20, 19–32. doi: 10.1016/j.devcel.2010.11.018

Bonev, B., Stanley, P., and Papalopulu, N. (2012). MicroRNA-9 modulates Hes1 ultradian oscillations by forming a double-negative feedback loop. *Cell Rep.* 2, 10–18. doi: 10.1016/j.celrep.2012.05.017

Buckley, N. J., Johnson, R., Zuccato, C., Bithell, A., and Cattaneo, E. (2010). The role of REST in transcriptional and epigenetic dysregulation in Huntington's disease. *Neurobiol. Dis.* 39, 28–39. doi: 10.1016/j.nbd.2010.02.003

Candiani, S., Moronti, L., De Pietri Tonelli, D., Garbarino, G., and Pestarino, M. (2011). A study of neural-related microRNAs in the developing amphioxus. *Evodevo* 2:15. doi: 10.1186/2041-9139-2-15

Choi, W.-Y., Giraldez, A. J., and Schier, A. F. (2007). Target protectors reveal dampening and balancing of Nodal agonist and antagonist by miR-430. *Science* 318, 271–274. doi: 10.1126/science.1147535

Christodoulou, F., Raible, F., Tomer, R., Simakov, O., Trachana, K., Klaus, S., et al. (2010). Ancient animal microRNAs and the evolution of tissue identity. *Nature* 463, 1084–1088. doi: 10.1038/nature08744

Clovis, Y. M., Enard, W., Marinaro, F., Huttner, W. B., and Tonelli, D. D. P. (2012). Convergent repression of Foxp2 3′UTR by miR-9 and miR-132 in embryonic mouse neocortex: implications for radial migration of neurons. *Development* 139, 3332–3342. doi: 10.1242/dev.078063

Cogswell, J. P., Ward, J., Taylor, I. A., Waters, M., Shi, Y., Cannon, B., et al. (2008). Identification of miRNA changes in Alzheimer's disease brain and CSF yields putative biomarkers and insights into disease pathways. *J. Alzheimers Dis.* 14, 27–41.

Coolen, M., Thieffry, D., Drivenes, Ø., Becker, T. S., and Bally-Cuif, L. (2012). miR-9 controls the timing of neurogenesis through the direct inhibition of antagonistic factors. *Dev. Cell* 22, 1052–1064. doi: 10.1016/j.devcel.2012.03.003

Dajas-Bailador, F., Bonev, B., Garcez, P., Stanley, P., Guillemot, F., and Papalopulu, N. (2012). microRNA-9 regulates axon extension and branching by targeting Map1b in mouse cortical neurons. *Nat. Neurosci.* doi: 10.1038/nn.3082. [Epub ahead of print].

Darnell, D. K., Kaur, S., Stanislaw, S., Konieczka, J. H., Konieczka, J. K., Yatskievych, T. A., et al. (2006). MicroRNA expression during chick embryo development. *Dev. Dyn.* 235, 3156–3165. doi: 10.1002/dvdy.20956

Delaloy, C., Liu, L., Lee, J.-A., Su, H., Shen, F., Yang, G.-Y., et al. (2010). MicroRNA-9 coordinates proliferation and migration of human embryonic stem cell-derived neural progenitors. *Cell Stem Cell* 6, 323–335. doi: 10.1016/j.stem.2010.02.015

Deo, M., Yu, J.-Y., Chung, K.-H., Tippens, M., and Turner, D. L. (2006). Detection of mammalian microRNA expression by in situ hybridization with RNA oligonucleotides. *Dev. Dyn.* 235, 2538–2548. doi: 10.1002/dvdy.20847

Ebert, M. S., and Sharp, P. A. (2012). Roles for microRNAs in conferring robustness to biological processes. *Cell* 149, 515–524. doi: 10.1016/j.cell.2012.04.005

Eda, A., Tamura, Y., Yoshida, M., and Hohjoh, H. (2009). Systematic gene regulation involving miRNAs during neuronal differentiation of mouse P19 embryonic carcinoma cell. *Biochem. Biophys. Res. Commun.* 388, 648–653. doi: 10.1016/j.bbrc.2009.08.040

Ferretti, E., De Smaele, E., Po, A., Di Marcotullio, L., Tosi, E., Espinola, M. S. B., et al. (2009). MicroRNA profiling in human medulloblastoma. *Int. J. Cancer* 124, 568–577. doi: 10.1002/ijc.23948

Georgi, S. A., and Reh, T. A. (2010). Dicer is required for the transition from early to late progenitor state in the developing mouse retina. *J. Neurosci.* 30, 4048–4061. doi: 10.1523/jneurosci.4982-09.2010

Haramati, S., Chapnik, E., Sztainberg, Y., Eilam, R., Zwang, R., Gershoni, N., et al. (2010). miRNA malfunction causes spinal motor neuron disease. *Proc. Natl. Acad. Sci. U S A* 107, 13111–13116. doi: 10.1073/pnas.1006151107

Hébert, S. S., Horré, K., Nicolaï, L., Papadopoulou, A. S., Mandemakers, W., Silahtaroglu, A. N., et al. (2008). Loss of microRNA cluster miR-29a/b-1 in sporadic Alzheimer's disease correlates with increased BACE1/beta-secretase expression. *Proc. Natl. Acad. Sci. U S A* 105, 6415–6420. doi: 10.1073/pnas.0710263105

Heimberg, A. M., Cowper-Sal-lari, R., Semon, M., Donoghue, P. C. J., and Peterson, K. J. (2010). From the cover: microRNAs reveal the interrelationships of hagfish, lampreys, and gnathostomes and the nature of the ancestral vertebrate. *Proc. Natl. Acad. Sci. U S A* 107, 19379–19383. doi: 10.1073/pnas.1010350107

Heller, G., Weinzierl, M., Noll, C., Babinsky, V., Ziegler, B., Altenberger, C., et al. (2012). Genome-wide miRNA expression profiling identifies miR-9-3 and miR-193a as targets for DNA methylation in non-small cell lung cancers. *Clin. Cancer Res.* 18, 1619–1629. doi: 10.1158/1078-0432.CCR-11-2450

Hisahara, S., Chiba, S., Matsumoto, H., Tanno, M., Yagi, H., Shimohama, S., et al. (2008). Histone deacetylase SIRT1 modulates neuronal differentiation by its nuclear translocation. *Proc. Natl. Acad. Sci. U S A* 105, 15599–15604. doi: 10.1073/pnas.0800612105

Huang, Z., Cheng, L., Guryanova, O. A., Wu, Q., and Bao, S. (2010). Cancer stem cells in glioblastoma–molecular signaling and therapeutic targeting. *Protein Cell* 1, 638–655. doi: 10.1007/s13238-010-0078-y

Jafar-Nejad, H., Acar, M., Nolo, R., Lacin, H., Pan, H., Parkhurst, S. M., et al. (2003). Senseless acts as a binary switch during sensory organ precursor selection. *Genes Dev.* 17, 2966–2978. doi: 10.1101/gad.1122403

Jeon, H. M., Sohn, Y. W., Oh, S. Y., Kim, S. H., Beck, S., Kim, S., et al. (2011). ID4 imparts chemoresistance and cancer stemness to glioma cells by derepressing miR-9*-mediated suppression of SOX2. *Cancer Res.* 71, 3410–3421. doi: 10.1158/0008-5472.can-11-2545

Jung, H.-J., Coffinier, C., Choe, Y., Beigneux, A. P., Davies, B. S. J., Yang, S. H., et al. (2012). Regulation of prelamin A but not lamin C by miR-9, a brain-specific microRNA. *Proc. Natl. Acad. Sci. U S A* 109, E423–E431. doi: 10.1073/pnas.1111780109

Kageyama, R., Ohtsuka, T., and Kobayashi, T. (2008). Roles of Hes genes in neural development. *Dev. Growth Differ.* 50(Suppl. 1), S97–S103. doi: 10.1111/j.1440-169x.2008.00993.x

Kapsimali, M., Kloosterman, W. P., de Bruijn, E., Rosa, F., Plasterk, R. H. A., and Wilson, S. W. (2007). MicroRNAs show a wide diversity of expression profiles in the developing and mature central nervous system. *Genome Biol.* 8:R173. doi: 10.1186/gb-2007-8-8-r173

Kiecker, C., and Lumsden, A. (2005). Compartments and their boundaries in vertebrate brain development. *Nat. Rev. Neurosci.* 6, 553–564. doi: 10.1038/nrn1702

Kim, J., Inoue, K., Ishii, J., Vanti, W. B., Voronov, S. V., Murchison, E., et al. (2007). A MicroRNA feedback circuit in midbrain dopamine neurons. *Science* 317, 1220–1224. doi: 10.1126/science.1140481

Kim, T. M., Huang, W., Park, R., Park, P. J., and Johnson, M. D. (2011). A developmental taxonomy of glioblastoma defined and maintained by MicroRNAs. *Cancer Res.* 71, 3387–3399. doi: 10.1158/0008-5472.CAN-10-4117

Krichevsky, A. M., King, K. S., Donahue, C. P., Khrapko, K., and Kosik, K. S. (2003). A microRNA array reveals extensive regulation of microRNAs during brain development. *RNA* 9, 1274–1281. doi: 10.1261/rna.5980303

Krichevsky, A. M., Sonntag, K.-C., Isacson, O., and Kosik, K. S. (2006). Specific microRNAs modulate embryonic stem cell-derived neurogenesis. *Stem Cells* 24, 857–864. doi: 10.1634/stemcells.2005-0441

La Torre, A., Georgi, S., and Reh, T. A. (2013). Conserved microRNA pathway regulates developmental timing of retinal neurogenesis. *Proc. Natl. Acad. Sci. U S A* 110, E2362–E2370. doi: 10.1073/pnas.1301837110

Lagos-Quintana, M., Rauhut, R., Yalcin, A., Meyer, J., Lendeckel, W., and Tuschl, T. (2002). Identification of tissue-specific microRNAs from mouse. *Curr. Biol.* 12, 735–739. doi: 10.1016/s0960-9822(02)00809-6

Lai, E. C., and Posakony, J. W. (1997). The bearded box, a novel 3′ UTR sequence motif, mediates negative post-transcriptional regulation of bearded and enhancer of split complex gene expression. *Development* 124, 4847–4856.

Lai, E. C., Tam, B., and Rubin, G. M. (2005). Pervasive regulation of Drosophila Notch target genes by GY-box-, Brd-box-, and K-box-class microRNAs. *Genes Dev.* 19, 1067–1080. doi: 10.1101/gad.1291905

Lai, E. C., Wiel, C., and Rubin, G. M. (2004). Complementary miRNA pairs suggest a regulatory role for miRNA:miRNA duplexes. *RNA* 10, 171–175. doi: 10.1261/rna.5191904

Laneve, P., Gioia, U., Andriotto, A., Moretti, F., Bozzoni, I., and Caffarelli, E. (2010). A minicircuitry involving REST and CREB controls miR-9-2 expression during human neuronal differentiation. *Nucleic Acids Res.* 38, 6895–6905. doi: 10.1093/nar/gkq604

Lau, P., and de Strooper, B. (2010). Dysregulated microRNAs in neurodegenerative disorders. *Semin. Cell Dev. Biol.* 21, 768–773. doi: 10.1016/j.semcdb.2010.01.009

Leucci, E., Zriwil, A., Gregersen, L. H., Jensen, K. T., Obad, S., Bellan, C., et al. (2012). Inhibition of miR-9 de-represses HuR and DICER1 and impairs Hodgkin lymphoma tumour outgrowth in vivo. Oncogene. Available at: http://www.ncbi.nlm.nih.gov/pubmed/22310293 [Accessed March 26, 2012].

Leucht, C., Stigloher, C., Wizenmann, A., Klafke, R., Folchert, A., and Bally-Cuif, L. (2008). MicroRNA-9 directs late organizer activity of the midbrain-hindbrain boundary. *Nat. Neurosci.* 11, 641–648. doi: 10.1038/nn.2115

Li, X., Cassidy, J. J., Reinke, C. A., Fischboeck, S., and Carthew, R. W. (2009). A microRNA imparts robustness against environmental fluctuation during development. *Cell* 137, 273–282. doi: 10.1016/j.cell.2009.01.058

Li, Y., Wang, F., Lee, J.-A., and Gao, F.-B. (2006). MicroRNA-9a ensures the precise specification of sensory organ precursors in Drosophila. *Genes Dev.* 20, 2793–2805. doi: 10.1101/gad.1466306

Li, Z., Lu, Y., Xu, X.-L., and Gao, F.-B. (2013). The FTD/ALS-associated RNA-binding protein TDP-43 regulates the robustness of neuronal specification through microRNA-9a in Drosophila. *Hum. Mol. Genet.* 22, 218–225. doi: 10.1093/hmg/dds420

Lim, L. P., Lau, N. C., Weinstein, E. G., Abdelhakim, A., Yekta, S., Rhoades, M. W., et al. (2003). The microRNAs of Caenorhabditis elegans. *Genes Dev.* 17, 991–1008. doi: 10.1101/gad.1074403

Lu, M.-H., Huang, C.-C., Pan, M.-R., Chen, H.-H., and Hung, W.-C. (2012). Prospero homeobox 1 promotes epithelial-mesenchymal transition in colon cancer cells by inhibiting E-cadherin via miR-9. *Clin. Cancer Res.* 18, 6416–6425. doi: 10.1158/1078-0432.ccr-12-0832

Ma, L., Young, J., Prabhala, H., Pan, E., Mestdagh, P., Muth, D., et al. (2010). miR-9, a MYC/MYCN-activated microRNA, regulates E-cadherin and cancer metastasis. *Nat. Cell Biol.* 12, 247–256. doi: 10.1038/ncb2024

Miska, E. A., Alvarez-Saavedra, E., Townsend, M., Yoshii, A., Sestan, N., Rakic, P., et al. (2004). Microarray analysis of microRNA expression in the developing mammalian brain. *Genome Biol.* 5:R68. doi: 10.1186/gb-2004-5-9-r68

Nissan, X., Blondel, S., Navarro, C., Maury, Y., Denis, C., Girard, M., et al. (2012). Unique preservation of neural cells in Hutchinson- Gilford progeria syndrome is due to the expression of the neural-specific miR-9 microRNA. *Cell Rep.* 2, 1–9. doi: 10.1016/j.celrep.2012.05.015

Nolo, R., Abbott, L. A., and Bellen, H. J. (2000). Senseless, a Zn finger transcription factor, is necessary and sufficient for sensory organ development in Drosophila. *Cell* 102, 349–362. doi: 10.1016/s0092-8674(00)00040-4

Otaegi, G., Pollock, A., Hong, J., and Sun, T. (2011). MicroRNA miR-9 modifies motor neuron columns by a tuning regulation of FoxP1 levels in developing spinal cords. *J. Neurosci.* 31, 809–818. doi: 10.1523/jneurosci.4330-10.2011

Packer, A. N., Xing, Y., Harper, S. Q., Jones, L., and Davidson, B. L. (2008). The bifunctional microRNA miR-9/miR-9* regulates REST and CoREST and is downregulated in Huntington's disease. *J. Neurosci.* 28, 14341–14346. doi: 10. 1523/jneurosci.2390-08.2008

Peláez, N., and Carthew, R. W. (2012). Biological robustness and the role of microRNAs: a network perspective. *Curr. Top. Dev. Biol.* 99, 237–255. doi: 10. 1016/b978-0-12-387038-4.00009-4

Prozorovski, T., Schulze-Topphoff, U., Glumm, R., Baumgart, J., Schröter, F., Ninnemann, O., et al. (2008). Sirt1 contributes critically to the redox-dependent fate of neural progenitors. *Nat. Cell Biol.* 10, 385–394. doi: 10.1038/ncb1700

Rajasethupathy, P., Fiumara, F., Sheridan, R., Betel, D., Puthanveettil, S. V., Russo, J. J., et al. (2009). Characterization of small RNAs in Aplysia reveals a role for miR-124 in constraining synaptic plasticity through CREB. *Neuron* 63, 803–817. doi: 10.1016/j.neuron.2009.05.029

Ramain, P., Khechumian, R., Khechumian, K., Arbogast, N., Ackermann, C., and Heitzler, P. (2000). Interactions between chip and the achaete/scute-daughterless heterodimers are required for pannier-driven proneural patterning. *Mol. Cell* 6, 781–790. doi: 10.1016/s1097-2765(00)00077-0

Rotkrua, P., Akiyama, Y., Hashimoto, Y., Otsubo, T., and Yuasa, Y. (2011). MiR-9 downregulates CDX2 expression in gastric cancer cells. *Int. J. Cancer* 129, 2611–2620. doi: 10.1002/ijc.25923

Schraivogel, D., Weinmann, L., Beier, D., Tabatabai, G., Eichner, A., Zhu, J. Y., et al. (2011). CAMTA1 is a novel tumour suppressor regulated by miR-9/9* in glioblastoma stem cells. *EMBO J.* 30, 4309–4322. doi: 10.1038/emboj.2011.301

Sempere, L. F., Freemantle, S., Pitha-Rowe, I., Moss, E., Dmitrovsky, E., and Ambros, V. (2004). Expression profiling of mammalian microRNAs uncovers a subset of brain-expressed microRNAs with possible roles in murine and human neuronal differentiation. *Genome Biol.* 5:R13. doi: 10.1186/gb-2004-5-3-r13

Senyuk, V., Zhang, Y., Liu, Y., Ming, M., Premanand, K., Zhou, L., et al. (2013). Critical role of miR-9 in myelopoiesis and EVI1-induced leukemogenesis. *Proc. Natl. Acad. Sci. U S A* 110, 5594–5599. doi: 10.1073/pnas.1302645110

Shibata, M., Kurokawa, D., Nakao, H., Ohmura, T., and Aizawa, S. (2008). MicroRNA-9 modulates Cajal-Retzius cell differentiation by suppressing Foxg1 expression in mouse medial pallium. *J. Neurosci.* 28, 10415–10421. doi: 10. 1523/jneurosci.3219-08.2008

Shibata, M., Nakao, H., Kiyonari, H., Abe, T., and Aizawa, S. (2011). MicroRNA-9 regulates neurogenesis in mouse telencephalon by targeting multiple transcription factors. *J. Neurosci.* 31, 3407–3422. doi: 10.1523/jneurosci.5085-10.2011

Shimojo, H., Ohtsuka, T., and Kageyama, R. (2008). Oscillations in notch signaling regulate maintenance of neural progenitors. *Neuron* 58, 52–64. doi: 10.1016/j. neuron.2008.02.014

Skeath, J. B., and Carroll, S. B. (1994). The achaete-scute complex: generation of cellular pattern and fate within the Drosophila nervous system. *FASEB J.* 8, 714–721. doi: 10.1016/0168-9525(92)90234-u

Stigloher, C., Chapouton, P., Adolf, B., and Bally-Cuif, L. (2008). Identification of neural progenitor pools by E(Spl) factors in the embryonic and adult brain. *Brain Res. Bull.* 75, 266–273. doi: 10.1016/j.brainresbull.2007.10.032

Takacs, C. M., and Giraldez, A. J. (2010). MicroRNAs as genetic sculptors: fishing for clues. *Semin. Cell Dev. Biol.* 21, 760–767. doi: 10.1016/j.semcdb.2010.02. 003

Tan, S.-L., Ohtsuka, T., González, A., and Kageyama, R. (2012). MicroRNA9 regulates neural stem cell differentiation by controlling Hes1 expression dynamics in the developing brain. *Genes Cells* 17, 952–961. doi: 10.1111/gtc.12009

Tozzini, E. T., Baumgart, M., Battistoni, G., and Cellerino, A. (2012). Adult neurogenesis in the short-lived teleost Nothobranchius furzeri: localization of neurogenic niches, molecular characterization and effects of aging. *Aging Cell* 11, 241–251. doi: 10.1111/j.1474-9726.2011.00781.x

Walker, J. C., and Harland, R. M. (2008). Expression of microRNAs during embryonic development of Xenopus tropicalis. *Gene Expr. Patterns. GEP* 8, 452–456. doi: 10.1016/j.gep.2008.03.002

Wheeler, B. M., Heimberg, A. M., Moy, V. N., Sperling, E. A., Holstein, T. W., Heber, S., et al. (2009). The deep evolution of metazoan microRNAs. *Evol. Dev.* 11, 50–68. doi: 10.1111/j.1525-142x.2008.00302.x

Wienholds, E., Kloosterman, W. P., Miska, E., Alvarez-Saavedra, E., Berezikov, E., de Bruijn, E., et al. (2005). MicroRNA expression in zebrafish embryonic development. *Science* 309, 310–311. doi: 10.1126/science.1114519

Wilting, S. M., Snijders, P. J. F., Verlaat, W., Jaspers, A., van de Wiel, M. A., van Wieringen, W. N., et al. (2013). Altered microRNA expression associated with chromosomal changes contributes to cervical carcinogenesis. *Oncogene* 32, 106–116. doi: 10.1038/onc.2012.20

Xu, X.-L., Zong, R., Li, Z., Biswas, M. H. U., Fang, Z., Nelson, D. L., et al. (2011). FXR1P but not FMRP regulates the levels of mammalian brain-specific microRNA-9 and microRNA-124. *J. Neurosci.* 31, 13705–13709. doi: 10. 1523/jneurosci.2827-11.2011

Yang, J.-S., and Lai, E. C. (2011). Alternative miRNA biogenesis pathways and the interpretation of core miRNA pathway mutants. *Mol. Cell* 43, 892–903. doi: 10. 1016/j.molcel.2011.07.024

Yoo, A. S., Staahl, B. T., Chen, L., and Crabtree, G. R. (2009). MicroRNA-mediated switching of chromatin-remodelling complexes in neural development. *Nature* 460, 642–646. doi: 10.1038/nature08139

Yoo, A. S., Sun, A. X., Li, L., Shcheglovitov, A., Portmann, T., Li, Y., et al. (2011). MicroRNA-mediated conversion of human fibroblasts to neurons. *Nature* 476, 228–231. doi: 10.1038/nature10323

Zhao, C., Sun, G., Li, S., and Shi, Y. (2009). A feedback regulatory loop involving microRNA-9 and nuclear receptor TLX in neural stem cell fate determination. *Nat. Struct. Mol. Biol.* 16, 365–371. doi: 10.1038/nsmb.1576

16

NanoCAGE analysis of the mouse olfactory epithelium identifies the expression of vomeronasal receptors and of proximal LINE elements

Giovanni Pascarella[1,2], Dejan Lazarevic[1,3], Charles Plessy[2], Nicolas Bertin[2], Altuna Akalin[4], Christina Vlachouli[1], Roberto Simone[1], Geoffrey J. Faulkner[5,6], Silvia Zucchelli[1,7], Jun Kawai[8], Carsten O. Daub[2], Yoshihide Hayashizaki[8], Boris Lenhard[4]*, Piero Carninci[2]* and Stefano Gustincich[1]*

[1] Area of Neuroscience, International School for Advanced Studies (SISSA), Trieste, Italy
[2] RIKEN Center for Life Science Technologies, Division of Genomic Technologies, Tsurumi-ku, Yokohama, Japan
[3] Cluster in Biomedicine (CBM), AREA Science Park, Trieste, Italy
[4] Bergen Center for Computational Science - Computational Biology Unit and Sars Centre for Marine Molecular Biology, University of Bergen, Bergen, Norway
[5] Cancer Biology Program, Mater Medical Research Institute, South Brisbane, QLD, Australia
[6] School of Biomedical Sciences, University of Queensland, Brisbane, QLD, Australia
[7] Department of Health Sciences, University of Eastern Piedmont "A. Avogadro," Novara, Italy
[8] RIKEN Preventive Medicine and Diagnosis Innovation Program, Wako, Saitama, Japan

Correspondence:
Boris Lenhard, Bergen Center for Computational Science - Computational Biology Unit and Sars Centre for Marine Molecular Biology, University of Bergen, Hoyteknologisenteret, Thormohlensgate 55, N-5008 Bergen, Norway
e-mail: boris.Lenhard@bccs.uib.no;
Piero Carninci, RIKEN Center for Life Science Technologies, Division of Genomic Technologies, 1-7-22 Suehiro-cho, Tsurumi-ku, Yokohama, Kanagawa 230-0045, Japan
e-mail: carninci@riken.jp;
Stefano Gustincich, The Giovanni Armenise-Harvard Foundation Laboratory, Area of Neuroscience, International School for Advanced Studies (SISSA), Via Bonomea 265, 34136 Trieste, Italy
e-mail: gustinci@sissa.it

By coupling laser capture microdissection to nanoCAGE technology and next-generation sequencing we have identified the genome-wide collection of active promoters in the mouse Main Olfactory Epithelium (MOE). Transcription start sites (TSSs) for the large majority of Olfactory Receptors (ORs) have been previously mapped increasing our understanding of their promoter architecture. Here we show that in our nanoCAGE libraries of the mouse MOE we detect a large number of tags mapped in loci hosting Type-1 and Type-2 Vomeronasal Receptors genes (V1Rs and V2Rs). These loci also show a massive expression of Long Interspersed Nuclear Elements (LINEs). We have validated the expression of selected receptors detected by nanoCAGE with *in situ* hybridization, RT-PCR and qRT-PCR. This work extends the repertory of receptors capable of sensing chemical signals in the MOE, suggesting intriguing interplays between MOE and VNO for pheromone processing and positioning transcribed LINEs as candidate regulatory RNAs for VRs expression.

Keywords: vomeronasal receptors, main olfactory epithelium, vomeronasal organ, VNO, MOE, V1Rs, V2Rs

INTRODUCTION

Next-generation sequencing technologies have reshaped our understanding of the molecular constituents of cells and their regulatory elements. The majority of the mammalian genome is transcribed generating a vast repertoire of transcripts that includes protein-coding RNAs and a surprisingly similar number of non-coding RNAs (ncRNAs), the latter category harboring transcripts that can greatly differ in size and biogenesis and whose biological activities remain largely unexplored (Carninci and Hayashizaki, 2007; Forrest and Carninci, 2009; Mercer et al., 2009; Washietl et al., 2012). Furthermore, the combination of technologies to isolate discrete cell types or tissues with the information gathered with modern sequencing platforms has critically improved the resolution of genome-wide transcriptional profiling thus revealing new scenarios in which biological paradigms had often to be adapted and reformulated. An increasing number of these observations leads to a serious challenge to the concept of functional "ectopic" expression suggesting that proteins with defined biochemical activities may exert their biological function or acquire some new ones in previously unnoticed cells and tissues.

Cap Analysis of Gene Expression (CAGE) technology was previously developed for the systematic analysis of Transcription Start Sites (TSSs) in eukaryotic cells and tissues (Shiraki et al.,

2003). It is based on sequencing cDNA copies of the 5′ends of mRNAs, of which the integrity is inferred by the presence of their cap. These sequences ("*tags*") are sufficiently long to be aligned in most cases at a single location in the genome. The first position of this alignment identifies a base pair where transcription is initiated defining a TSS. The number of times a given tag is represented in a library gives an estimate of the expression level of the corresponding transcript. To expand this analysis to tiny amounts of *ex vivo* tissue and to the polyA$^-$ fraction of RNAs we have developed nanoCAGE, a technology that miniaturizes the requirement of CAGE for RNA material to the nanogram range and which can be used on fixed tissues (Plessy et al., 2010). Using nanoCAGE we have previously shown that the well known oxygen carrier hemoglobin, previously believed to be specifically expressed in erythrocytes, is also selectively expressed in subtypes of dopaminergic neurons of the mesencephalon as well as in glial cells throughout the brain (Biagioli et al., 2009). Recently, we have used nanoCAGE to investigate the transcriptional landscape of the mouse Main Olfactory Epithelium (MOE) (Plessy et al., 2012).

The rodent olfactory system is composed by two major functional units, the MOE and the Vomeronasal Organ (VNO), and sensing of odor mixtures and pheromones are segregated into these two independent systems. Odorant detection in the MOE is mainly performed by Olfactory Sensory Neurons (OSNs) expressing Olfactory Receptors (ORs) while pheromones in VNO are revealed by two classes of Vomeronasal Sensory Neurons (VSNs) distinguished by the expression of a large repertory of Vomeronasal type-1 (V1Rs) and Vomeronasal type-2 Receptors (V2Rs) (Mombaerts, 2004; Zufall and Leinders-Zufall, 2007).

The extraordinary chemical diversity of olfactory ligands is matched in the mouse genome by more than 1100 intact OR genes (Buck and Axel, 1991; Zhang et al., 2007). With nanoCAGE we have confidently associated TSSs to 955 of them thereby defining a comprehensive picture of their promoter map at a single-base resolution (Plessy et al., 2012).

Here we show that further exploration of MOE nanoCAGE libraries reveals multiple evidences of transcription upstream of the annotated coding sequences for V1Rs and V2Rs. The expression of selected V1Rs and V2Rs has been validated by RT-PCR, RT-qPCR and *in situ* hybridization. Previous studies have highlighted the peculiar density of Repeat Elements (REs) and in particular Long Interspersed Nuclear Elements (LINE)s in V1Rs, V2Rs, and ORs loci (Kambere and Lane, 2009). Here we report that LINEs proximal to V1Rs and V2Rs are massively transcribed. These results significantly expand the potential repertory of chemoreceptors of the MOE and position transcribed LINE1 as candidate regulatory RNAs for VRs expression.

MATERIALS AND METHODS

NanoCAGE TECHNOLOGY AND PROTOCOL

For a detailed description of nanoCAGE please refer to Plessy et al. (2010).

ANIMALS, TISSUE PREPARATION, LASER CAPTURE MICRODISSECTION AND RNA QUALITY CONTROL FOR NanoCAGE

This study has been approved by the Ethics Committee of the International School for Advanced Studies. All animal procedures have been applied in compliance with the "Directive 86/609/EEC on the protection of Animals used for Experimental and other scientific purposes" (European Commission, 2010).

For the first MOE collection, two C57BL/6J mice (a p20 male and a p21 female) were sacrificed by inhalation of carbon dioxide. After decapitation, the skin and the jaw were removed from the heads and the samples were left overnight in ZincFix fixative (BD Biosciences, CA, USA) diluted in DEPC-treated water. After a 4 h cryoprotection step in a 30% sucrose/1x ZincFix solution the heads were included in Frozen section medium Neg-50 (Richard Allan scientific, MI, USA) and left on liquid nitrogen-iced isopentane for 2 min. The frozen blocks were brought into a cryostat (Microm International, Walldorf, Germany) and left at −21°C for 30–120 min. Serial coronal sections of mouse heads (16 mm) were cut with a clean blade, transferred on PEN-coated P.A.L.M. MembraneSlides (P.A.L.M. Microlaser Tehnologies, Germany) and immediately stored at −80°C. For the second MOE collection, three C57BL/6J mice (two p12 males and a p13 female) were processed as described above. The total number of slices obtained in the two collections was 100, with 3/4 sections on each glass slide. The MOE was collected from mouse head sections by laser capture microdissection. Before processing, slides were left at RT and air dried for 2 min. The MOE was morphologically identified, marked, microdissected and catapulted with a Zeiss P.A.L.M. laser microdissection and pressure catapulting (LM-PC) microscope (Carl Zeiss Inc., Germany) in P.A.L.M. tubes with adhesive caps (PALM Microlaser Technologies GmbH, Germany). After the harvest, 10 µl of lysis buffer (Stratagene, CA, USA) were added in each cap; the samples were left capsized at RT for 10 min, centrifuged at 6000 × g for 10 min and stored at −80°C. RNA was then extracted, DNase-treated and purified with Absolutely RNA Microprep kit (Stratagene, CA, USA) following manufacturer's instruction. After the elution step in nuclease-free water (Ambion, TX, USA) the concentration of the samples was measured with ND-1000 spectrophotometer; 500 pg of each sample were run on a 2100 Bioanalyzer (Agilent, CA, USA); samples with high RNA quality were pooled (26 out of 30 samples).

CONSERVATION-BASED MAPPING OF NanoCAGE TCs ON V1Rs AND V2Rs GENOMIC REGIONS

Most of the TSSs around V1Rs and V2Rs genes were mapping to repeats, mostly overlapping with LINE1, which is in accordance with the observation made by Kambere and Lane (Kambere and Lane, 2009).

For the mapping purposes, we have considered TCs that were not overlapping repeats. Many of the non-repeat TCs overlapped with the opossum and platypus conserved blocks and alongside the rat conserved blocks (**Table 3**). This was in agreement with the observation that the number and complexity of V1Rs and V2Rs in rodents, platypus and opossum are very similar to one another (Grus et al., 2005, 2007). We have clustered the conserved blocks on the upstream of V1Rs and V2Rs and looked for TCs overlapping with them. The mapping method is similar to the TC-to-OR genes mapping method used in (Plessy et al., 2012). However, since there are many TCs with opossum and platypus conservation, we added these species to the conserved block clusters. Conserved blocks from mouse (mm9) against the other species (rat, human, horse, dog, opossum and platypus) were clustered together if they were at least 4000 bp away. These clusters were mapped to upstream regions of vomeronasal genes. If upstream regions were overlapping with another refseq gene on the same strand, the upstream region clipped accordingly. Furthermore, if the conserved upstream region is longer than 15000 bp we clipped the region to 15000 bp from the gene start. The TCs (non-repeat overlapping) mapping to these conserved upstream regions were ranked by their expression and the TC with the highest expression mapped to the gene. All of the V1Rs and V2Rs genes were overlapping with a conserved upstream region. The median length of conserved upstream regions was 4478 bp. 30.2% of V2Rs and 53.1% of V1Rs mapped to a non-repeat TC overlapping a conserved block cluster

ANIMALS AND PREPARATION OF TISSUES FOR RT-PCR AND qRT-PCR NanoCAGE DATA VALIDATION

For RT-PCR, five adult C57B6/J mice (Charles River Laboratories International, Japan) were killed by carbon dioxide inhalation and decapitated; the MOE and the VNO were dissected from the heads, added with TRIzol reagent (Invitrogen, USA), immediately snap-frozen in liquid nitrogen and stored at −80°C.

For qRT-PCR, the MOE and VNO were dissected from P21 (2 males, 2 females) and P50 (2 males, 2 females) C57BL/6J mice (Charles River Laboriatories International, Japan) added with TRIzol reagent, immediately snap-frozen in liquid nitrogen and stored at −80°C. The quality of RNA samples was assessed with 2100 Bioanalyzer (Agilent Technologies, USA)

RT-PCR

First strand cDNA synthesis was performed as described elsewhere (Pifferi et al., 2006). PCR was carried out by adding 1 μl of first strand reaction to a mix containing 5u of Takara Taq DNA polymerase, 10× buffer, dNTPs mix 2.5mM each (all reagents from Takara, Japan), 50 pmol forward and reverse primers and nuclease-free water to a final volume of 50 μl. Forward exon-spanning primers were used to avoid unwanted amplification of residual genomic DNA.

qRT-PCR

cDNAs were synthesized as previously described (Pifferi et al., 2006). Quantitative real-time PCR experiments were performed with SYBR Premix Ex Taq II (Takara, Japan) in a volume of 10 μl on 384-wells plates using up to 30 ng of cDNA per reaction. Amplification and scanning were performed in a 7900HT Fast Real-Time PCR system (Applied Biosystems, USA). Standard curves with 3-points serial dilutions for each target were included on each plate to allow for inter-plate comparisons. RT- and PCR mix with no cDNA were included as negative controls.

After normalization with Gapdh *Ct* values, the inverse power of the normalized *Ct* values for each target were used to calculate the mean and the standard deviations plotted in the shown figures.

ANIMALS AND PREPARATION OF TISSUES FOR *IN SITU* HYBRIDIZATION

18–25 days old C57BL/6J mice were anesthetized with a 0.75 g/kg urethane solution injection and perfused intracardially with a 4% parafomaldehyde/PBS1x solution pH7.4 prepared in DEPC-treated water (PFA). After the perfusion mice were decapitated, the skin and the lower jaw were removed and the sample was put in the same PFA solution O/N at 4°C. Samples were decalcified for 12 h in a 0.5 M EDTA pH8.0/PBS1x solution prepared in DEPC-treated water. Cryoprotection was carried out in 10% sucrose/PBS1x for 2 h, 20% sucrose/PBS1x for 2 h and 30% sucrose/PBS1x 3 h to O/N at 4°C. Heads were included in Frozen section medium Neg-50 (Richard Allan scientific, MI, USA) and left on liquid nitrogen-iced isopentane for 2 min. The frozen blocks were left into a cryostat (Microm International, Walldorf, Germany) at −21°C for 30–120 min. Serial coronal sections of mouse heads (16 μm) were cut with a clean blade, and transferred on Superfrost Plus glass slides (Menzel-Glaser, Menzel GmbH and co KG, Germany) with a maximum number of three slices per slide. Sections were air-dried for 120 min and immediately used for hybridization or stored at −80°C.

BIOTIN-LABELED RIBOPROBES PREPARATION

PCR products were cloned in pGEM T-easy vector (Promega, WI, USA). 10 μg of each plasmid containing the specific PCR product were linearized with SacII (NEB) or with SalI (Promega) restriction enzymes for transcription with SP6 and T7 promoter, respectively. After an O/N incubation at 37°C, samples were cleaned with the PCR purification kit (Qiagen). For riboprobes transcription, 1 μg of each digested plasmid was added to a mix containing 2 μl of RNA BIO-labeling mix (Roche Applied Science, Germany), 20 units of SP6 or T7 RNA polymerases, 5× transcription buffer (both from Promega, WI, USA), 0.1 M DTT, 20 units of SuperaseIn RNase inhibitor (Ambion) and nuclease-free water (Ambion) in a volume of 20 μl. After 2 h of incubation at 37°C, the transcription reaction was stopped by adding 2 μl of 0.2 M pH 8.0 EDTA. RNA probes were precipitated by adding 1.25 μl of 4 M LiCl and 37.5 μl of absolute ethanol cooled at −20°C and stored for 2 h at −80°C. Samples were centrifuged at 20.000 × g for 30 min at 4°C and RNA pellets were washed once with 70% ethanol, briefly air-dried and resuspended in 50 μl of nuclease-free water with the addition of 20 units of Superase RNase inhibitor (Ambion).

IN SITU HYBRIDIZATION PROTOCOL

In situ hybridizations were carried out as previously described by Ishii et al. (2004). Please refer to Supplementary Data for details.

DETECTION OF BIOTIN-LABELED RNA PROBES

For the detection of BIO-labeled RNA probes Cy3-tyramide or Cy5-tyramide reactions (Perkin Elmer Life Sciences, Boston, MA) were used. Stainings were analyzed and acquired with a Leica TCS LSI confocal microscope or with a Leica DM6000B light microscope (Leica Microsystems GmbH, Germany). Images were resized with Photoshop CS3 software (Adobe Systems Incorporated, CA, USA). Please refer to Supplementary Data for details.

RESULTS

NanoCAGE DETECTS ACTIVE TRANSCRIPTION AT V1Rs AND V2Rs LOCI IN THE MOUSE MOE

The MOE was harvested with LCM from adjacent histological sections of C57BL/6J mice at 12 or 20–22 post-natal days. Samples were processed with zinc-fix, an optimal fixative for both tissue morphology and RNA integrity preservation. Two nanoCAGE libraries were synthesized from independent harvests and deeply sequenced using Illumina technology, yielding a total of 53,158,862 tags with a length of 25 bp and corresponding to the very 5′-end of MOE capped transcripts. 31,031,749 tags were confidently mapped to the mouse genome (Faulkner et al., 2008; Hashimoto et al., 2009). The mapped nanoCAGE tags were clustered and aggregated into Tag Clusters (TCs) (Carninci et al., 2006), and the data were unified in publicly accessible tracks that can be uploaded in UCSC Genome Browser (see Supplementary Data). This dataset displayed evidence for the expression of 87.5% of OR genes (955/1092), defining a comprehensive description of their TSSs and core promoters (Plessy et al., 2012).

When screened for the expression of additional candidate receptors for chemical sensing, the nanoCAGE libraries displayed multiple evidences of TCs mapping upstream of the annotated coding sequences for V1Rs genes and in close proximity to the 5′-end of V2Rs genes. We found TCs mapping upstream of 112/191 V1Rs and 96/123 V2Rs; the overall number of TCs mapping in V1Rs and V2Rs genes loci was 577 and 812, respectively, with an average TPM score of 0.53 and 0.12 (Supplementary Table S1). Furthermore, TCs were also associated to the 5′ TSS of core components of the vomeronasal transduction pathway such as *Gαo* (544 reads), *Gαi2* (64 reads), *Trpc2 isoform 1* (NM_011644, 261 reads) and *Trpc2 isoform 2* (NM_001109897, 243 reads); these data are summarized in Supplementary Table S2.

ANALYSIS OF TSSs ASSOCIATED TO V1Rs AND V2Rs EXPRESSION IN THE MOUSE MOE

The majority of TCs in proximity to V1Rs and V2Rs mapped on REs (**Table 1**) and more specifically on LINE1s (**Table 2** and Supplementary Table S3). Both young and ancestral LINE1 families were expressed.

A large portion of TCs not mapping on repeats (30.2% of V2Rs and 53.1% of V1Rs) overlapped with genomic regions conserved in opossum, platypus and rat genomes (**Table 3**). This is not surprising since number and genomic complexity of V1Rs and V2Rs in rodents, platypus and opossum are similar (Grus et al., 2007). We then sought to associate with confidence a particular TC to its downstream VR transcript, thus defining its TSS; for this analysis, only TCs not mapping to repeats were taken in consideration. We clustered the conserved regions of rat, platypus and opossum directly upstream of each VR gene. The resulting median length of these conserved sequences was 4478 bp; for V1Rs the median distance between the TCs selected by this association procedure and the annotated gene start was 3592 bp while for the V2Rs it was 842 bp (**Figure 1**). This was expected since most of the V1Rs are only annotated as single-exon open reading frames (ORFs) as in the case of ORs, whereas most V2Rs have annotated exon-intron structures that are defective of the untranslated regions (UTRs) at both the 5′ and 3′-ends. A detailed description of all the TCs mapping in V1Rs and V2Rs genes loci is presented in Supplementary Table S1.

Table 1 | Percentage of repeat and non-repeat overlapping TCs around V1Rs and V2Rs.

	% of CAGE TCs mapped in proximity of V1R and V2R genes	
VRs family	**Repeat overlapping**	**Non-repeat overlapping**
V1Rs	56.3% (325/577)	43.6% (252/577)
V2Rs	57.1% (464/812)	42.8% (348/812)

Table 2 | Classes of Repeat Elements overlapping with TCs mapping around V1R and V2R receptors.

	% repeats overlapping with TCs around Vomeronasal genes				
VRs family	**LINEs (%)**	**LTRs (%)**	**SINEs (%)**	**Simple_repeat (%)**	**Others (%)**
V1Rs	66.4	21.8	5.8	2.1	4.3
V2Rs	61.8	26.5	3.8	3.4	5.5

VALIDATION OF NanoCAGE DATA AND SINGLE TSSs BY RT-PCR

We validated the nanoCAGE data of selected genes by performing a standard RT-PCR starting from the same total RNA sample used for the synthesis of the nanoCAGE libraries. We amplified transcripts for the V2Rs family (*Vmn2r29*, *Vmn2r69*, and *Vmn2r95*), the V1Rs family (*Vmn1r51*, *Vmn1r50*, *Vmn1r10*) and the components of the vomeronasal transduction pathway (*Gαo*, *Gαi2*, and *Trpc2*); *Omp* was chosen as a positive control for its high expression in the MOE (**Figure 2A**). Because of the high level of intra-cluster homology, RT-PCRs for *Vmn2r29* and *Vmn2r95* amplified additional V2Rs including *Vmn2r30*, *Vmn2r31*, and *Vmn2r42* on chromosome 7 as well as *Vmn2r104* and *Vmn2r107* on chromosome 17. We also validated the expression of *Vmn2r26*, the only V2Rs that has been experimentally proven to bind a MHC class I peptide in the VNO (Leinders-Zufall et al., 2009) and for which nanoCAGE identified a sharp TSS mapped 105 bases upstream of the annotated Refseq gene. Cloning and sequencing confirmed the identity of all validated transcripts.

The transcription starting sites identified by nanoCAGE for receptors *Vmn1r228*, *Vmn2r3*, *Vmn2r69*, and *Vmn2r76* were confirmed by RT-PCRs with forward primers designed immediately downstream of the TSSs and reverse primers within the respective Refseq sequences. The sequence of the PCR products that confirms the TSS for *Vmn2r69* is shown uploaded in the UCSC Genome Browser as a representative example of validation in **Figure 2B**; the sequences of all the obtained amplicons are available in Supplementary Data.

IN SITU HYBRIDIZATION CONFIRMS THE EXPRESSION OF VRs IN A CONSISTENT NUMBER OF CELLS THROUGHOUT THE MOUSE MOE

To explore the identity of the cells expressing VRs transcripts we performed fluorescent *in situ* hybridization with specific

Table 3 | Percentages of non-repeat TCs overlapping with species-specific conserved blocks; a given TC can overlap with different species-specific blocks at the same time.

	% of conserved non-repeat TCs around VR genes						
VRs family (%)	**Rat (%)**	**Human (%)**	**Horse (%)**	**Dog (%)**	**Opossum (%)**	**Platypus (%)**	**Not conserved in these species (%)**
V1Rs	34.6	9.2	6.1	3.8	27.9	18.2	23.0
V2Rs	32.1	14.3	11.2	13.1	17.6	11.4	30.7

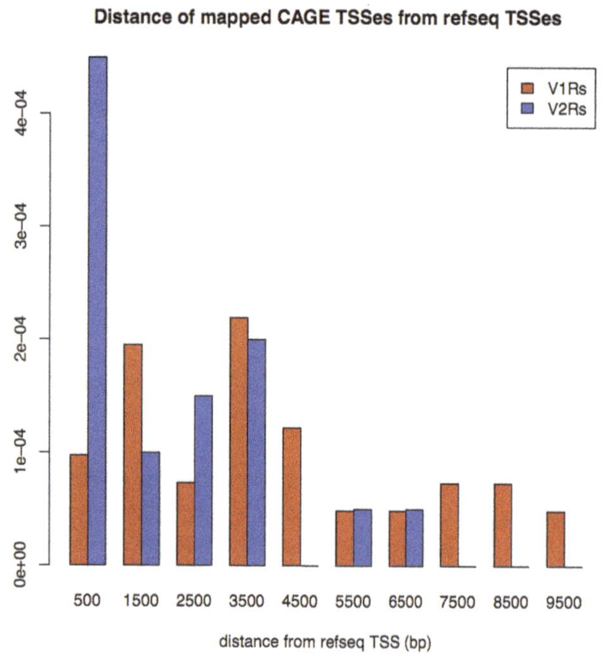

FIGURE 1 | Density of distances between mapped TCs identified by nanoCAGE and associated with VRs, and annotated TSS for RefSeq V1Rs and V2Rs. On the X-axis: Distance from RefSeq TSSs in basepairs; on the Y-axis: Frequency of mappings. The mean distance for V1Rs is higher than for V2Rs, in agreement with the observation that most of V1Rs genes are only annotated as single-exon ORFs whereas V2Rs genes have annotated exon-intron structures.

riboprobes synthesized from a selection of RT-PCR products. Sense and antisense probes were assayed on serial MOE cryosections of mice matching in age and sex those used for the construction of nanoCAGE libraries.

For the V1Rs family we investigated the expression of *Vmn1r201* on the basis of its sharp TSS identified by nanoCAGE. Due to high sequence homology, the antisense riboprobe for *Vmn1r201* was theoretically able to hybridize also to *Vmn1r215* and *Vmn1r218* mRNA, although for *Vmn1r218* no significant TSSs were detected in the nanoCAGE libraries. The *Vmn1r201* riboprobe decorated a discrete number of cells residing in the basal and middle layer of the epithelium with no zonal preference (**Figures 3A,B,D,E**).

For the V2Rs family we synthesized riboprobes for *Vmn2r26* and *Vmn2r69*. Due to the high level of homology among V2Rs genes, the antisense probe for *Vmn2r26* was able to hybridize to *Vmn2r19, Vmn2r23,* and *Vmn2r24*, sharing a homology rate ≥80%. All these V2Rs presented non-repeats mapping TCs in close proximity to the annotated RefSeq 5′ end. The riboprobe for *Vmn2r69* was specific for this receptor. *Vmn2r26* antisense riboprobe distinguished numerous cells in the middle layer as well as a group of cells located in the basal layer of the MOE; all of them displayed morphological features remarkably similar to those of the OSNs. *Vmn2r26*$^+$ cells were mainly localized in the central/dorsal turbinates of the MOE (**Figures 4A,B,D,E**).

The ISH results obtained with *Vmn2r69* riboprobe were comparable to those obtained for *Vmn2r26* in terms of cell morphology, while *Vmn2r69*$^+$ cells were only observed in dorsal turbinates (**Figures 5A,B,D,E**). Supplementary Figure S1 shows *in situ* hybridization results for *Vmn2r26* and *Vnm2r69* on dorsal/central turbinates of the MOE where the highest density of positive cells was observed. A complete count of *Vmn2r26*$^+$ and *Vmn2r69*$^+$ cells was performed in the whole MOE of two sexually mature 45-days old males C57BL/6J, resulting in a total of 543 and 332 positive cells, respectively.

The specificity of the *Vmn1r201, Vmn2r26,* and *Vmn2r69* antisense riboprobes was confirmed by the expected staining of numerous cells in the basal and upper layer of the VNO (**Figures 3C–F, 4C–F, 5C–F** respectively); the control sense probes for each target gene were extensively tested on serial sections of the MOE and the VNO, with no detectable signal in both tissues for all probes; a representative set of images for the negative controls is presented in Supplementary Figure S2.

VALIDATION OF EXPRESSION LEVELS OF *Vmn2r26* AND *Vmn2r69* IN THE MOE OF P21 AND P50 MICE BY qRT-PCR AND COMPARISON WITH EXPRESSION LEVELS OF SELECTED ORs

In order to confirm the reliability of nanoCAGE in detecting the expression of selected VRs genes we performed a real-time quantitative RT-PCR (qRT-PCR) on *OMP* (TPM = 157), an OR gene with an high expression level (*Olfr 110*, TPM = 22.7), three vomeronasal receptor genes (*Vmn1r201*, TPM = 0.18; *Vmn2r26*, TPM = 0.15; *Vmn2r69*, TPM = 0.22) and three OR genes with a low tag count comparable to the selected vomeronasal receptor targets (*Olfr480*, TPM = 0.25; *Olfr995*, TPM = 0.22; *Olfr1413*, TPM = 0.16) (**Figure 6**). qRT-PCR reactions were performed in triplicates on total RNA purified from dissections of the MOE and VNO of P21 (males $n = 5$ and females $n = 5$) and P50 (males $n = 5$ and females $n = 5$) C57BL/6J animals. As a negative control we performed qRT-PCR on the same targets using as a template total RNA purified from mouse liver. After copy numbers count and normalization with Gapdh *Ct* values, we were able to quantify mRNAs for *Olfr995*, *Olfr480, Olfr1413, Vmn2r26,* and *Vmn2r69* and to confirm that qRT-PCR data are consistent with the expression levels detected by nanoCAGE (Supplementary Figure S3). We were not able to detect the expression of *Vmn1r201* in P50 female mice. As

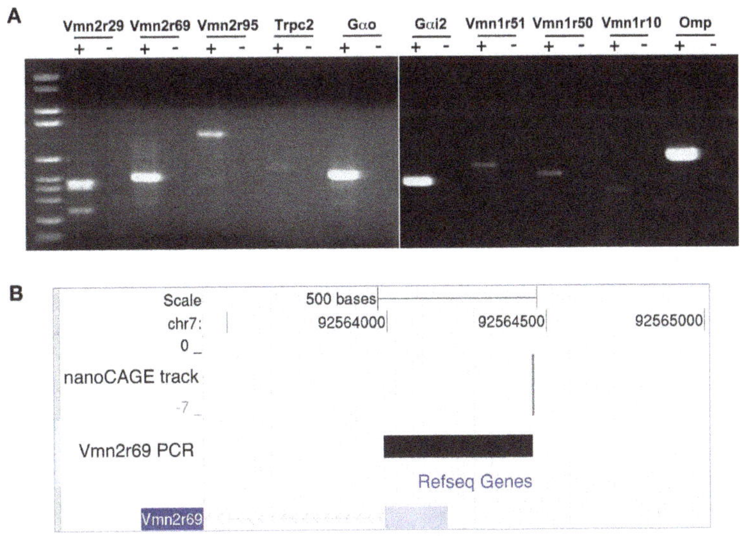

FIGURE 2 | Validation of nanoCAGE data by RT-PCR confirms the expression in the MOE of V1Rs, V2Rs, and key components of the pheromone transduction pathway. (A) RT-PCR validation was carried out starting from the same total RNA sample of the MOE used for the nanoCAGE workflow. V1Rs and V2Rs to be validated were chosen by interest or on the basis of their TPM score from the list of all expressed VRs detected by nanoCAGE. DNA molecular weight Marker VI is used as DNA ladder (Roche Applied Science). **(B)** The TSS of *Vmn2r69* identified by nanoCAGE was validated by RT-PCR with a forward primer designed in proximity of the TSSs and a reverse primer designed on the first exon. The sequence of the RT-PCR product is shown uploaded in the UCSC Genome Browser along with the nanoCAGE data.

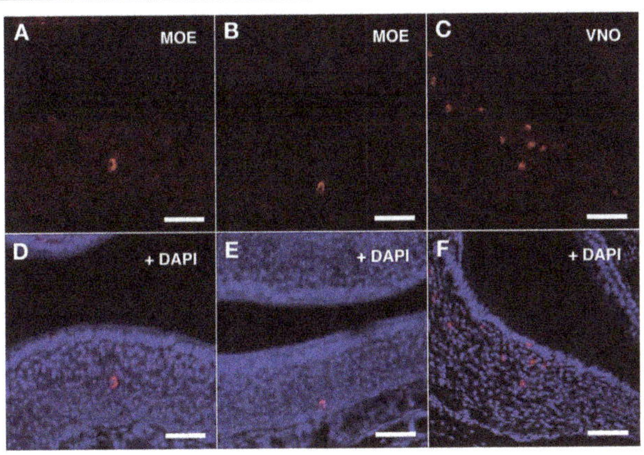

FIGURE 3 | *In situ* hybridization with *Vmn1r201* riboprobes on serial sections of the MOE. (A,B) Several cells throughout the MOE are revealed by the antisense *Vmn1r201* riboprobe. These cells are mainly found in the middle and basal layers of the MOE. The control sense probe for *Vmn1r201* did not display any detectable staining in the MOE or VNO. **(C)** The *Vmn1r201* antisense riboprobe hybridizes as expected with a high number of cells throughout the VNO. **(D–F)** Panels **(A–C)** merged with stained nuclei (DAPI). Scale bars: 60 μm.

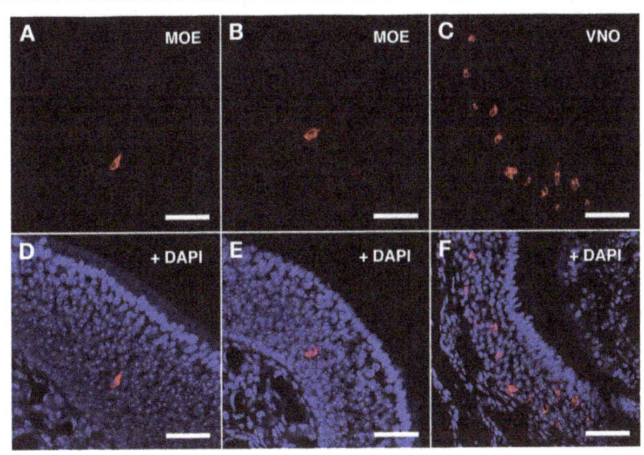

FIGURE 4 | *In situ* hybridization with *Vmn2r26* riboprobes on serial sections of the MOE. (A,B) The *Vmn2r26* antisense riboprobe hybridizes with a high number of cells throughout the MOE, mostly located in the basal and medial layers. **(C)** The *Vmn2r26* antisense riboprobe specifically stains a high number of cells throughout the VNO. **(D–F)** Panels **(A–C)** merged with stained nuclei (DAPI). Scale bars: **(A,B,D,E)** 50 μm; **(C,F)** 60 μm.

expected, we were not able to amplify any of the targets from liver RNA apart from Gapdh. We detected expression of *Olfr110*, *Olfr995*, and *Olfr1413* genes also in the VNO samples.

DISCUSSION

The traditional model of chemoreception in rodents considers MOE and VNO as two independent functional units, where sensing of odor mixtures and pheromones are segregated in independent detection systems (Mombaerts, 2004). In recent years, experimental evidences have suggested that these functional boundaries are uncertain since both structures can sense volatile plus non-volatile compounds and pheromonal plus non-pheromonal cues.

The activity of the VNO is not required for some olfactory-mediated instinctual behaviors (Dorries et al., 1997; Stowers and Logan, 2010). In turn, upon MOE selective ablation, male mice display a critical loss of interest toward female inspection and mounting, two behaviors classically attributed to the influence of pheromones (Yoon et al., 2005). Mouse models knocked out for the canonical mediators of OR signaling show impaired ability to fight and mate (Wang et al., 2006), unusual sexual behavior and lack of male-to-male aggressiveness (Wang and Storm, 2011). Neurons residing in MOE respond physiologically to compounds that have pheromonal characteristics leading to stereotyped behaviors including suckling, mate identification and male aggressiveness (Zufall and Leinders-Zufall, 2007; Stowers and Logan, 2010).

The existence of shared detection capabilities between VNO and MOE has been first suggested by the presence of 44 ORs in the VSNs; these ORs are canonically co-expressed with *Gαi2* and project their axons to the accessory olfactory bulb (Levai et al., 2006).

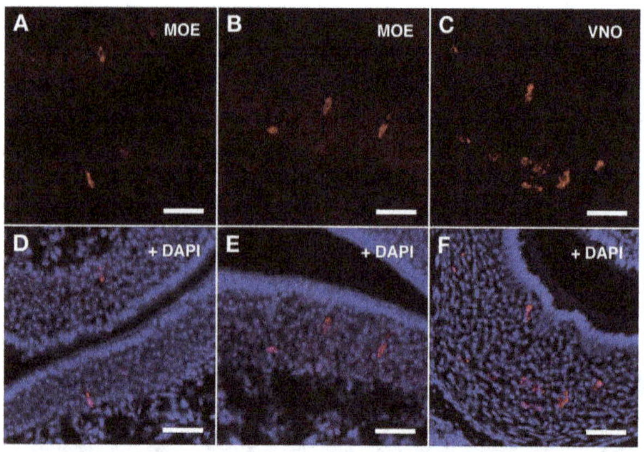

FIGURE 5 | *In situ* hybridization with *Vmn2r69* riboprobes on serial sections of the MOE. (A,B) Cells detected with the *Vmn2r69* riboprobe reside in the middle layer of the MOE, and are mostly found in dorsal turbinates. **(C)** The *Vmn2r69* antisense riboprobe hybridizes with a high number of cells in the VNO. **(D–F)** Panels **(A–C)** merged with stained nuclei (DAPI). Scale bars: 60 μm.

However, the molecular basis of pheromone sensing in MOE remains poorly understood although several evidences suggest that its receptors repertoire extends beyond ORs. A significant example is provided by the expression of several members of trace amine-associated receptors (*TAARs*) and guanylyl cyclase-D receptor (*GC-D*) in subsets of OSNs (Liberles and Buck, 2006; Zufall and Munger, 2010).

Intriguingly, two members of the murine V1Rd family, *V1rd17* and *V1rd20*, have been found expressed in MOE at embryonic and postnatal stages (Karunadasa et al., 2006). A custom microarray-based gene expression analysis has previously detected mRNAs for three V1Rs and two V1Rs, however their identity has not been disclosed (Zhang et al., 2010). A putative human pheromone receptor, *V1RL1*, has been identified by Southern blot analysis of RT-PCR products in human olfactory mucosa as well as in other human tissues (Rodriguez et al., 2000).

Both V1Rs and V2Rs are G protein-coupled receptors (GPCRs) but share little homology. The mouse genome contains 191 intact V1Rs genes with predicted short extracellular domain and no introns in the coding sequence (Zhang et al., 2010); conversely, the 123 intact V2Rs genes are structurally characterized by a predicted long and highly variable N-terminal and are encoded by multiple exons (Young and Trask, 2007; Zhang et al., 2010). The division between these two receptor families is also functional, since they are coupled to different α-subunits of the trimeric G protein (Gαi2 for VIRs and *Gαo* for V2Rs) and bind different sets of molecules (Berghard and Buck, 1996).

No evidence for the presence of additional V1Rs or of any V2Rs in MOE has been provided so far.

Here we have taken advantage of nanoCAGE (Plessy et al., 2010), a next-generation sequencing technology for unbiased 5′-end transcriptome profiling, to detect in the MOE consistent evidences of transcription that can be associated to a large

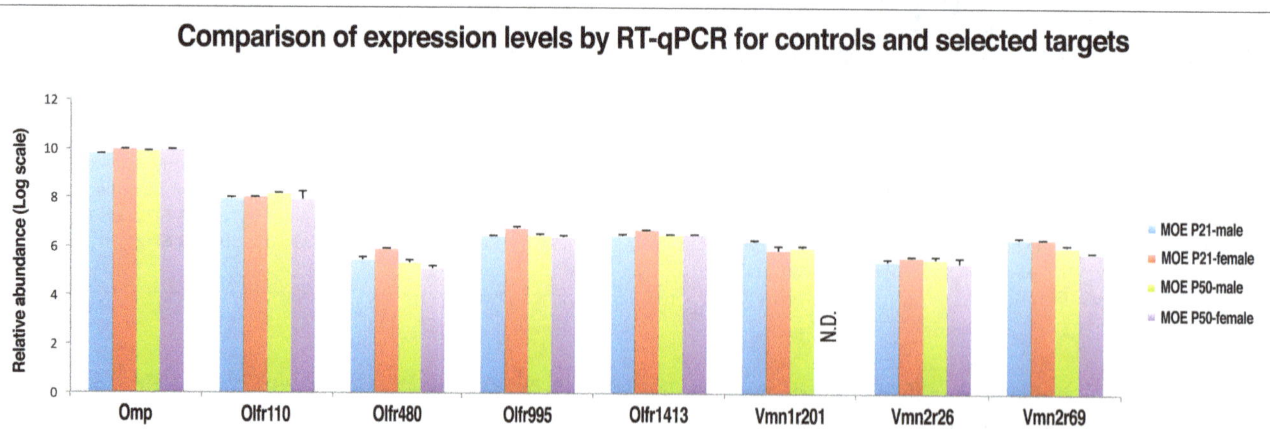

FIGURE 6 | Validation of nanoCAGE data by qRT-PCR confirms that the expression levels of selected VRs in the MOE of young and adult mice are comparable to the expression levels of ORs genes with similar tag counts in nanoCAGE libraries. The qRT-PCR validation was performed in triplicates on RNA purified from the dissected MOE and VNO of P21 (males $n = 5$, females $n = 5$) and P50 (males $n = 5$, females $n = 5$) C57BL/6J mice. All primers used were designed in an exon-spanning fashion; the *Ct* values of each target were normalized on Gapdh *Ct* values. The expression levels in the VNO and the copy number calculation are shown in Supplementary Figure S3.

number of V1Rs and V2Rs genes. NanoCAGE enables the quantitative measurement of transcripts expression level along with the precise definition of their TSSs from nanograms of total RNA obtained from fixed tissues. Being a single-nucleotide resolution technology, it greatly differs in terms of quantitative and qualitative output from microarray platforms or from PCR screenings based on degenerated oligonucleotides, as used so far to assess VRs expression in MOE. Furthermore, nanoCAGE was applied to RNA purified from tissue harvested by LCM (Plessy et al., 2012) to increase sensitivity for gene expression detection.

By multiple lines of evidence obtained from different experimental approaches we have proved that *Vmn1r201*, *Vmn2r26*, and *Vmn2r69* genes are expressed in the MOE by cells that reside in the basal and medial layers of the tissue and display morphological similarities with OSNs. Importantly, we have found that the absolute number of cells expressing these genes in the MOE of adult mice is comparable to what has been reported for *Vmn2r26* in the VNO (Del Punta et al., 2002; Leinders-Zufall et al., 2009). We have demonstrated by qRT-PCR that the expression levels of *Vmn2r26* and *Vmn2r69* in the MOE of sexually mature, adult mice are comparable to that of ORs with a similar total tags count in the nanoCAGE libraries.

Interestingly, *V2r1b* (*Vmn2r26* in the Refseq database) has been recently shown to respond to subpicomolar concentrations of MHC class I peptides in the VNO (Leinders-Zufall et al., 2009). Since the same class of non-volatile chemosignals is able to elicit physiological responses in the MOE (Spehr et al., 2006), our data suggests that *Vmn2r26* or additional highly homologous V2Rs may have a role in MHC class I peptides detection.

In the case of cells expressing *Vmn2r69*, we observed a spatial restriction in the dorsal turbinates of MOE suggesting the anatomical segregation of some V2Rs, as shown for several ORs. Interestingly, cells expressing *Vmn1r201* were much less abundant than those positive for *Vmn2r26* and *Vmn2r69* although consistently found in the MOE of all tested animals. It will be important to assess in details the identity of V1Rs- and V2Rs-expressing cells in the MOE by mapping their axonal projections.

NanoCAGE data have also revealed the expression of several V1Rs and V2Rs in addition to the ones we have validated. In some cases the low associated TPM scores suggest that a given VR may be expressed by a very restricted number of cells, as shown by the comparison of the DeepCAGE data with *in situ* hybridization for the hippocampus (Valen et al., 2009).

We have also detected relevant TSSs for several core components of the V1Rs- and V2Rs-associated chemo-transduction machinery including *Trpc2*, *Gαo*, and *Gαi2* that were then validated by RT-PCR from LCM-purified RNA. While they have been previously found expressed in the rodent MOE (Berghard and Buck, 1996), these observations have apparently attracted little attention.

These results strongly support the idea that transcripts from VRs loci are translated in signaling receptors. However, within the context of this work, we cannot exclude that some of V1Rs and V2Rs transcripts may not encode for VRs proteins but be non-coding RNA isoforms. A detailed analysis of transcript anatomy for every single gene will assess this important issue.

Interestingly, more than half of TCs upstream of V1Rs and V2Rs overlap with LINE1 transposable elements. The extraordinary content of LINE1 in V1Rs, V2Rs and ORs loci has been investigated for the first time by Kambere and Lane (2009). Focusing on V1Rs loci, the authors proposed an epigenetic role of LINE1 elements in the monoallelic expression of VR and OR genes on the basis of similar observations made on the inactivation mechanism of the X chromosome (Bailey et al., 2000).

Our analysis of MOE nanoCAGE data shows that LINE1s hosted in V1Rs and V2Rs loci are transcribed, thus adding a significant piece of information. Although we observe the transcription of members of active, young LINE1 families in both V1Rs and V2Rs loci (L1Md_A, L1Md_F, L1Md_F2, L1Md_F3, L1Md_Gf, L1Md_T) we do not confirm any preferential expression in comparison to ancestral, non-active ones (Supplementary Table S3). Several models can be proposed for how LINE1 elements can modulate the transcription of proximal VR genes. LINE1s present predominantly single-peak promoters that are active in somatic cells and exhibit far higher tissue specificity than conventional promoters, frequently driving transcription of nearby protein-coding genes. Along with the canonical 5′-sense promoter, LINE1s host a 5′-antisense promoter that in human cell lines is involved in the transcription of chimeric transcripts harboring partial sequences of sense and antisense downstream protein-coding mRNAs (Speek, 2001). An additional sense promoter is contained within the 3′ of LINE1s that may influence the local transcriptional activity of genes proximal to the insertion sites and even constitute alternative promoters for downstream sense protein-coding genes (Faulkner and Carninci, 2009; Faulkner et al., 2009). Alternatively, the presence of LINE1s may modulate nearby VR and OR genes expression through epigenetic mechanisms. In this context it is interesting that the GC-rich region of the LINE1 5′-sense promoter is a target for methylation and a potential trigger for seeding and spreading of heterochromatin (Zhang et al., 2012). The demethylation of this region can drive transcription of LINE1s and induce functional chromatin domains that may inhibit the influence of repressive chromatin modifications, a mechanism already described for the mouse growth hormone locus (Lunyak et al., 2007). In addition, small non-coding RNAs transcribed from LINE1s and other retrotransposons may also be involved in the regulation of local chromatin structure (Olovnikov et al., 2012).

Considering the sustained neurogenic capabilities of MOE and VNO throughout the lifespan of rodents (Dulac and Zakhary, 2004; Brann and Firestein, 2010) and the documented activation of LINE1s during adult neurogenesis (Muotri et al., 2005; Kuwabara et al., 2009), transcriptional activation of LINE1s in VRs and ORs loci may be involved in the neurogenesis and/or maturation of OSNs and VSNs. The 5′-UTR, ORF1, and ORF2 regions of mouse, rat and human LINE1s share conserved binding sites for Sox2/LEF which act as bi-directional promoters once transcribed during neurogenesis and can induce the transcriptional activation of proximal neuronal genes. Intriguingly, our nanoCAGE libraries show a pronounced expression of Sox2 in the MOE.

In summary, the application of next generation sequencing coupled to LCM-based tissue sampling is a powerful strategy to unveil unexpected transcription of protein coding genes and repetitive elements. While we and others are observing ORs expression outside of sites involved in olfactory chemoreception (Kang and Koo, 2012; Flegel et al., 2013; Foster et al., 2013; Li et al., 2013), evidences for VRs transcription in the central nervous system have been reported while drafting this manuscript (Ansoleaga et al., 2013; Garcia-Esparcia et al., 2013). Once again, these discoveries strongly suggest that our definition of "ectopic" expression needs to be revised and that a better understanding of its biological meaning is required for each case. V1Rs and V2Rs transcription in both chemosensory organs supports the possibility of a functional cross-talk between MOE and VNO posing interesting questions about their relative contribution to pheromone-triggered social behaviors in rodents.

AUTHORS CONTRIBUTIONS

Giovanni Pascarella, Charles Plessy, Dejan Lazarevic, Christina Vlachouli, Roberto Simone, Silvia Zucchelli performed the experiments, Charles Plessy, Jun Kawai, Carsten O. Daub, Yoshihide Hayashizaki, and Piero Carninci were involved in the large-scale data production, Charles Plessy, Nicolas Bertin, Altuna Akalin, Geoffrey J. Faulkner, Boris Lenhard analyzed the data, Giovanni Pascarella, Charles Plessy, Stefano Gustincich, and Piero Carninci wrote the manuscript, Stefano Gustincich and Piero Carninci designed the experiments and directed the project.

ACKNOWLEDGMENTS

We are indebted to all the members of Stefano Gustincich lab, especially Milena Pinto and Claudia Carrieri. We thank Prof. Anna Menini (SISSA, Italy) for helpful discussions and Alessandro Bonetti (RIKEN CLST, DGT) for help with qRT-PCR data analysis. This work was supported by a career developmental award from The Giovanni Armenise-Harvard Foundation to Stefano Gustincich, by a EU FP6 grant to the NFG consortium (Stefano Gustincich and Piero Carninci), a Grant-in-Aids for Scientific Research (A) No.20241047 to Piero Carninci. This work was also supported by a research grant for RIKEN Omics Science Center from the Japanese Ministry of Education, Culture, Sports, Science and Technology (MEXT) to Yoshihide Hayashizaki. Furthermore this work was realized with the contribution of the Italian Ministry of Foreign Affairs, "Direzione Generale per la Promozione e la Cooperazione Culturale" to Stefano Gustincich. Charles Plessy was supported by the Japanese Society for the Promotion of Science long-term fellowship number P05880.

REFERENCES

Ansoleaga, B., Garcia-Esparcia, P., Llorens, F., Moreno, J., Aso, E., and Ferrer, I. (2013). Dysregulation of brain olfactory and taste receptors in AD, PSP and CJD, and AD-related model. *Neuroscience* 248C, 369–382. doi: 10.1016/j.neuroscience.2013.06.034

Bailey, J. A., Carrel, L., Chakravarti, A., and Eichler, E. E. (2000). Molecular evidence for a relationship between LINE-1 elements and X chromosome inactivation: the Lyon repeat hypothesis. *Proc. Natl. Acad. Sci. U.S.A.* 97, 6634–6639. doi: 10.1073/pnas.97.12.6634

Berghard, A., and Buck, L. B. (1996). Sensory transduction in vomeronasal neurons: evidence for G alpha o, G alpha i2, and adenylyl cyclase II as major components of a pheromone signaling cascade. *J. Neurosci.* 16, 909–918.

Biagioli, M., Pinto, M., Cesselli, D., Zaninello, M., Lazarevic, D., Roncaglia, P., et al. (2009). Unexpected expression of alpha- and beta-globin in mesencephalic dopaminergic neurons and glial cells. *Proc. Natl. Acad. Sci. U.S.A.* 106, 15454–15459. doi: 10.1073/pnas.0813216106

Brann, H., and Firestein, S. (2010). Regeneration of new neuron is preserved in aged vomeronasal epithelia. *J. Neurosci.* 30, 15686–15694. doi: 10.1523/JNEUROSCI.4316-10.2010

Buck, L., and Axel, R. (1991). A novel multigene family may encode odorant receptors: a molecular basis for odor recognition. *Cell* 65, 175–187. doi: 10.1016/0092-8674(91)90418-X

Carninci, P., and Hayashizaki, Y. (2007). Noncoding RNA transcription beyond annotated genes. *Curr. Opin. Genet. Dev.* 17, 139–144. doi: 10.1016/j.gde.2007.02.008

Carninci, P., Sandelin, A., Lenhard, B., Katayama, S., Shimokawa, K., Ponjavic, J., et al. (2006). Genome-wide analysis of mammalian promoter architecture and evolution. *Nat. Genet.* 38, 626–635. doi: 10.1038/ng1789

Del Punta, K., Leinders-Zufall, T., Rodriguez, I., Jukam, D., Wysocki, C. J., Ogawa, S., et al. (2002). Deficient pheromone responses in mice lacking a cluster of vomeronasal receptor genes. *Nature* 419, 70–74. doi: 10.1038/nature00955

Dorries, K. M., Adkins-Regan, E., and Halpern, B. P. (1997). Sensitivity and behavioral responses to the pheromone androstenone are not mediated by the vomeronasal organ in domestic pigs. *Brain Behav. Evol.* 49, 53–62. doi: 10.1159/000112981

Dulac, C., Zakhary, L. (2004). "Stem cells of the olfactory epithelium," in *Handbook of Stem Cells*, Vol. 2 (Maryland Heights, MO: Academic Press), 233–244.

European Commission. (2010). Directive 2010/63/EU of the European Parliament and of the Council of 22 September 2010 on the protection of animals used for scientific purposes (Text with EEA relevance). *Official Journal L 276* 53, 33–79.

Faulkner, G. J., and Carninci, P. (2009). Altruistic functions for selfish DNA. *Cell Cycle* 8, 2895–2900. doi: 10.4161/cc.8.18.9536

Faulkner, G. J., Forrest, A. R., Chalk, A. M., Schroder, K., Hayashizaki, Y., Carninci, P., et al. (2008). A rescue strategy for multimapping short sequence tags refines surveys of transcriptional activity by CAGE. *Genomics* 91, 281–288. doi: 10.1016/j.ygeno.2007.11.003

Faulkner, G. J., Kimura, Y., Daub, C. O., Wani, S., Plessy, C., Irvine, K. M., et al. (2009). The regulated retrotransposon transcriptome of mammalian cells. *Nat. Genet.* 41, 563–571. doi: 10.1038/ng.368

Flegel, C., Manteniotis, S., Osthold, S., Hatt, H., and Gisselmann, G. (2013). Expression profile of ectopic olfactory receptors determined by deep sequencing. *PLoS ONE* 8:e55368. doi: 10.1371/journal.pone.0055368

Forrest, A. R., and Carninci, P. (2009). Whole genome transcriptome analysis. *RNA Biol.* 6, 107–112. doi: 10.4161/rna.6.2.7931

Foster, S. R., Roura, E., and Thomas, W. G. (2013). Extrasensory perception: odorant and taste receptors beyond the nose and mouth. *Pharmacol. Ther.* doi: 10.1016/j.pharmthera.2013.11.004. [Epub ahead of print].

Garcia-Esparcia, P., Schluter, A., Carmona, M., Moreno, J., Ansoleaga, B., Torrejon-Escribano, B., et al. (2013). Functional genomics reveals dysregulation of cortical olfactory receptors in Parkinson disease: novel putative chemoreceptors in the human brain. *J. Neuropathol. Exp. Neurol.* 72, 524–539. doi: 10.1097/NEN.0b013e318294fd76

Grus, W. E., Shi, P., and Zhang, J. (2007). Largest vertebrate vomeronasal type 1 receptor gene repertoire in the semiaquatic platypus. *Mol. Biol. Evol.* 24, 2153–2157. doi: 10.1093/molbev/msm157

Grus, W. E., Shi, P., Zhang, Y. P., and Zhang, J. (2005). Dramatic variation of the vomeronasal pheromone receptor gene repertoire among five orders of placental and marsupial mammals. *Proc. Natl. Acad. Sci. U.S.A.* 102, 5767–5772. doi: 10.1073/pnas.0501589102

Hashimoto, T., De Hoon, M. J., Grimmond, S. M., Daub, C. O., Hayashizaki, Y., and Faulkner, G. J. (2009). Probabilistic resolution of multi-mapping reads in massively parallel sequencing data using MuMRescueLite. *Bioinformatics* 25, 2613–2614. doi: 10.1093/bioinformatics/btp438

Ishii, T., Omura, M., and Mombaerts, P. (2004). Protocols for two- and three-color fluorescent RNA *in situ* hybridization of the main and accessory olfactory epithelia in mouse. *J. Neurocytol.* 33, 657–669. doi: 10.1007/s11068-005-3334-y

Kambere, M. B., and Lane, R. P. (2009). Exceptional LINE density at V1R loci: the Lyon repeat hypothesis revisited on autosomes. *J. Mol. Evol.* 68, 145–159. doi: 10.1007/s00239-008-9195-0

Kang, N., and Koo, J. (2012). Olfactory receptors in non-chemosensory tissues. *BMB Rep.* 45, 612–622. doi: 10.5483/BMBRep.2012.45.11.232

Karunadasa, D. K., Chapman, C., and Bicknell, R. J. (2006). Expression of pheromone receptor gene families during olfactory development in the mouse: expression of a V1 receptor in the main olfactory epithelium. *Eur. J. Neurosci.* 23, 2563–2572. doi: 10.1111/j.1460-9568.2006.04795.x

Kuwabara T., Hsieh J., Muotri A., Yeo G., Warashima M., Lie, D. C., et al. (2009). Wnt-mediated activation of NeuroD1 and retro-elements during adult neurogenesis. *Nat. Neurosci.* 12, 1097–105. doi: 10.1038/nn.2360

Leinders-Zufall, T., Ishii, T., Mombaerts, P., Zufall, F., and Boehm, T. (2009). Structural requirements for the activation of vomeronasal sensory neurons by MHC peptides. *Nat. Neurosci.* 12, 1551–1558. doi: 10.1038/nn.2452

Levai, O., Feistel, T., Breer, H., and Strotmann, J. (2006). Cells in the vomeronasal organ express odorant receptors but project to the accessory olfactory bulb. *J. Comp. Neurol.* 498, 476–490. doi: 10.1002/cne.21067

Li, J. J., Tay, H. L., Plank, M., Essilfie, A. T., Hansbro, P. M., Foster, P. S., et al. (2013). Activation of olfactory receptors on mouse pulmonary macrophages promotes monocyte chemotactic protein-1 production. *PLoS ONE* 8:e80148. doi: 10.1371/journal.pone.0080148

Liberles, S. D., and Buck, L. B. (2006). A second class of chemosensory receptors in the olfactory epithelium. *Nature* 442, 645–650. doi: 10.1038/nature05066

Lunyak, V. V., Prefontaine, G. G., Nunez, E., Cramer, T., Ju, B. G., Ohgi, K. A., et al. (2007). Developmentally regulated activation of a SINE B2 repeat as a domain boundary in organogenesis. *Science* 317, 248–251. doi: 10.1126/science.1140871

Mercer, T. R., Dinger, M. E., and Mattick, J. S. (2009). Long non-coding RNAs: insights into functions. *Nat. Rev. Genet.* 10, 155–159. doi: 10.1038/nrg2521

Mombaerts, P. (2004). Genes and ligands for odorant, vomeronasal and taste receptors. *Nat. Rev. Neurosci.* 5, 263–278. doi: 10.1038/nrn1365

Muotri, A. R., Chu, V. T., Marchetto, M. C., Deng, W., Moran, J. V., and Gage F. H. (2005). Somatic mosaicism in neuronal precursor cells mediated by L1 retrotransposition. *Nature* 435, 903–910. doi: 10.1038/nature03663

Olovnikov, I., Aravin, A. A., and Fejes Toth, K. (2012). Small RNA in the nucleus: the RNA-chromatin ping-pong. *Curr. Opin. Genet. Dev.* 22, 164–171. doi: 10.1016/j.gde.2012.01.002

Pifferi, S., Pascarella, G., Boccaccio, A., Mazzatenta, A., Gustincich, S., Menini, A., et al. (2006). Bestrophin-2 is a candidate calcium-activated chloride channel involved in olfactory transduction. *Proc. Natl. Acad. Sci. U.S.A.* 103, 12929–12934. doi: 10.1073/pnas.0604505103

Plessy, C., Bertin, N., Takahashi, H., Simone, R., Salimullah, M., Lassmann, T., et al. (2010). Linking promoters to functional transcripts in small samples with nanoCAGE and CAGEscan. *Nat. Methods* 7, 528–534. doi: 10.1038/nmeth.1470

Plessy, C., Pascarella, G., Bertin, N., Akalin, A., Carrieri, C., Vassalli, A., et al. (2012). Promoter architecture of mouse olfactory receptor genes. *Genome Res.* 22, 486–497. doi: 10.1101/gr.126201.111

Rodriguez, I., Greer, C. A., Mok, M. Y., and Mombaerts, P. (2000). A putative pheromone receptor gene expressed in human olfactory mucosa. *Nat. Genet.* 26, 18–19. doi: 10.1038/79124

Shiraki, T., Kondo, S., Katayama, S., Waki, K., Kasukawa, T., Kawaji, H., et al. (2003). Cap analysis gene expression for high-throughput analysis of transcriptional starting point and identification of promoter usage. *Proc. Natl. Acad. Sci. U.S.A.* 100, 15776–15781. doi: 10.1073/pnas.2136655100

Speek M. (2001). Antisense promoter of human L1 retrotransposon drives transcription of adjacent cellular genes. *Mol. Cell. Biol.* 21, 1973–1985. doi: 10.1128/MCB.21.6.1973-1985.2001

Spehr, M., Kelliher, K. R., Li, X. H., Boehm, T., Leinders-Zufall, T., and Zufall, F. (2006). Essential role of the main olfactory system in social recognition of major histocompatibility complex peptide ligands. *J. Neurosci.* 26, 1961–1970. doi: 10.1523/JNEUROSCI.4939-05.2006

Stowers, L., and Logan, D. W. (2010). Olfactory mechanisms of stereotyped behavior: on the scent of specialized circuits. *Curr. Opin. Neurobiol.* 20, 274–280. doi: 10.1016/j.conb.2010.02.013

Valen, E., Pascarella, G., Chalk, A., Maeda, N., Kojima, M., Kawazu, C., et al. (2009). Genome-wide detection and analysis of hippocampus core promoters using DeepCAGE. *Genome Res.* 19, 255–265. doi: 10.1101/gr.084541.108

Wang, Z., Balet Sindreu, C., Li, V., Nudelman, A., Chan, G. C., and Storm, D. R. (2006). Pheromone detection in male mice depends on signaling through the type 3 adenylyl cyclase in the main olfactory epithelium. *J. Neurosci.* 26, 7375–7379. doi: 10.1523/JNEUROSCI.1967-06.2006

Wang, Z., and Storm, D. R. (2011). Maternal behavior is impaired in female mice lacking type 3 adenylyl cyclase. *Neuropsychopharmacology* 36, 772–781. doi: 10.1038/npp.2010.211

Washietl, S., Will, S., Hendrix, D. A., Goff, L. A., Rinn, J. L., Berger, B., et al. (2012). Computational analysis of noncoding RNAs. *Wiley Interdiscip. Rev. RNA* 3, 759–778. doi: 10.1002/wrna.1134

Yoon, H., Enquist, L. W., and Dulac, C. (2005). Olfactory inputs to hypothalamic neurons controlling reproduction and fertility. *Cell* 123, 669–682. doi: 10.1016/j.cell.2005.08.039

Young, J. M., and Trask, B. J. (2007). V2R gene families degenerated in primates, dog and cow, but expanded in opossum. *Trends Genet.* 23, 212–215. doi: 10.1016/j.tig.2007.03.004

Zhang, X., De La Cruz, O., Pinto, J. M., Nicolae, D., Firestein, S., and Gilad, Y. (2007). Characterizing the expression of the human olfactory receptor gene family using a novel DNA microarray. *Genome Biol.* 8, R86. doi: 10.1186/gb-2007-8-5-r86

Zhang, X., Marcucci, F., and Firestein, S. (2010). High-throughput microarray detection of vomeronasal receptor gene expression in rodents. *Front. Neurosci.* 4:164. doi: 10.3389/fnins.2010.00164

Zhang, Y., Shu, J., Si, J., Shen, L., Estecio, M. R. H., and Issa J. P. (2012). Repetitive elements and enforced transcriptional repression co-operate to enhance DNA methylation spreading into a promoter CpG island. *Nucleic Acid Res.* 40, 7275–7268. doi: 10.1093/nar/gks429

Zufall, F., and Leinders-Zufall, T. (2007). Mammalian pheromone sensing. *Curr. Opin. Neurobiol.* 17, 483–489. doi: 10.1016/j.conb.2007.07.012

Zufall, F., and Munger, S. D. (2010). Receptor guanylyl cyclases in mammalian olfactory function. *Mol. Cell. Biochem.* 334, 191–197. doi: 10.1007/s11010-009-0325-9

17

The role of miRNA in motor neuron disease

Min Jeong Kye[1,2] * and Inês do Carmo G. Gonçalves[1,2]

[1] *Institute of Human Genetics, University of Cologne, Cologne, Germany*
[2] *Institute for Genetics, University of Cologne, Cologne, Germany*

***Correspondence:**
Min Jeong Kye, Institute of Human Genetics and Institute for Genetics, University of Cologne, 50931 Cologne, Germany
e-mail: min.kye@uk-koeln.de

microRNA is a subset of endogenous non-coding RNA. It binds to partially complementary sequences in mRNAs and inhibits mRNA translation by either blocking translational machinery or degrading mRNAs. It is involved in various cellular processes including cell cycle, development, metabolism, and synaptic plasticity. Dysregulation of miRNA expression and function is reported in various diseases including cancer, metabolic disorders as well as neurological disorders. In nervous system, miRNA related pathways play a very important role in development and function of neuronal cells. Moreover, numerous evidences suggest that dysregulated miRNA related pathways contribute to pathology of neurological disorders such as Alzheimer's disease, amyotrophic lateral sclerosis (ALS) and spinal muscular atrophy (SMA). Here, we review current knowledge about the role of miRNAs in motor neuron disorders, especially about two common diseases: SMA and ALS.

Keywords: microRNA, motor neurons, neuromuscular junction, spinal muscular atrophy, amyotrophic lateral sclerosis

INTRODUCTION

microRNAs (miRNAs) are endogenous non-coding single-stranded RNA molecules that play important roles in eukaryotic gene expression through posttranscriptional regulation (Bartel, 2009). It mainly binds to the 3′-untranslated region (3′-UTR) of messenger RNAs (mRNAs) from target protein-coding genes and leads to gene silencing by mRNA cleavage, translational repression and deadenylation (Huntzinger and Izaurralde, 2011). Functional studies indicate that miRNA plays a significant role in a broad range of cellular and developmental processes such as stem cell maintenance (Houbaviy et al., 2003), differentiation (Chen et al., 2004; Naguibneva et al., 2006), cell cycle (Hatfield et al., 2005), development (Hornstein et al., 2005), learning and memory formation (Gao et al., 2010), energy metabolism (Gao et al., 2009), and immune responses (Xiao et al., 2007). miRNAs can only function as part of ribonucleoprotein (RNP) complex called RNA induced silencing complex (RISC), which contains various proteins such as argonautes, fragile X mental retardation protein (FMRP), Dicer and monkey leukemia virus 10 (MOV10; Jin et al., 2004; Landthaler et al., 2008). Like miRNAs, RISC plays a crucial role in many cellular processes during development and cellular differentiation. For example, deletion of core protein of RISC, Ago2 leads to embryonic lethality in mouse (Morita et al., 2007). Similarly, ablation of *Dicer* or DiGeorge syndrome critical region gene 8 (*DGCR8*) also causes developmental arrest in murine embryonic stem cells (Bernstein et al., 2003; Wang et al., 2007). Although it is widely accepted that miRNAs are important for nervous system development and function, a little is known about the role of individual miRNAs in neuron at the moment.

BIOGENESIS AND DECAY OF miRNAs

The majority of characterized miRNAs are transcribed by RNA polymerase II from their own independent genes or introns of protein-coding genes (Krol et al., 2010). The primary transcript (pri-miRNAs) of miRNA is specifically recognized by microprocessor complex. The microprocessor complex is composed by nuclear ribonuclease III, Drosha, and its binding partner, DGCR8. In this complex, a double stranded RNA-binding protein, DGCR8 recognizes the stem-loop structure in pri-miRNA and Drosha cleaves the pri-miRNA into a ~70-nucleotide precursor form (pre-miRNA). Afterward, pre-miRNA is translocated to the cytoplasm by exportin 5 through the nuclear pore complex in a Ran guanosine triphosphate (RanGTP)-dependent process. In the cytoplasm, second RNaseIII containing protein complex cleaves pre-miRNA to ~20 bp miRNA/miRNA* duplex. This complex is composed of Dicer (RNaseIII), transactivation response RNA binding protein (TRBP), and protein activator of the interferon-induced protein kinase (PACT). One strand of the miRNA duplex is incorporated into the RISC as a mature miRNA (guide strand/miRNA), whereas the other strand (passenger strand/miRNA*) is degraded (Kim et al., 2009).

miRNA can only function in the RISC. The functional core proteins of RISC are mainly composed of Argonaute families (Ago1-4) and glycin-tryptophan protein of 182 kDa (GW182). In RISC, only Agonaute proteins show endonuclease enzymatic activity, which is responsible for mRNA silencing (Huntzinger and Izaurralde, 2011). GW182 proteins are also essential for the RISC function (Eulalio et al., 2008). It inhibits binding of poly-A binding protein (PABPC) to poly-A tail and induces deadenylation, decapping, and decay of mRNAs (Zekri et al., 2009). Additional proteins associated with RISC have been identified such as FMRP, MOV10, and Hu-Antigen R (HuR; Landthaler et al., 2008).

Expression of miRNAs seems to be tightly regulated by sophisticated mechanisms from the biogenesis to decay. Although it is not yet fully understood, the stability of mature miRNA is controlled by endogenous factors such as miRNA degrading enzymes and occupancy by target mRNAs. In animal cells, miRNA decay is carried out by the 5′-to-3′ exoribonuclease 1 and 2 (XRN1 and XRN2; Bail et al., 2010). Interestingly, it seems that binding to their target mRNAs can increase or decrease stability of miRNAs (Chatterjee et al., 2011; Iio et al., 2013). Additionally, environmental factors such as growth factors, cell cycle, and neuronal activity can influence on stability of miRNAs (Ruegger and Grosshans, 2012).

miRNA IN MOTOR NEURONS

Numerous studies have shown that miRNAs play an important role for nervous system development (Conaco et al., 2006; Akerblom et al., 2012; Zhu et al., 2013). Disturbing miRNA biogenesis pathway by deleting Dicer1 from spinal motor neurons in mouse caused spinal muscular atrophy (SMA) like phenotype (Haramati et al., 2010). More specifically, modifying miR-9 expression in developing motor neurons alters motor neuron subtype specification as well as columnar development of spinal cords in chick embryos (Otaegi et al., 2011a). In this model, miR-9 regulates expression of transcription factor, forkhead box P1 (*FoxP1*), which plays a crucial role for development and neuronal subtype differentiation in spinal cord (Otaegi et al., 2011b). Another interesting miRNA in motor neuron is miR-17-3p. This miRNA directly regulates mRNA translation of oligodendrocyte transcription factor 2 (*Olig2*), which is an important transcription factor for spinal motor neuron differentiation. The expression of miR-17-3p is repressed by sonic hedgehog (Shh), which results in elevated expression of *Olig2*. Thus, high amount of Shh will direct neuronal progenitors to differentiate toward motor neurons and decrease interneuron population. Additionally, deletion of miR-17~92 cluster from mouse embryos suggests that this cluster regulates differentiation of interneurons as well as motor neurons in early spinal cord development (Chen et al., 2011). **Table 1** summarizes motor neuron related miRNAs discussed in this review.

miRNAs are also important for axonal regeneration process in spinal motor neurons. Ablation of Dicer in sciatic nerve of mouse suggested that functional miRNAs are pivotal for nerve regeneration and axonal re-growth (Wu et al., 2012). In zebrafish, elevated expression of miR-133b after spinal cord injury represses mRNA translation of RhoA. This process promotes functional recovery of motor neuron axons after traumatic injury (Yu et al., 2011). Taken together, we can conclude that miRNAs play a significant role in various processes in motor neurons such as neuronal subtype specification, functional maintenance, and regeneration after injury.

miRNA AT THE NEUROMUSCULAR JUNCTION

miRNAs are differentially distributed in neuronal compartments such as soma and neurites (Kye et al., 2007). Numerous miRNAs are presented in axonal compartment and growth cones in cortical and sympathetic neurons (Natera-Naranjo et al., 2010; Sasaki et al., 2013). These data suggests that miRNAs can regulate mRNA translation at the axonal compartments. It seems that miRNAs play a significant role in motor neuron axons, especially at the neuromuscular junction (NMJ). Interestingly, in contrast to vertebrates, *Drosophila* mutant, who lacks one of the most abundant neuronal miRNA, miR-124 did not show any strong defect in neuronal production, differentiation, and NMJ morphology. However, the miR-124 *Drosophila* mutant showed shorter life span, impaired locomotion as well as increased presynaptic neurotransmitter release at the NMJ (Sun et al., 2012). Additionally, miR-8 is also reported as an important miRNA for pre-synaptic bouton formation at the *Drosophila* NMJ. Repeated neuronal activity represses the expression of miR-8, and it results in elevated neuronal mRNA translation and synaptic growth (Nesler et al., 2013). *Drosophila* mutants lacking miR-125 or let-7 expression also showed defects in NMJ phenotypes such as delayed maturation of NMJ, smaller size of NMJ, and abnormality in locomotion. Interestingly, these phenotypes are shown only during metamorphosis (Caygill and Johnston, 2008). This implies that miRNAs play a specific role for temporal and spatial regulation of gene expression during development. Another interesting miRNA is miR-310. It regulates synaptic homeostasis at the NMJ by regulating translation of kinesin super family member, Khc-73. miR-310 directly represses the translation of Khc-73 to control neurotransmitter release in motor neurons during larval stages (Tsurudome et al., 2010). Finally, function of miRNA at mammalian NMJ is described in a mouse model for neuromuscular disease, slow-channel congenital myasthenic syndrome (SCS). Axonal expression of miR-124 is elevated in this model compared to the wild type animals. miR-124 regulates mRNA translation of *Rab3a* in axon in response to amplified Ca^{2+}/calpain/cdk5/nitric oxide pathway in muscle cells. In consequence, the elevated expression of miR-124 and reduced expression of Rab3a proteins in nerve terminals decrease neurotransmitter release to the NMJ (Zhu et al., 2013). Taken together, we can conclude that miRNAs are important players for NMJ formation and function as well as maintaining synaptic homeostasis.

Recently, protein and nucleic acids containing vesicles (exosomes) have been suggested as a new molecular mechanism for communication between cells in nervous system (Sharma et al., 2013). They can transfer genetic molecules from donor cells to recipient cells, by which they can change physiology of recipient cells (Valadi et al., 2007). For example, cancer cells release more exosomes than healthy ones. In consequence, it changes physiology of surrounding cells to have more favorable conditions for their metastasis (Grange et al., 2011; Soldevilla et al., 2013). Moreover, various miRNAs are detected in exosomes released from neurons and muscle cells (Forterre et al., 2013; Fruhbeis et al., 2013). These findings strongly suggest that miRNA can function as a signaling molecule for intracellular communication at the NMJ.

TWO COMMON MOTOR NEURON DISEASES; SMA AND ALS

PROXIMAL SPINAL MUSCULAR ATROPHY

Spinal muscular atrophy is a genetically and clinically heterogeneous group of neuromuscular disorders characterized by progressive degeneration of lower alpha motor neurons in the anterior horn of spinal cord (Crawford and Pardo, 1996). Affected individuals exhibit proximal manifestation of muscle weakness and atrophy. With an incidence of 1:6000 ~ 1:10000 newborns and a carrier frequency of 1:35, proximal SMA is the leading hereditary cause of infant mortality (Wirth et al., 2006). Due to the highly variable disease severity, four clinical types of SMA are classified

Table 1 | The list of motor neuron related miRNAs discussed in this review.

miRNA	Findings	Target genes	Related disease/model organism	Reference
miR-8	Presynaptic bouton formation/synaptic growth	Lar and Wg	Fruit fly	Nesler et al. (2013)
miR-9	Motor neuron subtype specification/spinal cord development	FoxP1	Chick	Otaegi et al. (2011a,b)
	Dysregulated expression in motor neurons differentiated from embryonic stem cells		SMA/mouse	Haramati et al. (2010)
	Expression is elevated in induced stem cell derived neurons from ALS patient		ALS/cell line (Human)	Zhang et al. (2013)
	Axon growth	MAP1B	Mouse	Dajas-Bailador et al. (2012)
miR-17-3p	Spinal motor neuron differentiation	Olig2	Mouse	Chen et al. (2011)
miR17~92 cluster	Differentiation of interneuron and motor neurons		Mouse	Chen et al. (2011)
miR-21	Axonal regeneration	Sprouty2	Mouse	Strickland et al. (2011)
	Spinal cord injury	PTEN and FasL	Rat	Hu et al. (2013)
miR-23a, miR-29b, and miR-455	Expression is increased in skeletal muscle from ALS patients and it may cause dysregulation in mitochondrial gene expression	PGC1-α (miR-23a)	ALS/mouse	Russell et al. (2012)
miR-106	Regeneration of NMJ	HDAC4	ALS/mouse	Williams et al. (2009)
miR-124	Neurotransmitter release		Fruit fly	Sun et al. (2012)
	Neurotransmitter release at the NMJ	Rab3a	Slow-channel congenital myasthenic syndrome/mouse	Zhu et al. (2013)
miR-125 and let-7	NMJ phenotype, delayed maturation, smaller size, abnormal locomotion, reduced lifespan	Abrupt	Fruit fly	Caygill and Johnston (2008)
miR-132	Neuronal morphology and cognition	AChE and p250GAP	ALS/mouse	Edbauer et al. (2010), Shaltiel et al. (2013)
	Splicing of Tau	PTBP2	Tauopathies/mouse	Smith et al. (2011), Hebert et al. (2012)
miR-132, miR-143, and miR-558	Expression is dysregulated in TDP-43 deficient cells. Neurites outgrowth (miR-132)		ALS and FTLD (frontotemporal lobar degeneration)/cell line (mouse)	Kawahara and Mieda-Sato (2012)
miR-133b	Spinal cord regeneration	RhoA	Zebrafish	Yu et al. (2011)
miR-134	Neuronal development and dendritogenesis	Pumilio2	Mouse	Fiore et al. (2009)
miR-138	Axonal regeneration	SIRT1	Mouse	Liu et al. (2013)
miR-310	Neurotransmitter release at the NMJ	Khc-73	Fruit fly	Tsurudome et al. (2010)
miR-338-3p	Expression is elevated in ALS patients		ALS/human	De Felice et al. (2012)
miR-431	Axonal regeneration and outgrowth	Kremen1	Mouse	Wu and Murashov (2013)
miR-451	Dysregulated in immune cells (with many other miRNAs)		ALS/mouse	Butovsky et al. (2012)

based on the age of onset and achieved motor abilities: Type I SMA (Werdnig–Hoffmann), intermediate Type II SMA, mild Type III SMA (Kugelberg–Welander), and Type IV SMA (adult SMA; Pearn, 1980; Wirth et al., 2013).

Survival of motor neuron 1 (*SMN1*) is the major disease-determining gene of SMA. SMA is caused by homozygous deletion or mutation of *SMN1* (Lefebvre et al., 1995). This gene is located on the chromosomal region 5q11.2-13.3 in a segment of ~500 kb, which includes the telomeric *SMN1* and the similar but slightly different centromeric *SMN2*. *SMN2*, which is >99% identical to *SMN1*, has only a reduced capacity for correct splicing due to a single silent mutation in exon7. *SMN2* produces about 10% of full-length *SMN2* RNA that encodes a protein identical to the one from *SMN1*. *SMN2*, which can vary from one to six copies per genome, is the main modifier of SMA and influences on SMA severity. The severity of SMA can be affected by various genetic factors (Wirth et al., 2013). The human SMN protein is a 38 kDa protein, which forms multi-protein complex with its binding partners, seven Gemins (Gemin 2–8). Self-oligomerization of SMN creates the backbone of the complex (Battle et al., 2006). SMN is ubiquitously expressed and can be found in the nucleus as well as in the axons and dendrites of neurons (Cougot et al., 2008; Akten et al., 2011). In the nucleus, SMN is localized in subcellular structures called gems, where it interacts with a number of proteins that are essential for RNA processing and splicing (Pellizzoni et al., 1998). In the axons, SMN interacts with RNA-binding proteins, such as HuD, and plays a role in RNP trafficking for local mRNA translation (Akten et al., 2011; Fallini et al., 2011). SMN also binds to FMRP (Piazzon et al., 2008), KH-type splicing regulatory protein (KSRP; Tadesse et al., 2008) and fused in sarcoma (FUS; Yamazaki et al., 2012), which are important for miRNA biogenesis and function.

AMYOTROPHIC LATERAL SCLEROSIS

Amyotrophic lateral sclerosis (ALS) is a progressive neurodegenerative disorder, which leads to death within 2–3 years of onset. It is one of the most common motor neuron diseases occurring 1.7 ~ 2.3 out of 100,000 person per year in worldwide (Beghi et al., 2006). The symptom of ALS usually starts after age 50, but it can happen in younger age group. The disease manifests itself by onset of degeneration in specific subset of motor neurons. It progressively spreads to neighboring motor neurons and leads to atrophy of associated muscle tissues (Pratt et al., 2012). The genetic and environmental causes of ALS is still under investigation, but 90% of them are sporadic or from unknown genetic factors. So far only about 10% of the cases can be traced to genetic factors (Al-Chalabi et al., 2012). The most well known genetic cause of ALS is mutations in or deletion of Cu/Zn Super Oxide Dismutase 1 (*SOD1*; Rosen et al., 1993). Only recently, with advanced genomic screening tools, several other genes associated with ALS have been identified including TAR DNA-binding protein (*TDP-43*), *FUS*, ALS 2 (*ALS2*), neurofilament heavy peptide (*NEFH*; Al-Chalabi et al., 2012) and C9ORF72 (DeJesus-Hernandez et al., 2011; Renton et al., 2011). However, the cellular and pathological mechanisms causing ALS due to mutation or deletion of these genes are still under investigation.

miRNA IN MOTOR NEURON DISEASES

The role of miRNA and their target genes are intensively studied in cancer field. Studies in cancer cells suggest us that miRNA are involved in many different pathways and their dysregulation can cause various types of cancers (Esteller, 2011; Jansson and Lund, 2012). While the role of individual miRNAs in neurological disorders is not yet fully understood, there are growing evidences that miRNAs play a critical role in neurological disorders, such as miR-206/miR-153 in Alzheimer's disease (Lee et al., 2012; Liang et al., 2012), miR-34b/miR-9/miR-9* in Huntington's disease (Packer et al., 2008; Gaughwin et al., 2011), miR-128a/miR-24/let-7b in mood disorder (Zhou et al., 2009), miR-189 in Tourette's syndrome (Abelson et al., 2005), miR-9 in SMA (Haramati et al., 2010), miR-106/miR-338-3p/miR-451 in ALS (Williams et al., 2009; Butovsky et al., 2012; De Felice et al., 2012), miR-21/miR-431/miR-138 for axonal regeneration for sensory neurons (Strickland et al., 2011; Liu et al., 2013; Wu and Murashov, 2013), and miR-133b/miR-21 for spinal cord injury (Yu et al., 2011; Hu et al., 2013). However, pathological contribution of individual miRNAs to each of these diseases is still under investigation. Especially, our knowledge about the role of miRNAs in motor neuron diseases is very limited. This can be both due to the complexity of the nervous system and the technical difficulties of studying neurological disorders. In this section, we will focus on miRNA related dysregulation in two motor neuron diseases; SMA, and ALS.

miRNA IN SPINAL MUSCULAR ATROPHY PATHOLOGY

As it is mentioned above, SMN is a RNA binding protein, which forms a complex with other Gemin proteins, Gemin2-8 (Battle et al., 2006). Among the Gemins, Gemin3 and Gemin4 also bind to Ago2, which served the core protein in RISC and plays a role in miRNA biogenesis (Mourelatos et al., 2002). Moreover, numerous miRNAs bind to Gemin3 in human and murine neuronal cell lines (Dostie et al., 2003). From these reports, we can reason that the SMN complex is involved in miRNA biogenesis and/or function. In fact, expression of miRNAs such as miR-9 and miR-9* were dysregulated in murine embryonic stem cell derived motor neurons harboring a mutation causing SMA (Haramati et al., 2010). However, cellular mechanisms underlying in SMN mediated miRNA expression and/or function is not yet identified.

Dicer is an RNase playing a role in miRNA biogenesis pathway. The enzyme acts on the stem-loop shape of precursor miRNA (pre-miR) and creates a doubles stranded-miRNAs by cleaving the loop structure off from the pre-miR (Bernstein et al., 2001). It seems that a group of miRNAs get mature by Dicer, while other subset of miRNAs are processed by Ago2 (Cheloufi et al., 2010). Thus, deletion of either Dicer or Ago2 protein in cell may lead to severe impairments in miRNA biogenesis and function. In fact, deletion of Dicer in post-mitotic motor neuron causes motor neuron degeneration, similar to the neuromuscular phenotype observed in mouse model for SMA (Haramati et al., 2010).

miRNA IN AMYOTROPHIC LATERAL SCLEROSIS PATHOLOGY

Dysregulation in miRNA expression and miRNA-related pathways are also reported in ALS. The expression of miR-206, a skeletal muscle specific miRNA, was increased in muscle after denervation of sciatic nerve and its deficiency synergistically worsened disease progress in ALS mouse model harboring a disease causing mutation in superoxide dismutase, *SOD1*. In this study, the elevated expression of miR-206 after denervation promotes reinnervation process at the NMJ via regulating histone deacetylase 4 (*HDAC4*) and fibroblast growth factor (FGF) pathway (Williams et al., 2009).

This study is the first report suggesting the role of miRNA for nerve regeneration at the NMJ. Recently, additional report showed that the expression of miR-23a, miR-29b, and miR-455 are elevated in skeletal muscle tissues from ALS patients and this may cause dysregulation in mitochondrial gene expression (Russell et al., 2012). These findings hint us that dysregulated expression of miRNA in muscle cells significantly contributes to ALS pathology.

Another ALS associated gene, TAR DNA-binding protein-43 (TDP-43) is directly involved in miRNA pathway. TDP-43 is a component of the Dicer and Drosha complexes, which are important for miRNA biogenesis. TDP-43 selectively regulates pri-miRNA processing by binding to primary transcripts of specific miRNAs. It is reported that mutations in *TDP-43* gene causes differential expression of mature and functional miRNAs such as miR-132, miR-143 and miR-558 that in turn contribute to ALS pathology. Interestingly, TDP-43 deficiency caused impairment in neurite outgrowth in Neuro2a cells and it was rescued by over-expressing miR-132 (Kawahara and Mieda-Sato, 2012). Additionally, elevated expression of miR-9 is also observed in induced pluripotent stem cell-derived neurons from ALS patient harboring a mutation in *TDP-43* (Zhang et al., 2013). Together, these data suggest that TDP-43 is required for neuronal differentiation and neurite outgrowth via regulating miRNA biogenesis pathway and their expression.

Mutations in RNA binding protein FUS/TLS (FUS/translocated in liposarcoma) are also found in ALS patients (Kwiatkowski et al., 2009). Similar to TDP-43, FUS/TLS protein binds to pre-mRNA molecules and determines their fate via regulating splicing, transport, stability, and translation (Lagier-Tourenne et al., 2012). Recently, it has been shown that FUS/TLS promotes biogenesis of specific miRNAs via recruiting Drosha to primary miRNA transcripts. Among them, miRNAs with known function for synaptic plasticity and neuronal development such as miR-132, miR-134, and miR-9 were identified (Morlando et al., 2012). miR-9 regulates axon growth via direct regulation of microtubule-associated protein 1b (MAP1B) mRNA translation and miR-132 regulates neuronal morphology and growth by targeting various genes including acetylcholinesterase and Tau (Edbauer et al., 2010; Smith et al., 2011; Dajas-Bailador et al., 2012; Hebert et al., 2012; Shaltiel et al., 2013). miR-134 regulates neuronal development and dendritogenesis in response to neuronal activity (Fiore et al., 2009). These results suggest that mutations in FUS/TLS may lead to disturbance in miRNA biogenesis and function, which contributes to pathological phenotype observed in ALS patients.

In addition to it, miRNA expression in white blood cells from sporadic ALS patients exhibited distinct expression pattern during disease progress. miRNA profiling data from 14 patients and 14 controls showed that expression of miR-338-3p is increased and expression of seven other miRNAs is decreased in leukocyte from ALS patients (De Felice et al., 2012). Since bloods are more accessible than motor neurons from patients, this finding suggests that profiling of miRNA expression from bloods can be used as a diagnostic tool for ALS. Taken together, we can conclude that dysregulated miRNA expression contributes to the ALS pathology and profiling of the miRNA expression can serve as a tool for ALS diagnosis.

SUMMARY AND PERSPECTIVE

With current advanced genetic tools, genetic causes of motor neuron diseases are getting unveiled. However, pathogenesis of motor neuron disease is extremely complex and not yet fully understood. Due to this reason, efficient cure for motor neuron disease is currently unavailable. Interestingly, even though the genetic causes of the diseases are different, their cellular pathomechanisms share common traits; miRNA biogenesis and expression. Here, we reviewed current knowledge about the role of miRNA in two common motor neuron diseases, SMA and ALS. Dysregulated miRNA expression in neuromuscular system may lead to neurodegeneration and disease pathology. However, the question, how individual miRNAs contribute to development and maintenance of the NMJ and how their dysregulation may cause ALS or SMA, requires further investigation.

ACKNOWLEDGMENT

Our work is supported by Institute of Human Genetics, University of Cologne.

REFERENCES

Abelson, J. F., Kwan, K. Y., O'Roak, B. J., Baek, D. Y., Stillman, A. A., Morgan, T. M., et al. (2005). Sequence variants in SLITRK1 are associated with Tourette's syndrome. *Science* 310, 317–320. doi: 10.1126/science.1116502

Akerblom, M., Sachdeva, R., Barde, I., Verp, S., Gentner, B., Trono, D., et al. (2012). MicroRNA-124 is a subventricular zone neuronal fate determinant. *J. Neurosci.* 32, 8879–8889. doi: 10.1523/JNEUROSCI.0558-12.2012

Akten, B., Kye, M. J., Hao Le, T., Wertz, M. H., Singh, S., Nie, D., et al. (2011). Interaction of survival of motor neuron (SMN) and HuD proteins with mRNA cpg15 rescues motor neuron axonal deficits. *Proc. Natl. Acad. Sci. U.S.A.* 108, 10337–10342. doi: 10.1073/pnas.1104928108

Al-Chalabi, A., Jones, A., Troakes, C., King, A., Al-Sarraj, S., and Van Den Berg, L. H. (2012). The genetics and neuropathology of amyotrophic lateral sclerosis. *Acta Neuropathol.* 124, 339–352. doi: 10.1007/s00401-012-1022-4

Bail, S., Swerdel, M., Liu, H., Jiao, X., Goff, L. A., Hart, R. P., et al. (2010). Differential regulation of microRNA stability. *RNA* 16, 1032–1039. doi: 10.1261/rna.1851510

Bartel, D. P. (2009). MicroRNAs: target recognition and regulatory functions. *Cell* 136, 215–233. doi: 10.1016/j.cell.2009.01.002

Battle, D. J., Kasim, M., Yong, J., Lotti, F., Lau, C. K., Mouaikel, J., et al. (2006). The SMN complex: an assembly machine for RNPs. *Cold. Spring Harb. Symp. Quant. Biol.* 71, 313–320. doi: 10.1101/sqb.2006.71.001

Beghi, E., Logroscino, G., Chio, A., Hardiman, O., Mitchell, D., Swingler, R., et al. (2006). The epidemiology of ALS and the role of population-based registries. *Biochim. Biophys. Acta* 1762, 1150–1157. doi: 10.1016/j.bbadis.2006.09.008

Bernstein, E., Caudy, A. A., Hammond, S. M., and Hannon, G. J. (2001). Role for a bidentate ribonuclease in the initiation step of RNA interference. *Nature* 409, 363–366. doi: 10.1038/35053110

Bernstein, E., Kim, S. Y., Carmell, M. A., Murchison, E. P., Alcorn, H., Li, M. Z., et al. (2003). Dicer is essential for mouse development. *Nat. Genet.* 35, 215–217. doi: 10.1038/ng1253

Butovsky, O., Siddiqui, S., Gabriely, G., Lanser, A. J., Dake, B., Murugaiyan, G., et al. (2012). Modulating inflammatory monocytes with a unique microRNA gene signature ameliorates murine ALS. *J. Clin. Invest.* 122, 3063–3087. doi: 10.1172/JCI62636

Caygill, E. E., and Johnston, L. A. (2008). Temporal regulation of metamorphic processes in *Drosophila* by the let-7 and miR-125 heterochronic microRNAs. *Curr. Biol.* 18, 943–950. doi: 10.1016/j.cub.2008.06.020

Chatterjee, S., Fasler, M., Bussing, I., and Grosshans, H. (2011). Target-mediated protection of endogenous microRNAs in *C. elegans*. *Dev. Cell* 20, 388–396. doi: 10.1016/j.devcel.2011.02.008

Cheloufi, S., Dos Santos, C. O., Chong, M. M., and Hannon, G. J. (2010). A dicer-independent miRNA biogenesis pathway that requires Ago catalysis. *Nature* 465, 584–589. doi: 10.1038/nature09092

Chen, C. Z., Li, L., Lodish, H. F., and Bartel, D. P. (2004). MicroRNAs modulate hematopoietic lineage differentiation. *Science* 303, 83–86. doi: 10.1126/science.1091903

Chen, J. A., Huang, Y. P., Mazzoni, E. O., Tan, G. C., Zavadil, J., and Wichterle, H. (2011). Mir-17-3p controls spinal neural progenitor patterning by regulating Olig2/Irx3 cross-repressive loop. *Neuron* 69, 721–735. doi: 10.1016/j.neuron.2011.01.014

Conaco, C., Otto, S., Han, J. J., and Mandel, G. (2006). Reciprocal actions of REST and a microRNA promote neuronal identity. *Proc. Natl. Acad. Sci. U.S.A.* 103, 2422–2427. doi: 10.1073/pnas.0511041103

Cougot, N., Bhattacharyya, S. N., Tapia-Arancibia, L., Bordonne, R., Filipowicz, W., Bertrand, E., et al. (2008). Dendrites of mammalian neurons contain specialized P-body-like structures that respond to neuronal activation. *J. Neurosci.* 28, 13793–13804. doi: 10.1523/JNEUROSCI.4155-08.2008

Crawford, T. O., and Pardo, C. A. (1996). The neurobiology of childhood spinal muscular atrophy. *Neurobiol. Dis.* 3, 97–110. doi: 10.1006/nbdi.1996.0010

Dajas-Bailador, F., Bonev, B., Garcez, P., Stanley, P., Guillemot, F., and Papalopulu, N. (2012). microRNA-9 regulates axon extension and branching by targeting Map1b in mouse cortical neurons. *Nat. Neurosci.* doi: 10.1038/nn.3082 [Epub ahead of print].

De Felice, B., Guida, M., Coppola, C., De Mieri, G., and Cotrufo, R. (2012). A miRNA signature in leukocytes from sporadic amyotrophic lateral sclerosis. *Gene* 508, 35–40. doi: 10.1016/j.gene.2012.07.058

DeJesus-Hernandez, M., Mackenzie, I. R., Boeve, B. F., Boxer, A. L., Baker, M., Rutherford, N. J., et al. (2011). Expanded GGGGCC hexanucleotide repeat in noncoding region of C9ORF72 causes chromosome 9p-linked FTD and ALS. *Neuron* 72, 245–256. doi: 10.1016/j.neuron.2011.09.011

Dostie, J., Mourelatos, Z., Yang, M., Sharma, A., and Dreyfuss, G. (2003). Numerous microRNPs in neuronal cells containing novel microRNAs. *RNA* 9, 180–186. doi: 10.1261/rna.2141503

Edbauer, D., Neilson, J. R., Foster, K. A., Wang, C. F., Seeburg, D. P., Batterton, M. N., et al. (2010). Regulation of synaptic structure and function by FMRP-associated microRNAs miR-125b and miR-132. *Neuron* 65, 373–384. doi: 10.1016/j.neuron.2010.01.005

Esteller, M. (2011). Non-coding RNAs in human disease. *Nat. Rev. Genet.* 12, 861–874. doi: 10.1038/nrg3074

Eulalio, A., Huntzinger, E., and Izaurralde, E. (2008). GW182 interaction with Argonaute is essential for miRNA-mediated translational repression and mRNA decay. *Nat. Struct. Mol. Biol.* 15, 346–353. doi: 10.1038/nsmb.1405

Fallini, C., Zhang, H., Su, Y., Silani, V., Singer, R. H., Rossoll, W., et al. (2011). The survival of motor neuron (SMN) protein interacts with the mRNA-binding protein HuD and regulates localization of poly(A) mRNA in primary motor neuron axons. *J. Neurosci.* 31, 3914–3925. doi: 10.1523/JNEUROSCI.3631-10.2011

Fiore, R., Khudayberdiev, S., Christensen, M., Siegel, G., Flavell, S. W., Kim, T. K., et al. (2009). Mef2-mediated transcription of the miR379-410 cluster regulates activity-dependent dendritogenesis by fine-tuning Pumilio2 protein levels. *EMBO J.* 28, 697–710. doi: 10.1038/emboj.2009.10

Forterre, A., Jalabert, A., Chikh, K., Pesenti, S., Euthine, V., Granjon, A., et al. (2013). Myotube-derived exosomal miRNAs downregulate Sirtuin1 in myoblasts during muscle cell differentiation. *Cell Cycle* 13, 78–89. doi: 10.4161/cc.26808

Fruhbeis, C., Frohlich, D., Kuo, W. P., Amphornrat, J., Thilemann, S., Saab, A. S., et al. (2013). Neurotransmitter-triggered transfer of exosomes mediates oligodendrocyte-neuron communication. *PLoS Biol.* 11:e1001604. doi: 10.1371/journal.pbio.1001604

Gao, J., Wang, W. Y., Mao, Y. W., Graff, J., Guan, J. S., Pan, L., et al. (2010). A novel pathway regulates memory and plasticity via SIRT1 and miR-134. *Nature* 466, 1105–1109. doi: 10.1038/nature09271

Gao, P., Tchernyshyov, I., Chang, T. C., Lee, Y. S., Kita, K., Ochi, T., et al. (2009). c-Myc suppression of miR-23a/b enhances mitochondrial glutaminase expression and glutamine metabolism. *Nature* 458, 762–765. doi: 10.1038/nature07823

Gaughwin, P. M., Ciesla, M., Lahiri, N., Tabrizi, S. J., Brundin, P., and Bjorkqvist, M. (2011). Hsa-miR-34b is a plasma-stable microRNA that is elevated in pre-manifest Huntington's disease. *Hum. Mol. Genet.* 20, 2225–2237. doi: 10.1093/hmg/ddr111

Grange, C., Tapparo, M., Collino, F., Vitillo, L., Damasco, C., Deregibus, M. C., et al. (2011). Microvesicles released from human renal cancer stem cells stimulate angiogenesis and formation of lung premetastatic niche. *Cancer Res.* 71, 5346–5356. doi: 10.1158/0008-5472.CAN-11-0241

Haramati, S., Chapnik, E., Sztainberg, Y., Eilam, R., Zwang, R., Gershoni, N., et al. (2010). miRNA malfunction causes spinal motor neuron disease. *Proc. Natl. Acad. Sci. U.S.A.* 107, 13111–13116. doi: 10.1073/pnas.1006151107

Hatfield, S. D., Shcherbata, H. R., Fischer, K. A., Nakahara, K., Carthew, R. W., and Ruohola-Baker, H. (2005). Stem cell division is regulated by the microRNA pathway. *Nature* 435, 974–978. doi: 10.1038/nature03816

Hebert, S. S., Sergeant, N., and Buee, L. (2012). MicroRNAs and the regulation of Tau metabolism. *Int. J. Alzheimers Dis.* 2012, 406561. doi: 10.1155/2012/406561

Hornstein, E., Mansfield, J. H., Yekta, S., Hu, J. K., Harfe, B. D., McManus, M. T., et al. (2005). The microRNA miR-196 acts upstream of Hoxb8 and Shh in limb development. *Nature* 438, 671–674. doi: 10.1038/nature04138

Houbaviy, H. B., Murray, M. F., and Sharp, P. A. (2003). Embryonic stem cell-specific MicroRNAs. *Dev. Cell* 5, 351–358. doi: 10.1016/S1534-5807(03)00227-2

Hu, J. Z., Huang, J. H., Zeng, L., Wang, G., Cao, M., and Lu, H. B. (2013). Anti-apoptotic effect of microRNA-21 after contusion spinal cord injury in rats. *J. Neurotrauma* 30, 1349–1360. doi: 10.1089/neu.2012.2748

Huntzinger, E., and Izaurralde, E. (2011). Gene silencing by microRNAs: contributions of translational repression and mRNA decay. *Nat. Rev. Genet.* 12, 99–110. doi: 10.1038/nrg2936

Iio, A., Takagi, T., Miki, K., Naoe, T., Nakayama, A., and Akao, Y. (2013). DDX6 post-transcriptionally down-regulates miR-143/145 expression through host gene NCR143/145 in cancer cells. *Biochim. Biophys. Acta* 1829, 1102–1110. doi: 10.1016/j.bbagrm.2013.07.010

Jansson, M. D., and Lund, A. H. (2012). MicroRNA and cancer. *Mol. Oncol.* 6, 590–610. doi: 10.1016/j.molonc.2012.09.006

Jin, P., Zarnescu, D. C., Ceman, S., Nakamoto, M., Mowrey, J., Jongens, T. A., et al. (2004). Biochemical and genetic interaction between the fragile X mental retardation protein and the microRNA pathway. *Nat. Neurosci.* 7, 113–117. doi: 10.1038/nn1174

Kawahara, Y., and Mieda-Sato, A. (2012). TDP-43 promotes microRNA biogenesis as a component of the Drosha and Dicer complexes. *Proc. Natl. Acad. Sci. U.S.A.* 109, 3347–3352. doi: 10.1073/pnas.1112427109

Kim, V. N., Han, J., and Siomi, M. C. (2009). Biogenesis of small RNAs in animals. *Nat. Rev. Mol. Cell Biol.* 10, 126–139. doi: 10.1038/nrm2632

Krol, J., Loedige, I., and Filipowicz, W. (2010). The widespread regulation of microRNA biogenesis, function and decay. *Nat. Rev. Genet.* 11, 597–610. doi:10.1038/nrg2843

Kwiatkowski, T. J. Jr., Bosco, D. A., Leclerc, A. L., Tamrazian, E., Vanderburg, C. R., Russ, C., et al. (2009). Mutations in the FUS/TLS gene on chromosome 16 cause familial amyotrophic lateral sclerosis. *Science* 323, 1205–1208. doi: 10.1126/science.1166066

Kye, M. J., Liu, T., Levy, S. F., Xu, N. L., Groves, B. B., Bonneau, R., et al. (2007). Somatodendritic microRNAs identified by laser capture and multiplex RT-PCR. *RNA* 13, 1224–1234. doi: 10.1261/rna.480407

Lagier-Tourenne, C., Polymenidou, M., Hutt, K. R., Vu, A. Q., Baughn, M., Huelga, S. C., et al. (2012). Divergent roles of ALS-linked proteins FUS/TLS and TDP-43 intersect in processing long pre-mRNAs. *Nat. Neurosci.* 15, 1488–1497. doi: 10.1038/nn.3230

Landthaler, M., Gaidatzis, D., Rothballer, A., Chen, P. Y., Soll, S. J., Dinic, L., et al. (2008). Molecular characterization of human Argonaute-containing ribonucleoprotein complexes and their bound target mRNAs. *RNA* 14, 2580–2596. doi: 10.1261/rna.1351608

Lee, S. T., Chu, K., Jung, K. H., Kim, J. H., Huh, J. Y., Yoon, H., et al. (2012). miR-206 regulates brain-derived neurotrophic factor in Alzheimer disease model. *Ann. Neurol.* 72, 269–277. doi: 10.1002/ana.23588

Lefebvre, S., Burglen, L., Reboullet, S., Clermont, O., Burlet, P., Viollet, L., et al. (1995). Identification and characterization of a spinal muscular atrophy-determining gene. *Cell* 80, 155–165. doi: 10.1016/0092-8674(95)90460-3

Liang, C., Zhu, H., Xu, Y., Huang, L., Ma, C., Deng, W., et al. (2012). MicroRNA-153 negatively regulates the expression of amyloid precursor protein and amyloid precursor-like protein 2. *Brain Res.* 1455, 103–113. doi: 10.1016/j.brainres.2011.10.051

Liu, C. M., Wang, R. Y., Saijilafu, Jiao, Z. X., Zhang, B. Y., and Zhou, F. Q. (2013). MicroRNA-138 and SIRT1 form a mutual negative feedback loop to regulate mammalian axon regeneration. *Genes Dev.* 27, 1473–1483. doi: 10.1101/gad.209619.112

Morita, S., Horii, T., Kimura, M., Goto, Y., Ochiya, T., and Hatada, I. (2007). One Argonaute family member, Eif2c2 (Ago2), is essential for development and appears not to be involved in DNA methylation. *Genomics* 89, 687–696. doi: 10.1016/j.ygeno.2007.01.004

Morlando, M., Dini Modigliani, S., Torrelli, G., Rosa, A., Di Carlo, V., Caffarelli, E., et al. (2012). FUS stimulates microRNA biogenesis by facilitating co-transcriptional Drosha recruitment. *EMBO J.* 31, 4502–4510. doi: 10.1038/emboj.2012.319

Mourelatos, Z., Dostie, J., Paushkin, S., Sharma, A., Charroux, B., Abel, L., et al. (2002). miRNPs: a novel class of ribonucleoproteins containing numerous microRNAs. *Genes Dev.* 16, 720–728. doi: 10.1101/gad.974702

Naguibneva, I., Ameyar-Zazoua, M., Polesskaya, A., Ait-Si-Ali, S., Groisman, R., Souidi, M., et al. (2006). The microRNA miR-181 targets the homeobox protein Hox-A11 during mammalian myoblast differentiation. *Nat. Cell Biol.* 8, 278–284. doi: 10.1038/ncb1373

Natera-Naranjo, O., Aschrafi, A., Gioio, A. E., and Kaplan, B. B. (2010). Identification and quantitative analyses of microRNAs located in the distal axons of sympathetic neurons. *RNA* 16, 1516–1529. doi: 10.1261/rna.1833310

Nesler, K. R., Sand, R. I., Symmes, B. A., Pradhan, S. J., Boin, N. G., Laun, A. E., et al. (2013). The miRNA pathway controls rapid changes in activity-dependent synaptic structure at the *Drosophila melanogaster* neuromuscular junction. *PLoS ONE* 8:e68385. doi: 10.1371/journal.pone.0068385

Otaegi, G., Pollock, A., Hong, J., and Sun, T. (2011a). MicroRNA miR-9 modifies motor neuron columns by a tuning regulation of FoxP1 levels in developing spinal cords. *J. Neurosci.* 31, 809–818. doi: 10.1523/JNEUROSCI.4330-10.2011

Otaegi, G., Pollock, A., and Sun, T. (2011b). An optimized sponge for microRNA miR-9 affects spinal motor neuron development in vivo. *Front. Neurosci.* 5:146. doi: 10.3389/fnins.2011.00146

Packer, A. N., Xing, Y., Harper, S. Q., Jones, L., and Davidson, B. L. (2008). The bifunctional microRNA miR-9/miR-9* regulates REST and CoREST and is downregulated in Huntington's disease. *J. Neurosci.* 28, 14341–14346. doi: 10.1523/JNEUROSCI.2390-08.2008

Pearn, J. (1980). Classification of spinal muscular atrophies. *Lancet* 1, 919–922. doi: 10.1016/S0140-6736(80)90847-8

Pellizzoni, L., Kataoka, N., Charroux, B., and Dreyfuss, G. (1998). A novel function for SMN, the spinal muscular atrophy disease gene product, in pre-mRNA splicing. *Cell* 95, 615–624. doi: 10.1016/S0092-8674(00)81632-3

Piazzon, N., Rage, F., Schlotter, F., Moine, H., Branlant, C., and Massenet, S. (2008). In vitro and in cellulo evidences for association of the survival of motor neuron complex with the fragile X mental retardation protein. *J. Biol. Chem.* 283, 5598–5610. doi: 10.1074/jbc.M707304200

Pratt, A. J., Getzoff, E. D., and Perry, J. J. (2012). Amyotrophic lateral sclerosis: update and new developments. *Degener. Neurol. Neuromuscul. Dis.* 2012, 1–14.

Renton, A. E., Majounie, E., Waite, A., Simon-Sanchez, J., Rollinson, S., Gibbs, J. R., et al. (2011). A hexanucleotide repeat expansion in C9ORF72 is the cause of chromosome 9p21-linked ALS-FTD. *Neuron* 72, 257–268. doi: 10.1016/j.neuron.2011.09.010

Rosen, D. R., Siddique, T., Patterson, D., Figlewicz, D. A., Sapp, P., Hentati, A., et al. (1993). Mutations in Cu/Zn superoxide dismutase gene are associated with familial amyotrophic lateral sclerosis. *Nature* 362, 59–62. doi: 10.1038/362059a0

Ruegger, S., and Grosshans, H. (2012). MicroRNA turnover: when, how, and why. *Trends Biochem. Sci.* 37, 436–446. doi: 10.1016/j.tibs.2012.07.002

Russell, A. P., Wada, S., Vergani, L., Hock, M. B., Lamon, S., Leger, B., et al. (2012). Disruption of skeletal muscle mitochondrial network genes and miRNAs in amyotrophic lateral sclerosis. *Neurobiol. Dis.* 49C, 107–117. doi: 10.1016/j.nbd.2012.08.015

Sasaki, Y., Gross, C., Xing, L., Goshima, Y., and Bassell, G. J. (2013). Identification of axon-enriched microRNAs localized to growth cones of cortical neurons. *Dev. Neurobiol.* doi: 10.1002/dneu.22113 [Epub ahead of print].

Shaltiel, G., Hanan, M., Wolf, Y., Barbash, S., Kovalev, E., Shoham, S., et al. (2013). Hippocampal microRNA-132 mediates stress-inducible cognitive deficits through its acetylcholinesterase target. *Brain Struct. Funct.* 218, 59–72. doi: 10.1007/s00429-011-0376-z

Sharma, P., Schiapparelli, L., and Cline, H. T. (2013). Exosomes function in cell-cell communication during brain circuit development. *Curr. Opin. Neurobiol.* 23, 997–1004. doi: 10.1016/j.conb.2013.08.005

Smith, P. Y., Delay, C., Girard, J., Papon, M. A., Planel, E., Sergeant, N., et al. (2011). MicroRNA-132 loss is associated with tau exon 10 inclusion in progressive supranuclear palsy. *Hum. Mol. Genet.* 20, 4016–4024. doi: 10.1093/hmg/ddr330

Soldevilla, B., Rodriguez, M., San Millan, C., Garcia, V., Fernandez-Perianez, R., Gil-Calderon, B., et al. (2013). Tumor-derived exosomes are enriched in DeltaNp73, which promotes oncogenic potential in acceptor cells and correlates with patient survival. *Hum. Mol. Genet.* 23, 467–478. doi: 10.1093/hmg/ddt437

Strickland, I. T., Richards, L., Holmes, F. E., Wynick, D., Uney, J. B., and Wong, L. F. (2011). Axotomy-induced miR-21 promotes axon growth in adult dorsal root ganglion neurons. *PLoS ONE* 6:e23423. doi: 10.1371/journal.pone.0023423

Sun, K., Westholm, J. O., Tsurudome, K., Hagen, J. W., Lu, Y., Kohwi, M., et al. (2012). Neurophysiological defects and neuronal gene deregulation in *Drosophila* mir-124 mutants. *PLoS Genet.* 8:e1002515. doi: 10.1371/journal.pgen.1002515

Tadesse, H., Deschenes-Furry, J., Boisvenue, S., and Cote, J. (2008). KH-type splicing regulatory protein interacts with survival motor neuron protein and is misregulated in spinal muscular atrophy. *Hum. Mol. Genet.* 17, 506–524. doi: 10.1093/hmg/ddm327

Tsurudome, K., Tsang, K., Liao, E. H., Ball, R., Penney, J., Yang, J. S., et al. (2010). The *Drosophila* miR-310 cluster negatively regulates synaptic strength at the neuromuscular junction. *Neuron* 68, 879–893. doi: 10.1016/j.neuron.2010.11.016

Valadi, H., Ekstrom, K., Bossios, A., Sjostrand, M., Lee, J. J., and Lotvall, J. O. (2007). Exosome-mediated transfer of mRNAs and microRNAs is a novel mechanism of genetic exchange between cells. *Nat. Cell Biol.* 9, 654–659. doi: 10.1038/ncb1596

Wang, Y., Medvid, R., Melton, C., Jaenisch, R., and Blelloch, R. (2007). DGCR8 is essential for microRNA biogenesis and silencing of embryonic stem cell self-renewal. *Nat. Genet.* 39, 380–385. doi: 10.1038/ng1969

Williams, A. H., Valdez, G., Moresi, V., Qi, X., McAnally, J., Elliott, J. L., et al. (2009). MicroRNA-206 delays ALS progression and promotes regeneration of neuromuscular synapses in mice. *Science* 326, 1549–1554. doi: 10.1126/science.1181046

Wirth, B., Brichta, L., and Hahnen, E. (2006). Spinal muscular atrophy: from gene to therapy. *Semin. Pediatr. Neurol.* 13, 121–131. doi: 10.1016/j.spen.2006.06.008

Wirth, B., Garbes, L., and Riessland, M. (2013). How genetic modifiers influence the phenotype of spinal muscular atrophy and suggest future therapeutic approaches. *Curr. Opin. Genet. Dev.* 23, 330–338. doi: 10.1016/j.gde.2013.03.003

Wu, D., and Murashov, A. K. (2013). MicroRNA-431 regulates axon regeneration in mature sensory neurons by targeting the Wnt antagonist Kremen1. *Front. Mol. Neurosci.* 6:35. doi: 10.3389/fnmol.2013.00035

Wu, D., Raafat, A., Pak, E., Clemens, S., and Murashov, A. K. (2012). Dicer-microRNA pathway is critical for peripheral nerve regeneration and functional recovery in vivo and regenerative axonogenesis in vitro. *Exp. Neurol.* 233, 555–565. doi: 10.1016/j.expneurol.2011.11.041

Xiao, C., Calado, D. P., Galler, G., Thai, T. H., Patterson, H. C., Wang, J., et al. (2007). MiR-150 controls B cell differentiation by targeting the transcription factor c-Myb. *Cell* 131, 146–159. doi: 10.1016/j.cell.2007.07.021

Yamazaki, T., Chen, S., Yu, Y., Yan, B., Haertlein, T. C., Carrasco, M. A., et al. (2012). FUS-SMN protein interactions link the motor neuron diseases ALS and SMA. *Cell Rep.* 2, 799–806. doi: 10.1016/j.celrep.2012.08.025

Yu, Y. M., Gibbs, K. M., Davila, J., Campbell, N., Sung, S., Todorova, T. I., et al. (2011). MicroRNA miR-133b is essential for functional recovery after spinal cord injury in adult zebrafish. *Eur. J. Neurosci.* 33, 1587–1597. doi: 10.1111/j.1460-9568.2011.07643.x

Zekri, L., Huntzinger, E., Heimstadt, S., and Izaurralde, E. (2009). The silencing domain of GW182 interacts with PABPC1 to promote translational repression and degradation of microRNA targets and is required for target release. *Mol. Cell. Biol.* 29, 6220–6231. doi: 10.1128/MCB.01081-09

Zhang, Z., Almeida, S., Lu, Y., Nishimura, A. L., Peng, L., Sun, D., et al. (2013). Downregulation of MicroRNA-9 in iPSC-derived neurons of FTD/ALS patients with TDP-43 mutations. *PLoS ONE* 8:e76055. doi: 10.1371/journal.pone.0076055

Zhou, R., Yuan, P., Wang, Y., Hunsberger, J. G., Elkahloun, A., Wei, Y., et al. (2009). Evidence for selective microRNAs and their effectors as common long-term targets for the actions of mood stabilizers. *Neuropsychopharmacology* 34, 1395–1405. doi: 10.1038/npp.2008.131

Zhu, H., Bhattacharyya, B. J., Lin, H., and Gomez, C. M. (2013). Skeletal muscle calpain acts through nitric oxide and neural miRNAs to regulate acetylcholine release in motor nerve terminals. *J. Neurosci.* 33, 7308–7324. doi: 10.1523/JNEUROSCI.0224-13.2013

18

Elongation factor-2 phosphorylation in dendrites and the regulation of dendritic mRNA translation in neurons

Christopher Heise[1], Fabrizio Gardoni[2], Lorenza Culotta[1], Monica di Luca[2], Chiara Verpelli[1] and Carlo Sala[1,3]*

[1] CNR Institute of Neuroscience and Department of Biotechnology and Translational Medicine, University of Milan, Milan, Italy
[2] Department of Pharmacological and Biomolecular Sciences, University of Milan, Milan, Italy
[3] Neuromuscular Diseases and Neuroimmunology, Foundation Carlo Besta Neurological Institute, Milan, Italy

Correspondence:
Carlo Sala, CNR Institute of Neuroscience and Department of Biotechnology and Translational Medicine, University of Milan, Via Vanvitelli 32, 20129 Milan, Italy
e-mail: c.sala@in.cnr.it

Neuronal activity results in long lasting changes in synaptic structure and function by regulating mRNA translation in dendrites. These activity dependent events yield the synthesis of proteins known to be important for synaptic modifications and diverse forms of synaptic plasticity. Worthy of note, there is accumulating evidence that the eukaryotic Elongation Factor 2 Kinase (eEF2K)/eukaryotic Elongation Factor 2 (eEF2) pathway may be strongly involved in this process. Upon activation, eEF2K phosphorylates and thereby inhibits eEF2, resulting in a dramatic reduction of mRNA translation. eEF2K is activated by elevated levels of calcium and binding of Calmodulin (CaM), hence its alternative name calcium/CaM-dependent protein kinase III (CaMKIII). In dendrites, this process depends on glutamate signaling and N-methyl-D-aspartate receptor (NMDAR) activation. Interestingly, it has been shown that eEF2K can be activated in dendrites by metabotropic glutamate receptor (mGluR) 1/5 signaling, as well. Therefore, neuronal activity can induce local proteomic changes at the postsynapse by altering eEF2K activity. Well-established targets of eEF2K in dendrites include brain-derived neurotrophic factor (BDNF), activity-regulated cytoskeletal-associated protein (Arc), the alpha subunit of calcium/CaM-dependent protein kinase II (αCaMKII), and microtubule-associated protein 1B (MAP1B), all of which have well-known functions in different forms of synaptic plasticity. In this review we will give an overview of the involvement of the eEF2K/eEF2 pathway at dendrites in regulating the translation of dendritic mRNA in the context of altered NMDAR- and neuronal activity, and diverse forms of synaptic plasticity, such as metabotropic glutamate receptor-dependent-long-term depression (mGluR-LTD). For this, we draw on studies carried out both *in vitro* and *in vivo*.

Keywords: eEF2, eEF2K, translation, neurons, dendrites, synapses, synaptic plasticity

INTRODUCTION

The well conserved, ubiquitous eukaryotic Elongation Factor 2 kinase (eEF2K)/ eukaryotic Elongation Factor 2 (eEF2) pathway involves the phosphorylation and inactivation of eEF2 on Thr56 by eEF2K, thereby leading to an arrest of mRNA translation (Nairn et al., 1985; Mitsui et al., 1993; Ryazanov et al., 1997). Since eEF2K activity is regulated by calcium/CaM (Nairn et al., 1985; Mitsui et al., 1993), this pathway is of great interest to the field of neuroscience. Numerous papers have shown that dendritically localized eEF2K activity is altered by manipulating neuronal activity and glutamate signaling, owing to downstream events such as N-methyl-D-aspartate receptor (NMDAR) activation and subsequent increases in calcium levels (Marin et al., 1997; Scheetz et al., 2000; Lenz and Avruch, 2005; Maus et al., 2006; Sutton et al., 2007; Barrera et al., 2008; Autry et al., 2011), as well as metabotropic glutamate receptor (mGluR) activation (Park et al., 2008; Verpelli et al., 2010). Additionally, the eEF2K/eEF2 pathway is associated with diverse forms of synaptic plasticity (Chotiner et al., 2003; Kanhema et al., 2006; Davidkova and Carroll, 2007; Park et al., 2008; Seibt et al., 2012), most notably metabotropic glutamate receptor-dependent-long-term depression (mGluR-LTD), during which the pathway appears to regulate dendritic mRNA translation (Davidkova and Carroll, 2007; Park et al., 2008). Finally, while in general eEF2K activity and mRNA

Abbreviations: AMPAR, α-amino-3-hydroxy-5-methyl-4-isoxazolepropionic acid receptor; Arc, activity-regulated cytoskeletal-associated protein; BDNF, brain-derived neurotrophic factor; CaM, calmodulin; αCaMKII, alpha subunit of calcium/CaM-dependent protein kinase II; CaMKIII, calcium/CaM-dependent protein kinase III; cAMP, cyclic adenosine monophosphate; eEF2, eukaryotic Elongation Factor 2; eEF2K, eukaryotic Elongation Factor 2 Kinase; ERK, extracellular signal-regulated kinase; FMRP, fragile X mental retardation protein; GluR, glutamate receptor; LTD, long-term depression; LTP, long-term potentiation; MAP1B, microtubule-associated protein 1B; mGluR, metabotropic glutamate receptor; mGluR-LTD, metabotropic glutamate receptor-dependent-long-term depression; NMDAR, N-methyl-D-aspartate receptor; PI, phosphatase inhibitor; p70 S6K, p70S6 kinase; p90 RSK, p90 ribosomal S6 kinase; PKA, protein kinase A; SDS-PAGE, sodium dodecyl sulfate-polyacrylamide gel electrophoresis; TTX, tetrodotoxin.

translation are negatively correlated in dendrites (Scheetz et al., 2000; Sutton et al., 2007), for not well understood reasons the translation rate of certain proteins like microtubule-associated protein 1B (MAP1B), alpha subunit of calcium/CaM-dependent protein kinase II (αCaMKII), and activity-regulated cytoskeletal-associated protein (Arc) actually increases when eEF2K activity is elevated in the context of altered neuronal activity and synaptic plasticity paradigms (Scheetz et al., 2000; Chotiner et al., 2003; Davidkova and Carroll, 2007; Park et al., 2008; Autry et al., 2011). Since these upregulated proteins have well-known functions at the synapse and in synaptic plasticity (Zalfa et al., 2003; Davidkova and Carroll, 2007; Park et al., 2008; Dajas-Bailador et al., 2012; Lisman et al., 2012; Wibrand et al., 2012) this raises the exciting possibility that the eEF2K/eEF2 pathway may regulate mRNA translation dendritically in a more complex manner than elsewhere, especially during activity-dependent synaptic changes. This may have the purpose of implementing the kind of local proteomic modifications that are necessary for plastic changes to take place at the postsynapse, a conceivable scenario, considering that dendrites harbor the components that are necessary for protein translation (Asaki et al., 2003; Swanger and Bassell, 2013).

MANIPULATION OF N-METHYL-D-ASPARTATE RECEPTOR (NMDAR) SIGNALING AND NEURONAL ACTIVITY AFFECTS EUKARYOTIC ELONGATION FACTOR 2 KINASE (eEF2K)/EUKARYOTIC ELONGATION FACTOR 2 (eEF2) PATHWAY-DEPENDENT mRNA TRANSLATION IN DENDRITES

There are several studies which address an NMDAR-dependent eEF2K/eEF2 pathway activation and subsequent dendritic changes in mRNA translation. The NMDAR is an obvious target for manipulating the eEF2K/eEF2 pathway at dendrites since it is located at the postsynapse, is permeable to calcium and is a crucial element of several signaling pathways (Collingridge et al., 2004; Prybylowski et al., 2005; Kessels and Malinow, 2009; Traynelis et al., 2010). Similarly, the eEF2K/eEF2 pathway at dendrites may be activated by increased neuronal activity since it involves glutamate signaling, which in turn leads to an influx of calcium via glutamate receptors (GluRs) such as the NMDAR and the α-amino-3-hydroxy-5-methyl-4-isoxazolepropionic acid receptor (AMPAR) (Malenka and Bear, 2004; Bear et al., 2007; Major et al., 2013). Additionally, alterations in neuronal activity and associated glutamate signaling could trigger other forms of dendritic eEF2K/eEF2 pathway activation, e.g., due to stimulation of mGluRs (Davidkova and Carroll, 2007; Park et al., 2008) which will also be addressed in this article.

In one study (Scheetz et al., 2000), 30 s pulses of glutamate and NMDA were used to stimulate NMDARs in synaptoneurosomes (fractions with enrichment of functional synaptic components) prepared from the rat superior colliculus. The authors found that even though total protein synthesis was reduced several minutes after the pulse, the translation rate of αCaMKII was actually increased. Importantly, NMDAR activation also led to an increase of eEF2 phosphorylation, strongly suggesting the involvement of the eEF2K/eEF2 pathway. They also demonstrated that using cycloheximide, a substance that blocks translation elongation independently of eEF2, lead to very similar proteomic changes. The authors therefore propose the following sequence of events: "NMDAR-mediated Ca^{2+} influx into dendrites activates Ca^{2+}-dependent eEF2 kinase, which then phosphorylates eEF2. This phosphorylation might slow the local rate of protein translation, and elongation, rather than initiation, would consequently become the rate-limiting step in protein synthesis. Such a shift should favor upregulation of translation of abundant but poorly initiated transcripts such as αCaMKII in dendrites" (Scheetz et al., 2000). In another elegant study (Sutton et al., 2007), a microfluidic chamber was used which allows for the fluidic isolation of pre- and postsynaptic neurons. Application of tetrodotoxin (TTX) to the presynaptic compartment silenced presynaptic generation of action potentials while not interfering with miniature synaptic events/spontaneous neurotransmission. At the postsynaptic neuron a Green Fluorescent Protein (GFP) translation reporter was analyzed for 100 min after TTX application and interestingly an increase of eEF2 phosphorylation levels on Thr56 and a decrease of translation were reported as compared to baseline. Instead, applying TTX in addition with NMDAR blockers did not lead to this increase in phospho-eEF2 levels or decrease in translation, implying that NMDAR-mediated miniature excitatory synaptic events activate the eEF2K/eEF2 pathway and thereby lead to a decrease in translation. Additionally, using eEF2K inhibitors the authors were able to show that the decrease of translation that occurred during TTX treatment is due to activation of eEF2K, which is expected since eEF2K is the only known kinase regulating eEF2 (Nairn and Palfrey, 1987; Ryazanov et al., 1988; Mitsui et al., 1993; Dorovkov et al., 2002). The study concludes that the eEF2K/eEF2 pathway may act as a postsynaptic decoder of spontaneous and evoked neurotransmission (Sutton et al., 2007). A cautionary note, it is still unclear whether the available eEF2K inhibitors are well-suited to efficiently reduce eEF2 phosphorylation (Chen et al., 2011; Devkota et al., 2012), showing the need for the generation of new and efficient chemical compounds.

Two fascinating *in vivo* studies by Autry et al. (2011) and Nosyreva et al. (2013) used the NMDAR antagonist ketamine and eEF2K inhibitors to demonstrate that the eEF2K/eEF2 pathway regulates the expression of brain-derived neurotrophic factor (BDNF), a neurotrophin whose mRNA is found in dendrites (Tongiorgi et al., 1997, 2004; An et al., 2008) and is involved in numerous neuronal processes including synapse formation and synaptic plasticity (Reichardt, 2006). More specifically, they show that under resting conditions spontaneous glutamate release activates NMDARs which in turn engages eEF2K, resulting in the translational repression of BDNF. Consistently, acute administration of ketamine liberates BDNF expression and apparently alleviates depressive behavior in wildtype mice but not in eEF2K knockout mice, a fact that may prove to be useful in the context of major depressive disorder (Monteggia et al., 2013; Nosyreva et al., 2013). Importantly, the antidepressive effect appears to stem from BDNF-induced (presumably local) translation of AMPARs which become incorporated into the cell membrane and contribute to increased AMPAR-mediated synaptic transmission. In line with this fact, knockout mice for an AMPAR called GluA2 do not exhibit the antidepressive response induced by ketamin (Nosyreva et al., 2013). Interestingly, the finding that the (dendritically localized) eEF2K/eEF2 pathway leads to an activity-dependent upregulation of AMPAR currents also suggests that the activity of the eEF2K/eEF2 pathway may not only be dependent on network activity, but may itself determine the extent of network activity. Noteworthy, in opposition to the acute effect of ketamine, treatment with fluoxetine- another antidepressant- upregulates eEF2 phosphorylation in multiple brain regions only after chronic administration when antidepressive effects start taking place (Dagestad et al., 2006). This suggests that changes in eEF2K/eEF2 pathway-dependent mRNA translation enable not only acute but also chronic antidepressive effects, depending on the signaling cascade engaged by the antidepressant.

Most of the studies reviewed so far have implemented acute perturbation of NMDAR- and neuronal activity to look at eEF2K/eEF2-dependent changes of the dendritic proteome. Another interesting field of research revolves around the study of proteomic changes and associated events (such as changes in dendritic or spine morphology and synaptic transmission) which take place during prolonged modifications of network activity (Ehlers, 2003; Turrigiano and Nelson, 2004; Perez-Otano and Ehlers, 2005; Virmani et al., 2006; Turrigiano, 2008; Lazarevic et al., 2011). Two related studies (Piccoli et al., 2007; Verpelli et al., 2010) investigated the effect of prolonged changes in neuronal activity in primary neuronal cultures on the eEF2K/eEF2 pathway. The authors showed that increasing neuronal activity with bicuculline or lowering it with TTX for 48 h resulted in a dendritic increase of phosphorylation eEF2 on Thr56 or a decrease, respectively, strongly indicating an activation of eEF2K if neuronal networks are activated over longer periods of time (Verpelli et al., 2010). Verpelli et al. (2010) go on to show that activity dependent morphological changes of spine morphology depend on the presence of eEF2K, begging the question if there is a protein regulated by the eEF2K/eEF2 pathway that can account for the observed phenomenon. Indeed, the authors show that this protein is BDNF, whose mRNA translation is upregulated in dendrites in an eEF2K/eEF2 pathway-dependent fashion during long term bicuculline treatment. Interestingly, the bicuculline-induced increase of eEF2 phosphorylation and BDNF expression appears to depend on the activation of mGluRs rather than on the activation of AMPARs and NMDARs (Verpelli et al., 2010), suggesting that eEF2K activity can be modulated by a variety of GluRs.

Taken together, the data supports the notion that there are numerous ways of activating the dendritically localized eEF2K/eEF2-pathway, which can result from acute or prolonged stimulation of signaling elements like the NMDAR and mGluR (Nairn et al., 1985; Scheetz et al., 1997; Dorovkov et al., 2002; Chotiner et al., 2003; Davidkova and Carroll, 2007; Park et al., 2008; Verpelli et al., 2010; Autry et al., 2011; Tavares et al., 2012). Worthy of note, the proteomic changes induced by the activation eEF2K/eEF2 pathway can be quite diverse (and even opposite as in the case of BDNF and Arc), depending on which stimulation protocole is used. This may be due to the engagement of other signaling pathways but it may also mean that there is an extremely complex, protocole-specific eEF2K/eEF2 pathway-dependent change in the dendritic proteome which remains to be fully understood. For example, Im et al. (2009) show that the consolidation of fear memory involves an upregulation of BDNF and Arc synthesis in the hippocampus. However, hippocampal eEF2 phosphorylation is actually decreased during this process of memory consolidation, clearly contradicting the idea that a certain pool of proteins (like BDNF and Arc) is always positively correlated with an activation of the eEF2K/eEF2-pathway (Im et al., 2009). Lastly, a positive correlation between the activation of the eEF2K/eEF2 pathway and the translation rate of proteins may actually be unrelated in certain cases. For example, Panja et al. (2009) show that high frequency stimulation of neuronal populations leads to a phosphorylation of eEF2 and an increase Arc levels. However, the authors clearly show that in this experimental setting the activated eEF2K/eEF2 pathway is not responsible for the increase in Arc levels since pharmacologically blocking the pathway during the high frequency stimulation does not block the increase in Arc levels (Panja et al., 2009).

EUKARYOTIC ELONGATION FACTOR 2 KINASE (eEF2K)/EUKARYOTIC ELONGATION FACTOR 2 (eEF2) PATHWAY-DEPENDENT mRNA TRANSLATION IN DENDRITES IN THE CONTEXT OF SYNAPTIC PLASTICITY

Synaptic plasticity refers to a "modification of the strength or efficacy of synaptic transmission" due to neuronal activity and has been discussed as the molecular correlate of phenomena like learning and memory (Citri and Malenka, 2008; Ebert and Greenberg, 2013). Two well studied forms of synaptic plasticity are long-term potentiation (LTP) and long-term depression (LTD), which increase or decrease synaptic transmission efficacy or strength, respectively, and whose maintenance apparently requires general and dendritic protein synthesis (Malenka and Bear, 2004; Citri and Malenka, 2008; Turrigiano, 2008). Since neuronal activity, synaptic plasticity, and mRNA translation are related events, the question arises whether the eEF2K/eEF2 pathway and synaptic plasticity are functionally related. Indeed, this appears to be the case for at least three well-established forms of synaptic plasticity, namely mGluR-LTD, chemically-, and BDNF-induced LTP (Chotiner et al., 2003; Kanhema et al., 2006; Davidkova and Carroll, 2007; Park et al., 2008).

Arguably, the most well understood relationship exists between the eEF2K/eEF2 pathway and mGluR-LTD. This form of synaptic plasticity can be electrically or chemically induced by mGluR agonists, is protein synthesis dependent, involves group I mGluRs (mGluR1 and mGluR5), and apparently also involves AMPAR-endocytosis (Citri and Malenka, 2008). In a fascinating study Park et al. (2008) pooled *in vitro* and *in vivo* data to show that under resting conditions, inactive eEF2K associates with group I mGluRs but can be liberated from the physical interaction with these receptors when they are stimulated by ligands. Active eEF2K then inhibits global translation at dendrites by phosphorylating eEF2. However, dendritic Arc mRNA translation is upregulated, which under resting conditions is usually suppressed by fragile X mental retardation protein (FMRP). Newly translated Arc then induces AMPAR-endocytosis, thereby completing the process of mGluR-LTD (Park et al., 2008). The authors' notions are supported by their data showing that hippocampal slices of eEF2K-knockout mice do not exhibit mGluR-LTD, whereas previous work has shown that slices from FMRP-knockout mice exhibit exaggerated mGluR-LTD (Huber et al., 2002). Another study (Davidkova and Carroll, 2007), carried out in cultured neurons, also demonstrated that AMPAR-endocytosis following mGluR activation depends on the eEF2K/eEF2 pathway, since knocking down eEF2K abolishes this phenomenon. More specifically, after mGluR activation, eEF2K upregulates dendritic mRNA translation of MAP1B, which leads to the endocytosis of AMPAR, presumably because of an interaction of MAP1B and the AMPAR-associated protein Glutamate receptor-interacting protein 1.

The molecular basis of the relationship between the eEF2K/eEF2 pathway and LTP is less clear, even though the association visibly exists. It is also not clear whether this form of synaptic plasticity involves a dendritically or somatically located eEF2K/eEF2 pathway. The two forms of LTP that have been studied in this context are chemically-, and BDNF-induced LTP. Chemical LTP is induced by a combination of reagents (such as forskolin and tetraethylammonium) and depends on NMDARs, synaptic activity, cyclic adenosine monophosphate (cAMP)/adenylyl cyclase signaling, mRNA translation and gene expression (Chotiner et al., 2003; Zhao et al., 2012). BDNF-induced LTP also requires mRNA translation and gene expression but is induced by the infusion of BDNF (Kanhema et al., 2006). Interestingly, Chotiner et al. (2003) found that 1 h after induction of chemical LTP in the Cornu Ammonis area 1 of the mouse hippocampus protein synthesis was reduced but Arc mRNA translation was increased, reminiscent of the study of Scheetz et al. (Chotiner et al., 2003; Scheetz et al., 2000). As expected, eEF2 phosphorylation of Thr56 was increased which strongly indicates an activation of eEF2K in this experimental setting of chemical LTP. Since the increase of phosphorylation depended on cAMP/adenylyl cyclase activation and therefore engages protein kinase A (PKA) signaling (Voet et al., 2006), the authors hypothesize that eEF2K is activated during the induction of chemical LTP by PKA, which is known to phosphorylate and thereby activate eEF2K (Redpath and Proud, 1993a), resulting in the aforementioned changes in mRNA translation. Another study (Kanhema et al., 2006) addressed changes that are associated with BDNF-induced LTP. Among other things, the authors showed that inducing LTP by infusing BDNF into rat dentate gyrus lead to a transient phosphorylation of eEF2 on Thr56 in tissue homogenates, strongly suggesting an involvement of the eEF2K/eEF2 pathway in this form of synaptic plasticity. Worthy of note, the eEF2K/eEF2 pathway does not appear to be activated in dendrites during BDNF-induced LTP, but rather at non-synaptic sites, since the increase of eEF2 phosphorylation was not obtained when executing BDNF-induced LTP in synaptodendrosomes (fractions enriched in dendritic spine structures).

Importantly, the involvement of the eEF2K/eEF2 pathway is not limited to LTD and LTP, but instead has also been proven in the context of other forms of synaptic plasticity. One example of this is the participitation of the the eEF2K/eEF2 pathway in the context of monocular deprivation, which causes a reorganization of synapses and is a classical paradigm for inducing cortical synaptic plasticity. Seibt et al. (2012) showed that during sleep (when monocular deprivation-induced plasticity can occur) there is an increase of eEF2 phosphorylation and an increase in the translation of BDNF and Arc mRNA. These proteomic changes, which are presumably related to the activation of the eEF2K/eEF2 pathway, are necessary for synaptic plasticity to occur, indicating a strong involvement of the eEF2K/eEF2 pathway in the context of monocular deprivation-induced synaptic plasticity (Seibt et al., 2012). Curiously, eEF2 phosphorylation was observed in total lysates but not in synaptoneurosomes, indicating that in this specific experimental design for synaptic plasticity, the eEF2K/eEF2 pathway may not be engaged at the synapse but rather at the non-synaptic sites like in the soma. This result and the results of aforementioned work of Kanhema et al. (2006) suggest that not only the synaptically located eEF2K/eEF2 pathway, but also the somatically located eEF2K/eEF2 pathway may be important for synaptic plasticity to occur. In a further study, a connection between stress/sleep disruption were tied to the eEF2K/eEF2 pathway. More precisely, inducing stress by a combination of different factors like food deprivation, water deprivation etc., as well as sleep deprivation led to an upregulation of eEF2 phosphorylation levels in different parts of the brain, indicating a connection between the eEF2K/eEF2 pathway and these stressful events (Gronli et al., 2012). Since stress/sleep deprivation are known to impair plastic events at the synapse, this study highlights that there is, indeed, a strong and multifaceted link between the eEF2K/eEF2

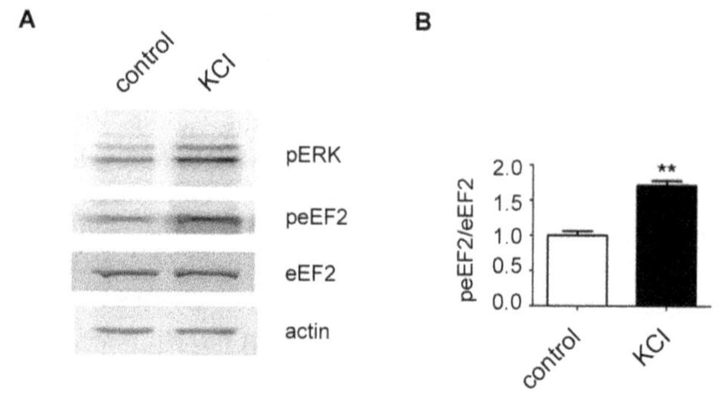

FIGURE 1 | Increase of eEF2 phosphorylation on Thr56 in neurons by KCL. (A) Western blot analysis of neuronal lysates reveals a strong upregulation of phosphorylated ERK and eEF2 upon KCL treatment. Neuronal cultures were prepared from day 18 rat embryos (Charles River) and plated at medium density (200 cells/mm^2) on 12-well plates and cultured with home-made B27 according to a protocole previously described (Romorini et al., 2004). At days *in vitro* 18, neurons were pretreated with TTX (1 μM) for 12 h and treated with KCL (55 mM) for 5 min. A strong increase of phosphorylated ERK on Thr202 and Tyr204 (pERK) and phosphorylated eEF2 on Thr56 (peEF2) can be appreciated. **(B)** Quantifications of normalized peEF2 band intensities (peEF2/eEF2) (vertical axis shows the mean fold change vs. control). Error bars are SEMs; ** $p <$ 0.01 vs. control (student's *t*-test).

pathway and synaptic plasticity, which is just beginning to be understood.

NEW INSIGHTS INTO THE ACTIVATION OF THE EUKARYOTIC ELONGATION FACTOR 2 KINASE (eEF2K)/EUKARYOTIC ELONGATION FACTOR 2 (eEF2) PATHWAY AND CALCIUM-DEPENDENT EUKARYOTIC ELONGATION FACTOR 2 KINASE (eEF2K) PHOSPHORYLATION IN NEURONS *IN VITRO*

In the course of this article several possibilities of activating the eEF2K/eEF2 pathway in neurons have been pointed out. We have found that a published protocol involving KCl, which leads to depolarization of neurons (Sala et al., 2000), can be utilized to increase eEF2 phosphorylation on Thr56 in primary neuronal cultures. For this, neurons were cultured as previously described (Romorini et al., 2004) and treated with KCl (55 mM) for 5 min at *days in vitro 18*. As expected, western blot analysis of lysates revealed a strong upregulation of phosphorylated extracellular signal-regulated kinase (ERK) on Thr202 and Tyr204 and, interestingly, a strong increase of phosphorylated eEF2 on Thr56 was also observed (**Figures 1A, B**). This is in line with the concept that depolarization of neurons and subsequent influx of calcium triggers eEF2K activation.

But what happens to the phosphorylation of eEF2K itself in neurons when it is activated by increasing levels of calcium? In this context, levels of eEF2K phosphorylation may be the result of calcium-dependent autophosphorylation (Mitsui et al., 1993; Redpath and Proud, 1993b; Pigott et al., 2012; Pyr Dit Ruys et al., 2012; Tavares et al., 2012), phosphorylation by another kinase, or dephosphorylation by a phosphatase. There are several identified upstream kinases of eEF2K such as PKA, p70S6 kinase (p70 S6K), and p90 ribosomal S6 kinase (p90 RSK) that regulate eEF2K phosphorylation in response to changes in cAMP-levels, ERK-signaling, and mammalian target of rapamycin-signaling, respectively (Redpath and Proud, 1993a; Wang et al., 2001; Browne et al., 2004; Browne and Proud, 2004; Lenz and Avruch, 2005). However, it has not been studied if the kinases upstream of eEF2K change their eEF2K-phosphorylation activity in response to increases in calcium levels though of course this is conceivable due to the broad effects of calcium signaling (Clapham, 2007;

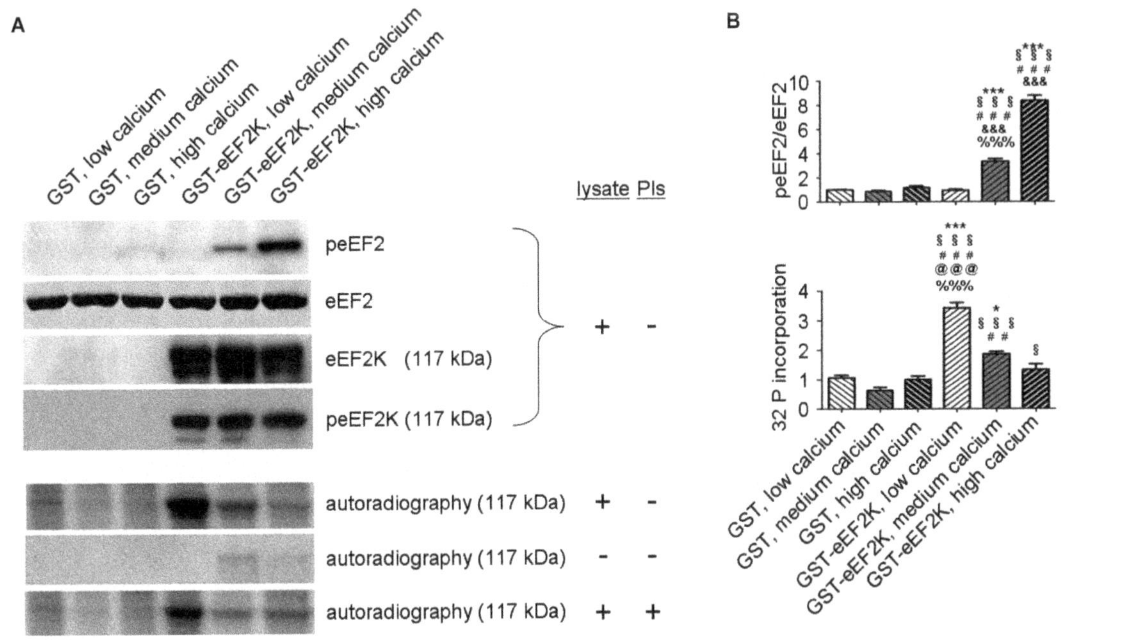

FIGURE 2 | eEF2K activity and total eEF2K phosphorylation are negatively correlated *in vitro*. (A) Phosphorylation assays with varying levels of freely available calcium and subsequent western blot and autoradiographical analysis reveal a negative correlation between eEF2K activity and total eEF2K phosphorylation. Assays were carried in a total volume of 60 μl for 30 min at 37°C and had the following final composition: GST or GST–eEF2K preparations (3–5 μg), rat brain lysate (30 μg) or double distilled water (condition "- lysate"), HEPES (20 mM) pH 7.4, $MgCl_2$ (10 mM), DTT (20 mM), ATP (100 μM; for subsequent western blot) or [γ-32P]ATP (100 μM; 5000 Ci/mmol; for subsequent autoradiography), and CaM (40 μg/ml). Depending on the group, ethylene glycol tetraacetic acid or $CaCl_2$ (1 mM each) was added to mimic low calcium and high calcium levels, respectively. For medium calcium levels double distilled water was used to arrive at the total volume of 60 μl. For the condition "+ PIs" phosphatase inhibitors were added to the mix. For western blot analysis, the reactions were terminated by addition of sample buffer, whereas autoradiography was carried out on pelleted GST-eEF2K (centrifugation at 500 g for 1 min followed by addition of sample buffer). Western blot analysis (top) was done after phosphorylation assays containing lysates but no PIs. Immunodetection was carried out against peEF2, eEF2, eEF2K at 117 kDa (corresponding to molecular weight of GST-eEF2K, view **Figure 3**), and peEF2K (Ser 366; phosphorylation site of p70 S6K and p90 RSK) at 117 kDa. Autoradiography analysis (bottom) was done after phosphorylation assays a) with lysate but without PIs, b) without lysate or PIs, and c) with lysate and PIs. **(B)** Quantifications of normalized peEF2 (peEF2/eEF2) band intensities and autoradiographical band intensities (32 P incorporation) of assay (with lysate but without PIs) at 117 kDa (vertical axis shows the mean fold change vs. GST, low calcium). Error bars are SEMs; *, **, and *** $p < 0.05$, 0.01, and 0.001 vs. GST, low calcium; § vs. GST, medium calcium; # vs. GST, high calcium; & vs. GST-eEF2K, low calcium; @ vs. GST-eEF2K, medium calcium; % vs. GST-eEF2K, high calcium (ANOVA and *post hoc* Tukey test).

Chuderland and Seger, 2008; Fortin et al., 2013). To address the question of how eEF2K phosphorylation changes in response to elevated levels of calcium we bacterially overexpressed eEF2K as a fusion protein with glutathione S-transferase (GST) and purified it as previously described (Tao et al., 2010; Pigott et al., 2012; Pyr Dit Ruys et al., 2012). The resulting GST-eEF2K ran at about 117 kDa in sodium dodecyl sulfate-polyacrylamide gel electrophoresis (SDS-PAGE; **Figure 3**). The fusion protein was then used for a phosphorylation assay with rat brain lysates in which the availability of calcium ions was manipulated. After this, a western blot analysis of eEF2 phosphorylation or an autoradiographical analysis of GST-eEF2K phosphorylation was carried out as previously described (Gardoni et al., 2001) with minor modifications. As expected, eEF2 phosphorylation increased with rising calcium levels (**Figure 2A**, top; **Figure 2B**), which suggests an intact catalytic activity of the purified GST-eEF2K. Interestingly, GST-eEF2K phosphorylation was higher in low calcium than in high calcium (**Figure 2A**, bottom; **Figure 2B**) and this is probably not due to autophosphorylation since eEF2K autophosphorylates itself preferentially when calcium levels are increased (Mitsui et al., 1993; Redpath and Proud, 1993b; Tavares et al., 2012). Accordingly, carrying out the assay in the absence of lysate did not yield the aforementioned trend in GST-eEF2K phosphorylation (**Figure 2A**, bottom). Instead, carrying out the assay with the addition of phosphatase inhibitors (PIs) lead to a comparable trend in GST-eEF2K phosphorylation (**Figure 2A**, bottom). Altogether, this suggests that the higher phosphorylation of GST-eEF2K in low calcium is most likely due to upstream (possibly calcium dependent) kinases of eEF2K though we can exclude p70 S6K and p90 RSK since their phosphorylation site Ser366 (Wang et al., 2001; Browne and Proud, 2004) does not exhibit a calcium-dependent profile (**Figure 2A**, top). Possibly, the responsible kinases affect their phosphorylation sites on eEF2K in a calcium-dependent manner in order to regulate its activity. This would be an additional way to control the eEF2K/eEF2 pathway (and therefore mRNA translation) in response to changes of intracellular calcium levels which would imply an even more complex regulation of the eEF2K/eEF2 pathway than is already known.

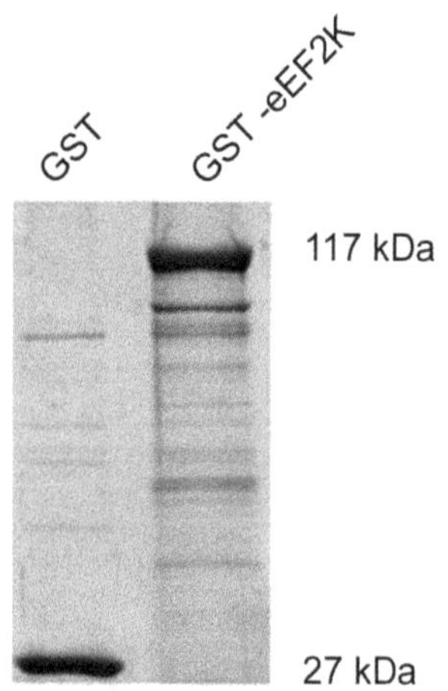

FIGURE 3 | Coomassie Brilliant Blue staining of GST-eEF2K reveals expected molecular weight of fusion protein. eEF2K was expressed as the fusion protein GST-eEF2K (kind gift of Professor Chris G. Proud, University of Southampton) in BL21 competent *Escherichia coli* and purified as previously described (Tao et al., 2010; Pigott et al., 2012; Pyr Dit Ruys et al., 2012). After SDS-PAGE, gels were stained with Coomassie Brilliant Blue.

CONCLUSION

Phosphorylation of eEF2 via eEF2K in dendrites is one way for neurons to regulate dendritic mRNA translation. In general, activation of the eEF2K/eEF2 pathway leads to a dramatic reduction of mRNA translation. This also holds true for the subcellular compartment of dendrites, but interestingly the mRNA translation rate of a small subset of synaptic proteins with well-known synaptic functions is increased. Since eEF2K activity can be altered by the state of neuronal activation, this suggests the intriguing possibility that the eEF2K/eEF2 pathway may be utilized by neurons to implement proteomic changes at dendrites to facilitate activity-dependent plastic changes at the synapse.

AUTHOR CONTRIBUTIONS

Christopher Heise wrote the text, planned and carried out the experiments; Fabrizio Gardoni corrected the text, provided expertise for the experiments, and carried out the autoradiography; Lorenza Culotta helped to carry out the experiments; Monica di Luca provided expertise and funding for the experiments; Chiara Verpelli corrected the text and helped in the organization of the GST-eEF2K DNA; Carlo Sala corrected the text, provided expertise and funding for the experiments.

ACKNOWLEDGMENTS

This work was financially supported by Comitato Telethon Fondazione Onlus, grant GGP11095, Fondazione CARIPLO project number 2012-0593, Italian Institute of Technology, Seed Grant, Ministry of Health in the frame of ERA-NET NEURON, PNR-CNR Aging Program 2012-2014. Christopher Heise was supported by SyMBaD (ITN Marie Curie, Grant Agreement no. 238608—7th Framework Programme of the EU).

REFERENCES

An, J. J., Gharami, K., Liao, G. Y., Woo, N. H., Lau, A. G., Vanevski, F., et al. (2008). Distinct role of long 3′ UTR BDNF mRNA in spine morphology and synaptic plasticity in hippocampal neurons. *Cell* 134, 175–187. doi: 10.1016/j.cell.2008.05.045

Asaki, C., Usuda, N., Nakazawa, A., Kametani, K., and Suzuki, T. (2003). Localization of translational components at the ultramicroscopic level at postsynaptic sites of the rat brain. *Brain Res.* 972, 168–176. doi: 10.1016/s0006-8993(03)02523-x

Autry, A. E., Adachi, M., Nosyreva, E., Na, E. S., Los, M. F., Cheng, P. F., et al. (2011). NMDA receptor blockade at rest triggers rapid behavioural antidepressant responses. *Nature* 475, 91–95. doi: 10.1038/nature10130

Barrera, I., Hernandez-Kelly, L. C., Castelan, F., and Ortega, A. (2008). Glutamate-dependent elongation factor-2 phosphorylation in Bergmann glial cells. *Neurochem. Int.* 52, 1167–1175. doi: 10.1016/j.neuint.2007.12.006

Bear, M. F., Connors, B. W., and Paradiso, M. A. (2007). *Neuroscience: Exploring the Brain.* 3rd Edn. Philadelphia, PA: Lippincott Williams & Wilkins.

Browne, G. J., Finn, S. G., and Proud, C. G. (2004). Stimulation of the AMP-activated protein kinase leads to activation of eukaryotic elongation factor 2 kinase and to its phosphorylation at a novel site, serine 398. *J. Biol. Chem.* 279, 12220–12231. doi: 10.1074/jbc.m309773200

Browne, G. J., and Proud, C. G. (2004). A novel mTOR-regulated phosphorylation site in elongation factor 2 kinase modulates the activity of the kinase and its binding to calmodulin. *Mol. Cell. Biol.* 24, 2986–2997. doi: 10.1128/mcb.24.7.2986-2997.2004

Chen, Z., Gopalakrishnan, S. M., Bui, M. H., Soni, N. B., Warrior, U., Johnson, E. F., et al. (2011). 1-Benzyl-3-cetyl-2-methylimidazolium iodide (NH125) induces phosphorylation of eukaryotic elongation factor-2 (eEF2: a cautionary note on the anticancer mechanism of an eEF2 kinase inhibitor. *J. Biol. Chem.* 286, 43951–43958. doi: 10.1074/jbc.M111.301291

Chotiner, J. K., Khorasani, H., Nairn, A. C., O'Dell, T. J., and Watson, J. B. (2003). Adenylyl cyclase-dependent form of chemical long-term potentiation triggers translational regulation at the elongation step. *Neuroscience* 116, 743–752. doi: 10.1016/s0306-4522(02)00797-2

Chuderland, D., and Seger, R. (2008). Calcium regulates ERK signaling by modulating its protein-protein interactions. *Commun. Integr. Biol.* 1, 4–5. doi: 10.4161/cib.1.1.6107

Citri, A., and Malenka, R. C. (2008). Synaptic plasticity: multiple forms, functions, and mechanisms. *Neuropsychopharmacology* 33, 18–41. doi: 10.1038/sj.npp.1301559

Clapham, D. E. (2007). Calcium signaling. *Cell* 131, 1047–1058. doi: 10.1016/j.cell.2007.11.028

Collingridge, G. L., Isaac, J. T., and Wang, Y. T. (2004). Receptor trafficking and synaptic plasticity. *Nat. Rev. Neurosci.* 5, 952–962. doi: 10.1038/nrn1556

Dagestad, G., Kuipers, S. D., Messaoudi, E., and Bramham, C. R. (2006). Chronic fluoxetine induces region-specific changes in translation factor eIF4E and eEF2 activity in the rat brain. *Eur. J. Neurosci.* 23, 2814–2818. doi: 10.1111/j.1460-9568.2006.04817.x

Dajas-Bailador, F., Bonev, B., Garcez, P., Stanley, P., Guillemot, F., and Papalopulu, N. (2012). microRNA-9 regulates axon extension and branching by targeting Map1b in mouse cortical neurons. *Nat. Neurosci.* doi: 10.1038/nn.3082. [Epub ahead of print].

Davidkova, G., and Carroll, R. C. (2007). Characterization of the role of microtubule-associated protein 1B in metabotropic glutamate receptor-mediated endocytosis of AMPA receptors in hippocampus. *J. Neurosci.* 27, 13273–13278. doi: 10.1523/jneurosci.3334-07.2007

Devkota, A. K., Tavares, C. D., Warthaka, M., Abramczyk, O., Marshall, K. D., Kaoud, T. S., et al. (2012). Investigating the kinetic mechanism of inhibition of elongation factor 2 kinase by NH125: evidence of a common in vitro artifact. *Biochemistry* 51, 2100–2112. doi: 10.1021/bi201787p

Dorovkov, M. V., Pavur, K. S., Petrov, A. N., and Ryazanov, A. G. (2002). Regulation of elongation factor-2 kinase by pH. *Biochemistry* 41, 13444–13450. doi: 10.1021/bi026494p

Ebert, D. H., and Greenberg, M. E. (2013). Activity-dependent neuronal signalling and autism spectrum disorder. *Nature* 493, 327–337. doi: 10.1038/nature11860

Ehlers, M. D. (2003). Activity level controls postsynaptic composition and signaling via the ubiquitin-proteasome system. *Nat. Neurosci.* 6, 231–242. doi: 10.1038/nn1013

Fortin, D. A., Srivastava, T., Dwarakanath, D., Pierre, P., Nygaard, S., Derkach, V. A., et al. (2013). Brain-derived neurotrophic factor activation of CaM-kinase kinase via transient receptor potential canonical channels induces the translation and synaptic incorporation of GluA1-containing calcium-permeable AMPA receptors. *J. Neurosci.* 32, 8127–8137. doi: 10.1523/JNEUROSCI.6034-11.2012

Gardoni, F., Bellone, C., Cattabeni, F., and Di Luca, M. (2001). Protein kinase C activation modulates alpha-calmodulin kinase II binding to NR2A subunit of N-methyl-D-aspartate receptor complex. *J. Biol. Chem.* 276, 7609–7613. doi: 10.1074/jbc.m009922200

Gronli, J., Dagestad, G., Milde, A. M., Murison, R., and Bramham, C. R. (2012). Post-transcriptional effects and interactions between chronic mild stress and acute sleep deprivation: regulation of translation factor and cytoplasmic polyadenylation element-binding protein phosphorylation. *Behav. Brain Res.* 235, 251–262. doi: 10.1016/j.bbr.2012.08.008

Huber, K. M., Gallagher, S. M., Warren, S. T., and Bear, M. F. (2002). Altered synaptic plasticity in a mouse model of fragile X mental retardation. *Proc. Natl. Acad. Sci. U S A* 99, 7746–7750. doi: 10.1073/pnas.122205699

Im, H. I., Nakajima, A., Gong, B., Xiong, X., Mamiya, T., Gershon, E. S., et al. (2009). Post-training dephosphorylation of eEF-2 promotes protein synthesis for memory consolidation. *PLoS One* 4:e7424. doi: 10.1371/journal.pone.0007424

Kanhema, T., Dagestad, G., Panja, D., Tiron, A., Messaoudi, E., Havik, B., et al. (2006). Dual regulation of translation initiation and peptide chain elongation during BDNF-induced LTP in vivo: evidence for compartment-specific translation control. *J. Neurochem.* 99, 1328–1337. doi: 10.1111/j.1471-4159.2006.04158.x

Kessels, H. W., and Malinow, R. (2009). Synaptic AMPA receptor plasticity and behavior. *Neuron* 61, 340–350. doi: 10.1016/j.neuron.2009.01.015

Lazarevic, V., Schone, C., Heine, M., Gundelfinger, E. D., and Fejtova, A. (2011). Extensive remodeling of the presynaptic cytomatrix upon homeostatic adaptation to network activity silencing. *J. Neurosci.* 31, 10189–10200. doi: 10.1523/JNEUROSCI.2088-11.2011

Lenz, G., and Avruch, J. (2005). Glutamatergic regulation of the p70S6 kinase in primary mouse neurons. *J. Biol. Chem.* 280, 38121–38124. doi: 10.1074/jbc.c500363200

Lisman, J., Yasuda, R., and Raghavachari, S. (2012). Mechanisms of CaMKII action in long-term potentiation. *Nat. Rev. Neurosci.* 13, 169–182. doi: 10.1038/nrn3192

Major, G., Larkum, M. E., and Schiller, J. (2013). Active properties of neocortical pyramidal neuron dendrites. *Annu. Rev. Neurosci.* 36, 1–24. doi: 10.1146/annurev-neuro-062111-150343

Malenka, R. C., and Bear, M. F. (2004). LTP and LTD: an embarrassment of riches. *Neuron* 44, 5–21. doi: 10.1016/j.neuron.2004.09.012

Marin, P., Nastiuk, K. L., Daniel, N., Girault, J. A., Czernik, A. J., Glowinski, J., et al. (1997). Glutamate-dependent phosphorylation of elongation factor-2 and inhibition of protein synthesis in neurons. *J. Neurosci.* 17, 3445–3454.

Maus, M., Torrens, Y., Gauchy, C., Bretin, S., Nairn, A. C., Glowinski, J., et al. (2006). 2-Deoxyglucose and NMDA inhibit protein synthesis in neurons and regulate phosphorylation of elongation factor-2 by distinct mechanisms. *J. Neurochem.* 96, 815–824. doi: 10.1111/j.1471-4159.2005.03601.x

Mitsui, K., Brady, M., Palfrey, H. C., and Nairn, A. C. (1993). Purification and characterization of calmodulin-dependent protein kinase III from rabbit reticulocytes and rat pancreas. *J. Biol. Chem.* 268, 13422–13433.

Monteggia, L. M., Gideons, E., and Kavalali, E. T. (2013). The role of eukaryotic elongation factor 2 kinase in rapid antidepressant action of ketamine. *Biol. Psychiatry* 73, 1199–1203. doi: 10.1016/j.biopsych.2012.09.006

Nairn, A. C., Bhagat, B., and Palfrey, H. C. (1985). Identification of calmodulin-dependent protein kinase III and its major Mr 100,000 substrate in mammalian tissues. *Proc. Natl. Acad. Sci. U S A* 82, 7939–7943. doi: 10.1073/pnas.82.23.7939

Nairn, A. C., and Palfrey, H. C. (1987). Identification of the major Mr 100,000 substrate for calmodulin-dependent protein kinase III in mammalian cells as elongation factor-2. *J. Biol. Chem.* 262, 17299–17303.

Nosyreva, E., Szabla, K., Autry, A. E., Ryazanov, A. G., Monteggia, L. M., and Kavalali, E. T. (2013). Acute suppression of spontaneous neurotransmission drives synaptic potentiation. *J. Neurosci.* 33, 6990–7002. doi: 10.1523/JNEUROSCI.4998-12.2013

Panja, D., Dagyte, G., Bidinosti, M., Wibrand, K., Kristiansen, A. M., Sonenberg, N., et al. (2009). Novel translational control in Arc-dependent long term potentiation consolidation in vivo. *J. Biol. Chem.* 284, 31498–31511. doi: 10.1074/jbc.M109.056077

Park, S., Park, J. M., Kim, S., Kim, J. A., Shepherd, J. D., Smith-Hicks, C. L., et al. (2008). Elongation factor 2 and fragile X mental retardation protein control the dynamic translation of Arc/Arg3.1 essential for mGluR-LTD. *Neuron* 59, 70–83. doi: 10.1016/j.neuron.2008.05.023

Perez-Otano, I., and Ehlers, M. D. (2005). Homeostatic plasticity and NMDA receptor trafficking. *Trends Neurosci.* 28, 229–238. doi: 10.1016/j.tins.2005.03.004

Piccoli, G., Verpelli, C., Tonna, N., Romorini, S., Alessio, M., Nairn, A. C., et al. (2007). Proteomic analysis of activity-dependent synaptic plasticity in hippocampal neurons. *J. Proteome Res.* 6, 3203–3215. doi: 10.1021/pr0701308

Pigott, C. R., Mikolajek, H., Moore, C. E., Finn, S. J., Phippen, C. W., Werner, J. M., et al. (2012). Insights into the regulation of eukaryotic elongation factor 2 kinase and the interplay between its domains. *Biochem. J.* 442, 105–118. doi: 10.1042/BJ20111536

Prybylowski, K., Chang, K., Sans, N., Kan, L., Vicini, S., and Wenthold, R. J. (2005). The synaptic localization of NR2B-containing NMDA receptors is controlled by interactions with PDZ proteins and AP-2. *Neuron* 47, 845–857. doi: 10.1016/j.neuron.2005.08.016

Pyr Dit Ruys, S., Wang, X., Smith, E. M., Herinckx, G., Hussain, N., Rider, M. H., et al. (2012). Identification of autophosphorylation sites in eukaryotic elongation factor-2 kinase. *Biochem. J.* 442, 681–692. doi: 10.1042/BJ20111530

Redpath, N. T., and Proud, C. G. (1993a). Cyclic AMP-dependent protein kinase phosphorylates rabbit reticulocyte elongation factor-2 kinase and induces calcium-independent activity. *Biochem. J.* 293(Pt. 1), 31–34.

Redpath, N. T., and Proud, C. G. (1993b). Purification and phosphorylation of elongation factor-2 kinase from rabbit reticulocytes. *Eur. J. Biochem.* 212, 511–520. doi: 10.1111/j.1432-1033.1993.tb17688.x

Reichardt, L. F. (2006). Neurotrophin-regulated signalling pathways. *Philos. Trans. R. Soc. Lond. B Biol. Sci.* 361, 1545–1564. doi: 10.1098/rstb.2006.1894

Romorini, S., Piccoli, G., Jiang, M., Grossano, P., Tonna, N., Passafaro, M., et al. (2004). A functional role of postsynaptic density-95-guanylate kinase-associated protein complex in regulating Shank assembly and stability to synapses. *J. Neurosci.* 24, 9391–9404. doi: 10.1523/jneurosci.3314-04.2004

Ryazanov, A. G., Shestakova, E. A., and Natapov, P. G. (1988). Phosphorylation of elongation factor 2 by EF-2 kinase affects rate of translation. *Nature* 334, 170–173. doi: 10.1038/334170a0

Ryazanov, A. G., Ward, M. D., Mendola, C. E., Pavur, K. S., Dorovkov, M. V., Wiedmann, M., et al. (1997). Identification of a new class of protein kinases represented by eukaryotic elongation factor-2 kinase. *Proc. Natl. Acad. Sci. U S A* 94, 4884–4889. doi: 10.1073/pnas.94.10.4884

Sala, C., Rudolph-Correia, S., and Sheng, M. (2000). Developmentally regulated NMDA receptor-dependent dephosphorylation of cAMP response element-binding protein (CREB) in hippocampal neurons. *J. Neurosci.* 20, 3529–3536.

Scheetz, A. J., Nairn, A. C., and Constantine-Paton, M. (1997). N-methyl-D-aspartate receptor activation and visual activity induce elongation factor-2 phosphorylation in amphibian tecta: a role for N-methyl-D-aspartate receptors in controlling protein synthesis. *Proc. Natl. Acad. Sci. U S A* 94, 14770–14775. doi: 10.1073/pnas.94.26.14770

Scheetz, A. J., Nairn, A. C., and Constantine-Paton, M. (2000). NMDA receptor-mediated control of protein synthesis at developing synapses. *Nat. Neurosci.* 3, 211–216. doi: 10.1038/72915

Seibt, J., Dumoulin, M. C., Aton, S. J., Coleman, T., Watson, A., Naidoo, N., et al. (2012). Protein synthesis during sleep consolidates cortical plasticity in vivo. *Curr. Biol.* 22, 676–682. doi: 10.1016/j.cub.2012.02.016

Sutton, M. A., Taylor, A. M., Ito, H. T., Pham, A., and Schuman, E. M. (2007). Postsynaptic decoding of neural activity: eEF2 as a biochemical sensor coupling miniature synaptic transmission to local protein synthesis. *Neuron* 55, 648–661. doi: 10.1016/j.neuron.2007.07.030

Swanger, S. A., and Bassell, G. J. (2013). Dendritic protein synthesis in the normal and diseased brain. *Neuroscience* 232C, 106–127. doi: 10.1016/j.neuroscience.2012.12.003

Tao, H., Liu, W., Simmons, B. N., Harris, H. K., Cox, T. C., and Massiah, M. A. (2010). Purifying natively folded proteins from inclusion bodies using sarkosyl, Triton X-100 and CHAPS. *Biotechniques* 48, 61–64. doi: 10.2144/000113304

Tavares, C. D., O'Brien, J. P., Abramczyk, O., Devkota, A. K., Shores, K. S., Ferguson, S. B., et al. (2012). Calcium/calmodulin stimulates the autophosphorylation of elongation factor 2 kinase on Thr-348 and Ser-500 to regulate its activity and calcium dependence. *Biochemistry* 51, 2232–2245. doi: 10.1021/bi201788e

Tongiorgi, E., Armellin, M., Giulianini, P. G., Bregola, G., Zucchini, S., Paradiso, B., et al. (2004). Brain-derived neurotrophic factor mRNA and protein are targeted to discrete dendritic laminas by events that trigger epileptogenesis. *J. Neurosci.* 24, 6842–6852. doi: 10.1523/jneurosci.5471-03.2004

Tongiorgi, E., Righi, M., and Cattaneo, A. (1997). Activity-dependent dendritic targeting of BDNF and TrkB mRNAs in hippocampal neurons. *J. Neurosci.* 17, 9492–9505.

Traynelis, S. F., Wollmuth, L. P., McBain, C. J., Menniti, F. S., Vance, K. M., Ogden, K. K., et al. (2010). Glutamate receptor ion channels: structure, regulation and function. *Pharmacol. Rev.* 62, 405–496. doi: 10.1124/pr.109.002451

Turrigiano, G. G. (2008). The self-tuning neuron: synaptic scaling of excitatory synapses. *Cell* 135, 422–435. doi: 10.1016/j.cell.2008.10.008

Turrigiano, G. G., and Nelson, S. B. (2004). Homeostatic plasticity in the developing nervous system. *Nat. Rev. Neurosci.* 5, 97–107. doi: 10.1038/nrn1327

Verpelli, C., Piccoli, G., Zibetti, C., Zanchi, A., Gardoni, F., Huang, K., et al. (2010). Synaptic activity controls dendritic spine morphology by modulating eEF2-dependent BDNF synthesis. *J. Neurosci.* 30, 5830–5842. doi: 10.1523/JNEUROSCI.0119-10.2010

Virmani, T., Atasoy, D., and Kavalali, E. T. (2006). Synaptic vesicle recycling adapts to chronic changes in activity. *J. Neurosci.* 26, 2197–2206. doi: 10.1523/jneurosci.4500-05.2006

Voet, D., Voet, J. G., and Pratt, C. W. (2006). *Fundamentals of Biochemistry: Life at the Molecular Level.* 2nd Edn. Hoboken, NJ: Wiley.

Wang, X., Li, W., Williams, M., Terada, N., Alessi, D. R., and Proud, C. G. (2001). Regulation of elongation factor 2 kinase by p90(RSK1) and p70 S6 kinase. *Embo J.* 20, 4370–4379. doi: 10.1093/emboj/20.16.4370

Wibrand, K., Pai, B., Siripornmongcolchai, T., Bittins, M., Berentsen, B., Ofte, M. L., et al. (2012). MicroRNA regulation of the synaptic plasticity-related gene Arc. *PLoS One* 7:e41688. doi: 10.1371/journal.pone.0041688

Zalfa, F., Giorgi, M., Primerano, B., Moro, A., Di Penta, A., Reis, S., et al. (2003). The fragile X syndrome protein FMRP associates with BC1 RNA and regulates the translation of specific mRNAs at synapses. *Cell* 112, 317–327. doi: 10.1016/s0092-8674(03)00079-5

Zhao, S., Studer, D., Chai, X., Graber, W., Brose, N., Nestel, S., et al. (2012). Structural plasticity of spines at giant mossy fiber synapses. *Front. Neural Circuits* 6:103. doi: 10.3389/fncir.2012.00103

19

miR-7 and miR-153 protect neurons against MPP$^+$-induced cell death via upregulation of mTOR pathway

Apostolia Fragkouli and Epaminondas Doxakis *

Lab of Molecular and Cellular Neuroscience, Center for Basic Research, Biomedical Research Foundation of the Academy of Athens, Athens, Greece

Correspondence:
Epaminondas Doxakis, Lab of Molecular and Cellular Neuroscience, Center for Basic Research, Biomedical Research Foundation of the Academy of Athens, Soranou Efesiou 4, Athens 11527, Greece
e-mail: edoxakis@bioacademy.gr

Differential expression of microRNAs (miRs) in the brain of patients with neurodegenerative diseases suggests that they may have key regulatory roles in the development of these disorders. Two such miRs, miR-7, and miR-153 have recently been shown to target α-synuclein, a protein critically involved in the pathological process of Parkinson's disease. By using a well-established in culture Parkinson's disease model that of neurotoxin 1-Methyl-4-Phenyl-Pyridinium (MPP$^+$), we examined whether miR-7 and miR-153 display neuroprotective properties. Herein, we demonstrate that treatment of cortical neurons with MPP$^+$ induced a dose-dependent cell death with apoptotic characteristics. This was reflected in altered intracellular signaling characterized by increased levels of activated kinases p38MAPK and ERK1/2 and reduced levels of activated AKT, p70S6K, and SAPK/JNK. Overexpression of miR-7 or miR-153 by adenoviral transduction protected cortical neurons from MPP$^+$-induced toxicity, restored neuronal viability and anti-apoptotic BCL-2 protein levels while attenuated activation of caspase-3. Moreover, both miR-7 and miR-153 interfered with MPP$^+$-induced alterations in intracellular signaling pathways in a partially overlapping manner; specifically, they preserved activation of mTOR and SAPK/JNK signaling pathways in the MPP$^+$-treated neurons, while miR-153 also attenuated MPP$^+$-induced activation of p38MAPK. No major effects were observed in the rest of signaling cascades or proteins investigated. Furthermore, the neuroprotective effect of miR-7 and miR-153 was alleviated when MPP$^+$ was co-administered with rapamycin. Taken together, our results suggest that miR-7 and miR-153 protect neurons from cell death by interfering with the MPP$^+$-induced downregulation of mTOR signaling.

Keywords: Parkinson's disease, miR-7, miR-153, MPP$^+$, neuron, neuroprotection, rapamycin, mTOR

INTRODUCTION

Parkinson's disease (PD) is a heterogeneous neurodegenerative disorder that affects 1% of the population aged over 65. It perturbs both dopaminergic (substantia nigra pars compacta) and non-dopaminergic (locus coeruleous, raphe nuclei, nucleus basalis of Meynert, hypothalamus, pedunculopontine nucleus) neuronal systems. Our current understanding of the disease points toward a variety of genetic, cellular, and environmental factors that independently or in combination cause progressive neurodegeneration. These factors lead to oxidative stress, abnormal protein degradation, autophagy, reduced protein synthesis, and altered signal transduction that combined induce neuronal death. Which of these mechanisms is more important to PD pathogenesis and progression remains unknown (Obeso et al., 2010). So far, epidemiological data and therapeutic studies using neuroprotective substances such as caffeine, nicotine, ginsenosides, flavonoids, vitamins, and growth factors have pointed out that drugs directed against a single molecular target are likely to be ineffective in treating the disease while agents with multiple pharmacological targets appear more suitable. Consistently, treatments with generic neuroprotective factors and various combinations of approved drugs are now vigorously explored (reviewed in Seidl and Potashkin, 2011; Mythri et al., 2012; Rodnitzky, 2012; Santos, 2012; Kordower and Bjorklund, 2013).

microRNAs (miRs) are a class of highly conserved small, about 22 nucleotides in length, non-coding endogenous RNA molecules that act to inhibit protein expression by partially hybridizing to complementary sequences, in mainly the 3′ UTR, of target RNA transcripts (reviewed in Doxakis, 2013). Each miR is estimated to regulate multiple target mRNAs, and the combinatorial action of miRs is expected to regulate the expression of hundreds of mRNAs. They display a wide variety of expression patterns and many are differentially expressed during development or disease (reviewed in Wienholds and Plasterk, 2005). With respect to PD, it has been shown that two miRs, miR-34, and miR-133, are significantly reduced in affected brain regions relative to controls (reviewed in Mouradian, 2012). Moreover, we and others have reported that two additional miRs, miR-7, and miR-153, target α-synuclein, a protein critically involved in both familial and sporadic pathological processes of PD (Junn et al., 2009; Doxakis, 2010). Importantly, miR-7 and miR-153 are neuron-enriched and show highest levels of expression in murine midbrain (Doxakis, 2010). In addition, miR-7 levels are down-regulated in the midbrain of mice intraperitoneally injected with the PD neurotoxin, MPTP (Junn et al., 2009) while miR-153 has been shown to regulate amyloid β precursor protein (APP) expression and its levels are significantly reduced in Alzheimer's disease brains (Liang et al., 2007; Long et al., 2012). Finally, both miR-7 and miR-153 have been known to modulate intracellular signaling by targeting upstream components of the AKT pathway (Kefas et al., 2008; Fang et al., 2012; Song et al., 2012; Sanchez et al., 2013; Wang et al., 2013; Wu et al., 2013).

1-methyl-4-phenyl-1,2,3,6-tetrahydropyridine (MPTP) is a neurotoxin that was discovered accidentally in exposed humans. Young drug addicts developed an idiopathic parkinsonian syndrome after intravenous self-administration of a synthetic heroin with this contaminant (Davis et al., 1979; Langston et al., 1983). Significantly, most of the biochemical, neuropathological, and clinical characteristics observed, corresponded to the cardinal symptoms of human PD with the exemption of the formation of Lewy bodies (Langston et al., 1983; Ballard et al., 1985). At the molecular level, MPTP is transformed into its toxic derivative 1-methyl-4-phenylpyridinium ion (MPP^+) by the enzyme MAO-B in astrocytes (Langston et al., 1984; Nicklas et al., 1985). Today, MPTP and MPP^+ represent the most relevant and frequently used parkinsonian toxins for animal and *in culture* PD models, respectively. A number of studies have, thus far, indicated that inhibition of complex I of the mitochondria electron transport chain, elevation of oxidative stress, activation of pro-apoptotic ERK-1/2 and p38 MAPK and suppression of pro-survival AKT and mTOR signaling pathways contribute to MPP^+-induced cell death (Mizuno et al., 1987; Deguil et al., 2007; Karunakaran et al., 2008; Cui et al., 2011).

Based on the above, our current study was undertaken to evaluate the ability of miR-7 and miR-153 to prevent MPP^+-induced toxicity in neurons and delineate the underlying mechanism. Our results demonstrate that miR-7 and miR-153 could protect cortical neurons against MPP^+-induced death by preserving the activation of the downstream master integrating signaling pathway of mTOR. We argue that these findings may have important therapeutic preclinical applications for PD.

MATERIALS AND METHODS

ETHICS STATEMENT

All rodent tissues were obtained in accordance with European Union (2003/65/CE) guidelines regarding the use of laboratory animals. Experimental protocols were approved by the Institutional Animal Care and Use Committee of BRFAA and the Veterinary Services of Attica prefecture (K/2134).

ANTIBODIES

The rabbit polyclonal antibodies phospho-S6 ribosomal protein (Ser240/244 CST#2215), phospho-eEF2k (Ser366, CST#3691), phospho-p70 S6 kinase (Thr389, CST#9234), phospho-AKT (Ser473, CST#9271), phospho-ERK1/2 (Thr202/Tyr204, CST# 9101), phospho-p38 (Thr180/Tyr182, CST#4511), phospho-SAPK/JNK (Thr183/Tyr185, CST#4668), phospho-GSK3β (Ser9, CST#), phospho-Mapkapk2 (Thr334, CST#3007), S6 ribosomal protein (CST#2217), p70 S6 kinase (CST#9202), AKT (CST# 9272), ERK1/2 (CST#9102), p38 (CST#9212), SAPK/JNK (CST# 92588), and cleaved caspase-3 (Asp175, CST#9664) were purchased from Cell Signaling Technologies (Beverly, MA, USA). The mouse monoclonal IgG antibodies against BAX (sc-493) and BCL-2 (sc-7382) were purchased from Santa Cruz Biotechnology (Santa Cruz, CA, USA). The anti-GAPDH (GT239) monoclonal antibody was purchased from Genetex (Irvine, CA, USA). The mouse (CST#7076) and rabbit (CST#7074) HRP-conjugated secondary antibodies were from Cell Signaling Technologies.

GENERATION OF DNA CONSTRUCTS

The construction of pcDNA6.2-GW/EmGFP- scramble/pri-miR-7/pri-miR-153 and pri-miR-7/153 plasmids has been described previously (Doxakis, 2010). The entry plasmids pENTR/EmGFP-scramble/pri-miR-7/pri-miR-153 and pri-miR-7/153 were constructed by inserting the EmGFP-pri-miR cassettes from the pcDNA6.2-GW/EmGFP-pri-miR plasmids into the XhoI/NotI sites of the pENTR Gateway plasmid (Life Technologies, Carlsbad, CA, USA). Using LR clonase II enzyme (Life Technologies) the EmGFP-pri-miR cassettes were, subsequently, transferred by LR recombination from the pENTR plasmid into the pAd5 destination adenoviral vector (Life Technologies). All pAd5/EmGFP-pri-miR vectors were verified by sequencing before use.

ADENOVIRAL PRODUCTION

pAd5/EmGFP-pri-miR vectors were digested with the PacI enzyme, to lineralize DNA, before transfecting into HEK293A producer cell line in 12-well plates by using Lipofectamine 2000 according to the manufacturer's instructions (Life Technologies). Two days later, cells were trypsinized and transferred onto 10 cm dishes. Culture media were replaced with fresh every 2–3 days until visible regions of cytopathic effect were observed (typically 5–8 days post-transfection). Adenovirus-containing cells and media were harvested when approximately 50% of cells were detached from dish. Crude lysates were prepared by 3 freeze/thaw cycles followed by centrifugation at 3000 rpm for 15 min. To amplify viral stock, 1% of crude adenoviral stocks were used to infect freshly-plated HEK293A cells. Infections were allowed to proceed until 80–90% of the cells have rounded up and were floating (typically 2 days later). High-titer viral stocks were, once again, prepared by 3 freeze/thaw cycles followed by centrifugation at 3000 rpm for 15 min. Adenoviral titers were determined by standard viral plaque assays. Titers were approximately 5×10^8 infectious units per ml.

NEURON CULTURE AND TRANSDUCTION

Dissociated, embryonic day 16 murine cortical neurons (>95% pure, 9×10^5 cells/ml), were grown in Neurobasal/DMEM 1:1 medium (Life Technologies) with $0.5 \times$ B-27 supplement (Life Technologies), 5% heat-inactivated horse serum and Glutamax (Life Technologies) in poly-L-lysine (SIGMA, St-Louis, USA) coated culture plates in the absence of trophic factors (Doxakis et al., 2004). Neurons were transduced by adenoviruses at multiplicity of infection (MOI) 40 at 6–7 days after plating and lysed 48 h post-transduction.

PHARMACOLOGICAL TREATMENTS

MPP^+ (SIGMA) and rapamycin (SIGMA) were dissolved at the stock concentration of 100 mM in distilled water and tissue culture grade dimethylsulfoxide (DMSO, Applichem, Darmstadt, Germany), respectively. All experiments were initiated at day 7 or 8 after plating when all of the neurons had developed extensive neurite outgrowths. In the case of transduced neurons all pharmacological treatments were performed 24 h post-transduction. In MPP^+ experiments, neurons were treated with 5–50 μM MPP^+ for 24 h before analysis while in mTOR experiments, neurons were treated with 20 or 50 nM rapamycin for either 1 h (for signal transduction analysis) or 24 h (for cell viability analysis). When neuronal cultures were co-treated with MPP^+ and rapamycin, the later compound was added 1 h earlier.

METHYL THIAZOL TETRAZOLIUM (MTT) ASSAY

MTT assay, a measure of mitochondrial dehydrogenase activity in live cells, was performed in neurons cultured in 96-well poly-L-lysine coated plates. Once the different treatments have been completed, 10 μl of MTT (Applichem) solution in PBS (5 mg/ml) was added to each well and the plate was placed back to incubator for a further 1.5 h. The MTT formazan precipitants formed by live cells were, subsequently, dissolved in 150 μl DMSO and the absorbance was measured at 570 nm by an ELISA microplate reader (ELx800, Bio-Tek Instruments, Winooski, VT, USA).

IMMUNOBLOTTING

Immunoblotting was used to assay the protein levels of various intracellular signaling components in 8–9 days old cultures of cortical neurons transduced and/or treated with pharmacological compounds. Neurons were harvested in a lysis buffer containing 25 mM Tris pH 7.5, 150 mM NaCl, 1 mM EDTA, 1%Triton X-100, phosphatase (PhosSTOP®, Roche Applied Sciences, Penzberg, Bavaria, Germany) and protease (Complete®, Roche Applied Sciences) inhibitor cocktails. Cellular protein content was determined by the Bradford assay (Biorad, Hercules, CA, USA). Equal amounts of cell extracts were supplemented with 6x SDS sample buffer (375 mM Tris pH6.8, 10% SDS, 50% glycerol, 10% β-mercaptoethanol, 0.03% bromophenol blue), boiled for 5 min and subjected to SDS-PAGE under reducing conditions on 10 or 12% polyacrylamide gels, depending on the molecular mass of the proteins under examination. After electrophoresis, the resolved proteins were transferred to Protran® nitrocellulose membrane (Whatman, Kent, UK) by electroblotting. Subsequently membranes were saturated for 1 h at room temperature in 5% non-fat milk/0.1% Tween-20 in TBS and incubated at overnight at 4°C in 5% non-fat milk/TBS containing the primary antibody. All primary antibodies were used at 1:1000 dilution as recommended by vendors. The following day, membranes were washed in TBS, incubated for 1 h at room temperature in 5% non-fat milk/TBS containing the appropriate HRP-conjugated secondary antibody, washed in TBS and finally developed using the Western Lighting Plus ECL reagents (PerkinElmer, Waltham, MA, USA) according to the manufacturer's instructions. To ensure equal loading, following film exposure membranes were washed in 0.1% Tween-20 in TBS (TBST), incubated for 30 min at 50°C in stripping buffer (2% SDS, 0.8% mercaptoethanol, 62.5 mM Tris-HCl pH6.8), extensively washed in TBST and after saturation reprobed with the appropriate primary antibodies. Each sample was tested in duplicate and samples obtained from three or four independent experiments were used for analysis. Densitometric analysis of immunoblotting images was performed using the image analysis software Image J, NIH USA.

STATISTICAL ANALYSIS

Mean values were derived from three to five independent experiments performed in duplicate. The effect of treatment on the different parameters examined was assessed using One-Way ANOVA with treatment as independent factor. Bonferroni *post-hoc* analysis was performed where applicable. Significance was defined as $p < 0.05$. All statistical analyses were performed using the SPSS software (Release 10.0.1, SPSS, Chicago, IL, USA).

RESULTS

MPP+ TREATMENT INDUCED APOPTOSIS IN CORTICAL NEURONS IN A CONCENTRATION-DEPENDENT MANNER, ACCOMPANIED BY ALTERATIONS IN ALL MAJOR INTRACELLULAR SIGNALING CASCADES

In order to study the mechanism of MPP^+-induced cell death in our experimental system, 7 days old primary cultures of cortical neurons were treated with various concentrations of MPP^+ for 24 h. Neuronal viability was, initially, monitored using the MTT assay. As shown in **Figure 1A**, a 24-h treatment with MPP^+ induced cytotoxicity in a concentration-dependent manner; loss of viability extended from 7 to 67% with MPP^+ concentrations ranging between 5 and 50 μM. Statistical analysis revealed a significant effect of MPP^+ treatment [$F_{(5, 35)} = 45.662$, $P < 0.001$ and *post-hoc*] at 10, 20, 30, and 50 μM, but not 5 μM, of MPP^+.

Subsequently, the protein levels of the apoptotic-related factors BCL-2, BAX and cleaved caspase-3 were assayed by immunoblot analysis. Consistent with the loss in cell viability, levels of BCL-2, a major pro-survival protein, were significantly reduced by 20, 30, and 48% in cortical neurons treated for 24 h with 10, 20, and 30 μM of MPP^+, respectively [$F_{(3, 11)} = 23.699$, $P < 0.001$ and *post-hoc*; **Figure 1B**]. In contrast, a dose-dependent increase was observed in protein levels of cleaved caspase-3, an important effector caspase. More specifically, compared to untreated controls, primary cortical neurons treated for 24 h with 10, 20 and 30 μM of MPP^+ displayed a significant 3.2-, 6.5-, and 11.3-fold increase of cleaved caspase-3 levels, respectively [$F_{(3, 11)} = 52.150$, $P < 0.001$ and *post-hoc*; **Figure 1C**]. In our experimental system, the levels of BAX, a major pro-apoptotic factor, were not significantly altered (data not shown). Collectively, these data indicate that MPP^+ induced a dose-dependent neuronal death that displayed apoptotic features.

It is well established that cell apoptosis and survival are regulated by intracellular signaling cascades; thus, activation by phosphorylation of the major signaling effectors was next examined in the same experimental system. As shown in **Figures 2A,B**, and consistent with previous studies (Junyent et al., 2010; Cui et al., 2011; Hashimoto et al., 2012), the levels of phosphorylated AKT, a major pro-survival kinase, were significantly reduced by ~30% in cortical neurons treated with 20 and 30 μM of MPP^+ [$F_{(3, 15)} = 10.932$, $P = 0.001$ and *post-hoc*], whereas levels of phosphorylated p38 MAPK, a major pro-apoptotic kinase, were significantly

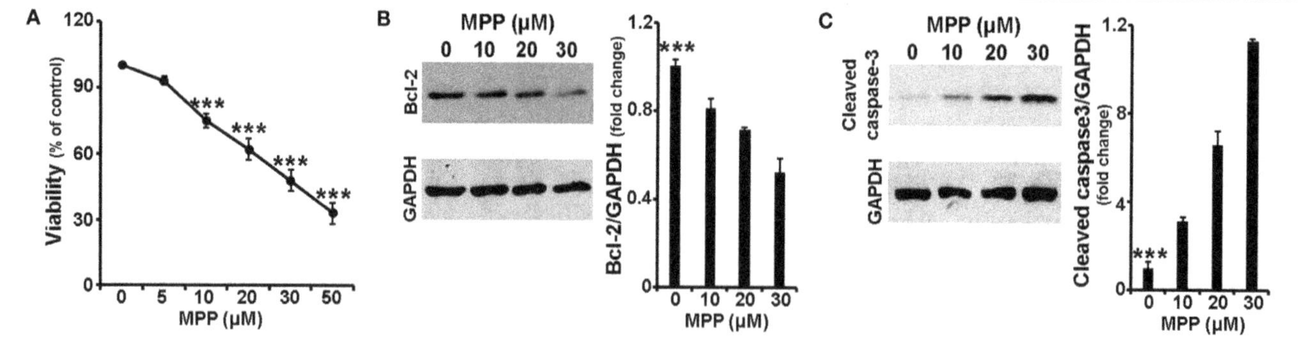

FIGURE 1 | MPP$^+$ induced neurotoxicity in cortical neurons. Seven-day primary cortical neurons were treated with various concentrations of MPP$^+$ for 24 h. **(A)** Cell viability following dose-dependent treatments was assayed by measuring MTT reduction by live neurons. Note that a significant reduction in neuronal viability was observed upon treatment with 10, 20, 30, and 50 μM, but not 5 μM, of MPP$^+$. **(B,C)** Equal amounts of total protein from lysates of cortical neurons cultured for 24 h in the presence of 10, 20, and 30 μM MPP$^+$ were analyzed on 12% SDS-PAGE and immunoblotted with antibodies specific for BCL-2 **(B)** and cleaved caspase-3 **(C)**. To ensure equal loading, membranes were re-probed against GAPDH. Note that compared to untreated controls, primary cortical neurons treated for 24 h with MPP$^+$ displayed a dose-dependent decrease of BCL-2 protein levels, as well as a dose-dependent increase of cleaved caspase-3 protein levels. Quantification of the results in **(B,C)** was performed by scanning densitometry. Bars in all the presented graphs depict mean ± s.e.m. ***$P \leq 0.001$.

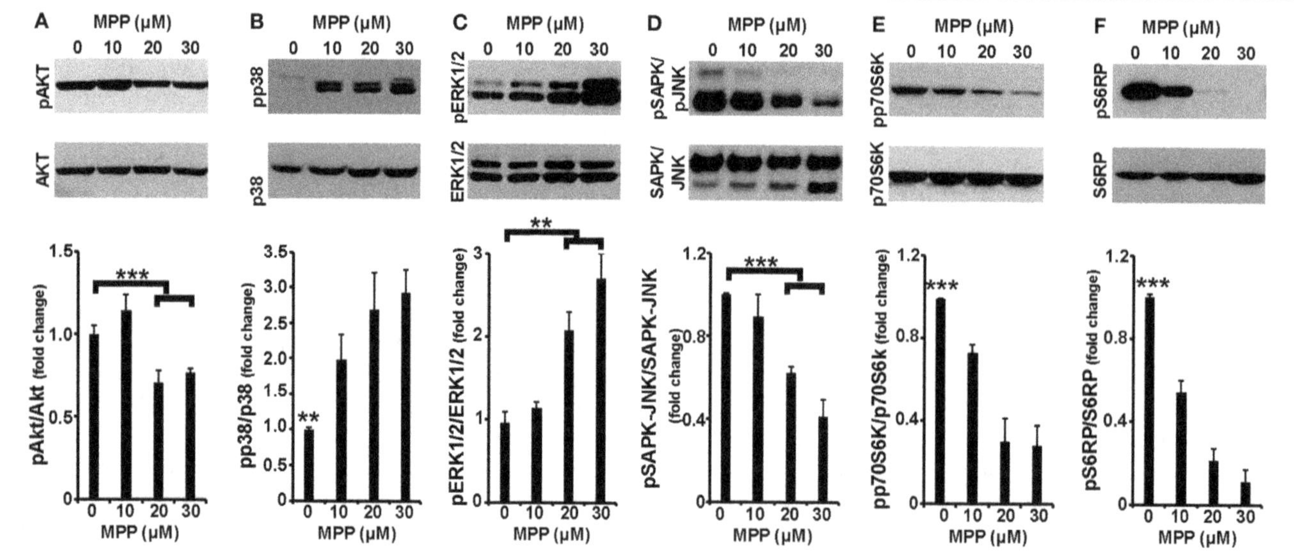

FIGURE 2 | Cortical neurons treated with MPP$^+$ displayed alterations in all major intracellular signaling cascades. Seven-day primary cortical neurons were treated with 10, 20, and 30 μM MPP$^+$ for 24 h. Equal amounts of total protein from lysates of cortical neurons were analyzed on 10% SDS-PAGE and immunoblotted with antibodies specific for phosphorylated forms of AKT **(A)**, p38 MAPK **(B)**, ERK1/2 **(C)**, JNK/SAPK **(D)**, p70S6K **(E)**, as well as for the phosphorylated forms of p70S6K substrate S6RP **(F)**. To ensure equal loading membranes were re-probed against AKT, p38 MAPK, ERK1/2, JNK/SAPK, p70S6K, and S6RP, respectively. Quantification of the results was performed by scanning densitometry. Bars in the graph depict mean ± s.e.m. Note that MPP$^+$-treatment changed the phosphorylation status of all the major signaling kinases examined in a concentration dependent manner. **$P \leq 0.01$, ***$P \leq 0.001$.

increased at all MPP$^+$ concentrations applied [$F_{(3, 15)} = 5.996$, $P = 0.01$ and *post-hoc*]. Similar results were observed in the levels of phosphorylated GSK-3β and MAPKAPK-2, downstream effectors of AKT and p38 MAPK, respectively (data not shown). Moreover, cortical neurons treated for 24 h with 20 or 30 μM, but not 10 μM, of MPP$^+$ displayed significant alterations in the levels of phosphorylated ERK1/2, a dubious MAPK, as well as of phosphorylated stress-induced kinases SAPK/JNK; levels of phosphorylated ERK1/2 were up-regulated by 110 and 170% [$F_{(3, 11)} = 11.806$, $P < 0.01$ and *post-hoc*; **Figure 2C**] and those of phosphorylated SAPK/JNK were down-regulated by 38 and 60% [$F_{(3, 15)} = 33.699$, $P < 0.001$ and *post-hoc*; **Figure 2D**] at 20 and 30 μM of MPP$^+$, respectively. Finally, as shown in **Figure 2E**, in our experimental system MPP$^+$ treatment also significantly reduced the phosphorylation status of the mTOR effector p70S6 kinase, even when applied at 10 μM; this reduction extended from 27% at 10 μM to 72% at 30 μM of MPP$^+$ [$F_{(3, 15)} = 20.701$, $P < 0.001$ and *post-hoc*]. Similar reductions were also observed in the levels of activated S6RP [$F_{(3, 15)} = 60.445$, $P < 0.001$ and *post-hoc*; **Figure 2F**] and of activated eEF2K [$F_{(3, 11)} = 18.310$, $P = 0.001$ and *post-hoc*; data not shown], two p70S6K substrates which mediate translation and cell growth (reviewed in Laplante and Sabatini, 2013). It is therefore evident that in cortical neurons, a 24-h treatment with MPP^+ leads to changes in the phosphorylation status of all major signaling kinases, in a concentration-dependent manner.

OVER-EXPRESSION OF miR-7 AND/OR miR-153 IN CORTICAL NEURONS ATTENUATED MPP+-INDUCED NEUROTOXICITY

It has been shown that miR-7 and miR-153 target α-synuclein, a protein critically involved in PD pathogenesis (Junn et al., 2009; Doxakis, 2010) and most importantly that miR-7 levels are down-regulated in the midbrain of mice intraperitoneally injected with the PD neurotoxin, MPTP (Junn et al., 2009). Therefore, in order to evaluate possible neuroprotective effects of miR-7 and/or miR-153 against MPP^+ insult, 6- to 7-day old primary cortical neurons were transduced with adenoviral particles expressing scramble miR, miR-7, miR-153, or both of these two miRs, miR-7/153. It should be noted that irrespective of the adenoviral particles used, overall adenoviral infection of primary cortical neurons affected cell viability, whereas adenoviral over-expression of miR-7 and/or miR-153 had no effect on neuronal viability compared to adenoviral expression of scramble miR (**Supplemental Figure 1**). Thus, in order to avoid any confounding effects due to the infection *per se*, all subsequent comparisons were performed between primary neurons transduced with adenoviral particles expressing a scramble miR and primary neurons transduced with adenoviral particles expressing the miR(s) of interest. Twenty four hours post-transduction, cortical neurons were exposed to MPP^+ concentrations ranging between 5 and 50 μM and left *in culture* for additional 24 h. Neuronal viability was then monitored by the MTT assay. As shown in **Figure 3A** and similar to uninfected neuronal cultures (see **Supplemental Figure 2**) in the scramble miR transduced cultures loss of viability extended from 10 to 62% with MPP^+ concentrations ranging between 5 and 50 μM. Statistical analysis revealed a significant effect of MPP^+ treatment [$F_{(5, 29)} = 48.968$, $P < 0.001$ and *post-hoc*] at 10, 20, 30, and 50 μM, but not 5 μM, of MPP^+. In contrast, neuronal viability in miR-7 or miR-153 transduced cultures was not impaired when treated with 5, 10, or 20 μM of MPP^+ and it was only reduced at the higher concentrations applied i.e., 30 and 50 μM [miR-7: $F_{(5, 29)} = 32.948$, $P < 0.001$ and *post-hoc*; miR-153: $F_{(5, 29)} = 24.816$, $P < 0.001$ and *post-hoc*; **Figure 3A**]. Interestingly, in neuronal cultures transduced with adenoviral particles expressing both miR-7/153 neuronal viability was only impaired upon 24-h treatment with 50 μM MPP^+ [$F_{(5, 29)} = 11.803$, $P < 0.001$ and *post-hoc*; **Figure 3A**], Nevertheless, even at the highest concentration applied, compared to scramble miR transduced control cultures, neuronal cultures transduced with both miR-7/153 displayed an approximately 2-fold increase in neuronal viability upon 24-h treatment with 50 μM MPP^+ [$F_{(3, 19)} = 11.444$, $P < 0.001$ and *post-hoc*; **Figure 3A**].

Finally, as depicted in **Figures 3B,C**, compared to scramble miR transduced untreated controls, only scramble-transduced cortical neurons displayed a significant decrease in the levels of anti-apoptotic BCL-2 [$F_{(4, 14)} = 4.567$, $P < 0.05$ and *post-hoc*], accompanied by a significant increase of cleaved caspase-3 levels [$F_{(4, 14)} = 10.438$, $P = 0.001$ and *post-hoc*], upon 24-h treatment with 10 μM of MPP^+. No such changes were observed among scramble-transduced untreated controls and MPP^+-treated neuronal cultures transduced with miR-7, miR-153, or miR-7/153 adenoviruses, suggesting that over-expression of miR-7 and miR-153 in cortical neurons attenuated both the MPP^+-induced down-regulation of pro-survival BCL-2 protein and activation of the pro-apoptotic caspase-3.

miR-7 AND miR-153 ACTIVATED p70S6K SIGNALING CASCADE IN PRIMARY CORTICAL NEURONS AND ATTENUATED THE EFFECTS OF RAPAMYCIN ON mTOR SIGNALING AND CELL VIABILITY

Given a number of studies that show that miR-7 and miR-153 modulate intracellular signaling (Kefas et al., 2008; Fang et al., 2012; Song et al., 2012; Sanchez et al., 2013; Wang et al., 2013, Wu

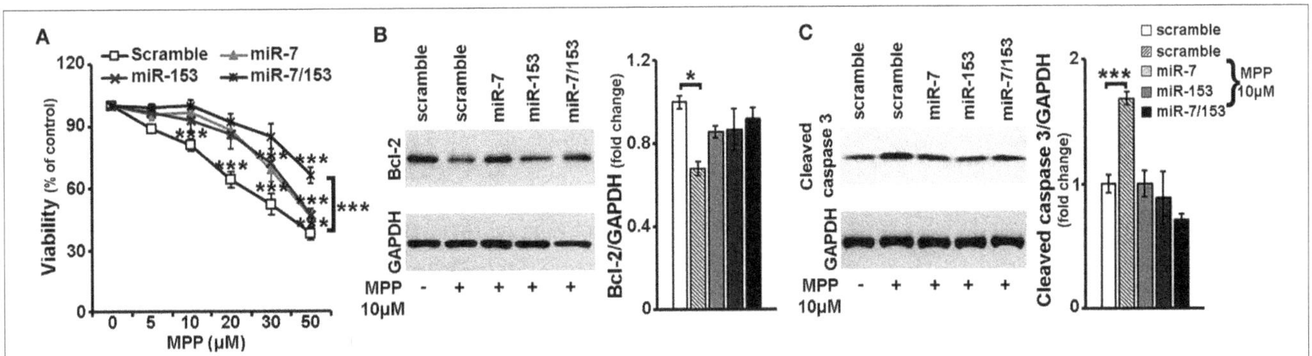

FIGURE 3 | Neuroprotective effects of miR-7 and miR-153 against MPP^+-toxicity. Six to seven days old primary cortical neurons were transduced with adenoviral particles expressing scramble miR, miR-7, miR-153, or both miR-7/153. After 24 h, transduced neurons were exposed for additional 24 h to various concentrations of MPP^+. **(A)** Neuronal viability following MPP^+-treatment was monitored by the MTT assay. Note that over-expression of miR-7 and/or miR-153 attenuated MPP^+-induced cell death. **(B,C)** Equal amounts of total protein from lysates of transduced cortical neurons cultured for 24 h in the presence of 10 μM MPP^+ were analyzed on 12% SDS-PAGE and immunoblotted with antibodies specific for BCL-2 **(B)** and cleaved caspase-3 **(C)**. To ensure equal loading membranes were re-probed against GAPDH. Quantification of the results was performed by scanning densitometry. Note that compared to scramble-transduced untreated controls, only scramble-transduced cortical neurons displayed significant changes in BCL-2 and cleaved caspase-3 protein levels. Bars in all the depicted graphs correspond to mean ± s.e.m. *$P \leq 0.05$, ***$P \leq 0.001$.

et al., 2013) in non-neuronal cells, we next investigated whether these miRs affect the activation of the major intracellular signaling cascades in neurons. Therefore, 6–7 days old primary cortical neurons were transduced with adenoviral particles expressing scramble miR, miR-7, or miR-153, and the activation of signaling kinases was assessed 48 h later by immunoblotting. As depicted in **Figure 4A**, overexpression of miR-7 or miR-153 in cortical neurons did not affect the phosphorylation status of pro-survival kinase AKT or of the pro-apoptotic p38 MAPK and similar results were also observed in the levels of phosphorylated GSK-3β and MAPKAPK-2, downstream effectors of AKT and p38 MAPK, respectively (data not shown). Finally, no significant change was either observed in the levels of phosphorylated ERK1/2 or those of activated stress-induced kinases SAPK/JNK (**Figure 4A**).

Markedly, in the same experimental system, both miR-7 and miR-153 appeared to induce p70S6 kinase signaling downstream of the mTOR signaling cascade. More specifically, levels of phosphorylated p70S6K were significantly up-regulated by 45 and 52% in cortical neurons transduced with adenoviral particles expressing miR-7 and miR-153, respectively [ANOVA: $F_{(2, 14)} = 8.056$, $P < 0.01$ and *post-hoc*; **Figure 4B**]. Consistent with the above, phosphorylation of p70S6K substrates S6RP and eEF2K was also significantly increased; levels of phosphorylated S6RP were up-regulated by 89 and 83% [ANOVA: $F_{(2, 11)} = 20.084$, $P < 0.001$ and *post-hoc*; **Figure 4C**], whereas levels of phosphorylated eEF2K were increased by 36 and 62% [ANOVA: $F_{(2, 11)} = 7.475$, $P < 0.05$ and *post-hoc*; data not shown] upon overexpression of miR-7 and miR-153, respectively. The latter mTOR downstream activation by miR-7 or miR-153 is unlikely to be attributed to an unspecific scramble miR effect, since transduction with adenoviral particles expressing scramble miR appeared to have no effect on the phosphorylation of p70S6K and of its substrate S6RP compared to transduced empty control neurons (**Supplemental Figure 3**). Taken together the latter observations suggest that miR-7 and miR-153 may activate the mTOR signaling cascade.

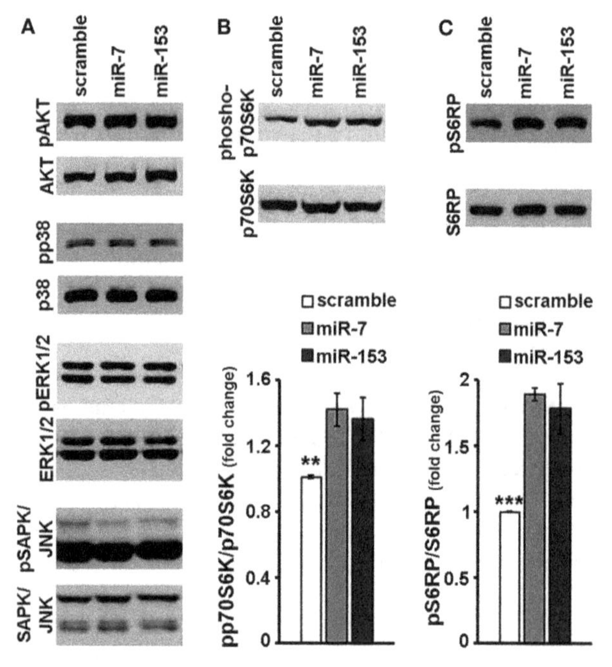

FIGURE 4 | miR-7 and miR-153 activated p70S6K signaling cascade in cortical neurons. Six to seven days old primary cortical neurons were transduced with adenoviral particles expressing scramble miR, miR-7, or miR-153 and were lysed 48 h post-transduction. **(A)** Equal amounts of total protein from lysates of cortical neurons were analyzed on 10% SDS-PAGE and immunoblotted with antibodies specific for phosphorylated forms of AKT, p38 MAPK, ERK1/2 SAPK/JNK. To ensure equal loading membranes were re-probed against AKT, p38 MAPK, ERK1/2, and SAPK/JNK, respectively. **(B,C)** Equal amounts of total protein from lysates of cortical neurons were analyzed on 10% SDS-PAGE and immunoblotted with antibodies specific for phosphorylated forms of p70S6K **(B)** as well as for the phosphorylated forms of p70S6K substrate, S6RP **(C)**. To ensure equal loading, membranes were re-probed against p70S6K and S6RP, respectively. Quantification of the results was performed by scanning densitometry. Bars in the graph depict mean ± s.e.m. Note that compared to scramble-transduced controls, primary cortical neurons transduced with miR-7 or miR-153 expressing adenoviruses displayed a significant increase only in the levels of phosphorylated forms of p70S6K and S6RP. $^{**}P \leq 0.01$, $^{***}P \leq 0.001$.

To further explore the latter hypothesis, 6–7 days old primary cortical neurons were again transduced with adenoviral particles expressing scramble miR, miR-7, or miR-153 and left *in culture* for additional 48 h. One hour before harvest, cultures were supplemented with 20 nM rapamycin, a potent mTORC1 (and mTORC2 at higher doses and long-term treatment) inhibitor (Sarbassov et al., 2006; Rosner and Hengstschlager, 2008; Chen et al., 2010) and levels of phosphorylated mTORC1 effector p70S6K and its phosphorylated substrates S6RP and eEF2K were determined. As shown in **Figure 5A**, irrespective of the adenovirus used, 1-h rapamycin treatment resulted to a significant decrease in the levels of phosphorylated p70S6K [ANOVA: $F_{(3, 11)} = 36.857$, $P < 0.001$ and *post-hoc*]; nevertheless, primary cortical neurons transduced with miR-7 or miR-153 sustained phosphorylated p70S6K levels at more than 2-fold higher than scramble miR-transduced controls (*post-hoc*, $P < 0.01$). Consistently, overexpression of miR-7 and miR-153 attenuated the effect of rapamycin on the phosphorylation of S6RP [ANOVA: $F_{(3, 11)} = 71.638$, $P < 0.001$ and *post-hoc*; **Figure 5B**], and of eEF2K [ANOVA: $F_{(3, 11)} = 65.623$, $P < 0.001$ and *post-hoc*; **Figure 5B**], More specifically, compared to scramble-transduced rapamycin-treated controls, primary cortical neurons transduced with miR-7 or miR-153 and treated with rapamycin displayed significantly increased levels of phosphorylated S6RP (4.7- and 5.4-fold increase in the case of miR-7, miR-153 overexpression, respectively; *post-hoc*, $P < 0.001$), as well as of phosphorylated eEF2K (by 90% for miR-7 and 65% for miR-153, *post-hoc*, $P < 0.001$). It appears, therefore, that miR-7 and miR-153 may act as "activators" of mTOR signaling pathway.

Given that mTOR signaling pathway is a downstream regulator of neuronal survival (see also **Supplemental Figure 4**), we next wanted to examine whether overexpression of miR-7 and/or miR-153 is able to interfere with the effect of mTOR signaling inhibition on cell survival. In order to address this, 6–7 days old primary cortical neurons were transduced with adenoviral particles expressing scramble miR, miR-7, or miR-153, supplemented with 20 nM rapamycin 24 h post-transduction, and left *in*

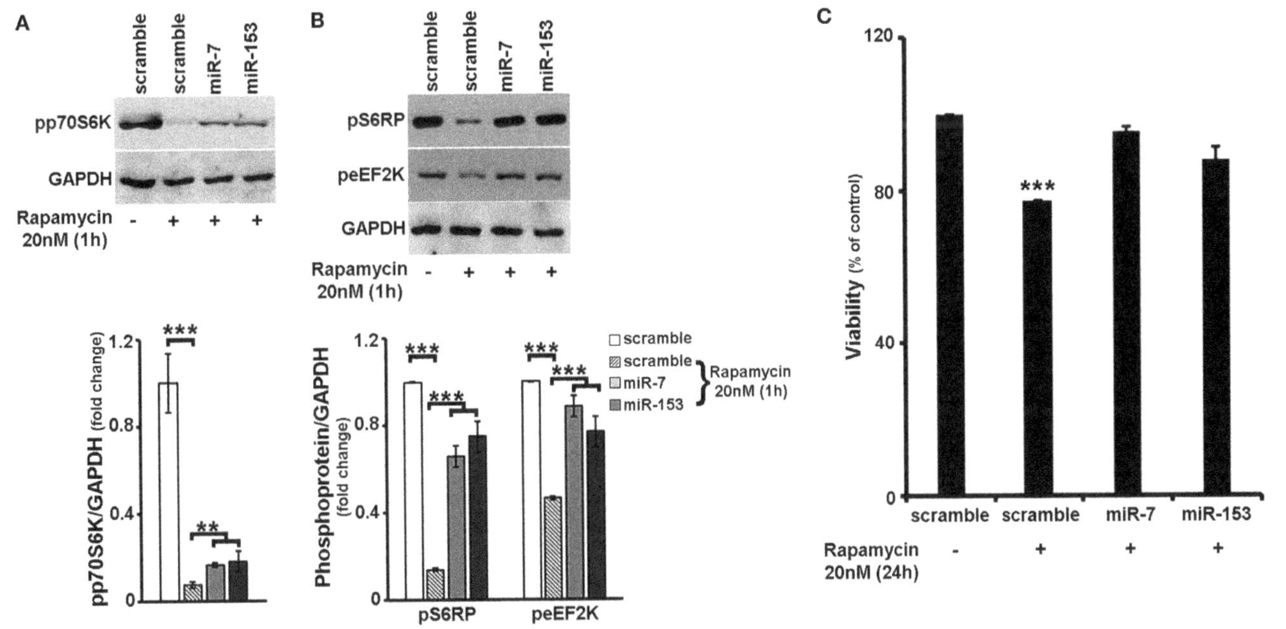

FIGURE 5 | Overexpression of miR-7 or miR-153 attenuated the effects of rapamycin in cortical neurons. (A,B) Six to seven days old primary cortical neurons were transduced with adenoviral particles expressing scramble miR, miR-7, or miR-153 and left *in culture* for additional 48 h. One hour before harvest, cultures were supplemented with 20 nM rapamycin. Equal amounts of total protein from lysates of cortical neurons were analyzed on 10% SDS-PAGE and immunoblotted with antibodies specific for phosphorylated forms of p70S6K, S6RP, and eEF2K. To ensure equal loading, membranes were re-probed against GAPDH. Quantification of the results was performed by scanning densitometry. Note that overexpression of miR-7, as well as that of miR-153 attenuated the effect of rapamycin on the phosphorylation of all proteins examined. **(C)** Six to seven days old primary cortical neurons were transduced with the same adenoviral particles and after 24 h were exposed to 20 nM of rapamycin for an additional of 24 h. Neuronal viability following 24-h treatment with rapamycin was monitored by the MTT assay. Note that overexpression of miR-7 and/or miR-153 attenuated rapamycin-induced cell death. Bars in all the presented graphs depict mean ± s.e.m. **$P \leq 0.01$, ***$P \leq 0.001$.

culture for an additional 24 h. Neuronal viability was monitored using the MTT assay. As depicted in **Figure 5C**, a 24-h treatment with rapamycin reduced significantly the viability of scramble-transduced neuronal cultures to 77% [ANOVA: $F_{(3,\ 11)} = 32.804$, $P < 0.001$ and *post-hoc*], a reduction that was comparable to the one observed in untransduced cortical neuronal cultures (**Supplemental Figure 4**). In contrast, viability of miR-7-, or miR-153- transduced neuronal cultures was not significantly impaired, providing further support that these two miRs sustain mTOR signaling in neurons.

OVEREXPRESSION OF miR-7 AND/OR miR-153 IN CORTICAL NEURONS ATTENUATED MPP$^+$-INDUCED NEUROTOXICITY VIA UPREGULATION OF mTOR PATHWAY

Our results so far suggest that miR-7 and miR-153 are able to induce rapamycin-sensitive mTOR downstream signaling, which appeared significantly impaired in cortical neurons upon MPP$^+$ treatment. Therefore, in order to evaluate whether miR-7 and/or miR-153 exert their neuroprotective effect through upregulation of mTOR signaling pathway, 6- to 7- day old primary cortical neurons were again transduced with adenoviral particles expressing scramble miR, miR-7, or miR-153, as well as with an adenoviral construct expressing both of these two miRs. Twenty four hours post-transduction, cortical neurons were exposed to 10 μM of MPP$^+$ and the activation of p70S6K and its substrates was assessed 24 h later by immunoblotting. As shown in **Figures 6A,B**, compared to scramble-transduced untreated controls, 24-h treatment with 10 μM of MPP$^+$ induced a significant decrease in the levels of phosphorylated p70S6K [$F_{(4,\ 14)} = 5.072$, $P < 0.05$ and *post-hoc*] and of its phosphorylated substrate S6RP [$F_{(4,\ 14)} = 5.241$, $P < 0.05$ and *post-hoc*] in only the scramble-transduced cortical neurons; overexpression of miR-7 or miR-153 attenuated the MPP$^+$-induced reduction in the activation of p70S6K and its downstream targets, while overexpression of both miRs restored their phosphorylation status to that of scramble-transduced untreated controls. To further explore the possibility that sustained mTOR downstream signaling activation underlies the neuroprotective effects of miR-7 and miR-153, 20 nM of rapamycin was co-administered with 10 μM MPP$^+$ in these neuronal cultures. As shown in **Figure 6C**, in scramble miR-transduced cultures all treatments lead to a significant reduction in neuronal viability [$F_{(3,\ 11)} = 25.244$, $P < 0.001$ and *post-hoc*]. In contrast, in miR-7, miR-153, or miR-7/153 -transduced cultures, neuronal viability was significantly impaired only when MPP$^+$ was co-administered with rapamycin [miR-7: $F_{(3,\ 11)} = 41.253$, $P < 0.001$ and *post-hoc*; miR-153: $F_{(3,\ 11)} = 14.061$, $P = 0.001$ and *post-hoc*, miR-7/153: $F_{(3,\ 11)} = 26.653$, $P < 0.001$ see **Figure 6C**]. Taken together the above results suggest that miR-7 and/or miR-153 induced activation of mTOR pathway largely mediates their neuroprotective effect against MPP$^+$ toxicity in cortical neurons.

Finally, in order to explore whether miR-7 and/or miR-153 interfere with MPP$^+$-induced changes in other than mTOR

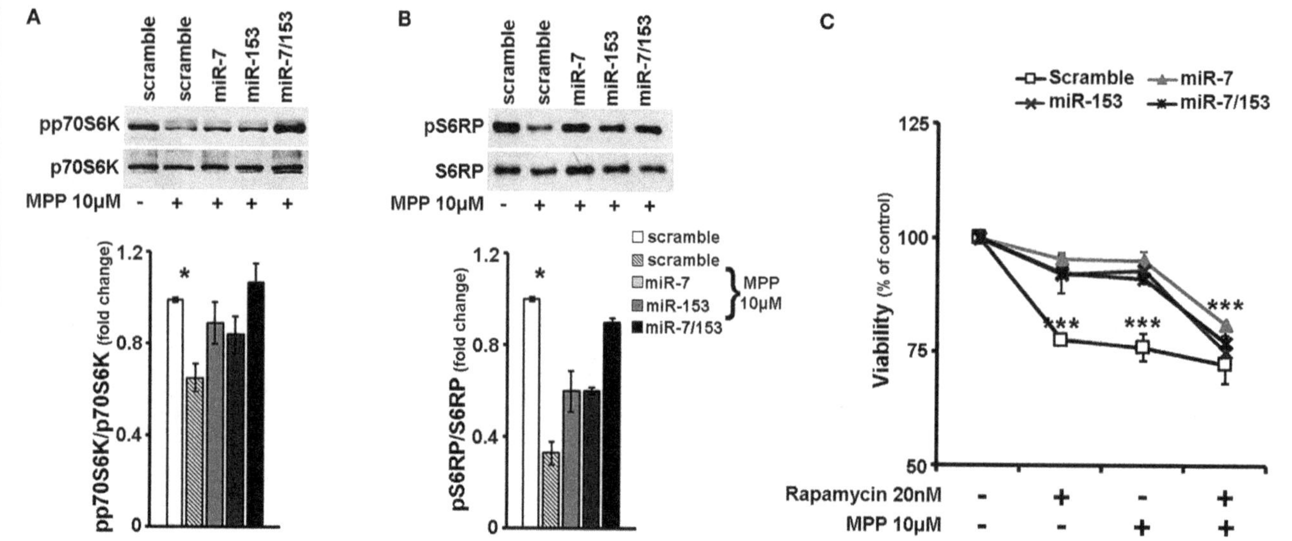

FIGURE 6 | miR-7 and/or miR-153 attenuated MPP+-induced neurotoxicity via upregulation of rapamycin sensitive mTOR pathway. (A,B) Six to seven days old primary cortical neurons were transduced with adenoviral particles expressing scramble miR, miR-7, miR-153, or both miR-7/153. After 24 h, transduced neurons were exposed for additional 24 h to 10 μM of MPP+. Equal amounts of total protein from lysates of transduced cortical neurons cultured for 24 h in the presence of 10 μM MPP+ were analyzed on 10% SDS-PAGE and immunoblotted with antibodies specific for phosphorylated forms of p70S6K **(A)** and S6RP **(B)**. To ensure equal loading membranes were re-probed against p70S6K and S6RP, respectively. Note that overexpression of miR-7 and/or miR-153 attenuated the effect of MPP+ on the phosphorylation of all proteins examined. Quantification of the results was performed by scanning densitometry. **(C)** Six to seven days old cultures of primary cortical neurons were transduced as described above, and 24 h later were exposed to 20 nM of rapamycin, 10 μM of MPP+, or both. Neuronal viability was monitored 24 h post-exposure by the MTT assay. Note that in the presence of rapamycin, overexpression of miR-7 and/or miR-153 failed to protect cortical neurons against MPP+-induced cell death. Bars in all presented graphs depict mean ± s.e.m. $^{*}P < 0.05$, $^{***}P \leq 0.001$.

intracellular signaling cascades, the phosphorylation status of other major signaling effectors was examined in cortical neurons transduced with scramble miR, miR-7, miR-153, or miR-7/153 adenoviruses and treated for 24 h with 10 μM MPP^+. As shown in **Figure 7A**, in MPP^+-treated cortical neurons overexpression of both miR-7/153, but not that of miR-7 or miR-153 alone, attenuated the MPP^+-induced reduction in the levels of phosphorylated AKT [$F_{(4, 24)} = 12.314$, $P = 0.01$ and *post-hoc*]. Interestingly, miR-153, but not miR-7 or miR-7/153, attenuated the MPP^+-induced activation of pro-apoptotic p38 MAPK [$F_{(4, 24)} = 12.978$, $P = 0.01$ and *post-hoc*; **Figure 7B**]. Finally, overexpression of miR-7 and/or miR-153 had no significant effect on the phosphorylation status of ERK1/2 (**Figure 7C**), but resulted in a significant increase of phosphorylated SAPK/JNK levels to above control levels [$F_{(4, 24)} = 15.894$, $P < 0.001$ and *post-hoc*; **Figure 7D**]. It, therefore, appears that miR-7 and/or miR-153 alter the intracellular response of cortical neurons to MPP^+ insult and thus interfere with MPP^+-induced neurotoxicity.

DISCUSSION

The mechanisms underlying chronic neurodegeneration in PD remain obscure. An emerging hypothesis is that neuronal systems deteriorate and eventually degenerate due to failure of intrinsic cellular pathways that mediate neuronal homeostasis. This failure maybe due to lack of external neurotrophic support or to mutations in intrinsic factors such as the PARK genes that modify intracellular signaling (reviewed in Wang et al., 2012). Thus, far, a great number of studies have indicated that neurotrophic factors or herbal extracts protect neurons from PD insults by enhancing pro-survival and/or decreasing pro-apoptotic signaling pathways (Nakaso et al., 2008; Wang et al., 2010; Cui et al., 2011; Zhang et al., 2011; Bao et al., 2012; Hashimoto et al., 2012). In addition, manipulation of specific intracellular signaling cascades by either overexpressing or inhibiting signaling protein kinases has revealed that they modulate most PD neurotoxin effects (Malagelada et al., 2006; Zhu et al., 2007, 2012; Nakaso et al., 2008; Cui et al., 2011; Bao et al., 2012; Piao et al., 2012). Most importantly, these findings phenocopy data from the analysis of human postmortem PD brains that show decreased phosphorylation of pro-survival and enhanced activation of pro-apoptotic pathways (Zhu et al., 2002, 2003; Malagelada et al., 2006; Timmons et al., 2009; Reinhardt et al., 2013).

Previous work from our group has shown that mir-7 and mir-153 significantly regulate the expression of α-synuclein, a protein encoded by the gene SNCA that belongs to the PARK gene family (Doxakis, 2010). A-synuclein plays a seminal role in neurodegeneration and has been shown, among others, to affect signaling by modulating neurotrophin BDNF expression and AKT activity (Yuan et al., 2010; Chung et al., 2011). Based on the intrinsic property of miRs to regulate the expression of multiple proteins and possibly the activation of signaling cascades, in the present study we wished to investigate if miR-7 and miR-153 protect neurons exposed to PD insults via altering intracellular signaling. Thus, we evaluated whether overexpression of mir-7 and/or mir-153 could prevent MPP^+-induced toxicity in cortical neurons. Cortical neurons were selected because they are directly

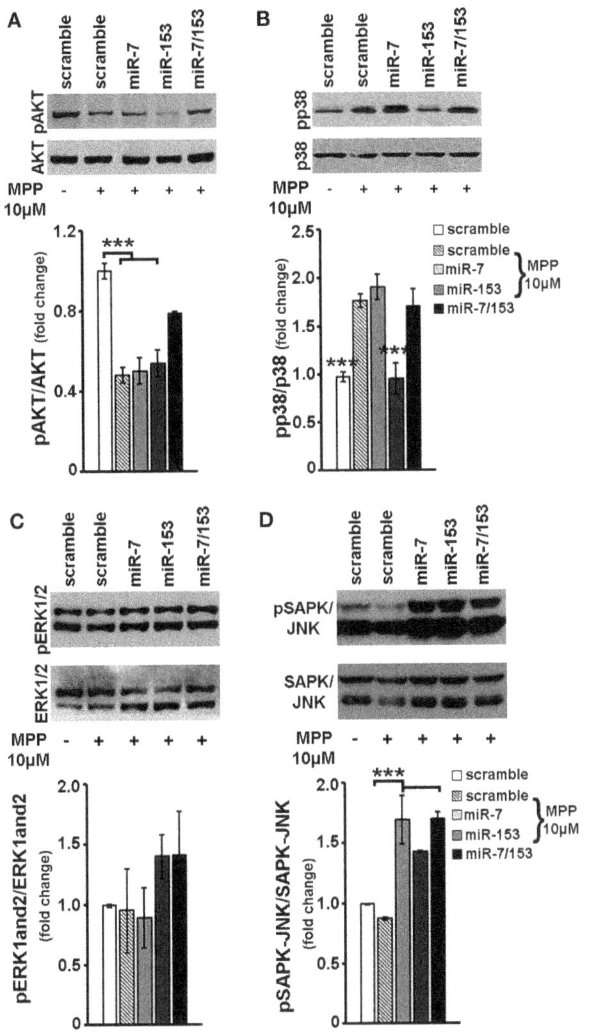

FIGURE 7 | Effect of miR-7 and/or mir-153 overexpression on AKT, p38, ERK-1/2, and SAPK/JNK signaling in MPP+-treated cortical neurons. Six to seven days old primary cortical neurons were transduced with adenoviral particles expressing scramble miR, miR-7, miR-153, or both miR-7/153. After 24 h, transduced neurons were exposed for additional 24 h to 10 μM of MPP+. Equal amounts of total protein from lysates of transduced cortical neurons cultured for 24 h in the presence of 10 μM MPP+ were analyzed on 10% SDS-PAGE and immunoblotted with antibodies specific for phosphorylated forms of AKT **(A)**, p38 MAPK **(B)**, ERK1/2 **(C)**, and SAPK/JNK **(D)**. To ensure equal loading membranes were re-probed against AKT, p38 MAPK, ERK1/2, and SAPK/JNK, respectively. Quantification of the results was performed by scanning densitometry. Bars in all the presented graphs depict mean ± s.e.m. Note that miR-7, miR-153, or miR-7/153 altered in an opposite way MPP+-induced changes in intracellular signaling cascades. *** $P < 0.001$.

affected in PD by showing progressive pathology (Trojanowski et al., 1998; Braak et al., 2006) and they can be isolated in great numbers relative free of glial cells. MPP+, on the other hand, is a widely used neurotoxin that reproduces the neuronal dysfunction of PD both *in vivo* and in different cell systems *in vitro*. MPP+ enters cells through the dopamine re-uptake system, present in dopaminergic neurons; however, at higher concentrations it can enter all cell types by passive diffusion (Reinhard et al., 1990) and/or by the extraneuronal monoamine transporter (Russ et al., 1996). The mechanism of MPP+ toxicity in cells is rather ubiquitous and involves inhibition of the mitochondrial respiratory chain, elevation of oxidative stress and alteration of intracellular signaling. The vulnerability of neurons to MPP+ is modified by microglia numbers in the vicinity of neurons, neurotrophic support, glutathione, or superoxide dismutase content (antioxidant capacity), the content of redox active molecules or elements (such as dopamine or iron), the ratio of anti-apoptotic vs. pro-apoptotic BCL-2 family proteins and basal levels of phosphorylated signaling kinases (Lawson et al., 1990; Kim et al., 2000; Zigmond et al., 2002; Wu et al., 2003; Zecca et al., 2004; Willis et al., 2007). Noteworthy, modulation of intracellular signaling pathways has been shown to mediate most of the MPP+ effects in neurons indicating that signaling cascades are downstream of MPP+ targets and/or can reverse pro-apoptotic effects (Nakaso et al., 2008; Wang et al., 2010; Cui et al., 2011; Bao et al., 2012; Hashimoto et al., 2012; Piao et al., 2012).

Based on the above, we initially characterized the molecular mechanisms underlying MPP+-induced neuronal death in cortical neurons since most studies have been carried out in dividing neuroblastoma cells and/or were limited to two or three signaling pathways. Hence, the levels of apoptosis-related BCL-2 family members and the major signaling pathways, AKT, ERK-1/2, p38, SAPK/JNK, and mTOR were determined. Consistent with previous studies, we found that MPP+-induced neurotoxicity displayed apoptotic characteristics, as documented by the reduced levels of BCL-2 and the increased levels of cleaved caspase-3, and was accompanied by enhanced activities of the pro-apoptotic p38 and ERK-1/2 MAPK signaling pathways as well as by reduced activation of pro-survival AKT and p70S6K kinases (Deguil et al., 2007; Junyent et al., 2010; Cui et al., 2011; Bao et al., 2012; Hashimoto et al., 2012; Rodriguez-Blanco et al., 2012). Finally, contrary to most other findings (Wang et al., 2010; Zhang et al., 2011; Hashimoto et al., 2012; Rodriguez-Blanco et al., 2012), and with the exception of a single study (Sun and Chang, 2003), activation of the SAPK/JNK kinase was suppressed in a dose-dependent manner by MPP+ treatment of cortical neurons.

Subsequently, the effect of miR-7 and miR-153 overexpression in neurons was determined. We found that miR overexpression did not, overall, alter neuronal viability or the activity of AKT, ERK-1/2, p38, and SAPK/JNK signaling pathways. However, a significant upregulation of mTORC1 downstream signaling was observed by the overexpression of both miRs, as evident by the increased levels of phosphorylated p70S6K and its downstream targets S6RP and eEF2K. mTOR complexes (mTORC1/2) serve as central regulators of cell metabolism, growth and survival by integrating intracellular (energy status, oxygen, and amino acids) and extracellular signals (growth factors) (Wu et al., 2004; Takei et al., 2009; reviewed in Swiech et al., 2008; Laplante and Sabatini, 2013). Mutant mTOR embryos lack telencephalon and die by midgestation, an effect that is phenocopied by the mTOR inhibitor, rapamycin, validating the importance of this pathway in brain development (Hentges et al., 2001). In cultured neurons, mTORC1, the best studied mTOR complex, has been shown to regulate soma size, dendrite axonal growth, dendrite development, and regeneration (Campbell and Holt, 2001; Jaworski et al., 2005; Kumar et al., 2005; Tavazoie et al., 2005; Verma et al., 2005; Li et al., 2008; Park et al., 2008). Our finding that the activation of mTOR downstream effectors was significantly increased in cortical neurons over-expressing miR-7 or miR-153, suggests that these two miRs may act as "activators" of mTOR signaling pathway. The latter hypothesis is further supported by our observations showing that overexpression of miR-7 or miR-153 in primary neurons is able to attenuate the effects of rapamycin on both the activation of mTOR downstream effectors and neuronal viability.

Probing the effect of miR-7 and miR-153 overexpression in MPP^+-treated neurons, we revealed that they could, either alone or together, significantly protect neurons from cell death. We reasoned that this was due to enhanced mTOR signaling as this was the only pathway that was upregulated by the overexpression of both miRs. Consistent with the latter hypothesis, overexpression of miR-7 and/or miR-153 attenuated the MPP^+-induced reduction on the activation of p70S6K and its downstream targets, whereas treatment of transduced neurons with rapamycin abolished the pro-survival effects of miR-7 and miR-153 upon MPP^+ exposure.

To further explore the modulation of intracellular signaling by miR-7 and miR-153 overexpression in MPP^+-treated neurons, the activation of the remaining pathways was also determined. It should be noted that compared to untransduced cortical neurons, transduced primary cortical neurons used in the present study appeared less resistant to MPP^+-treatment and therefore displayed a more robust intracellular response to the same MPP^+ concentration i.e., 10 μM; this is likely to be attributed to the adenoviral transduction, given that it comprises an additional, to that of MPP^+, insult for the cortical neurons. Taking the latter observation into account, herein we found that the activity of AKT which is known to activate mTORC1 by alleviating the inhibition induced by TSC2 and PRAS40 proteins (Dan et al., 2002; Inoki et al., 2002; Manning et al., 2002; Vander Haar et al., 2007; Zhu et al., 2007), was not restored by either miR-7 or miR-153; however, overexpressing both miR-7 and miR-153 significantly relieved the suppression of AKT activation by MPP^+, likely by having overlapping or additive effects on their targets. In addition, the finding that AKT was activated at Ser473, known to be mediated by mTORC2 complex (Sarbassov et al., 2005), may indicate that mTORC2 signaling is also contributing to the survival of neurons transduced by both miRs. p38 is a stress kinase that has been linked to neuro-inflammation and MPP^+-mediated apoptosis (Karunakaran et al., 2008; Thomas et al., 2008b). It should be noted that miR-153, but not miR-7, significantly prevented the activation of p38 by MPP^+ which may have partly contributed to its pro-survival effects in cortical neurons. Overexpressing miR-7 and miR-153 together alleviated the negative effect of miR-153 on p38 phosphorylation indicating that miR-7 targets may block mir-153 responses on p38 signaling pathway activation. The role of ERK-1/2 activation in neuronal survival is context-specific; some reports show positive or negative input on survival after induction by growth factors, glutamate, or okadaic acid (Runden et al., 1998; Bonni et al., 1999; Satoh et al., 2000; Stanciu et al., 2000; Cui et al., 2011) while others implicate it in MPP^+- and 6-hydroxydopamine- induced mitophagy/autophagy and cell death (Zhu et al., 2007, 2012). In the present study, neither miR-7 nor miR-153 overexpression significantly changed ERK-1/2 phosphorylation in the MPP^+-treated neurons. SAPK/JNK is a kinase with an indispensable role in microtubule stability in neurons. It stimulates dendrite formation, axodendritic length, axonal regeneration, mediates fast axonal transport, and contributes to the regulation of synaptic plasticity (Bjorkblom et al., 2005; Chen et al., 2005; Zhu et al., 2005; Tararuk et al., 2006; Thomas et al., 2008a; Morfini et al., 2009; Barnat et al., 2010; Podkowa et al., 2010). At the same time it has been linked to stress-induced apoptosis in different pathological conditions as a result of its inhibition of autophagy and the induction of pro-apoptotic BCL-2 family members (Jia et al., 2006; Hubner et al., 2008; Xu et al., 2011). In our cell culture system, miR-7 and miR-153 overexpression significantly lifted SAPK/JNK activation in the MPP^+-treated neurons. Overexpression of both miRs together did not further induce SAPK/JNK activation indicating that they modulate a similar target group. Additional experiments will be required to determine if the effect of miR-7 and miR-153 overexpression on SAPK/JNK phosphorylation partly negates their neuroprotective responses via mTOR signaling, and/or maintains the axodendritic growth of neurons which is impaired by MPP^+-induced microtubule dysfunction (Cartelli et al., 2010) and/or negates MPP^+-induced ERK-1/2-mediated enhanced autophagy in neurons.

Taken together, our data suggest that miR-7 and miR-153 protect neurons against MPP^+-induced toxicity via upregulation of mTOR downstream targets. In addition, we show that miR-7 and miR-153 modulate the signaling pathways of SAPK/JNK and p38 in MPP^+-treated cells, however, their effect on neuronal viability maybe less important. Given also our previous study showing that miR-7 and miR-153 regulate α-synuclein expression, it appears these two miRs may prove good therapeutic candidates for the treatment of PD. Evidence from successful medical interventions based on miRs has already been shown in cornerstone studies to lower plasma cholesterol levels in rodents and primates (Krutzfeldt et al., 2005; Elmen et al., 2008a,b). Currently, a large number of miRs are studied in preclinical and clinical settings by biotechnology companies (Lindow and Kauppinen, 2012). In future, it will be important to characterize the effect of miR-7 and miR-153 on neurite outgrowth and synaptogenesis and test if they can support neurons treated with other PD neurotoxins.

ACKNOWLEDGMENTS

We thank Paulos Alexakos for excellent veterinary assistance. Epaminondas Doxakis has received funding from the Greek General Secretariat for Research and Technology (Grant IDs 09Syn-12-876 and 12RUS-11-65).

SUPPLEMENTARY MATERIAL

Supplemental Figure 1 | Overexpression of miR-7 or miR-153 has no effect on neuronal viability. (A) Six to seven days old primary cortical neurons were left untreated or were transduced with adenoviral particles expressing scramble miR, miR-7, miR-153, or both miR-7153 and neuronal viability was assayed by MTT reduction 48 h later. It should be noted that overall adenoviral infection of primary cortical neurons affected cell viability [$F_{(4,\ 19)} = 2.979$, *$P = 0.05$ and *post-hoc*]; nevertheless, no significant difference was observed among transduced primary neurons, i.e., those transduced with adenoviral particles expressing a scramble miR or the miR (s) of interest. **(B)** Six to seven days old primary cortical neurons were left untreated or were transduced with the same adenoviral particles and lysed 48 h later. Equal amounts of total protein from lysates of cortical neurons were analyzed on 12% SDS-PAGE and immunoblotted with antibodies specific for BCL-2 and cleaved caspase-3. To ensure equal loading membranes were re-probed against GAPDH. Compared to scramble-transduced controls, primary cortical neurons transduced with miR-7, miR-153, or miR-7/153 displayed no significant change on either BCL-2 or cleaved caspase-3 protein levels; it should be noted that a statistically insignificant increase in the levels of cleaved caspase-3 was observed among transduced and untransduced primary neurons.

Supplemental Figure 2 | MMP$^+$ treatment induced neurotoxicity and alterations in major signaling cascades in both untransduced and scramble miR transduced cortical neurons in a similar manner. (A) Six to seven days old primary cortical neurons were left untreated or were transduced with adenoviral particles expressing scramble miR. After 24 h, neuronal cultures were exposed for additional 24 h to various concentrations of MPP$^+$. Cell viability following dose-dependent treatments was assayed by measuring MTT reduction by live neurons. Note that similar significant reductions in neuronal viability was observed in both untransduced and scramble miR transduced neurons upon treatment with 10, 20, 30, and 50 μM, but not 5 μM, of MPP$^+$. **(B,C)** Six to seven days old primary cortical neurons were left untreated or were transduced with adenoviral particles expressing scramble miR. After 24 h, neuronal cultures were exposed for additional 24 h to 10 μM of MPP$^+$. Equal amounts of total protein from lysates of cortical neurons were analyzed on 10% SDS-PAGE and immunoblotted with antibodies specific for phosphorylated forms of AKT, p38 MAPK, p70S6K, SAPK/JNK, and ERK1/2. To ensure equal loading membranes were re-probed against AKT, p38 MAPK, p70S6K, SAPK/JNK, and ERK1/2, respectively. Note that in contrast to untransduced neurons, scramble miR transduced neurons displayed significant reduction of phosphorylated AKT levels even at 10 μM of MPP$^+$. No difference was observed in the phosphorylation status of the other major signaling kinases examined among untransduced and scramble miR transduced neurons upon treatment with 10 μM of MPP$^+$. ***$P < 0.001$.

Supplemental Figure 3 | Adenoviral overexpression of miR-7 and miR-153 in cortical neurons, but not of scramble miR, activated p70S6K signaling cascade. Six to seven days old primary cortical neurons were transduced with empty adenoviral particles or adenoviral particles expressing scramble miR, miR-7, or miR-153 and were lysed 48 later. Equal amounts of total protein from lysates of untransduced and transduced cortical neurons were analyzed on 10% SDS-PAGE and immunoblotted with antibodies specific for phosphorylated forms of p70S6K **(A)** and S6RP **(B)**. To ensure equal loading, membranes were re-probed against GAPDH. Note that no difference was observed in the levels of phosphorylated p70S6K and S6RP between transduced empty control and scramble miR transduced cortical neurons.

Supplemental Figure 4 | Rapamycin induced neurotoxicity in cortical neurons. Seven-day primary cortical neurons were treated with various concentrations of rapamycin and MPP$^+$ for 24 h. Cell viability following dose-dependent treatments was assayed by measuring MTT reduction by live neurons. Note that a significant ~20% reduction in neuronal viability was observed upon treatment with rapamycin at concentrations 20–50 nM [$F_{(4,\ 14)} = 20.852$, $P < 0.001$]. No synergistic effect was observed among rapamycin and MPP$^+$. ***$P < 0.001$.

REFERENCES

Ballard, P. A., Tetrud, J. W., and Langston, J. W. (1985). Permanent human parkinsonism due to 1-methyl-4-phenyl-1,2,3,6-tetrahydropyridine (MPTP): seven cases. *Neurology* 35, 949–956. doi: 10.1212/WNL.35.7.949

Bao, X. Q., Kong, X. C., Qian, C., and Zhang, D. (2012). FLZ protects dopaminergic neuron through activating protein kinase B/mammalian target of rapamycin pathway and inhibiting RTP801 expression in Parkinson's disease models. *Neuroscience* 202, 396–404. doi: 10.1016/j.neuroscience.2011.11.036

Barnat, M., Enslen, H., Propst, F., Davis, R. J., Soares, S., and Nothias, F. (2010). Distinct roles of c-Jun N-terminal kinase isoforms in neurite initiation and elongation during axonal regeneration. *J. Neurosci.* 30, 7804–7816. doi: 10.1523/JNEUROSCI.0372-10.2010

Bjorkblom, B., Ostman, N., Hongisto, V., Komarovski, V., Filen, J. J., Nyman, T. A., et al. (2005). Constitutively active cytoplasmic c-Jun N-terminal kinase 1 is a dominant regulator of dendritic architecture: role of microtubule-associated protein 2 as an effector. *J. Neurosci.* 25, 6350–6361. doi: 10.1523/JNEUROSCI.1517-05.2005

Bonni, A., Brunet, A., West, A. E., Datta, S. R., Takasu, M. A., and Greenberg, M. E. (1999). Cell survival promoted by the Ras-MAPK signaling pathway by transcription-dependent and -independent mechanisms. *Science* 286, 1358–1362. doi: 10.1126/science.286.5443.1358

Braak, H., Rub, U., Schultz, C., and Del Tredici, K. (2006). Vulnerability of cortical neurons to Alzheimer's and Parkinson's diseases. *J. Alzheimers Dis.* 9, 35–44.

Campbell, D. S., and Holt, C. E. (2001). Chemotropic responses of retinal growth cones mediated by rapid local protein synthesis and degradation. *Neuron* 32, 1013–1026. doi: 10.1016/S0896-6273(01)00551-7

Cartelli, D., Ronchi, C., Maggioni, M. G., Rodighiero, S., Giavini, E., and Cappelletti, G. (2010). Microtubule dysfunction precedes transport impairment and mitochondria damage in MPP$^+$ -induced neurodegeneration. *J. Neurochem.* 115, 247–258. doi: 10.1111/j.1471-4159.2010.06924.x

Chen, J. T., Lu, D. H., Chia, C. P., Ruan, D. Y., Sabapathy, K., and Xiao, Z. C. (2005). Impaired long-term potentiation in c-Jun N-terminal kinase 2-deficient mice. *J. Neurochem.* 93, 463–473. doi: 10.1111/j.1471-4159.2005.03037.x

Chen, X. G., Liu, F., Song, X. F., Wang, Z. H., Dong, Z. Q., Hu, Z. Q., et al. (2010). Rapamycin regulates Akt and ERK phosphorylation through mTORC1 and mTORC2 signaling pathways. *Mol. Carcinog.* 49, 603–610. doi: 10.1002/mc.20628

Chung, J. Y., Lee, S. J., Lee, S. H., Jung, Y. S., Ha, N. C., Seol, W., et al. (2011). Direct interaction of alpha-synuclein and AKT regulates IGF-1 signaling: implication of Parkinson disease. *Neurosignals* 19, 86–96. doi: 10.1159/000325028

Cui, W., Li, W., Han, R., Mak, S., Zhang, H., Hu, S., et al. (2011). PI3-K/Akt and ERK pathways activated by VEGF play opposite roles in MPP$^+$-induced neuronal apoptosis. *Neurochem. Int.* 59, 945–953. doi: 10.1016/j.neuint.2011.07.005

Dan, H. C., Sun, M., Yang, L., Feldman, R. I., Sui, X. M., Ou, C. C., et al. (2002). Phosphatidylinositol 3-kinase/Akt pathway regulates tuberous sclerosis tumor suppressor complex by phosphorylation of tuberin. *J. Biol. Chem.* 277, 35364–35370. doi: 10.1074/jbc.M205838200

Davis, G. C., Williams, A. C., Markey, S. P., Ebert, M. H., Caine, E. D., Reichert, C. M., et al. (1979). Chronic Parkinsonism secondary to intravenous injection of meperidine analogues. *Psychiatry Res.* 1, 249–254. doi: 10.1016/0165-1781(79)90006-4

Deguil, J., Jailloux, D., Page, G., Fauconneau, B., Houeto, J. L., Philippe, M., et al. (2007). Neuroprotective effects of pituitary adenylate cyclase-activating polypeptide (PACAP) in MPP$^+$-induced alteration of translational control in Neuro-2a neuroblastoma cells. *J. Neurosci. Res.* 85, 2017–2025. doi: 10.1002/jnr.21318

Doxakis, E. (2010). Post-transcriptional regulation of alpha-synuclein expression by mir-7 and mir-153. *J. Biol. Chem.* 285, 12726–12734. doi: 10.1074/jbc.M109.086827

Doxakis, E. (2013). Principles of miRNA-Target Regulation in Metazoan Models. *Int. J. Mol. Sci.* 14, 16280–16302. doi: 10.3390/ijms140816280

Doxakis, E., Huang, E. J., and Davies, A. M. (2004). Homeodomain-interacting protein kinase-2 regulates apoptosis in developing sensory and sympathetic neurons. *Curr. Biol.* 14, 1761–1765. doi: 10.1016/j.cub.2004.09.050

Elmen, J., Lindow, M., Schutz, S., Lawrence, M., Petri, A., Obad, S., et al. (2008a). LNA-mediated microRNA silencing in non-human primates. *Nature* 452, 896–899. doi: 10.1038/nature06783

Elmen, J., Lindow, M., Silahtaroglu, A., Bak, M., Christensen, M., Lind-Thomsen, A., et al. (2008b). Antagonism of microRNA-122 in mice by systemically administered LNA-antimiR leads to upregulation of a large set of predicted target mRNAs in the liver. *Nucleic Acids Res.* 36, 1153–1162. doi: 10.1093/nar/gkm1113

Fang, Y., Xue, J. L., Shen, Q., Chen, J., and Tian, L. (2012). MicroRNA-7 inhibits tumor growth and metastasis by targeting the phosphoinositide 3-kinase/Akt pathway in hepatocellular carcinoma. *Hepatology* 55, 1852–1862. doi: 10.1002/hep.25576

Hashimoto, R., Yu, J., Koizumi, H., Ouchi, Y., and Okabe, T. (2012). Ginsenoside Rb1 Prevents MPP(+)-Induced Apoptosis in PC12 Cells by Stimulating Estrogen Receptors with Consequent Activation of ERK1/2, Akt and Inhibition of SAPK/JNK, p38 MAPK. *Evid. Based Complement. Alternat. Med.* 2012, 693717. doi: 10.1155/2012/693717

Hentges, K. E., Sirry, B., Gingeras, A. C., Sarbassov, D., Sonenberg, N., Sabatini, D., et al. (2001). FRAP/mTOR is required for proliferation and patterning during embryonic development in the mouse. *Proc. Natl. Acad. Sci. U.S.A.* 98, 13796–13801. doi: 10.1073/pnas.241184198

Hubner, A., Barrett, T., Flavell, R. A., and Davis, R. J. (2008). Multisite phosphorylation regulates Bim stability and apoptotic activity. *Mol. Cell* 30, 415–425. doi: 10.1016/j.molcel.2008.03.025

Inoki, K., Li, Y., Zhu, T., Wu, J., and Guan, K. L. (2002). TSC2 is phosphorylated and inhibited by Akt and suppresses mTOR signalling. *Nat. Cell Biol.* 4, 648–657. doi: 10.1038/ncb839

Jaworski, J., Spangler, S., Seeburg, D. P., Hoogenraad, C. C., and Sheng, M. (2005). Control of dendritic arborization by the phosphoinositide-3′-kinase-Akt-mammalian target of rapamycin pathway. *J. Neurosci.* 25, 11300–11312. doi: 10.1523/JNEUROSCI.2270-05.2005

Jia, G., Cheng, G., Gangahar, D. M., and Agrawal, D. K. (2006). Insulin-like growth factor-1 and TNF-alpha regulate autophagy through c-jun N-terminal kinase and Akt pathways in human atherosclerotic vascular smooth cells. *Immunol. Cell Biol.* 84, 448–454. doi: 10.1111/j.1440-1711.2006.01454.x

Junn, E., Lee, K. W., Jeong, B. S., Chan, T. W., Im, J. Y., and Mouradian, M. M. (2009). Repression of alpha-synuclein expression and toxicity by microRNA-7. *Proc. Natl. Acad. Sci. U.S.A.* 106, 13052–13057. doi: 10.1073/pnas.0906 277106

Junyent, F., Alvira, D., Yeste-Velasco, M., de la Torre, A. V., Beas-Zarate, C., Sureda, F. X., et al. (2010). Prosurvival role of JAK/STAT and Akt signaling pathways in MPP^+-induced apoptosis in neurons. *Neurochem. Int.* 57, 774–782. doi: 10.1016/j.neuint.2010.08.015

Karunakaran, S., Saeed, U., Mishra, M., Valli, R. K., Joshi, S. D., Meka, D. P., et al. (2008). Selective activation of p38 mitogen-activated protein kinase in dopaminergic neurons of substantia nigra leads to nuclear translocation of p53 in 1-methyl-4-phenyl-1,2,3,6-tetrahydropyridine-treated mice. *J. Neurosci.* 28, 12500–12509. doi: 10.1523/JNEUROSCI.4511-08.2008

Kefas, B., Godlewski, J., Comeau, L., Li, Y., Abounader, R., Hawkinson, M., et al. (2008). microRNA-7 inhibits the epidermal growth factor receptor and the Akt pathway and is down-regulated in glioblastoma. *Cancer Res.* 68, 3566–3572. doi: 10.1158/0008-5472.CAN-07-6639

Kim, W. G., Mohney, R. P., Wilson, B., Jeohn, G. H., Liu, B., and Hong, J. S. (2000). Regional difference in susceptibility to lipopolysaccharide-induced neurotoxicity in the rat brain: role of microglia. *J. Neurosci.* 20, 6309–6316.

Kordower, J. H., and Bjorklund, A. (2013). Trophic factor gene therapy for Parkinson's disease. *Mov. Disord.* 28, 96–109. doi: 10.1002/mds.25344

Krutzfeldt, J., Rajewsky, N., Braich, R., Rajeev, K. G., Tuschl, T., Manoharan, M., et al. (2005). Silencing of microRNAs *in vivo* with antagomirs. *Nature* 438, 685–689. doi: 10.1038/nature04303

Kumar, V., Zhang, M. X., Swank, M. W., Kunz, J., and Wu, G. Y. (2005). Regulation of dendritic morphogenesis by Ras-PI3K-Akt-mTOR and Ras-MAPK signaling pathways. *J. Neurosci.* 25, 11288–11299. doi: 10.1523/JNEUROSCI.2284-05.2005

Langston, J. W., Ballard, P., Tetrud, J. W., and Irwin, I. (1983). Chronic Parkinsonism in humans due to a product of meperidine-analog synthesis. *Science* 219, 979–980. doi: 10.1126/science.6823561

Langston, J. W., Irwin, I., Langston, E. B., and Forno, L. S. (1984). 1-Methyl-4-phenylpyridinium ion (MPP+): identification of a metabolite of MPTP, a toxin selective to the substantia nigra. *Neurosci. Lett.* 48, 87–92. doi: 10.1016/0304-3940(84)90293-3

Laplante, M., and Sabatini, D. M. (2013). Regulation of mTORC1 and its impact on gene expression at a glance. *J. Cell Sci.* 126, 1713–1719. doi: 10.1242/jcs.125773

Lawson, L. J., Perry, V. H., Dri, P., and Gordon, S. (1990). Heterogeneity in the distribution and morphology of microglia in the normal adult mouse brain. *Neuroscience* 39, 151–170. doi: 10.1016/0306-4522(90)90229-W

Li, Y. H., Werner, H., and Puschel, A. W. (2008). Rheb and mTOR regulate neuronal polarity through Rap1B. *J. Biol. Chem.* 283, 33784–33792. doi: 10.1074/jbc.M802431200

Liang, Y., Ridzon, D., Wong, L., and Chen, C. (2007). Characterization of microRNA expression profiles in normal human tissues. *BMC Genomics* 8:166. doi: 10.1186/1471-2164-8-166

Lindow, M., and Kauppinen, S. (2012). Discovering the first microRNA-targeted drug. *J. Cell Biol.* 199, 407–412. doi: 10.1083/jcb.201208082

Long, J. M., Ray, B., and Lahiri, D. K. (2012). MicroRNA-153 physiologically inhibits expression of amyloid-beta precursor protein in cultured human fetal brain cells and is dysregulated in a subset of Alzheimer disease patients. *J. Biol. Chem.* 287, 31298–31310. doi: 10.1074/jbc.M112.366336

Malagelada, C., Ryu, E. J., Biswas, S. C., Jackson-Lewis, V., and Greene, L. A. (2006). RTP801 is elevated in Parkinson brain substantia nigral neurons and mediates death in cellular models of Parkinson's disease by a mechanism involving mammalian target of rapamycin inactivation. *J. Neurosci.* 26, 9996–10005. doi: 10.1523/JNEUROSCI.3292-06.2006

Manning, B. D., Tee, A. R., Logsdon, M. N., Blenis, J., and Cantley, L. C. (2002). Identification of the tuberous sclerosis complex-2 tumor suppressor gene product tuberin as a target of the phosphoinositide 3-kinase/akt pathway. *Mol. Cell* 10, 151–162. doi: 10.1016/S1097-2765(02)00568-3

Mizuno, Y., Sone, N., and Saitoh, T. (1987). Effects of 1-methyl-4-phenyl-1,2,3,6-tetrahydropyridine and 1-methyl-4-phenylpyridinium ion on activities of the enzymes in the electron transport system in mouse brain. *J. Neurochem.* 48, 1787–1793. doi: 10.1111/j.1471-4159.1987.tb05737.x

Morfini, G. A., You, Y. M., Pollema, S. L., Kaminska, A., Liu, K., Yoshioka, K., et al. (2009). Pathogenic huntingtin inhibits fast axonal transport by activating JNK3 and phosphorylating kinesin. *Nat. Neurosci.* 12, 864–871. doi: 10.1038/nn.2346

Mouradian, M. M. (2012). MicroRNAs in Parkinson's disease. *Neurobiol. Dis.* 46, 279–284. doi: 10.1016/j.nbd.2011.12.046

Mythri, R. B., Harish, G., and Bharath, M. M. (2012). Therapeutic potential of natural products in Parkinson's disease. *Recent. Pat. Endocr. Metab. Immune Drug Discov.* 6, 181–200. doi: 10.2174/187221412802481793

Nakaso, K., Ito, S., and Nakashima, K. (2008). Caffeine activates the PI3K/Akt pathway and prevents apoptotic cell death in a Parkinson's disease model of SH-SY5Y cells. *Neurosci. Lett.* 432, 146–150. doi: 10.1016/j.neulet.2007.12.034

Nicklas, W. J., Vyas, I., and Heikkila, R. E. (1985). Inhibition of NADH-linked oxidation in brain mitochondria by 1-methyl-4-phenyl-pyridine, a metabolite of the neurotoxin, 1-methyl-4-phenyl-1,2,5,6-tetrahydropyridine. *Life Sci.* 36, 2503–2508. doi: 10.1016/0024-3205(85)90146-8

Obeso, J. A., Rodriguez-Oroz, M. C., Goetz, C. G., Marin, C., Kordower, J. H., Rodriguez, M., et al. (2010). Missing pieces in the Parkinson's disease puzzle. *Nat. Med.* 16, 653–661. doi: 10.1038/nm.2165

Park, K. K., Liu, K., Hu, Y., Smith, P. D., Wang, C., Cai, B., et al. (2008). Promoting axon regeneration in the adult CNS by modulation of the PTEN/mTOR pathway. *Science* 322, 963–966. doi: 10.1126/science.1161566

Piao, Y., Kim, H. G., Oh, M. S., and Pak, Y. K. (2012). Overexpression of TFAM, NRF-1 and myr-AKT protects the MPP(+)-induced mitochondrial dysfunctions in neuronal cells. *Biochim. Biophys. Acta* 1820, 577–585. doi: 10.1016/j.bbagen.2011.08.007

Podkowa, M., Zhao, X., Chow, C. W., Coffey, E. T., Davis, R. J., and Attisano, L. (2010). Microtubule stabilization by bone morphogenetic protein receptor-mediated scaffolding of c-Jun N-terminal kinase promotes dendrite formation. *Mol. Cell Biol.* 30, 2241–2250. doi: 10.1128/MCB.01166-09

Reinhard, J. F. Jr., Daniels, A. J., and Painter, G. R. (1990). Carrier-independent entry of 1-methyl-4-phenylpyridinium (MPP+) into adrenal chromaffin cells as a consequence of charge delocalization. *Biochem. Biophys. Res. Commun.* 168, 1143–1148. doi: 10.1016/0006-291X(90)91148-L

Reinhardt, P., Schmid, B., Burbulla, L. F., Schondorf, D. C., Wagner, L., Glatza, M., et al. (2013). Genetic correction of a LRRK2 mutation in human iPSCs links parkinsonian neurodegeneration to ERK-dependent changes in gene expression. *Cell Stem Cell* 12, 354–367. doi: 10.1016/j.stem.2013.01.008

Rodnitzky, R. L. (2012). Upcoming treatments in Parkinson's disease, including gene therapy. *Parkinsonism Relat. Disord.* 18(Suppl. 1), S37–S40. doi: 10.1016/S1353-8020(11)70014-1

Rodriguez-Blanco, J., Martin, V., Garcia-Santos, G., Herrera, F., Casado-Zapico, S., Antolin, I., et al. (2012). Cooperative action of JNK and AKT/mTOR in 1-methyl-4-phenylpyridinium-induced autophagy of neuronal PC12 cells. *J. Neurosci. Res.* 90, 1850–1860. doi: 10.1002/jnr.23066

Rosner, M., and Hengstschlager, M. (2008). Cytoplasmic and nuclear distribution of the protein complexes mTORC1 and mTORC2: rapamycin triggers dephosphorylation and delocalization of the mTORC2 components rictor and sin1. *Hum. Mol. Genet.* 17, 2934–2948. doi: 10.1093/hmg/ddn192

Runden, E., Seglen, P. O., Haug, F. M., Ottersen, O. P., Wieloch, T., Shamloo, M., et al. (1998). Regional selective neuronal degeneration after protein phosphatase inhibition in hippocampal slice cultures: evidence for a MAP kinase-dependent mechanism. *J. Neurosci.* 18, 7296–7305.

Russ, H., Staust, K., Martel, F., Gliese, M., and Schomig, E. (1996). The extraneuronal transporter for monoamine transmitters exists in cells derived from human central nervous system glia. *Eur. J. Neurosci.* 8, 1256–1264. doi: 10.1111/j.1460-9568.1996.tb01294.x

Sanchez, N., Gallagher, M., Lao, N., Gallagher, C., Clarke, C., Doolan, P., et al. (2013). MiR-7 triggers cell cycle arrest at the G1/S transition by targeting multiple genes including Skp2 and Psme3. *PLoS ONE* 8:e65671. doi: 10.1371/journal.pone.0065671

Santos, C. M. (2012). New agents promote neuroprotection in Parkinson's disease models. *CNS Neurol. Disord. Drug Targets* 11, 410–418. doi: 10.2174/187152712800792820

Sarbassov, D. D., Ali, S. M., Sengupta, S., Sheen, J. H., Hsu, P. P., Bagley, A. F., et al. (2006). Prolonged rapamycin treatment inhibits mTORC2 assembly and Akt/PKB. *Mol. Cell* 22, 159–168. doi: 10.1016/j.molcel.2006.03.029

Sarbassov, D. D., Guertin, D. A., Ali, S. M., and Sabatini, D. M. (2005). Phosphorylation and regulation of Akt/PKB by the rictor-mTOR complex. *Science* 307, 1098–1101. doi: 10.1126/science.1106148

Satoh, T., Nakatsuka, D., Watanabe, Y., Nagata, I., Kikuchi, H., and Namura, S. (2000). Neuroprotection by MAPK/ERK kinase inhibition with U0126 against oxidative stress in a mouse neuronal cell line and rat primary cultured cortical neurons. *Neurosci. Lett.* 288, 163–166. doi: 10.1016/S0304-3940(00)01229-5

Seidl, S. E., and Potashkin, J. A. (2011). The promise of neuroprotective agents in Parkinson's disease. *Front. Neurol.* 2:68. doi: 10.3389/fneur.2011.00068

Song, L., Duan, P., Guo, P., Li, D., Li, S., Xu, Y., et al. (2012). Downregulation of miR-223 and miR-153 mediates mechanical stretch-stimulated proliferation of venous smooth muscle cells via activation of the insulin-like growth factor-1 receptor. *Arch Biochem. Biophys.* 528, 204–211. doi: 10.1016/j.abb.2012.08.015

Stanciu, M., Wang, Y., Kentor, R., Burke, N., Watkins, S., Kress, G., et al. (2000). Persistent activation of ERK contributes to glutamate-induced oxidative toxicity in a neuronal cell line and primary cortical neuron cultures. *J. Biol. Chem.* 275, 12200–12206. doi: 10.1074/jbc.275.16.12200

Sun, D. S., and Chang, H. H. (2003). Differential regulation of JNK in caspase-3-mediated apoptosis of MPP(+)-treated primary cortical neurons. *Cell Biol. Int.* 27, 769–777. doi: 10.1016/S1065-6995(03)00165-3

Swiech, L., Perycz, M., Malik, A., and Jaworski, J. (2008). Role of mTOR in physiology and pathology of the nervous system. *Biochim. Biophys. Acta* 1784, 116–132. doi: 10.1016/j.bbapap.2007.08.015

Takei, N., Kawamura, M., Ishizuka, Y., Kakiya, N., Inamura, N., Namba, H., et al. (2009). Brain-derived neurotrophic factor enhances the basal rate of protein synthesis by increasing active eukaryotic elongation factor 2 levels and promoting translation elongation in cortical neurons. *J. Biol. Chem.* 284, 26340–26348. doi: 10.1074/jbc.M109.023010

Tararuk, T., Ostman, N., Li, W., Bjorkblom, B., Padzik, A., Zdrojewska, J., et al. (2006). JNK1 phosphorylation of SCG10 determines microtubule dynamics and axodendritic length. *J. Cell Biol.* 173, 265–277. doi: 10.1083/jcb.200511055

Tavazoie, S. F., Alvarez, V. A., Ridenour, D. A., Kwiatkowski, D. J., and Sabatini, B. L. (2005). Regulation of neuronal morphology and function by the tumor suppressors Tsc1 and Tsc2. *Nat. Neurosci.* 8, 1727–1734. doi: 10.1038/nn1566

Thomas, G. M., Lin, D. T., Nuriya, M., and Huganir, R. L. (2008a). Rapid and bi-directional regulation of AMPA receptor phosphorylation and trafficking by JNK. *EMBO J.* 27, 361–372. doi: 10.1038/sj.emboj.7601969

Thomas, T., Timmer, M., Cesnulevicius, K., Hitti, E., Kotlyarov, A., and Gaestel, M. (2008b). MAPKAP kinase 2-deficiency prevents neurons from cell death by reducing neuroinflammation–relevance in a mouse model of Parkinson's disease. *J. Neurochem.* 105, 2039–2052. doi: 10.1111/j.1471-4159.2008.05310.x

Timmons, S., Coakley, M. F., Moloney, A. M., and O'Neill, C. (2009). Akt signal transduction dysfunction in Parkinson's disease. *Neurosci. Lett.* 467, 30–35. doi: 10.1016/j.neulet.2009.09.055

Trojanowski, J. Q., Goedert, M., Iwatsubo, T., and Lee, V. M. (1998). Fatal attractions: abnormal protein aggregation and neuron death in Parkinson's disease and Lewy body dementia. *Cell Death Differ.* 5, 832–837. doi: 10.1038/sj.cdd.4400432

Vander Haar, E., Lee, S. I., Bandhakavi, S., Griffin, T. J., and Kim, D. H. (2007). Insulin signalling to mTOR mediated by the Akt/PKB substrate PRAS40. *Nat. Cell Biol.* 9, 316–323. doi: 10.1038/ncb1547

Verma, P., Chierzi, S., Codd, A. M., Campbell, D. S., Meyer, R. L., Holt, C. E., et al. (2005). Axonal protein synthesis and degradation are necessary for efficient growth cone regeneration. *J. Neurosci.* 25, 331–342. doi: 10.1523/JNEUROSCI.3073-04.2005

Wang, G., Pan, J., and Chen, S. D. (2012). Kinases and kinase signaling pathways: potential therapeutic targets in Parkinson's disease. *Prog. Neurobiol.* 98, 207–221. doi: 10.1016/j.pneurobio.2012.06.003

Wang, L., Yang, H. J., Xia, Y. Y., and Feng, Z. W. (2010). Insulin-like growth factor 1 protects human neuroblastoma cells SH-EP1 against MPP^{+}-induced apoptosis by AKT/GSK-3beta/JNK signaling. *Apoptosis* 15, 1470–1479. doi: 10.1007/s10495-010-0547-z

Wang, Y., Liu, J., Liu, C., Naji, A., and Stoffers, D. A. (2013). MicroRNA-7 regulates the mTOR pathway and proliferation in adult pancreatic beta-cells. *Diabetes* 62, 887–895. doi: 10.2337/db12-0451

Wienholds, E., and Plasterk, R. H. (2005). MicroRNA function in animal development. *FEBS Lett.* 579, 5911–5922. doi: 10.1016/j.febslet.2005.07.070

Willis, S. N., Fletcher, J. I., Kaufmann, T., van Delft, M. F., Chen, L., Czabotar, P. E., et al. (2007). Apoptosis initiated when BH3 ligands engage multiple Bcl-2 homologs, not Bax or Bak. *Science* 315, 856–859. doi: 10.1126/science.1133289

Wu, D. C., Teismann, P., Tieu, K., Vila, M., Jackson-Lewis, V., Ischiropoulos, H., et al. (2003). NADPH oxidase mediates oxidative stress in the 1-methyl-4-phenyl-1,2,3,6-tetrahydropyridine model of Parkinson's disease. *Proc. Natl. Acad. Sci. U.S.A.* 100, 6145–6150. doi: 10.1073/pnas.0937239100

Wu, X., Reiter, C. E., Antonetti, D. A., Kimball, S. R., Jefferson, L. S., and Gardner, T. W. (2004). Insulin promotes rat retinal neuronal cell survival in a p70S6K-dependent manner. *J. Biol. Chem.* 279, 9167–9175. doi: 10.1074/jbc.M312397200

Wu, Z., He, B., He, J., and Mao, X. (2013). Upregulation of miR-153 promotes cell proliferation via downregulation of the PTEN tumor suppressor gene in human prostate cancer. *Prostate* 73, 596–604. doi: 10.1002/pros.22600

Xu, P., Das, M., Reilly, J., and Davis, R. J. (2011). JNK regulates FoxO-dependent autophagy in neurons. *Genes Dev.* 25, 310–322. doi: 10.1101/gad.1984311

Yuan, Y., Sun, J., Zhao, M., Hu, J., Wang, X., Du, G., et al. (2010). Overexpression of alpha-synuclein down-regulates BDNF expression. *Cell. Mol. Neurobiol.* 30, 939–946. doi: 10.1007/s10571-010-9523-y

Zecca, L., Youdim, M. B., Riederer, P., Connor, J. R., and Crichton, R. R. (2004). Iron, brain ageing and neurodegenerative disorders. *Nat. Rev. Neurosci.* 5, 863–873. doi: 10.1038/nrn1537

Zhang, K., Ma, Z., Wang, J., Xie, A., and Xie, J. (2011). Myricetin attenuated MPP(+)-induced cytotoxicity by anti-oxidation and inhibition of MKK4 and JNK activation in MES23.5 cells. *Neuropharmacology* 61, 329–335. doi: 10.1016/j.neuropharm.2011.04.021

Zhu, J. H., Guo, F., Shelburne, J., Watkins, S., and Chu, C. T. (2003). Localization of phosphorylated ERK/MAP kinases to mitochondria and autophagosomes in Lewy body diseases. *Brain Pathol.* 13, 473–481. doi: 10.1111/j.1750-3639.2003.tb00478.x

Zhu, J. H., Gusdon, A. M., Cimen, H., van Houten, B., Koc, E., and Chu, C. T. (2012). Impaired mitochondrial biogenesis contributes to depletion of functional mitochondria in chronic MPP^+ toxicity: dual roles for ERK1/2. *Cell Death Dis.* 3, e312. doi: 10.1038/cddis.2012.46

Zhu, J. H., Horbinski, C., Guo, F., Watkins, S., Uchiyama, Y., and Chu, C. T. (2007). Regulation of autophagy by extracellular signal-regulated protein kinases during 1-methyl-4-phenylpyridinium-induced cell death. *Am. J. Pathol.* 170, 75–86. doi: 10.2353/ajpath.2007.060524

Zhu, J. H., Kulich, S. M., Oury, T. D., and Chu, C. T. (2002). Cytoplasmic aggregates of phosphorylated extracellular signal-regulated protein kinases in Lewy body diseases. *Am. J. Pathol.* 161, 2087–2098. doi: 10.1016/S0002-9440(10)64487-2

Zhu, Y., Pak, D., Qin, Y., McCormack, S. G., Kim, M. J., Baumgart, J. P., et al. (2005). Rap2-JNK removes synaptic AMPA receptors during depotentiation. *Neuron* 46, 905–916. doi: 10.1016/j.neuron.2005.04.037

Zigmond, M. J., Hastings, T. G., and Perez, R. G. (2002). Increased dopamine turnover after partial loss of dopaminergic neurons: compensation or toxicity? *Parkinsonism Relat. Disord.* 8, 389–393. doi: 10.1016/S1353-8020(02)00019-6

20

Increased microRNA-34c abundance in Alzheimer's disease circulating blood plasma

Shephali Bhatnagar[1], Howard Chertkow[2,3,4,5], Hyman M. Schipper[2,4,5], Zongfei Yuan[1], Vikranth Shetty[1], Samantha Jenkins[1], Timothy Jones[1] and Eugenia Wang[1]*

[1] Advanced Genomic Technology, LLC, Louisville, KY, USA
[2] Department of Neurology and Neurosurgery, McGill University, Montreal, QC, Canada
[3] Memory Clinic, Department of Medicine, Jewish General Hospital, Montreal, QC, Canada
[4] Bloomfield Centre for Research in Aging, Lady Davis Institute, Montreal, QC, Canada
[5] Division of Geriatric Medicine and Department of Clinical Neurosciences, Jewish General Hospital, Montreal, QC, Canada

Correspondence:
Eugenia Wang, Advanced Genomic Technology, 5100 US Highway 42, Suite 433, Louisville, KY 40241, USA
e-mail: ewangagt@gmail.com

Circulating microRNAs, present either in the cellular component, peripheral blood mononuclear cells (PBMC), or in cell-free plasma, have emerged as biomarkers for age-dependent systemic, disease-associated changes in many organs. Previously, we have shown that microRNA (miR)-34a is increased in circulating PBMC of Alzheimer's disease (AD) patients. In the present study, we show that this microRNA's sister, miR-34c, exhibits even greater increase in both cellular and plasma components of AD circulating blood samples, compared to normal age-matched controls. Statistical analysis shows the accuracy of levels of miR-34c assayed by receiver operating characteristic (ROC) analysis: the area under the curve is 0.99 ($p < 0.0001$) and the 95% confidence level extends from 0.97 to 1. Pearson correlation between miR-34c levels and mild and moderate AD, as defined by the mini-mental state examination (MMSE), shows an r-value of −0.7, suggesting a relatively strong inverse relationship between the two parameters. These data show that plasma levels of microRNA 34c are much more prominent in AD than those of its sister, miR-34a, or than its own level in PBMC. Transfection studies show that miR-34c, as does its sister miR-34a, represses the expression of several selected genes involved in cell survival and oxidative defense pathways, such as Bcl2, SIRT1, and others, in cultured cells. Taken together, our results indicate that increased levels of miR-34c in both PBMC and plasma may reflect changes in circulating blood samples in AD patients, compared to age-matched normal controls.

Keywords: peripheral blood mononuclear cells (PBMC), plasma microRNA, miR-34a, miR-34c

INTRODUCTION

Recently, microRNAs found in circulating blood, especially in cell-free plasma, have been noted functionally for intercellular and/or inter-organ communication. Circulating plasma microRNAs seem to be largely released from the cellular compartment, i.e., peripheral blood mononuclear cells (PBMC), either associated with specific protein or lipid molecules, or released in vesicles known as exosomes, with some portion derived from the cell debris of apoptotic bodies (Smalheiser, 2007; De Smaelea et al., 2010; Etheridge et al., 2011). Not surprisingly, differentially expressed plasma microRNAs have been noted as powerful biomarkers for several central nervous system disorders, from bipolar disorder to schizophrenia, Huntington's disease and Alzheimer's disease (AD) (Gaughwin et al., 2011; Rong et al., 2011; Suarez-Gomez et al., 2011; Geekiyanage et al., 2012; Sheinerman et al., 2012; Shi et al., 2012). Our own work has shown that lead microRNAs are differentially regulated in PBMC of AD patients compared with age-matched controls (Schipper et al., 2007; Maes et al., 2010). Therefore, unique microRNAs offer another aspect, in addition to specific transcriptome and serum protein profiling: blood biomarker discovery, for instance for AD.

Among many microRNAs, the miR-34 family, composed of three members, miR-34a, -34b, and -34c, is relatively well-understood. MicroRNA-34b, a plasma biomarker for Huntington disease (Gaughwin et al., 2011), and its sister, miR-34c, are linked as a bi-cistronic transcriptional unit (Liang et al., 2009); together with the other sister, miR-34a, they participate functionally in at least two signaling pathways: (1) Bcl2 for cell survival/apoptosis; and (2) SIRT1 deacetylase for p53 or neuroprotection signaling. SIRT1, p53, and miR-34a are involved in a positive feedback loop for miR-34a expression: acetylated p53 binds the promoter to activate this microRNA's transcription (He et al., 2007; Yamakuchi et al., 2008). Increased miR-34a suppresses SIRT1 expression, thereby diminishing its deacetylation of p53, leading to an increase in acetylated p53 transcriptional activity, resulting in the

Abbreviations: miR or miRNA, microRNA; AD, Alzheimer's disease; NEC, normal elderly control; MMSE, Mini-Mental State Examination; MMSE score (4–9), severe group; MMSE score (10–20), moderate group; MMSE score (21–24), mild group; Bcl2, B-cell lymphoma 2; SIRT1, sirtuin1; Psen1, presenilin-1.

continued up-regulation of this microRNA (Yamakuchi et al., 2008).

Many reports, including our own work in aged mice, observe parallel changes during aging between differentially regulated circulating microRNAs and changes in the central nervous system (Li et al., 2011a). During aging, accumulating oxidative stress-activated p53 may tilt the balance toward age-dependent increase of miR-34a, observed in the brains of old rats and mice (Li et al., 2011b,c); and a reduction in age-dependent increase in miR-34a in brain has been observed in calorie-restricted mice (Khanna et al., 2011). In animal models of AD, increased miR-34a levels are observed in brains of mouse models bearing both the APP^{swe} and presenilin transgenes (Wang et al., 2009). MicroRNA 34-c, a sister of miR-34a, is also observed in the hippocampal region of AD animal models to be functionally connected to cognitive decline, because inhibition of this microRNA rescues memory impairment in AD transgenic mice, with corresponding regained SIRT1 levels (Zovoilis et al., 2011). These results suggest that increased expression of miR-34a and -34c may repress SIRT1 and Bcl2 expression, one of the many underlying causes for dysregulation of oxidative defense and neuronal cell survival in the brain of AD transgenic animals.

The main objective of this study is to test the hypothesis that unique microRNA changes in AD patients, specifically those of the microRNA-34 family, can be identified in circulating blood samples in both the cellular component, PBMC, and cell-free plasma. To test this hypothesis, we have expanded beyond our previous observation of increased miR-34a in PBMC of AD patients (Schipper et al., 2007) to include also miR-34c in our study of specimens of both blood components. Here, we report that miR-34c in circulating plasma and PBMC indeed exhibits increased levels of expression in AD patients, compared with age-matched normal elderly controls (NEC). Transfection study shows that miR-34c, similar to reported findings for miR-34a, functionally represses Bcl2, SIRT1, and other proteins, all key genes whose decreases are functionally associated with weakened oxidative defense and cell survival.

MATERIALS AND METHODS

SUBJECTS AND CLINICAL EVALUATION

Informed consent was obtained from all participants, following the Institutional Review Board protocol approved by the Sir Mortimer B. Davis Jewish General Hospital (JGH) Research Ethics Committee. Blood samples were obtained from subjects at the Memory Clinic at the JGH, from 110 AD patients (age: 56–90) and 123 NEC (age: 61–90) without cognitive impairment. NEC were recruited by newspaper advertisements and public lectures, scored less than 4 on the Subjective Memory Scale of Schmand (Schmand et al., 1996), lacked other medical or neurological illnesses, and scored within 1 standard deviation (SD) of age and education means on memory screening tests. These consist of scores of 26 or more on the Montreal Cognitive Assessment (MoCA) (Nasreddine et al., 2005), a Mini-Mental State Examination (MMSE) scoring 25 or above (Folstein et al., 1975), and normal range scores on the delayed paragraph recall component of the Logical Memory Test of the WAIS-R (Wechsler, 2008). Patients with sporadic late onset AD were screened and assessed at the JGH McGill University Memory Clinic in Montréal; the diagnosis was made according to standard NINCDS-ADRDS criteria (McKhann et al., 1984), and conformed to the more recent revised criteria for probable AD as well (McKhann et al., 2011). Severity of dementia was stratified according to MMSE results: mild (21–24), moderate (10–20), or severe (4–9).

BLOOD COLLECTION AND ISOLATION AND QUALITY EVALUATION OF RNA SAMPLES

Approximately 30 ml of blood per donor was collected in EDTA vacutainers, and processed to isolate the plasma and PBMC fractions, using Ficoll-Plaque Plus (GE Healthcare, Piscataway, NJ). PBMC and plasma samples, stored in RNAlater buffer solution (Ambion, Austin, TX), were processed for RNA and protein isolation by Trizol/chloroform and centrifugation, to separate the upper RNA-containing aqueous phase from the lower proteinaceous phase, for isolation of microRNA from the plasma specimens, as previously described (Li et al., 2011a). Prior to RNA isolation, 0.625 ng of synthetic miRNA-39 from *Caenorhabditis elegans* (cel-miRNA-39) was added to the Trizol as a spike-in control for purification efficiency and cDNA synthesis quality validation during qPCR assays, as described below (Kroh et al., 2010) (Exiqon, #203203). RNA integrity was assessed using a Nanodrop spectrophotometer (Thermo Fischer Scientific, Barrington, IL) and Agilent 2100 bioanalyzer (Agilent Technologies, Waldbronn, Germany).

TAQMAN MicroRNA REAL TIME qPCR

Plasma microRNAs were used to generate cDNA using the Taqman® MicroRNA Reverse Transcription Kit (Applied Biosystems, Carlsbad, CA), with specific miRNA stem-loop primers for miR-34a, -34b, -34c, and -16, by MultiScribe Reverse Transcriptase; the reactions were carried out in a GeneAmp PCR System 9700 (Applied Biosystems). These cDNA samples were processed to assess mature miRNA levels by real time polymerase chain reactions (qPCR) using the Taqman® Universal PCR Master Mix kit (Applied Biosystems). The qPCR was conducted in a 7500 real time PCR system (Applied Biosystems) under the following conditions: 95°C 10 min, 60 cycles of 95°C 15 s, and 60°C 1 min. The levels of mature cel-miR-39 mRNA were measured using individual TaqMan microRNA Assays (Applied Biosystems) according to the manufacturer's instructions (Exiqon, #203203); cel-miR-39 was used to normalize miRNA levels. A mean Ct was calculated for *C. elegans* miRNA for each sample, followed by calculating the median of all mean *C. elegans* synthetic miRNA Cts, taking all samples into consideration. Then a normalization factor was calculated for each sample by subtracting the mean *C. elegans* synthetic miRNA Ct of the sample of interest from the median value calculated earlier. This normalization factor was then integrated into the calculation of the raw Ct value obtained for each sample, which was further normalized by reference to Ct values for miR-16.

WESTERN BLOT ANALYSES

Western blot analyses were performed as previously described (Bates et al., 2010; Li et al., 2011c), using an actin band for transfection cell lysates, to check equal loading across all lanes (Pendyala et al., 2010). The antibodies used were mouse anti-Bcl2 (1:1000, 692, Abcam Inc., Cambridge, MA), rabbit anti-Psen1 (1:500, 71181;Abcam), rabbit anti-Onecut2 (1:500, 28466;Abcam), rabbit anti-SIRT1 (1:500, 110304;Abcam), and rabbit anti-β-actin (1:1000, 8226;Abcam). Goat anti-mouse (31403, Thermo Fischer Scientific, Barrington, IL) was used for Bcl2 (1:2000), and goat anti-rabbit (31460, Thermo Scientific) for β-actin, SIRT1, Psen1, and Onecut2 (1:1000) as secondary antibodies. Intensities of antibody reactive bands were detected by Enhanced Chemiluminescence (ECL), (Pierce Biotechnology, Rockford, IL), and quantified by densitometry using ImageJ software (Public domain, NIH, USA).

CONSTRUCTION OF hsa34a AND hsa34c GFP RECOMBINANTS, AND FUNCTIONAL TARGET SUPPRESSION STUDY

Micro-34a and -34c were amplified from DNA purified from human embryonic kidney cells (HEK 293 cell line; ATCC# CRL 1573) with the following primers:

miR-34a forward 5′-tctagaGAG TCC CCT CCG GAT GCC GTG,
reverse 5′-ggatccCCA CCC ACCG TGG CGC AG, 229 bp;
miR-34c forward 5′-tctagaAGC CCC TCC ATC CAT GTA ACG GT,
reverse 5′-ggatccAAC ACC CCT CTT CCC CAC GCA, 328 bp.

Amplified PCR products were purified and cloned by the Qiagen PCR Cloning kit (Qiagen, Valencia, CA), and subcloned into the pCDH-CMV-MCS-EF1-copGFP vector (System Biosciences, Mountain View, CA), which was then used for functional assays by transfecting human embryonic kidney cells (HEK 293), as previously described (Bates et al., 2010).

STATISTICAL ANALYSES

All statistical analyses were performed using MS Excel 2010, SPSS 17.0 statistical software package (IBM), or SAS version 9.2 (SAS Institute Inc., Cary, NC). Student's *t*-test and one-way analysis of variance (ANOVA) were performed to determine significant differences for two-way or more than two groups. For multiple comparisons, Fisher's Least Significant Difference (LSD) test was used, following one-way ANOVA, in order to assign statistical significance, and then the Scheffé test was applied to reduce Type 1 errors. Levels of miR-34c, miR-34b, and miR-34a were normalized with regard to miR-16, as recommended by the manufacturer as well as a previous report of Huntington disease plasma biomarker discovery (Gaughwin et al., 2011), as a reference gene, using the comparative Delta Ct method. The ΔCt value is the difference between the Ct of the target microRNA and that of the reference microRNA (ΔCt = Ct miR34× − Ct miR16). To include the spike-in results in this calculation, the Ct values were first normalized against *Cel-39* and then against miR-16, according to the equation: normalizing factor = median ($Avg.Ct^{Celall} - Avg.Ct^{Celsample}$); normalized $Ct^{sample} = Ct^{sample}$ + normalizing factor (Livak and Schmittgen, 2001). Correlation between MMSE scores and expression levels of miR-34c and miR-34a in AD and NEC patients was calculated using the Pearson correlation coefficient (r) (Taylor, 1990); a correlation coefficient value of 0.8 or above indicates strong correlation, whereas a value around 0.5 is indicative of moderate correlation.

Receiver-Operating Characteristic (ROC) curves were used to determine the accuracy of the test differentiating AD from NEC individuals for miR-34c and miR-34a in age-matched cohorts (Zweig and Campbell, 1993; Fawcett, 2006). We calculated the sensitivity, specificity and accuracy as follows;

Sensitivity = TP/(TP + FN) = (Number of true positive assessments)/(Number of all positive assessments);
Specificity = TN/(TN + FP) = (Number of true negative assessments)/(Number of all negative assessments)
Accuracy = (TN + TP)/(TN + TP + FN + FP) = (Number of correct assessments)/(Number of all assessments)

A true positive (TP) is defined as an individual showing concordance between disease presence and a diagnostic test result, while a true negative (TN) represents disease absence with test result also negative. Contrary to these scenarios is discordance between these two categories: i.e., a false positive (FP) is defined as disease absence in an individual whose diagnostic test is positive, and a false negative (FN) characterizes disease presence in an individual whose diagnostic test is negative. All four counts, i.e., TP, TN, FP, and FN, were calculated with a cut-off point base (Li and Chung, 2013).

RESULTS

SELECTION OF SAMPLES FOR BEST RNA QUALITY, AND CONTROLS FOR CALCULATION OF miR-34a AND miR-34c LEVELS

From blood samples of 110 AD patients and 123 NEC, only 78 AD and 85 plasma specimens were selected to meet our requirements for RNA integrity: a single peak of small RNA in the 4–40 nucleotide (nt) range (Figure 1S). The age range for the AD group is between 56 and 90, with an average age of 80; the NEC cohort is between 61 and 90, with an average of 72 (**Table 1**). Our cohort's cognitive ability, assessed by the MMSE, is as reported in the literature (Sharp and Gatz, 2011), i.e., lower scores are linked with fewer years of education in AD individuals (Figure 2S). Our recruitment program for normal control individuals is limited by the fact that many are in their 60 s. In order to achieve an age-matched study design, we further selected from the AD and NEC groups such that the age range of both subcohorts lies between 76–90; the average age for the former is 82, and the latter 80 (**Table 1**).

To optimize the accuracy of quantitative PCR assays, we used two control steps: (a) quality control for the cDNA synthesis step with *C. elegans* Cel 39 spike-in; and (b) using miR-16 to standardize baseline level determination. **Figures 1A–D** shows similar levels of miR-34a and miR-34c with and without spike-in experiments in both AD and NEC plasma samples. These results suggest that the protocol established for miR-34a and miR-34c qPCR assays is stringent, providing optimal quality cDNA synthesis with minimal putative RT-RNA inhibitions. An additional standardized control is selecting appropriate microRNAs with no changes

Table 1 | Plasma specimens from the entire cohorts of Alzheimer's disease (AD) and normal elderly control (NEC) individuals, selected after RNA quality control, with age range, average age with standard deviation (SD), and sample size (N) for acceptable RNA in the entire cohort and age-matched cohorts.

	Original	Acceptable RNA			Age-matched		
	N	Age range	Avg (*SD*)	*N*	Age range	Avg (*SD*)	*N*
AD	110	56–90	80 (6.17)	78	76–90	82 (4.11)	25
NEC	123	61–90	72 (1.31)	85	76–90	80 (3.26)	27

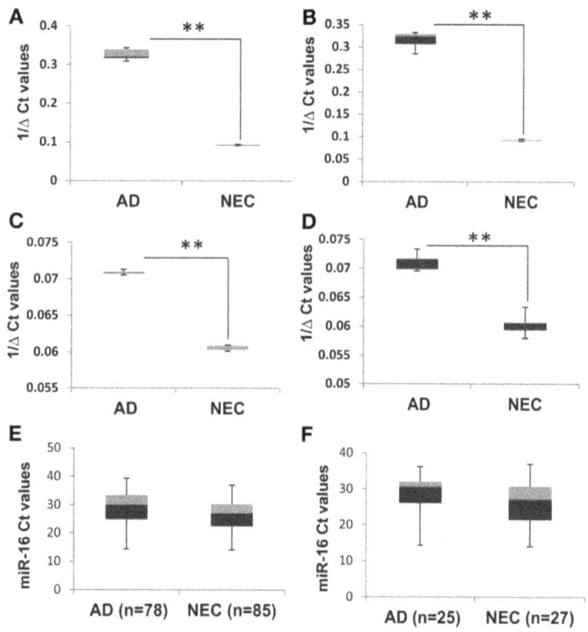

FIGURE 1 | Box plot representation of data from spike-in experiment with AD and NEC samples, miR-34c, with spike-in (A) and without spike-in (B) of *Cel-39*; and miR-34a with spike-in (C) and without spike-in (D). These figures show that levels of miR-34a and miR-34c are similar with and without spike-in experiments in both Alzheimer disease (AD) and normal elderly control (NEC) plasma samples. The Ct values of miR-16 in AD and NEC samples are represented as box plots in the whole population **(E)** and age-matched cohorts **(F)**. These figures indicate that levels of miR-34a and miR-34c are of the same range in both total and age-matched cohorts among both AD and NEC plasma samples. Student's *t*-test was used to determine statistical significance; $^{**}P < 0.01$.

between AD and control group blood samples. We followed the manufacturer's recommendation, as well as reports by Kroh et al. (2010) and Gaughwin et al. (2011) to use miR-16 as the control for each individual qPCR assay. However, since miR-16 is an abundant microRNA associated with red blood cells, even minimal hemolysis can cause unreliable qPCR results, as shown by Müller et al. (2014) in cerebrospinal fluid (CSF) qPCR assays. In this context, we evaluated miR-16 levels in all samples used in our study, as shown in **Figures 1E,F**, and found that in both total and age-matched cohorts, levels of this microRNA are similar between the AD and NEC cohorts. Thus, miR-16 levels are not differentially regulated between AD and NEC plasma samples in our study, and can serve as a standard.

EXPRESSION LEVELS OF miR-34a AND miR-34c IN PLASMA SAMPLES OF AD PATIENTS AND NORMAL ELDERLY CONTROLS (NEC)

Our initial study of quantitative reverse transcription PCR (qPCR) analyses of transcript levels of miR-34a and -34c in plasma samples of AD and NEC was performed with the entire cohorts (**Table 1**). When miR-34c levels were analyzed, NEC individuals were distributed in a close cluster around the median levels of the box plots, while AD specimens were distributed over a wider scatter span, with significantly wider SD range (**Figures 2A,B**). Similar wide spreads of AD values while NEC samples are clustered were also observed with miR-34a levels (**Figures 2C,D**). **Table 2** shows the wide distribution and high SD indices for both microRNAs in the AD group. To address the concern that higher AD microRNA values could be due to the older age group used, we next selected from our cohorts NEC individuals age-matched to AD counterparts, as listed in **Table 1**.

Figures 3A,B shows box plots and distribution of individual values for miR-34c in the two age-matched subcohorts. Clearly, the majority of AD plasma specimens in the age-matched control study exhibit higher miR-34c levels than do normal controls; **Table 3** shows 1/deltaCt values in the 0.20–0.53 range for AD, and 0.05–0.22 for NEC plasma specimens. When levels of miR-34a were analyzed, however, the range of distribution is not differentially expressed between the AD and NEC groups, with more spread-out distribution for both groups, as well as significant overlapping ranges, by both box plot and scatter plots (**Figures 3C,D; Table 3**). Levels of miR-34b were evaluated in the same age-matched subcohorts of the AD and NEC groups in plasma; the results show no significant difference between the two groups (Figure 3S, Table 1S). The box plot presentation of inverted ΔCt values from AD and NEC groups shows no change, indicating that the level of miR-34b does not change in the AD group compared to NEC.

Accuracy in differentiating AD ($n = 25$) and NEC ($n = 27$) individuals by miR-34c levels in plasma specimens was further tested by ROC curves (**Figure 4**). The area under the miR-34c curve is 0.99 ($p < 0.0001$), essentially 1.0, indicating perfect accuracy of the data; 95% confidence interval values fall in the range of 0.97–1.0. The ROC curve shows that miR-34c level is an excellent test for AD, with 94% accuracy, 92% sensitivity, and 96% specificity (**Table 4**). The area under the ROC curve for miR-34a is 0.81 ($p = 0.0001$), indicating a fairly good test; the 95% confidence interval lies between 0.69 and 0.93. The sensitivity is 84%, and specificity is 74% (**Figure 4, Table 4**). The area under the ROC curve, sensitivity, specificity and accuracy were calculated for a cut-off point chosen using the coordinates of ROC curves with balanced levels of high sensitivity and specificity.

miR-34c LEVELS IN MODERATE AND MILD AD COMPARED WITH AGE-MATCHED NORMAL ELDERLY CONTROLS

In our age-matched AD cohort, only two patients were evaluated by the MMSE in the severe stage, with scores in the range 4–9. **Figures 5A,B** show that when these two individuals' samples are excluded from our analysis, miR-34c levels in samples

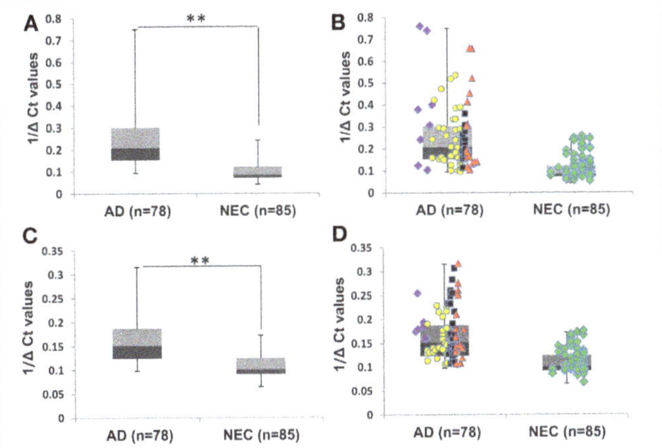

FIGURE 2 | Transcript levels of miR-34a and miR-34c in plasma samples of Alzheimer's disease (AD) patients and normal elderly controls (NEC). (A) Comparison of plasma levels of miR-34c in the whole population of AD patients ($n = 78$) with the NEC cohort ($n = 85$). **(B)** Distributions of individuals' levels of miR-34c along the box plot. NEC individuals were distributed in a close cluster around the median levels of the box plots, whereas AD specimens were distributed over a wider range with higher standard deviation. **(C)** Box plot representation of comparison in plasma levels of miR-34a in the whole population of AD patients ($n = 78$) with the NEC cohort ($n = 85$). **(D)** Individual miR-34a values along the box plot are less wide spread in the AD group as compared to those for miR-34c and a tight cluster for NEC is also observed. The data are plotted as inverse ΔCt derived from qPCR analysis. Data points of Mini-Mental Status Examination (MMSE) score ranges are: ◆ severe AD (score 4–9), ○ moderate AD (score 10–20), ■ mild AD (score 21–24), ▲ AD outlier (score 25–29), ◆ NEC (score 25–30). Student's *t*-test was used to determine statistical significance; $^{**}P < 0.01$.

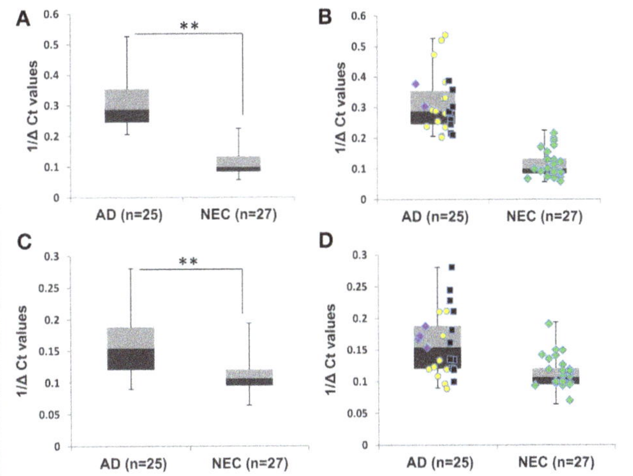

FIGURE 3 | Transcript levels of miR-34a and miR-34c in plasma samples of age-matched cohorts of Alzheimer's disease (AD) patients and normal elderly controls (NEC). (A) Plasma level comparison of miR-34c in the age-matched cohort of AD patients ($n = 25$) with the NEC cohort ($n = 27$). AD plasma samples in the age-matched cohort showed higher miR-34c levels than controls. **(B)** Distribution of individuals' levels of miR-34c along the box plot; NEC individuals were distributed in a close cluster around the median of the box plots, while AD patients were distributed over a wider range with greater standard deviation. **(C)** Comparison of plasma levels of miR-34a in age-matched cohorts of AD patients ($n = 25$) with the NEC cohort ($n = 27$). miR-34a levels were distributed in a range that is not differentially expressed between AD and NEC groups, with more spread-out distribution for both groups, as well as significant overlapping ranges, by both box and scatter plots. Distributing individuals along the box plot, NEC were distributed in a close cluster around the median levels of the box plots, whereas AD specimens were distributed over a wider range with higher standard deviation. Data points represent Mini-Mental Status Examination (MMSE) score as follows, (◆) severe AD (4–9), (○) moderate AD (10–20), (■) mild AD (21–24), and (◆) NEC (25–30). **(D)** Representation of individual miR-34a levels along the box plot for the range of distribution between AD and NEC groups. The data are plotted as inverse ΔCt derived from qPCR analysis. Student's *t*-test was used to determine statistical significance; $^{**}P < 0.01$.

Table 2 | Plasma microRNA 1/deltaCt level ranges in Alzheimer disease (AD) patients and normal elderly controls (NEC) with standard deviation *(SD)* and median, for miR-34c and miR-34a in the whole cohorts.

Whole cohort	miR-34c		miR-34a	
	Range (*SD*)	Median	Range (*SD*)	Median
AD	0.09–0.75 (0.15)	0.21	0.09–0.32 (0.05)	0.15
NEC	0.04–0.24 (0.05)	0.08	0.06–0.17 (0.02)	0.1

Table 3 | Ranges of 1/deltaCt levels of plasma microRNAs in Alzheimer disease (AD) patients and normal elderly controls (NEC), with standard deviation *(SD)* and median, for miR-34c and miR-34a in age-matched subcohorts.

Age-matched cohort	miR-34c		miR-34a	
	Range (*SD*)	Median	Range (*SD*)	Median
AD	0.20–0.53 (0.09)	0.29	0.08–0.28 (0.05)	0.15
NEC	0.05–0.22 (0.05)	0.1	0.06–0.19 (0.03)	0.11

from moderate and mild stages, with MMSE scores in 10–20 or 21–24 ranges respectively, remain higher than NEC controls. **Table 5** shows that levels of miR-34c expression are not only distinct between the moderate and NEC groups, but also between the mild group and normal controls, with the former in the range of 0.21–0.38, while the latter shows 0.05–0.22 1/deltaCt values. Similar separation between mild AD patients and the normal control group is not observed for levels of miR-34a in this age-matched cohort study, due to overlapping ranges between these two groups (**Table 5**).

We investigated further the relationship between MMSE and miR-34c levels, by calculating Pearson's correlation *r*-value of miR-34c levels and MMSE scores for moderate and mild AD and age-matched control cohorts. **Figure 6A** shows an *r*-value of −0.72, suggesting a strong inverse correlation between the expression levels of miR-34c and the two cognitive assessment groups. This inverse correlation between MMSE scores and miR-34c levels, i.e., lower scores and higher levels, as shown for the three groups, was not observed for miR-34a expression, with an r coefficient score of −0.34 (**Figure 6B**). Likewise, when Pearson's correlation was computed for only the moderate and mild clinical groups without NEC, the *r*-value is very low. These results

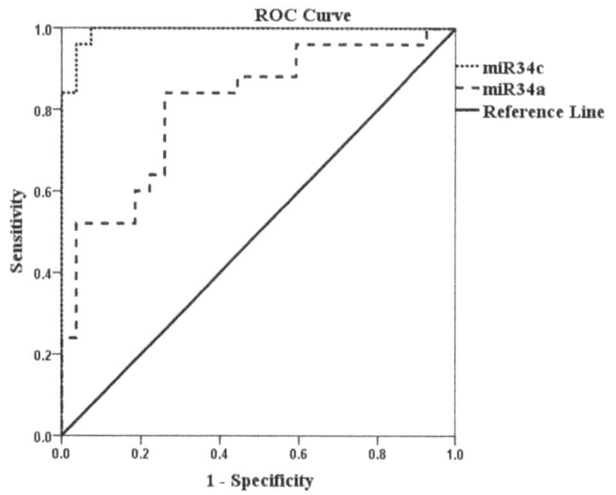

FIGURE 4 | Receiver Operation Characteristic (ROC) curves representing AD diagnostic tests by miR-34c and miR-34a in age-matched cohorts. The Receiver Operation Characteristic (ROC) curve for miR-34c (•····) is an excellent test since the area under the curve is 0.99 ($p < 0.0001$), number of samples for AD = 25 and NEC = 27. The area under the Receiver Operation Characteristic (ROC) for miR-34a (----) is 0.81 ($p = 0.0001$) which is a good/fair test, number of samples for AD = 25 and NEC = 27. Sensitivity and specificity are reported based on a cut-off point chosen using the coordinates of Receiver Operation Characteristic (ROC) curves with balanced levels of high sensitivity and specificity. The diagonal line represents a reference line showing zero sensitivity and zero specificity (—).

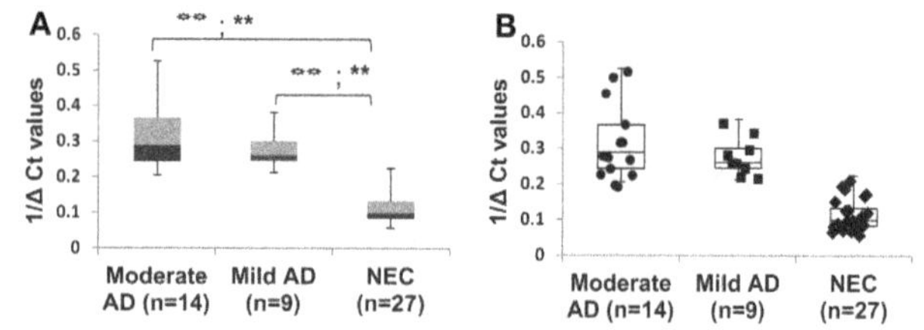

FIGURE 5 | Differential expression of miR-34c in plasma from patients with mild and moderate severity of Alzheimer's disease (AD), compared with normal elderly controls (NEC) in age-matched cohorts. AD patients were grouped by mild and moderate severity according to their Mini-Mental Status Examination (MMSE) scores. **(A)** Percentile distribution of samples within the various stages of AD and NEC, plotted against inverse ΔCt for individuals of age-matched cohorts. The levels of miR-34c are higher in samples from moderate (●) and mild (■) clinical groups, with MMSE scores in the range of 10–20 or 21–24, respectively, than NEC (◆) controls in the range of 25–30. **(B)** Data points added to illustrate the distribution of individuals within each group of the age-matched cohorts. We observe NEC to be in a close cluster around the median, whereas AD patients are scattered in a wider range in both moderate and mild groups. Both the LSD test (higher type 1 Error) and the Scheffé test (higher stringency) were used to determine statistical significance. The statistical significance level for the LSD test is represented with the symbol (∞), and for Scheffé test is represented with the symbol (*). ∞$P < 0.01$, **$P < 0.01$.

Table 4 | Receiver Operating Characteristic (ROC) curve parameters for plasma miR-34c and -34a among age-matched subcohorts.

ROC curve	miR-34c	miR-34a
Area under curve (AUC)	0.99 ($p < 0.0001$)	0.81 ($p = 0.0001$)
Sensitivity	0.92	0.84
Specificity	0.96	0.74
Accuracy	0.94	0.79

Table 5 | 1/deltaCt levels of plasma miR-34c and -34a by clinical category of mild and moderate Alzheimer's disease (AD) and in age-matched normal elderly controls (NEC): range with standard deviation (*SD*) and median.

	miR-34c		miR-34a	
	Range (*SD*)	Median	Range (*SD*)	Median
NEC	0.05–0.22 (0.05)	0.1	0.06–0.19 (0.02)	0.1
Mild AD	0.21–0.38 (0.06)	0.26	0.10–0.28 (0.06)	0.16
Moderate AD	0.20–0.53 (0.11)	0.29	0.09–0.21 (0.04)	0.12

suggests no relationship between MMSE scores and the levels of the two microRNA expression when comparing the moderate and mild groups between themselves (Figure 4S).

INCREASED EXPRESSION OF miR-34c IN CELLULAR COMPONENTS OF AD BLOOD SAMPLES

The observation of increased miR-34c expression in AD plasma prompted us to determine the level of expression of this microRNA in the cellular compartment, i.e., PBMCs of age-matched cohorts of AD and NEC samples. Increased miR-34c levels were observed in PBMC samples of AD blood specimens, compared to normal controls (**Figure 7A**), with a similar increase for miR-34a in AD over normal controls (**Figure 7B**). However, as shown in **Table 6**, as observed in the plasma samples, there is scant range overlap for miR-34c levels between AD and age-matched controls; this is not true for miR-34a levels between the two groups. Interestingly, the miR-34a levels assayed here as validation for our previous study (Schipper et al., 2007) show the same range of fold changes, i.e., ~3-fold increase in AD samples beyond normal controls (Figure 5S).

FUNCTIONAL ANALYSIS OF THE REPRESSION OF TARGET PROTEINS BY OVEREXPRESSING miRs -34a AND -34c IN CULTURED CELLS

We next investigated whether miR-34c represses the same targets as reported for its sister, miR-34a (He et al., 2007; Yamakuchi et al., 2008), by transfection studies in cultures of human embryonic kidney cells (HEK 293) overexpressing these microRNAs. Only cultures with >98% of cells showing green fluorescence positivity for the green fluorescence protein gene (GFP) were used in our functional assays. Our results with these transfection experiments show repression of Psen1, Bcl2, Sirt1, and Onecut2 by miR-34a ranging from ~11% to 27%, with the latter being the most affected (**Figures 8A–C, Table 7**). A more pronounced impact is observed by miR-34c, with repression ranging from ~16 to 40% (**Figures 8A,B,D, Table 7**). Co-transfection with both miRNAs induced further repression of all four target proteins, from ~32 to 46% (**Figures 8A,B,E, Table 7**). In all analyses, repression levels were evaluated by comparing transfected and

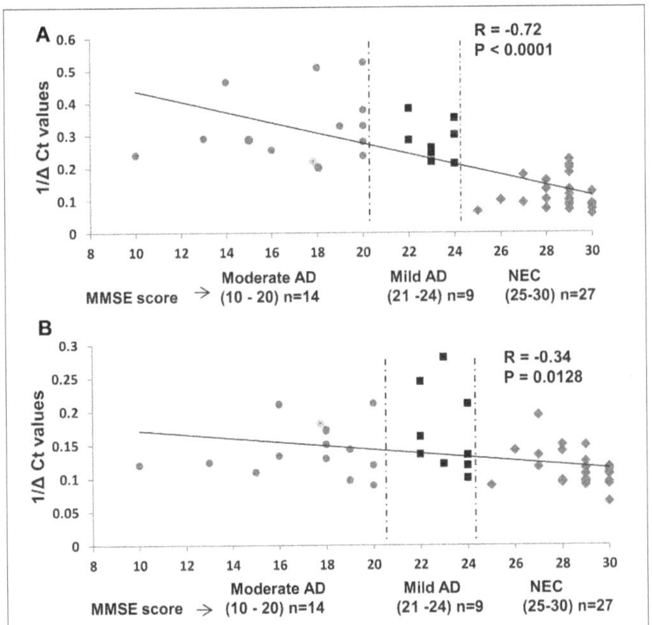

FIGURE 6 | Relationship between expression levels of miR-34c and miR-34a in plasma with Mini-Mental Status Examination (MMSE) scores in selected samples of age-matched groups. (A) Plasma expression levels of miR-34c represented by inverse ΔCt, plotted against corresponding MMSE scores. A high Pearson correlation coefficient value of −0.72 indicates a strong correlation between MMSE scores and 1/deltaCt values, $P < 0.0001$. **(B)** Expression levels of miR-34a in plasma of AD and NEC individuals represented by inverse ΔCt, plotted against corresponding MMSE scores. A low Pearson correlation coefficient value of −0.34 indicates a weak correlation between the MMSE scores and 1/deltaCt values, $P = 0.012$. Data points of Mini-Mental Status Examination (MMSE) score are shown as follows: (●) moderate AD (score 10–20), (■) mild AD (score 21–24), and (◆) NEC (score 25–30).

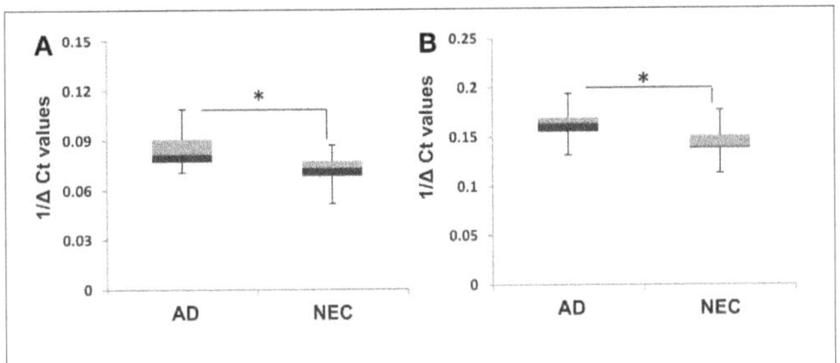

FIGURE 7 | Box plot representation of transcript levels of miR-34a and miR-34c in peripheral blood mononuclear cell (PBMC) samples from Alzheimer's disease (AD) patients and normal elderly controls (NEC). Comparison of levels of miR-34c **(A)** and miR-34a **(B)** in AD patients with that of the NEC cohort in PBMCs, showing increased transcript levels for both microRNAs in the former group, compared to normal controls. Student's *t*-test was used to determine statistical significance; $^{*}P < 0.05$.

scrambled control cultures, with repression of actin observed at ~0%. These observations suggest that miR-34c is a stronger suppressor of target gene expression than miR-34a, and that Onecut2 is the most repressed among the target proteins.

DISCUSSION

Members of the microRNA-34 family are present in most tissues, including PBMC. Our previous study reported miR-34a as a lead microRNA from array profiling and validated by qPCR assays, showing a 2.5-fold increase in PBMC isolated from AD specimens (Schipper et al., 2007). The present study shows that this microRNA's sister, miR-34c, is even more prominently increased in both PBMC and plasma fractions of AD blood samples over age-matched NEC. Most importantly, the majority of miR-34c levels among mild AD patients, determined by mini-mental state examination (MMSE), are elevated beyond those of normal controls. In addition, inclusion of patients with moderate degrees of AD dementia with mild and normal counterparts in our study shows a relatively strong inverse relationship between MMSE scores and levels of this microRNA among the three groups. Levels of miR-34b, the bicistronic sister of miR-34c, are not significantly different between AD and NEC age-matched controls. Thus, our results reported here will serve as future leads to identify key microRNA abundance, such as miR-34c, as noninvasive indicators for plasma changes associated with AD.

Table 6 | 1/deltaCt level ranges, with standard deviation (SD) and median, of microRNAs in PBMC from Alzheimer's disease (AD) patients and age-matched normal elderly controls (NEC), for miR-34c and miR-34a.

PBMC	miR-34c		miR-34a	
	Range (*SD*)	Median	Range (*SD*)	Median
AD	0.07–0.11 (0.01)	0.08	0.13–0.19 (0.01)	0.16
NEC	0.05–0.08 (0.01)	0.07	0.11–0.17 (0.02)	0.14

Age-matched circulating blood microRNA studies like ours by design suffer several limitations, such as: (1) restriction of obtaining gene expression changes at a particular snap-shot time window; and (2) inability to link with changes of the same gene expression in individuals' brains. The first limitation cannot be addressed by small scale studies like ours, but rather in large consortium studies such as the Alzheimer's Disease Neuroimaging Initiative (ADNI) study of the National Institute on Aging, USA, with longitudinal blood sample collection linking plasma and CSF analysis study, and MRI imaging of brain changes in the same individuals. However, most of these studies are centered on the analysis of protein changes, with some focus on Tau and Aβ as biomarkers (O'Bryant et al., 2011; Toledo et al., 2011, 2013). Other studies such as Müller et al. (2014) have limited sample size because such samples are only available from a very few centers where longitudinal *ante mortem* blood or CSF samples are collected along with follow-up acquisition of autopsy brain specimens. Comparative studies between *ante-mortem* blood samples and *post mortem* autopsy will emerge in future studies, yielding results elucidating the relationships between plasma biomarkers and brain pathology structural changes, including but not limited to amyloid plaques and Tau-associated tangle formation.

To identify body fluid-associated microRNA biomarkers for neurodegeneration, standardization of the sample collection protocol and quality control of RNA isolation are two obvious quality control criteria in any study of this kind. Although we have established meticulous procedures for collecting blood samples and further processing to PBMC and plasma fractions, a significant portion, ~20%, of the RNA fractions isolated from these

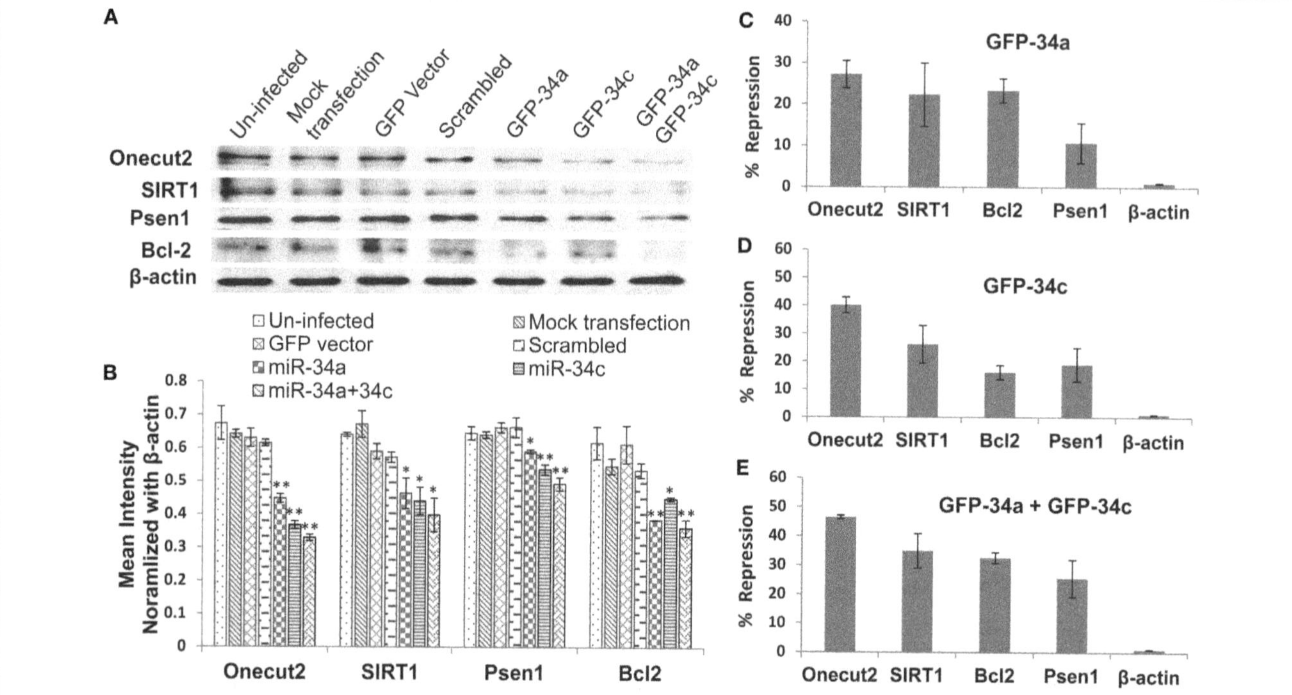

FIGURE 8 | Repression of expression of selected candidate target genes of miR-34a and miR-34c by transfection analysis. Human embryonic kidney (HEK 293) cultures were transfected with green fluorescence protein (GFP) expression vectors containing sequences encoding miR-34a, miR-34c, or a scrambled sequence. Controls included un-infected cultures, mock transfected cultures, cells transfected with either GFP vector alone or carrying a computer-generated scrambled sequence. **(A)** Western blot analysis of cell lysates probed for SIRT1, Onecut2, Presenilin-1, Bcl2, and β-actin proteins; **(B)** Graphic representation of a comparison of band intensities between the various treatments; image intensities of Western blotted bands were normalized against the β-actin band, which is constant throughout. Graphic representation showing percent of repression, estimated using scrambled controls for comparison (panels **C–E**): transfection with miR-34a **(C)**; miR-34c **(D)**; miR-34a and miR-34c **(E)**. One-way ANOVA followed by LSD test was used to determine statistical significance; $^{*}P < 0.05$, $^{**}P < 0.01$.

Table 7 | Levels of miR-34a and miR-34c repression of four target genes' expression.

	miR-34a *vs.* scrambled	miR-34c *vs.* scrambled	miR-34a + 34c *vs.* scrambled
Protein	**Mean % repression (*SD*)**	**Mean % repression (*SD*)**	**Mean % repression (*SD*)**
Onecut2	27.15 (3.34)	40.13 (2.85)	46.42 (0.63)
SIRT1	22.28 (7.68)	26.09 (6.78)	34.89 (5.92)
Bcl2	23.27 (2.87)	16.06 (2.48)	32.57 (1.85)
Psen1	10.69 (4.8)	18.89 (5.94)	25.54 (6.39)
β-actin	0	0	0

*Percent repression of target proteins in HEK 293 cells transfected with miR-34a, miR-34c, or both miRNAs. The repression levels shown here represent protein band intensities, after normalization against β-actin band intensities, when cultures transfected by microRNA are compared with those transfected by scrambled controls. As shown in **Figure 8**, the % change of β-actin levels between cultures transfected by the microRNAs of interest and by the scrambled controls is ~0. Mean % repression with standard deviation (SD) of each miR for each protein is tabulated.*

samples were unacceptable because of poor RNA integrity. Even among the 70–80 samples with good RNA quality, we had to narrow our study to 25 AD and 27 NEC as shown in **Table 1**, in order to satisfy age-matched criteria for our study. With samples from these two subcohorts, as in most neurodegenerative studies, before proceeding to qPCR assays of a particular microRNA of interest, we implemented quality control to insure the cDNA synthesis part of the assays by incorporating *Cel 39* spike-in in the step of RNA isolation.

Besides the above issues, selection of reference microRNAs for determination of microRNA levels of expression is crucial for studies of blood samples of neuronal disorders. We use miR-16 as our reference microRNA, following the report by Gaughwin et al. (2011), who used it as the reference microRNA to show that miR-34b is elevated in the plasma of Huntingdon mutation gene carriers, prior to disease manifestation. Interestingly, our study with this microRNA shows that miR-34b levels do not differ significantly in plasma specimens between AD patients and NEC. A recent study by Müller et al. (2014) shows that miR-16 and miR-146 are increased in AD in both hippocampus and cerebrospinal fluid (CSF). However, this report also suggests that miR-16, a major red blood cell microRNA (Kirschner et al., 2011, 2013; McDonald et al., 2011), may be contaminatedby hemolysis in CSF samples; even as little as 100 μl of erythrocytes added skews the qPCR results (Müller et al., 2014). In addition, several other microRNAs reported so far as unchanged in AD tissue have been used as references to determine levels of microRNAs of interest

(Geekiyanage et al., 2012; Sheinerman et al., 2012; Sheinerman and Umansky, 2013). Notwithstanding all these reports, no unifying approach of selecting appropriate reference controls has yet been reached. At present we are limited to the use of miR-16 as the reference, based on the rationale that we found no significant variance in it among our samples, as shown in **Figures 1E,F**.

The widespread variance in levels of both miR-34c and its sister, miR-34a in AD plasma compared with the tight NEC cluster range, shown in **Figures 1–4**, clearly suggests individual variability in the control of these microRNAs' expression. From our small age-matched cohorts, miR-34c levels may be a better candidate than miR-34a and miR-34b for future large-scale study as a blood-based biomarker, simply because its expression in most mild AD patients shows higher levels than most NEC. The ROC analyses performed for both miR-34c and miR-34a 1/deltaCt values in age-matched cohorts proved the former to be an excellent discriminant (AUC = 0.99), whereas the latter was merely fairly good (AUC = 0.81). However, these results suggest the need of further research with larger cohorts, to stringently validate our results of sensitivity using miR-34c as a diagnostic biomarker for plasma samples. Likewise, the inverse correlation, observed only when the moderate and mild groups are compared with their NEC between cognitive scoring and levels of expression of miR-34c in plasma also needs future studies with larger cohorts to define their true relationship. Nevertheless, our findings open the possibility that plasma microRNAs, along with other biomarkers, may be fertile ground for future research linking cognitive decline with changes of gene expression in blood samples.

The increased miR-34c in AD plasma may derive from PBMC, where miR-34c is also increased. As reported, microRNAs present in the circulating plasma may be found either in the encapsulated vesicles known as exosomes, or in lipid- or protein-associated free particulates (Smalheiser, 2007; Etheridge et al., 2011). Reports so far are inconclusive as to what proportion of plasma microRNAs are associated with the former vs. the latter components. Future comparative studies of PBMC, exosomal and free-form miR-34c will reveal the relationship among these three components of AD circulating blood specimens responsible for this microRNA's increased expression.

MicroRNA-34c, as reported for its sister, miR-34a (He et al., 2007; Yamakuchi et al., 2008) and as shown in **Figure 8**, represses Bcl2, SIRT1, Psen1, and Onecut2, all associated with cellular survival and oxidative defense signaling (Clotman et al., 2005; Goodall et al., 2013). This led us to suggest that increased miR-34c may be one of many factors contributing to an overall systemic weakening of stress defense and cell survival, as suggested in our model presented in **Figure 9**. Life-long cumulative oxidative stress induction of p53 up-regulation may activate the expression of this microRNA, with a steadily increasing trend during aging (Li et al., 2011b,c). In AD, this oxidative stress may be further enhanced, manifested in brain as well as perhaps system-wide, reflected in circulating blood by both PBMC and plasma (Maes et al., 2010; Goodall et al., 2013). Future culture experiments in PBMC isolated from AD patients compared with those from normal counterparts will allow us to investigate whether these cells with increased miR-34c levels are indeed prone to apoptotic death, and whether plasma from the same samples stimulates stress and apoptotic signaling in neighboring cells.

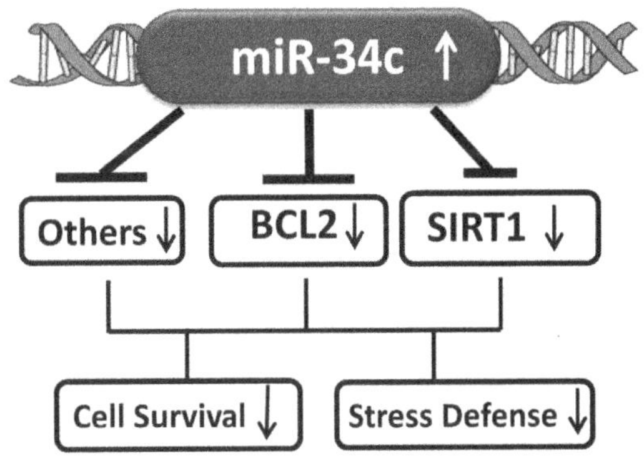

FIGURE 9 | A model suggesting that increased circulating miR-34c expression represses targets involved in oxidative stress and cell survival signaling pathways.

In conclusion, data presented here indicate that levels of miR-34c significantly increase in plasma samples of sporadic AD. Future studies with larger age-matched cohorts will validate these results, and reveal whether this microRNA change is characteristic of sporadic AD as a biomarker criterion, and further comparative studies will elucidate whether it is a common biomarker shared among various neurodegenerative disorders, associated with the decline of oxidative defense and cell survival in neuronal dysfunction.

DISCLOSURE STATEMENT

Howard Chertkow is supported by operating grants from the Canadian Institutes for Health Research (CIHR) and the Fonds de la recherche en santé du Québec (FRSQ). Dr. Chertkow sits on an adjudication board for clinical trials for Bristol Myers Squibb, and has been a speaker and Advisory Board member for Pfizer Canada. Hyman M. Schipper is supported by operating grants from the Canadian Institutes for Health Research (CIHR), and has served as consultant to Osta Biotechnologies, Molecular Biometrics, Inc., TEVA Neurosciences, and Caprion Pharmaceuticals. Eugenia Wang is on entrepreneurial leave from the University of Louisville, with 51% of her effort committed to Advanced Genomic Technology, LLC, a start-up company in Louisville, Kentucky; her other 49% is at the University of Louisville, as the Gheens Endowed Chair on Aging and Professor of Biochemistry and Molecular Biology. Shephali Bhatnagar, Zongfei Yuan, Vikranth Shetty, Samantha Jenkins, Timothy Jones, and Eugenia Wang are employees of Advanced Genomic Technology.

ACKNOWLEDGMENTS

This work was supported by a Small Business Innovation Research (SBIR) grant (R44AG035410) from the National Institute on Aging of the U.S. National Institutes of Health to Advanced Genomic Technology, LLC. The authors thank

Adrienne Liberman, Linda Eizenstat, Carmela Galindez, Alexandra Lyninger, Orchid Lin, Nathaniel Shelburne, Victor Whitehead, and Ljlal Yazdani for technical assistance. We thank the staff of the JGH Memory Clinic for support and organization of sample collection, and Chris Hosein and Shelley Solomon for outstanding organization of the clinical collections; Mr. Alan N. Bloch proof-read the article.

REFERENCES

Bates, D. J., Li, N., Liang, R., Sarojini, H., An, J., Masternak, M. M., et al. (2010). MicroRNA regulation in Ames dwarf mouse liver may contribute to delayed aging. *Aging Cell* 9, 1–18. doi: 10.1111/j.1474-9726.2009.00529.x

Clotman, F., Jacquemin, P., Plumb-Rudewiez, N., Pierreux, C. E., Van der Smissen, P., Dietz, H. C., et al. (2005). Control of liver cell fate decision by a gradient of TGFβ signaling modulated by Onecut transcriptional factors. *Genes Dev.* 19, 1849–1854. doi: 10.1101/gad.340305

De Smaelea, E., Ferrettia, E., and Gulinoa, A. (2010). MicroRNAs as biomarkers for CNS cancer and other disorders. *Brain Res.* 1338, 100–111. doi: 10.1016/j.brainres.2010.03.103

Etheridge, A., Lee, I., Hood, L., Galas, D., and Wang, K. (2011). Extracelluar microRNA: a new source of biomarkers. *Mutat. Res.* 717, 85–90. doi: 10.1016/j.mrfmmm.2011.03.004

Fawcett, T. (2006). An introduction to ROC analysis. *Pattern Recognit. Lett.* 27, 861–874. doi: 10.1016/j.patrec.2005.10.010

Folstein, M., Folstein, S., and McHugh, S. (1975). Mini-Mental State: a practical method for grading the cognitive status of patients for the clinician. *J. Psychiatr. Res.* 12, 189–198. doi: 10.1016/0022-3956(75)90026-6

Gaughwin, P. M., Ciesla, M., Lahiri, N., Tabrizi, S. J., Brundin, P., and Björkqvist, M. (2011). Hsa-miR-34b is a plasma-stable microRNA that is elevated in pre-manifest Huntington's disease. *Hum. Mol. Genet.* 20, 2225–2237. doi: 10.1093/hmg/ddr111

Geekiyanage, H., Jicha, G. A., Nelson, P. T., and Chan C. (2012). Blood serum miRNA: non-invasive biomarkers for Alzheimer's disease. *Exp. Neurol.* 235, 491–496. doi: 10.1016/j.expneurol.2011.11.026

Goodall, E. E., Heath, P. R., Bandmann, O., Kirby, J., and Shaw, P. J. (2013). Neuronal dark matter: the emerging role of microRNA in neurodegeneration. *Front. Cell. Neurosci.* 7:178. doi: 10.3389/fncel.2013.00178

He, L., He, X. Y., Lowe, S. W., and Hannon, G. J. (2007). microRNAs join the p53 network – another piece in the tumour-suppression puzzle. *Nat. Rev. Cancer* 7, 819–882. doi: 10.1038/nrc2232

Khanna, A., Muthusamy, S., Liang, R., Sarojini, H., and Wang, E. (2011). Gain of survival signaling by down-regulation of three key miRNAs in brain of calorie-restricted mice. *Aging* 3, 223–236.

Kirschner, M. B., Edelman, J. J. B., Kao, S. C. -H., Vallely, M. P., van Zandwijk, N., and Reid, G. (2013). The impact of hemolysis on cell-free microRNA biomarkers. *Front. Genet.* 4:94. doi: 10.3389/fgene.2013.00094

Kirschner, M. B., Kao, S. C., Edelman, J. J., Armstrong, N. J., Vallely, M. P., van Zandwijk, N., et al. (2011). Haemolysis during sample preparation alters microRNA content of plasma. *PLoS ONE* 6:e24145. doi: 10.1371/journal.pone.0024145

Kroh, E. M., Parkin, R. K., Mitchell, P. S., and Tewari, M. (2010). Analysis of circulating microRNA biomarkers in plasma and serum using quantitative reverse transcription-PCR (qRT-PCR). *Methods* 50, 298–301. doi: 10.1016/j.ymeth.2010.01.032

Li, G., and Chung, W. Y. (2013). Detection of driver drowsiness using wavelet analysis of heart rate variability and a support vector machine classifier. *Sensors* 13, 16494–16511. doi: 10.3390/s131216494

Li, X., Khanna, A., Li, N., and Wang, E. (2011a). Circulatory miR-34a as an RNA-based, noninvasive biomarker for brain aging. *Aging* 3, 985–1002.

Li, N., Bates, D. J., An, J., and Wang, E. (2011b). Up-regulation of key microRNAs and the inverse down-regulation of their potential target genes of oxidative phosphorylation during aging in mouse brains. *Neurobiol. Aging* 32, 944–955. doi: 10.1016/j.neurobiolaging.2009.04.020

Li, N., Muthusamy, S., Liang, R., Sarojini, H., and Wang, E. (2011c). Increased expression of miR-34a and miR-93 in rat liver during aging and their impact on the expression of Mgstl and Sirtl. *Mech. Ageing Dev.* 132, 75–85. doi: 10.1016/j.mad.2010.12.004

Liang, R., Bates, D. J., and Wang, E. (2009). Epigenetic control of microRNA expression and aging. *Curr. Genomics* 10, 184–193. doi: 10.2174/138920209788185225

Livak, K. J., and Schmittgen, T. D. (2001). Analysis of relative gene expression data using real-time quantitative PCR and the $2^{-\Delta\Delta CT}$ method. *Methods* 25, 402–408. doi: 10.1006/meth.2001.1262

Maes, O. C., Chertkow, H. M., Wang, E., and Schipper, H. M. (2010). MicroRNA: Implications for Alzheimer's disease and other human CNS disorders. *Curr. Genomics* 10, 154–168. doi: 10.2174/138920209788185252

McDonald, J. S., Milosevic, D., Reddi, H. V., Grebe, S. K., and Algeciras-Schimnich, A. (2011). Analysis of circulating microRNA: preanalytical and analytical challenges. *Clin. Chem.* 57, 833–840. doi: 10.1373/clinchem.2010.157198

McKhann, G., Drachman, D., Folstein, M., Katzman, R., Price, D., and Stadlan, E. M. (1984). Clinical diagnosis of Alzheimer's disease: report of the NINCDS-ADRDA work group under the auspices of Department of Health and Human Services Task Force on Alzheimer's disease. *Neurology* 34, 939–944. doi: 10.1212/WNL.34.7.939

McKhann, G. M., Knopman, D. S., Chertkow, H., Hyman, B. T., Jack, C. R. Jr, Kawas, C. H., et al. (2011). The diagnosis of dementia due to Alzheimer's disease: recommendation from the National Institute on Aging-Alzheimer's Association workgroups on diagnostic guidelines for Alzheimer's disease. *Alzheimers Dement* 7, 263–269. doi: 10.1016/j.jalz.2011.03.005

Müller, M., Kuiperij, H. B., Claassen, J. A., Küsters, B., and Verbeek, M. M. (2014). MicroRNAs in Alzheimer's disease: differential expression in hippocampus and cell-free cerebrospinal fluid. *Neurobiol. Aging* 35, 152–158. doi: 10.1016/j.neurobiolaging.2013.07.005

Nasreddine, Z. S., Phillips, N. A., Bédirian, V., Charbonneau, S., Whitehead, V., Collin, I., et al. (2005). The Montréal Cognitive Assessment, MoCA: a brief screening tool for mild cognitive impairment. *J. Am. Geriatr. Soc.* 53, 695–699. doi: 10.1111/j.1532-5415.2005.53221.x

O'Bryant, S. E., Xiao, G., Barber, R., Huebinger, R., Wilhelmsen, K., Edwards, M., et al. (2011). A blood based screening tool for Alzheimer's disease that spans serum and plasma: Findings from TARC and ADNI. *PLoS ONE* 6:e28092. doi: 10.1371/journal.pone.0028092

Pendyala, G., Trauger, S. A., Siuzdak, G., and Fox, H. S. (2010). Quantitative plasma proteomic profiling identifies the vitamin E binding protein afamin as a potential pathogenic factor in SIV induced CNS disease. *J. Proteome Res.* 9, 352–358. doi: 10.1021/pr900685u

Rong, H., Liu, T. B., Yang, K. J., Yang, H. C., Wu, D. H., Liao, C. P., et al. (2011). MicroRNA-134 plasma levels before and after treatment for bipolar mania. *J. Psychiatr. Res.* 45, 92–95. doi: 10.1016/j.jpsychires.2010.04.028

Schipper, H. M., Maes, O. C., Chertkow, H. M., and Wang, E. (2007). MicroRNA expression in Alzheimer blood mononuclear cells. *Gene Regul. Syst. Bio.* 1, 263–274.

Schmand, B., Jonker, C., Hooijer, C., and Lindeboom, J. (1996). Subjective memory complaints may announce dementia. *Neurology* 46, 121–125. doi: 10.1212/WNL.46.1.121

Sharp, E., and Gatz, M. (2011). The relationship between education and dementia: an updated systematic review. *Alzheimer Dis. Assoc. Disord.* 25, 289–304. doi: 10.1097/WAD.0b013e318211c83c

Sheinerman, K. S., Tsivinsky, V. G., Crawford, F., Mullan, M. J., Abdullah, L., and Umansky, S. R. (2012). Plasma microRNA biomarkers for detection of mild cognitive impairment. *Aging* 4, 590–605.

Sheinerman, K. S., and Umansky, S. R. (2013). Circulating cell-free microRNA as biomarkers for screening, diagnosis, and monitoring of neurodegenerative disease and other neurologic pathologies. *Front. Cell. Neurosci.* 7:150. doi: 10.3389/fncel.2013.00150

Shi, W., Du, J., Qi, Y., Liang, G., Wang, T., Li, S., et al. (2012). Aberrant expression of serum miRNA in schizophrenia. *J. Psychiatr. Res* 46, 198–204. doi: 10.1016/j.jpsychires.2011.09.010

Smalheiser, N. R. (2007). Exosomal transfer of proteins and RNAs at synapses in the nervous system. *Biol. Direct* 2:35. doi: 10.1186/1745-6150-2-35

Suarez-Gomez, M., Alejandre-Duran, E., and Ruiz-Rubio, M. (2011). MicroRNAs in bipolar disorder: diagnostic and therapeutic applications. *Rev. Neurol.* 53, 91–98.

Taylor, R. (1990). Interpretation of the correlation coefficient: a basic review. *JDMS* 1, 35–39.

Toledo, J. B., Da, X., Bhatt, P., Wolk, D. A., Arnold, S. E., Shaw, L. M., et al. (2013). Relationship between plasma analytes and SPARE-AD defined brain atrophy patterns in ADNI. *PLoS ONE* 8:e55531. doi: 10.1371/journal.pone.0055531

Toledo, J. B., Vanderstichele, H., Figurski, M., Aisen, P. S., Petersen, R. C., Weiner, M. W., et al. (2011). Factors affecting Aβ plasma levels and their utility as biomarkers in ADNI. *Acta Neuropathol.* 122, 401–413. doi: 10.1007/s00401-011-0861-8

Wang, X., Liu, P., Zhu, H., Xu, Y., Ma, C., Dai, X., et al. (2009). miR-34a, a microRNA up-regulated in a double transgenic mouse model of Alzheimer's disease, inhibits Bcl2 translation. *Brain Res. Bull.* 80, 268–273. doi: 10.1016/j.brainresbull.2009.08.006

Wechsler D. (2008). *Wechsler Memory Scale, 4th Edn.* San Antonio, TX: Pearson.

Yamakuchi, M., Ferlito, M., and Lowenstein, C. J. (2008). miR-34a repression of SIRT1 regulates apoptosis. *Proc. Natl. Acad. Sci. U.S.A.* 105, 13421–13426. doi: 10.1073/pnas.0801613105

Zovoilis, A., Agbemenyah, H. Y., Agis-Balboa, R. C., Stilling, R. M., Edbauer, D., Rao, P., et al. (2011). microRNA-34c is a novel target to treat dementias. *EMBO J.* 30, 4299–4308. doi: 10.1038/emboj.2011.327

Zweig, M. H., and Campbell, G. (1993). Receiver-operating characteristic (ROC) plots: a fundamental evaluation tool in clinical medicine. *Clin. Chem.* 39, 561–577.

Permissions

All chapters in this book were first published by Frontiers; hereby published with permission under the Creative Commons Attribution License or equivalent. Every chapter published in this book has been scrutinized by our experts. Their significance has been extensively debated. The topics covered herein carry significant findings which will fuel the growth of the discipline. They may even be implemented as practical applications or may be referred to as a beginning point for another development.

The contributors of this book come from diverse backgrounds, making this book a truly international effort. This book will bring forth new frontiers with its revolutionizing research information and detailed analysis of the nascent developments around the world.

We would like to thank all the contributing authors for lending their expertise to make the book truly unique. They have played a crucial role in the development of this book. Without their invaluable contributions this book wouldn't have been possible. They have made vital efforts to compile up to date information on the varied aspects of this subject to make this book a valuable addition to the collection of many professionals and students.

This book was conceptualized with the vision of imparting up-to-date information and advanced data in this field. To ensure the same, a matchless editorial board was set up. Every individual on the board went through rigorous rounds of assessment to prove their worth. After which they invested a large part of their time researching and compiling the most relevant data for our readers.

The editorial board has been involved in producing this book since its inception. They have spent rigorous hours researching and exploring the diverse topics which have resulted in the successful publishing of this book. They have passed on their knowledge of decades through this book. To expedite this challenging task, the publisher supported the team at every step. A small team of assistant editors was also appointed to further simplify the editing procedure and attain best results for the readers.

Apart from the editorial board, the designing team has also invested a significant amount of their time in understanding the subject and creating the most relevant covers. They scrutinized every image to scout for the most suitable representation of the subject and create an appropriate cover for the book.

The publishing team has been an ardent support to the editorial, designing and production team. Their endless efforts to recruit the best for this project, has resulted in the accomplishment of this book. They are a veteran in the field of academics and their pool of knowledge is as vast as their experience in printing. Their expertise and guidance has proved useful at every step. Their uncompromising quality standards have made this book an exceptional effort. Their encouragement from time to time has been an inspiration for everyone.

The publisher and the editorial board hope that this book will prove to be a valuable piece of knowledge for researchers, students, practitioners and scholars across the globe.

List of Contributors

Sandrine Galetti, Robert K. Maeda and François Karch
Department of Genetics and Evolution, University of Geneva, Geneva, Switzerland

Maheshwar Gummalla
Department of Genetics and Evolution, University of Geneva, Geneva, Switzerland
Institute of Biochemistry, University of Medicine – University of Göttingen, Göttingen, Germany

Archana N. Iyer and Marie-Laure Baudet
Center for Integrative Biology, University of Trento, Trento, Italy

Anaïs Bellon
Department of Physiology, Development and Neuroscience, University of Cambridge, Cambridge, UK

Paola Gavazzo and Massimo Vassalli
Institute of Biophysics, National Research Council (CNR), Genoa, Italy

Delfina Costa
Department of Experimental Medicine, University of Genoa, Genoa, Italy

Aldo Pagano
Department of Experimental Medicine, University of Genoa, Genoa, Italy
IRCCS Azienda Ospedaliera Universitaria San Martino-IST, Genoa, Italy

Elisabetta Maffioletti and Massimo Gennarelli
Genetic Unit, IRCCS Centro S. Giovanni di Dio Fatebenefratelli, Brescia, Italy
Department of Molecular and Translational Medicine, University of Brescia, Brescia, Italy

Daniela Tardito
Dipartimento di Scienze Farmacologiche e Biomolecolari, Università degli Studi di Milano, Milano, Italy

Luisella Bocchio-Chiavetto
Neuropsychopharmacology Unit, IRCCS Centro S. Giovanni di Dio Fatebenefratelli, Brescia, Italy

Alon Simchovitz and Hermona Soreq
Laboratory of Molecular Neuroscience, Department of Biological Chemistry, The Edmond and Lily Safra Center of Brain Science, The Hebrew University of Jerusalem, Jerusalem, Israel

Alessandro Guffanti
Laboratory of Molecular Neuroscience, Department of Biological Chemistry, The Edmond and Lily Safra Center of Brain Science, The Hebrew University of Jerusalem, Jerusalem, Israel
Bioinformatics, Genomnia srl, Milano, Italy

Floriana Della Ragione, Miriam Gagliardi, Maurizio D'Esposito and Maria R. Matarazzo
Functional Genomics and Epigenomics Laboratory, Institute of Genetics and Biophysics "ABT," Consiglio Nazionale delle Ricerche, Naples, Italy
Laboratorio di Genomica e di Epigenomica, Istituto di Ricovero e Cura a Carattere Scientifico Neuromed, Pozzilli, Italy

Balagopal Pai, Taweeporn Siripornmongcolchai, Birgitte Berentsen, Ashraf Pakzad, Karin Wibrand and Clive R. Bramham
Department of Biomedicine and K.G. Jebsen Centre for Research on Neuropsychiatric Disorders, University of Bergen, Bergen

Ståle Pallesen
Department of Psychosocial Science, University of Bergen, Bergen, Norway

Maciej Pajak
Institute for Adaptive and Neural Computation, School of Informatics, University of Edinburgh, Edinburgh, UK

T. Ian Simpson
Institute for Adaptive and Neural Computation, School of Informatics, University of Edinburgh, Edinburgh, UK
Biomathematics and Statistics Scotland, JCMB, Edinburgh, UK

Eva Terzibasi Tozzini, Aurora Savino, Roberto Ripa and Giorgia Battistoni
Laboratorio di Biologia, Scuola Normale Superiore, Pisa, Italy

Mario Baumgart
Fritz Lipmann Institute for Age Research, Leibniz Institute, Jena, Germany

Alessandro Cellerino
Laboratorio di Biologia, Scuola Normale Superiore, Pisa, Italy
Fritz Lipmann Institute for Age Research, Leibniz Institute, Jena, Germany

Sara Elramah, Marc Landry and Alexandre Favereaux
Interdisciplinary Institute for Neuroscience, UMR 5297, University of Bordeaux, Bordeaux, France
Interdisciplinary Institute for Neuroscience, UMR 5297, Centre National de la Recherche Scientifique, Bordeaux

Manuel Nieto-Diaz, David Reigada, Teresa Muñoz-Galdeano, Marcos Caballero-López, Rosa Navarro-Ruiz, Ángela del Águila and Rodrigo M. Maza
Molecular Neuroprotection Group, Experimental Neurology Unit, Hospital Nacional de Parapléjicos (Servicio de Salud de Castilla-La Mancha), Toledo, Spain

Francisco J. Esteban
Departamento de Biología Experimental, Facultad de Ciencias Experimentales y de la Salud, Universidad de Jaén, Jaén, Spain

MónicaYunta
Unidad de Patología Mitocondrial, Unidad Funcional de Investigación en Enfermedades Crónicas, Instituto de Salud Carlos III, Madrid, Spain

Chetan J. Gadgil
CSIR-National Chemical Laboratory, Chemical Engineering and Process Development Division, Pune, India

K. V. Venkatesh
Department of Chemical Engineering, Indian Institute of Technology Bombay, Mumbai, India

Ashwani Choudhary, Mayuresh A. Sarangdhar and Beena Pillai
Functional Genomics, CSIR-Institute of Genomics and Integrative Biology, Delhi, India

Bharat R. Iyengar
CSIR-National Chemical Laboratory, Chemical Engineering and Process Development Division, Pune, India
Department of Chemical Engineering, Indian Institute of Technology Bombay, Mumbai, India

Hui Chiu, Amel Alqadah and Chieh Chang
Division of Developmental Biology, Cincinnati Children's Hospital Research Foundation, Cincinnati, OH, USA

Simona Maciotta
Stem Cell Laboratory, Department of Pathophysiology and Transplantation, Centro Dino Ferrari, Università degli Studi di Milano, Fondazione IRCCS Cà Granda Ospedale Maggiore Policlinico, Milan, Italy
Diabetes Research Institute, University of Miami Miller School of Medicine, Miami, FL, USA

Mirella Meregalli and Yvan Torrente
Stem Cell Laboratory, Department of Pathophysiology and Transplantation, Centro Dino Ferrari, Università degli Studi di Milano, Fondazione IRCCS Cà Granda Ospedale Maggiore Policlinico, Milan, Italy

Christian Barbato, Silvia Pezzola, Cinzia Caggiano, Martina Antonelli, Paola Frisone, Maria Teresa Ciotti and Francesca Ruberti
Institute of Cell Biology and Neurobiology (IBCN), National Research Council (CNR), Rome, Italy

Marion Coolen, Shauna Katz and Laure Bally-Cuif
Zebrafish Neurogenetics Team, Laboratory of Neurobiology and Development, Institute of Neurobiology Alfred Fessard, CNRS, Gif-sur-Yvette, France

Christina Vlachouli, Stefano Gustincich and Roberto Simone
Area of Neuroscience, International School for Advanced Studies (SISSA), Trieste, Italy

Charles Plessy, Nicolas Bertin, Piero Carninci and Carsten O. Daub
RIKEN Center for Life Science Technologies, Division of Genomic Technologies, Tsurumi-ku, Yokohama, Japan

Giovanni Pascarella
Area of Neuroscience, International School for Advanced Studies (SISSA), Trieste, Italy
RIKEN Center for Life Science Technologies, Division of Genomic Technologies, Tsurumi-ku, Yokohama, Japan

Dejan Lazarevic
Area of Neuroscience, International School for Advanced Studies (SISSA), Trieste, Italy
Cluster in Biomedicine (CBM), AREA Science Park, Trieste, Italy

Altuna Akalin
Bergen Center for Computational Science - Computational Biology Unit and Sars Centre for Marine Molecular Biology, University of Bergen, Bergen, Norway

Geoffrey J. Faulkner
Cancer Biology Program, Mater Medical Research Institute, South Brisbane, QLD, Australia
School of Biomedical Sciences, University of Queensland, Brisbane, QLD, Australia

Silvia Zucchelli
Area of Neuroscience, International School for Advanced Studies (SISSA), Trieste, Italy
Department of Health Sciences, University of Eastern Piedmont "A. Avogadro," Novara, Italy

Jun Kawai and Yoshihide Hayashizaki
RIKEN Preventive Medicine and Diagnosis Innovation Program, Wako, Saitama, Japan

Min Jeong Kye and Inês do Carmo G. Gonçalves
Institute of Human Genetics, University of Cologne, Cologne, Germany
Institute for Genetics, University of Cologne, Cologne, Germany

Christopher Heise, Lorenza Culotta and Chiara Verpelli
CNR Institute of Neuroscience and Department of Biotechnology and Translational Medicine, University of Milan, Milan, Italy

Fabrizio Gardoni and Monica di Luca
Department of Pharmacological and Biomolecular Sciences, University of Milan, Milan, Italy

Carlo Sala
CNR Institute of Neuroscience and Department of Biotechnology and Translational Medicine, University of Milan, Milan, Italy
Neuromuscular Diseases and Neuroimmunology, Foundation Carlo Besta Neurological Institute, Milan, Italy

Apostolia Fragkouli and Epaminondas Doxakis
Lab of Molecular and Cellular Neuroscience, Center for Basic Research, Biomedical Research Foundation of the Academy of Athens, Athens, Greece

Shephali Bhatnagar, Zongfei Yuan, Vikranth Shetty, Samantha Jenkins, Timothy Jones and Eugenia Wang
Advanced Genomic Technology, LLC, Louisville, KY, USA

Howard Chertkow
Department of Neurology and Neurosurgery, McGill University, Montreal, QC, Canada
Memory Clinic, Department of Medicine, Jewish General Hospital, Montreal, QC, Canada
Bloomfield Centre for Research in Aging, Lady Davis Institute, Montreal, QC, Canada
Division of Geriatric Medicine and Department of Clinical Neurosciences, Jewish General Hospital, Montreal, QC, Canada

Hyman M. Schipper
Department of Neurology and Neurosurgery, McGill University, Montreal, QC, Canada
Bloomfield Centre for Research in Aging, Lady Davis Institute, Montreal, QC, Canada
Division of Geriatric Medicine and Department of Clinical Neurosciences, Jewish General Hospital, Montreal, QC, Canada

Index

www.ingramcontent.com/pod-product-compliance
Lightning Source LLC
LaVergne TN
LVHW082211200926
848484LV00008B/2239
* 9 7 9 8 8 8 7 4 0 2 7 8 9 *